# ADVANCES IN CANCER THERAPY

Edited by **Hala Gali-Muhtasib**

**Advances in Cancer Therapy**
Edited by Hala Gali-Muhtasib

**Published by InTech**

Janeza Trdine 9, 51000 Rijeka, Croatia



**Publishing Process Manager** Masa Vidovic

**Technical Editor** Teodora Smiljanic

**Cover Designer** InTech Design Team

Additional hard copies can be obtained from orders@intechopen.com

Advances in Cancer Therapy, Edited by Hala Gali-Muhtasib
p. cm.
978-953-307-703-1

For EU product safety concerns:
IN TECH d.o.o., Prolaz Marije Krucifikse Kozulić 3, 51000 Rijeka, Croatia,
info@intechopen.com or visit our website at intechopen.com.

# Meet the editor

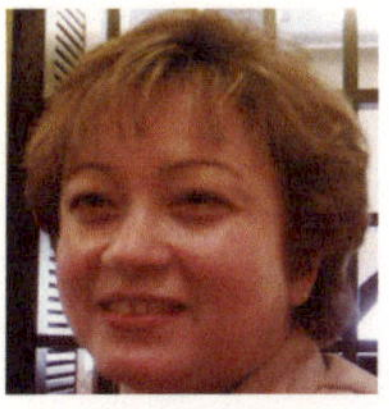

Hala Gali-Muhtasib obtained her PhD in Biology in 1990 after which she was awarded a postdoctoral research fellowship in the Anticancer Drug Laboratory in Manhattan, KS. In 1993 she accepted a research associate position at the Department of Physiology and Biophyscis, Case Western Reserve University School of Medicine, Cleveland, OH. She then joined AUB in 1994 as an Assistant Professor and was promoted to full Professor in 2004. H. Gali-Muhtasib has published more than 65 manuscripts in peer-reviewed international journals and 11 book chapters. Her research interests are in the field of cancer chemoprevention and chemotherapy, particularly in what relates to the study of plant-derived compounds, hypoxic cytotoxic agents, anti-angiogenic drugs and radiation modifier compounds in an attempt to study the interplay between tumor hypoxia, radiosensitization and angiogenesis. Her efforts have been directed towards understanding the cellular and molecular mechanisms of action of various anticancer agents using cellular biology techniques as well as an emerging array of molecular technologies. She has been honored with three research achievement awards; the Suad al-Sabbah prize in 2003, the Abdul Hameed Shoman prize for Young Arab Researchers in 2004 and the ISESCO prize in Biology in 2008.

# Contents

# Preface

The book "Advances in Cancer Therapy" is a new addition to the Intech collection of books and aims at providing scientists and clinicians with a comprehensive overview of the state of current knowledge and latest research findings in the area of cancer therapy. For this purpose research articles, clinical investigations and review papers that are thought to improve the readers' understanding of cancer therapy developments and/or to keep them up to date with the most recent advances in this field have been included in this book. With cancer being one of the most serious diseases of our times, I am confident that this book will meet the patients', physicians' and researchers' needs.

The participating authors have been selected from diverse countries based solely on their expertise and the appropriateness of their work to the book's topics listed in the table of contents. The authors have all willingly accepted our invitation to submit their chapters for review of their quality. The proposed drafts, consisting of original drafts only, were revised by the book's editor before making the final decision of acceptance or refusal. At this point of the process, some chapters were directly accepted or rejected, while others were sent back for revision according to the editor's recommendations to be later accepted after ensuring that they fulfill all the criteria of selection.

The publication here presented is unique in its content that covers various subjects from alternative traditional medicine, specifically natural compounds' therapeutic potentials to nanotechnology advances and applications in cancer treatment. All information presented is organized, clear and based on solid scientific facts. This book is therefore destined to all cancer researchers or therapists and it also represents a valuable addition to any scientific library.

With this book compilation the readers will not only find an overview of the big picture of cancer targets and targeting methods that are currently known, but also be aware of exactly where we stand today in the curing of cancer and what needs to be done further. Hopefully, this will all be accomplished during a pleasant enjoyable reading of this simply written book accessible to all.

**Dr. Hala Gali-Muhtasib**
Department of Biology, American University of Beirut,
Lebanon

# Part 1

## New Modalities of Cancer Treatment

1

# May Mast Cells Have Any Effect in New Modalities of Cancer Treatment?

Öner Özdemir
*Ministry of Health, İstanbul Medeniyet University*
*Göztepe Research / Training Hospital, Kadıköy*
*Republic of Turkey*

## 1. Introduction

Multifunctional mast cells (MC) have been recently reported as effectors in the human innate and even adaptive immune system, besides their known roles in allergic disorders. First in vivo observations in the 1950`s suggested their possible role as anti-tumor cells around certain solid tumors and questioned their interactions with tumor cells (Prior, 1953). Later, in vitro murine mast cell cytotoxicity (MCC) against murine tumor cells was described in 1981 (Henderson, 1981; Ghiara, 1985; Richards 1988). However, to the best of our knowledge, there is no reported data on in vitro human MCC against human tumor cells. Current in vivo observations and implications from human pathological specimens are also very controversial. Moreover, there is still difficulty in obtaining and maintaining human MCs in cultures since they have low expansion potential. These facts have hampered in vitro human MC studies up to the last decades of the 20th century. The recent use of methylcellulose media for in vitro human MC cultures increased the knowledge and data strongly supporting an increasing role of MC as effector elements of innate immunity (Leskinen, 2003; Marshall, 2004; Della Rovere, 2009; Özdemir, 2007, 2011).

Ambiguous and mounting evidence also indicates that MCs accumulate around tumors and could either promote or inhibit tumor growth, most likely depending on environmental conditions. Presently, believers in the inhibitory role of MCs assume them to be inhibitors of tumor development through their cytotoxic pro-necrolytic/-apoptotic granules (Wagelie-Steffen, 1998; Leskinen, 2003; Kataoka, 2004; Pardo, 2007; Heikkilä, 2008). In fact, the MC has been long believed to have natural cytotoxicity against murine TNF-α sensitive tumor cells in the long term incubations (>24h), by either TNF-α dependent or independent pathways. TNF-α independent pathways like cathepsin G, NO, serine proteases, peroxidases, $H_2O_2$ etc. were also assumed to contribute to MCC (Henderson, 1981; Ghiara, 1985; Richards 1988). Moreover, in vitro murine MCC has been well demonstrated against TNF-α-sensitive murine WEHI-164 and L929 tumor cells. Murine MCC seems to be different from natural killer (NK) cytotoxicity by means of acting in long term against unusual targets such as WEHI-164 and L929 with different mediators like peroxidases (Henderson, 1981; Ghiara, 1985; Richards 1988). Moreover, the last decade of research demonstrates that MC granules have pro-apoptotic characteristics (Wagelie-Steffen, 1998; Leskinen, 2003; Kataoka, 2004; Pardo, 2007; Heikkilä, 2008). Chymase was shown to induce apoptosis, and apoptotic pathway mediators such as FasL and granzyme B expressions were detected in mice and cultured MCs; respectively (Wagelie-Steffen, 1998; Leskinen, 2003; Kataoka, 2004; Pardo, 2007; Heikkilä, 2008). Thus, except for perforin (Pardo, 2007), MCs indeed have been proven to have all components of short and long-term cell-mediated cytotoxicity, which consist of the secretory pathway (via soluble TNF-α, chymase, serine proteases granzyme-B/-H), and non-secretory pathway (the death receptors Fas L and membranous TNF-α) (Özdemir, 2006, 2007, 2011).

Nonetheless, some researchers still consider MC as an enhancer of tumor development through their angiogenic effects, causing invasiveness and metastasis of tumor tissue (Özdemir, 2006). Some MC mediators such as heparin, IL-8 and tryptase are known to be responsible for angiogenesis (Ribatti, 2000). Yet, neither these mediators are the only known elements responsible from neoangiogenesis, nor are MCs the only resource. MCs also have a vast array of mediators, some of which have promoting, and others inhibitory effects on angiogenesis besides malignancies (Özdemir, 2006). The same researchers consistently based their theories on pathological specimen observations, showing an association between increased MCD and the worst prognosis in some cancers such as endometrial cancer, leukemia as well as lymphomas (Ribatti, 2009; Molin, 2002). Our correspondences against this conviction have been well documented in recent literature (Özdemir, 2006).

As summarized above, in this chaotic literature environment, our aim in this study was to investigate human MCC against NK- and lymphokine activated killer (LAK)-sensitive/ resistant human leukemia-lymphoma cells in short and long term coincubations by our established flow cytometric (FCM) cytotoxicity methods (Özdemir, 2003, 2007, 2011).

## 2. Material and methods

### 2.1 Mast cell (effector) development in methylcellulose and maintenance in suspension culture

A colony forming unit (CFU) -Mast was produced in vitro by our modified method (Özdemir, 2007, 2011). From several discarded patient samples, human bone marrow (BM) mononuclear cells (≥5x104) were obtained and suspended in 0.3 ml Iscove's Modified Dulbecco's Medium (IMDM) containing %1 Fetal Bovine Serum (FBS) after Ficoll (Sigma, St. Louis, MO). Cells were put into 3 ml serum-free methylcellulose medium [MethoCult™ SFBIT H4236, StemCell Technologies, British Columbia, Canada], supplemented with 200 ng/ml of SCF, 50 ng/ml of IL-6 and 1ng/ml of IL-3 (only at the beginning). All cytokines were purchased from Biosource, Camarillo, CA. We inoculated 0.3 ml of the mixed medium in the 12-well plate with a 16 gauge blunt needle and placed into an incubator. Every two weeks, the cells were fed with 0.3 ml new medium including 100 ng/ml of SCF and 50 ng/ml of IL-6. Thirty or more cells were scored as CFU-Mast in situ on an inverted microscope after 4 weeks. Before culturing in suspension, MCs are retrieved from only CFU-Mast`s in the medium and dissolved with >2-fold volume of phosphate buffer solution including FBS %10 at 6th weeks. Cells are centrifuged at 250xG for 5 minutes. They are suspended and cultured in complete IMDM supplemented with 100 ng/ml of SCF, 50 ng/ml of IL-6 and 2% FBS in 25cm$^2$ flask up to 8th weeks. The culture was started with ≤10$^4$ cells/ml and accumulated up to ≤2x10$^6$ cells/ml. The suspension culture was hemi-depleted every week and supplemented with 100 ng/ml of SCF and 50 ng/ml of IL-6.

### 2.2 Staining for verification of effector mast cells

Verification of MCs was done by May-Grunwald-Giemsa, Wright-Giemsa, acid Toluidine Blue staining and immunophenotyping on FCM. In brief, a colony was lifted with Eppendorf micropipette and spun down at 600 rpm for 5 minutes in the $4^{th}$ and $6^{th}$ week. Viability was checked with a trypan blue exclusion test. Cells from colonies were stained with May-Grunwald-Giemsa and Wright-Giemsa for verification purposes (Fig.1A1-4). MCs were fixated with a Carnoy solution and incubated for 2 minutes with acid toluidine blue to confirm their tryptase content as well. Furthermore, MCs were immunophenotyped for all related markers in FCM at $4^{th}$-$8^{th}$ weeks (Fig.1B1-3, Table 1). All monoclonal antibodies (mAb) were purchased from Immunotech, Inc. (Westbrook, ME).

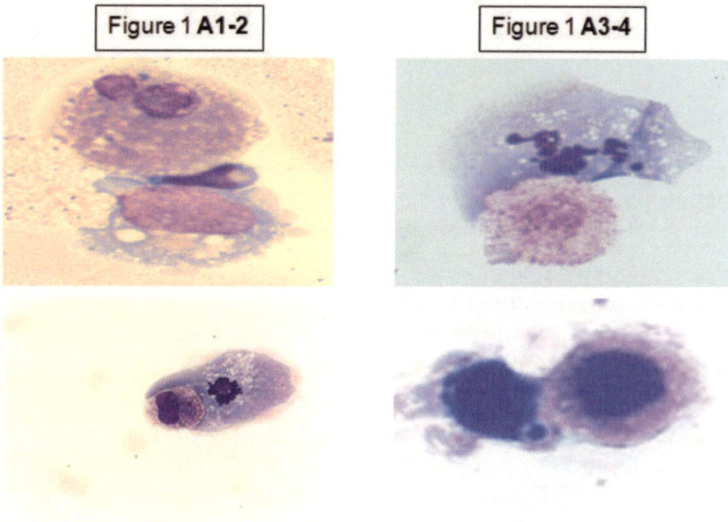


Fig. 1. A1- 4. Wright- Giemsa slides are showing conjugate formation between mast cell and both tumor cells (effector-target doublets). A1-2 show conjugate formation between mast and Daudi cells. A3-4 depict conjugate formation between mast and Raji cells.

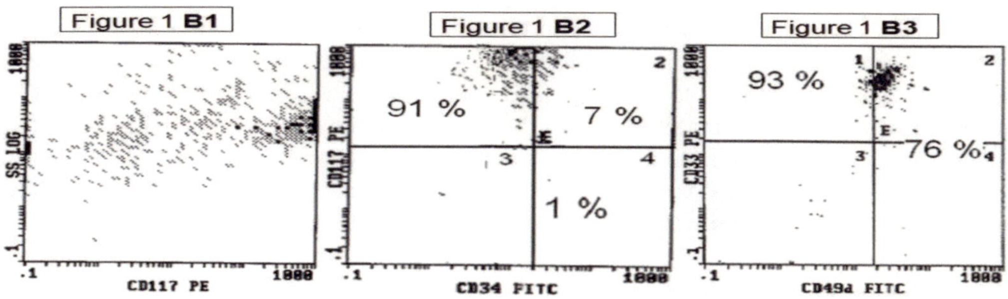


Fig. 1. B1- 3. Phenotyping of 4- week- old human bone marrow -derived mast cells on flow cytometry is shown in a representative sample. B1 shows CD117 (c-kit) expression vs. SS (granularity) of mast cells. B2 demonstrates ≥98% of cells already stained with CD117 and became CD34 negative. B3 illustrates 93% of cells stained with CD33 and 76% of cells were positive for CD49d. [The human effector (mast) cells produced from bone marrow were absolutely negative for CD19 in this study.]

| *Surface Marker Expressions* | *4th-week* | *6th-week* | *8th-week* |
|---|---|---|---|
| CD14 | 0 % | 0 % | 0 % |
| CD15 | 93 % | 3 % | 2 % |
| CD19 | 0 % | 0 % | 0 % |
| CD33 | 93 % | 25 % | 19 % |
| CD34 | 7 % | 1 % | 1 % |
| CD38 | 0 % | 0 % | 0 % |
| CD44 | 93 % | 85 % | 84 % |
| CD45 | 0 % | 0 % | 0 % |
| CD49d | 76 % | 12 % | 11 % |
| CD117 (c-kit) | 91 % | 95 % | 98 % |
| HLA-DR | 0 % | 0 % | 0 % |

Table 1. The phenotypic characterizations of 4- to 8- week-old human bone marrow- derived mast cells by flow cytometry in representative samples are shown.

### 2.3 Target lymphoma and leukemia cells

The human malignant B-lymphoblastoid cell lines such as Daudi/ Raji and erythroleukemia cell line K562, known as "LAK- sensitive" and "reference cells" in cytotoxicity studies, were utilized in this study. In several experiments we also utilized LAK- resistant human acute myeloid leukemia (AML) cell lines (HL-60, DAMI and Meg-01) and discarded AML patient samples were used. All cell lines were obtained from ATCC (Manassas, VA) and maintained in RPMI 1640 culture media, supplemented with 10% FBS. Before coincubation, target and effector cell viability were determined by the trypan blue exclusion test; a viability of 90% was required to proceed.

### 2.4 Assessment of human MCC on FCM

Cytotoxicity was assessed by two different FCM cytotoxicity techniques utilizing DIOC18 or mAb staining for target cell labeling (Özdemir, 2007, 2011). The basic strategy of two-color FCM assay involves labeling target cells with a fluorescent membrane dye DIOC18, in addition to staining with PI, to identify dead cells. Alternatively, a new three-color FCM approach called as "flow cytometric mast cell-mediated cytotoxicity assay (FCM-MCMCA) " , which entails target cell marking with specific mAb (CD19) and with AnnV/PI colabeling to identify apoptotic/dead target cells, was used for some tumor cells. Briefly, we performed the following stepwise approach for analyzing the samples:

### 2.5 Pre-labeling target leukemia cells with DIOC18

A stock solution was prepared by dissolving DIOC18 (Sigma, St. Louis, MO) in DMSO (2 mg/ml) overnight with agitation. The target cells ($10^6$cells/ ml) were incubated with 10μg/ml of DIOC18 (final concentration) in 1 ml of PBS containing %3 FBS for 45 minutes at incubator. Then, target cells were washed with PBS three times to get rid of dye remnant. DIOC18 pre-labeling before coincubation was done for K562, Meg-01, HL-60, DAMI cells and the patient samples (Fig.1C1-E3).

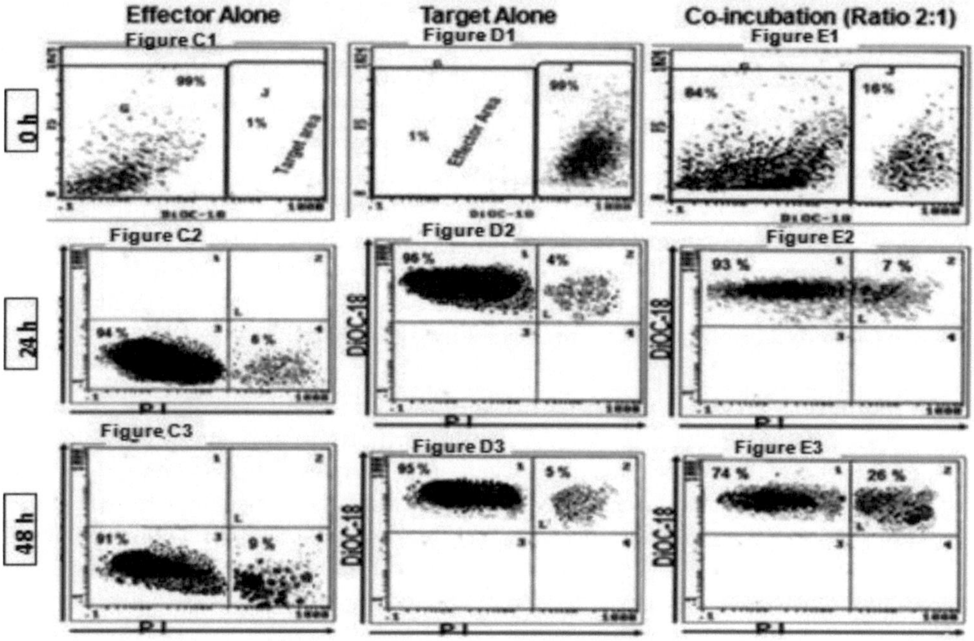


Fig. 1. C1- E3: Target cell (DAMI) death is shown by new flow cytometric assay at 24h and 48h in a representative sample. Identification of effector and target cells in alone/coincubation samples using target cell labeling (DIOC18) and cell size characteristics (FS) is shown in histograms at the first row. Spontaneous death and cytotoxicity evaluation of the cell populations alone or in co-incubation samples are shown with the rectilinear boxes of related histograms at the second and third rows. C1 shows location of effector-mast cell. Since effector cells are not pre-stained with DIOC18, they are DIOC18 negative and in a different area (Region G). C2 and C3 demonstrate the change in viability of effector cell alone population (DIOC18−/PI− viable cells: 94% and 91%; respectively) at 24h/48h. Spontaneous deaths in these effector alone samples are 6% and 9%; respectively. These histograms are obtained after gating on region G of a corresponding sample. D1 shows the target-DAMI cell population from target alone tube. As expected, target cells are very well-marked with DIOC18 (Region J). D2 and D3 depict the viability of the target population alone (DIOC18+/PI− viable cells: 96% and 95%; respectively) at 24h and 48h. Spontaneous deaths in these samples are 4% and 5%; respectively. These histograms are obtained after gating on region J of a corresponding sample. E1 obtained from an experiment where mast cells are co-incubated with DIOC18-positive DAMI cells at 2:1 effector/ target ratio. In this co-incubation sample; effector/target gatings are defined according to the target/effector alone (control) tubes. E2 depicts decrease in viability of previously gated target cells in J region of a corresponding co-incubation sample, 7% of them are stained with PI+ indicating necrotic killing (Region L2). In this representative sample, DAMI cell viability slightly decreased from 96% in the control to 93% after 24h co-incubation. The 4% of spontaneous death increased up to 7% with cytotoxicity mediated by mast cells during 24h co-incubation. E3 shows obvious decrease in viability of previously gated target DAMI cells, as 26% of them are dead. In this representative sample, DAMI cell viability further decreased from 95% to 74% throughout 48h co-incubation. The necrotic populations increased from a corresponding 5% of spontaneous death to 26% kill mediated by mast cell cytotoxicity in the co-incubated sample.

### 2.6 Coincubation

A few sets of human BM-derived MCs at 8th weeks of age, without any stimulation (PMA etc.) and human tumor targets were coincubated at certain effector/target ratios (1:1, 2:1, 4:1, 5:1) short-term and long-term. Human MCs were coincubated in vitro with human LAK-sensitive (K562, Daudi, Raji cells) and LAK- resistant tumor targets (Meg-01, HL-60, DAMI and patient cells) for the evaluation of human MCC. Tubes were centrifuged at 115xG for 5 minutes and incubated at 37°C in 5% $CO_2$ for short- (2h) and long-term (up to 48h) period. Although MCC is well-known to take place after long-term incubation (>18h), 2h and 48h coincubation times were selected so as not to miss any possible cytotoxicity. And these experiments were repeated several times with a few sets of MC colonies on different times. Samples were tested in duplicates for reproducibility and reliability.

### 2.7 Target lymphoma cell labeling with mAb and detection of death after coincubation

Labeling target cells were done by two different methods in this study. As mentioned earlier, the first one is DIOC18 prelabeling for leukemia samples, which is being done before coincubation. The second technique is based on marking the lymphoma targets such as Daudi and Raji cells after co-incubation with 10µl of mouse anti-human PE conjugated CD19 mAb (Immunotech, Westbrook, ME) for 20 minutes before staining for detection of death.

Detection of apoptosis/death in target cells in mAb labeling technique was done by staining with AnnexinV (AnnV) and propidium iodide (PI) (TACS™ AnnexinV-FITC; R&D Systems, Minneapolis, MN) for 20 minutes before FCM acquisition. AnnV+ and/or PI+ events were analyzed from gating on the events in the target population of the control as well as coincubation samples. Ann V+ events represent early apoptotic population, AnnV+/ PI+ dead (late apoptotic or necrotic) cells (Fig.1F1-I2). In the DIOC18 prelabeling method, counterstaining with the nuclear dye PI (R&D Systems, Minneapolis, MN) of target cells was also done for 20 minutes before acquisition to discriminate between live and dead target cells. PI+ events represent dead cell population in FCM (Fig.1C1-E3).

### 2.8 FCM acquisition and running

FCM was performed using an EPICS-XL MCL (multicarousel) (Coulter, Miami, FL) equipped with an argon laser (15 mW) source operating at 488 nm. The emission of three fluorochromes was recorded through specific band pass filters: 525 nm for FITC (FL1), 575 nm for PE (FL2), 620 nm for fluorospheres (FL3), and 675 nm for PI (FL4). The instrument was set for 4-color analysis. As the emission spectra of the three different dyes utilized in this bioassay interfere with one another, appropriate electronic compensations were adjusted by running individual cell populations stained with each dye consecutively through the EPICS. Once the compensations had been set, a gating was done on forward scatter (FS) (ordinate) versus log-scale fluorescence of mAb CD19 or DIOC18 (abscissa), to separate target cells from effector cells (Fig.1C1-I2). The FS gating was especially helpful for separating bigger DAMI and Meg-01 target cells from effector MCs. The log-scale fluorescence (CD19 or DIOC18) of abscissa was well enough to separate targets from effectors besides the aid of FS gatings. The different cell populations (target, effector and coincubated cells) were gated on with the help of isotype control samples. To measure target-cell death and apoptosis, CD19-/DIOC18- positive events were gated on, and analysis of log green fluorescence (AnnV) and/or log red fluorescence (PI) was performed depend on the cytotoxicity technique ( Fig.1C1-I2).

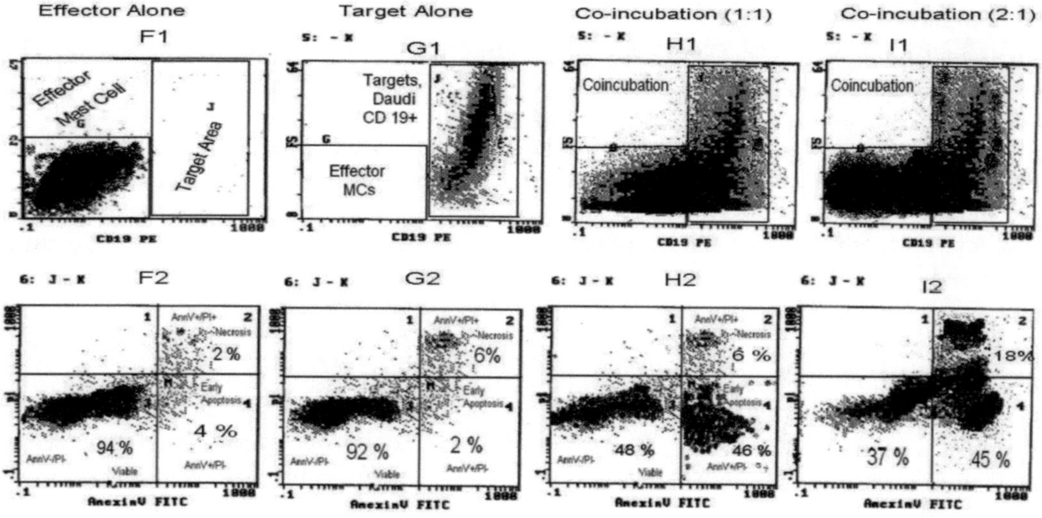


Fig. 1. F1- I2. Target (Daudi) cell kill, caused by mast cell- mediated cytotoxicity, is demonstrated by flow cytometric mast cell -mediated cytotoxicity assay (FCM-MCMCA) at 12h in a representative sample. Quadrant gating and determination of populations in fig. 1F1- H2 were defined by control samples consisting of target/effector alone tubes. The histograms in fig. 1G2-H2 were achieved from gating accordingly on target cell populations. 1F1 shows location of effector-mast cell in the histograms of FCM-MCMCA. Effector cells are seen as CD19 negative (effector alone sample). 1F2 demonstrates spontaneous kill in effector cell population in control tube. 1G1 shows target-tumor cells location. As expected, the target cell population is well-marked with CD19 in the histogram and there is no effector cell (target alone sample) in the tube. 1G2 shows spontaneous kill in the target cell population of the control sample. It shows 92% viable (Annexin-/ PI-) target (Daudi) cells with total 8% spontaneous killing including early apoptotic plus necrotic kill. 1H1 demonstrates co-incubated effector and target cells at 1:1 ratio after 12h (co-incubation sample). It reveals the changes in the target cell population in the quadrant J of the fig. 1G1 in coincubated samples after cytotoxic kill. Compared to fig. 1G1, decrease in size and amount of the target cell population of 1H1 indicates killing due to mast cell -mediated cytotoxicity. Effector cells in this sample are not stained with CD19 and they are in a different area. However; it is hard to say anything about conjugate formation between target and effector cells (effector-target doublets) in the co-incubation sample, and it seems probable that it is happening earlier. The doublets probably form and immediately dissolve during the beginning of this process. Thus, there is no reflection of conjugate formation in fig. 1H1. 1H2 histogram of co-incubation sample was acquired after gating on the population in the quadrant J of fig. 1H1 and reflects the alterations in that co-incubated target population after cytotoxic kill. It depicts obvious decrease in viability of the target cells from 92% to 48%. It shows increased death up to 52 %, which 6 % of killing was necrotic-late apoptotic (Annexin+/PI+) and 46 % of killing was early apoptotic (Annexin+/PI-). Obviously, decline in viability of the target cell population from 92% to 48% strongly reveals significant killing due to human mast cell- mediated cytotoxicity in vitro. Similarly, 1I1 shows further decrease in size and amount of the target cell population of 1G1 and 1H1 due to augmented cytotoxic kill at 2:1 ratio. And 1I2 demonstrates a decrease in viability of the target cell population from 92% to 37%, but death increased up to 53% at a higher ratio.

### 2.9 FCM data analysis

An average of 10,000 total events and 3,000 target cells were collected per sample. The gating for the target cells was based on the target-alone analysis and kept constant throughout all tubes to avoid exaggeration of the counts due to apoptotic body contamination. Cytotoxicity calculations were based on viable populations in target-alone (control) and co-culture (coincubated) tube analysis results. Viable target-cell percentage was determined, and calculations were based on the control-tube (target alone) values. Apoptotic and/or necrotic death happening in control tubes were identified as spontaneous, but those killed in coincubated tubes were identified as cytotoxic killing. We expressed the MCC as percentage based cytotoxicity:

### 2.10 Percentage based cytotoxicity (%, PC)

As mentioned, we defined MCC occurring in co-culture tube (coincubated sample) as percent (%, PC) cytotoxicity. And cytotoxicity calculations were based on viable populations in target-alone (control) and co-culture tube analysis results.

$$\text{Percent Cytotoxicity (PC)}=\frac{[\text{Control-viable cell\%}]-[\text{Coincubation-viable cell\%}]}{[\text{Control-viable cell\%}]}$$

Our in vitro experiments were repeated several times (n=27) with a few sets of MC colonies. Samples were tested in duplicates for reproducibility and reliability (mean coefficients of variation (CV) of 1.1% (95% CI, 0.8- 1.7%); r2=0.93, and $p<0.001$).

### 2.11 Comparison with chromium- $^{51}Cr$ release assay (CRA)

A standard assay was performed as previously described (Özdemir, 2007). Briefly, the assay is a standard 4h CRA using target cells that have been prelabeled with 100 µCi 51Cr (Perkin Elmer, Boston, MA) for 1h. Several concentrations of MCs were added to a fixed number of target cells (5,000) in a round bottom microtiter plate to a total volume of 0.2 ml. Following the 4h incubation, 0.1 ml of the supernatant was carefully harvested and counted on a scintillation counter (Packard, Downers Grove, IL). Maximum release was determined from wells including target cells and 10% sodium dodecyl sulfate in the medium. The PC was calculated using the following equation: $(E-S)/(M-S)\times 100$, where E is the experimental counts/minute, S is the spontaneous counts/minute and M is the maximum counts/minute. In the end, when we used some sets of our experimental data in comparing FCM cytotoxicity assays with CRA results, there was a significant correlation for PC (n=58; r= 0.95; $P<0.001$), similar to our earlier studies (Özdemir, 2007, 2011).

### 2.12 Cell staining with Wright/Giemsa for light microscopy

At the end of the coincubation period, the sample was gently mixed and 10µl was used to prepare slides at room temperature without cytospinning. The slides were then stained with Wright/Giemsa. Conjugate formations between some tumor cells and MCs were seen (Fig.1A1-A4).

### 2.13 Statistical analysis

Unless otherwise specified, all data are presented as means±SEM. The significance of differences between spontaneous and cytotoxic kill was determined using the paired

Student's t-test and/or Wilcoxon test. Correlations were estimated by Pearson correlation coefficients. Significance was considered as ≤0.05. All statistics were done using the Statistical Package for Social Sciences (SPSS-13 for Windows; Chicago, IL).

## 3. Results

This study demonstrated MCC against tumor cells by using human cells instead of murine effector/target cells. In vitro MCC against various tumor cells at different E:T ratios (1:1-5:1) was measured by FCM-MCMCA and DIOC18 methods on various periods (Table 2A-D).

| **Pecentage Based Mast Cell- Mediated Cytotoxicity (%, PC)** | | | | |
|---|---|---|---|---|
| **Cell characteristics** | | **%, PC on Coincubation Times** | | |
| **LAK-sensitive** | **Death Type** | **2h** | **18h** | **48h** |
| Effector (**Mast**) control/alone | Spontaneous | 2±1 | 1±1 | 3±1 |
| Target (**K562**) control | Spontaneous | 3±1 | 5±1 | 5±1 |
| Coincubation (5:1) | Cytotoxic | 4±2 | 7±1 | 18±2 |
| | N= | (3) | (9) | (9) |
| | P= | NS | NS | NS |
| **LAK-resistant** | **Death Type** | **2h** | **18h** | **48h** |
| Effector control /alone | Spontaneous | 1±1 | 2±1 | 3±1 |
| Target (**DAMI**) control | Spontaneous | 2±1 | 5±1 | 7±1 |
| Coincubation (5:1) | Cytotoxic | 9±1 | 19±2 | 24±2 |
| | N= | (3) | (9) | (9) |
| | P | NS | NS | NS |
| Effector control | Spontaneous | 2±1 | 3±1 | 3±1 |
| Target (**Meg-01**) control | Spontaneous | 1±0 | 5±1 | 8±1 |
| Coincubation (5:1) | Cytotoxic | 7±1 | 20±2 | 27±4 |
| | N= | (3) | (9) | (9) |
| | P= | NS | 0.059 | **0.031** |
| Effector control | Spontaneous | 3±1 | 4±1 | 4±1 |
| Target (**HL-60**) control | Spontaneous | 5±1 | 8±1 | 11±2 |
| Coincubation (5:1) | Cytotoxic | 6±2 | 18±1 | 39±3 |
| | N= | (3) | (9) | (9) |
| | P= | NS | 0.050 | **0.011** |
| Effector control | Spontaneous | 1±1 | 3±1 | 4±1 |
| Target (**Patients`**) control | Spontaneous | 2±1 | 8±1 | 13±1 |
| Coincubation (5:1) | Cytotoxic | 5±1 | 20±1 | 22±2 |
| | N= | (6) | (9) | (9) |
| | P= | NS | NS | NS |

The death/killings (percentage based cytotoxicity) in this table reflect the death at a 5:1 ratio in this study. Spontaneous kill reflects the death in target or effector alone tubes. Cytotoxic death shows the target cell death by only mast cell- mediated cytotoxicity in coincubation sample. The percentage based cytotoxicity was calculated according to the given formula in the methods. All values are given as mean±SEM. P values reflect the significance of differences between spontaneous and mast cell mediated cytotoxic killing. N denotes the number of experiments were repeated in each series. NS means not significant.

Table 2A. In vitro human mast cell -mediated cytotoxicity measured by DIOC18 method against different human tumor cells is shown.

| Percentage Based Human Mast Cell- Mediated Cytotoxicity (%, PC) | | | | |
|---|---|---|---|---|
| Cell characteristics | | %, PC on Coincubation Times | | |
| **LAK-sensitive** | **Death Type** | **2h** | **12h** | **24h** |
| Effector (**Mast**) control | Spontaneous | 3 ± 1 | 4 ± 1 | 5 ± 2 |
| Target (**Daudi**) control | Spontaneous | 2 ± 1 | 3 ± 1 | 6 ± 2 |
| Coincubation (1:1) | Cytotoxic | 21 ± 2 | 49 ± 2 | 53 ± 3 |
| | N= | (9) | (9) | (9) |
| | P= | **0.048** | **0.009** | **0.005** |
| Effector control/alone | Spontaneous | 4±1 | 3 ± 2 | 4 ± 2 |
| Target (Daudi) control/alone | Spontaneous | 4±1 | 3 ± 1 | 5 ± 2 |
| Coincubation (2:1) | Cytotoxic | 31±1 | 57± 2 | 63 ± 3 |
| | N= | (3) | (9) | (9) |
| | P= | **0.039** | **0.001** | **0.001** |
| Effector control | Spontaneous | 4±1 | 3 ± 2 | 4 ± 2 |
| Target (Daudi) control | Spontaneous | 2±1 | 4 ± 1 | 6 ± 2 |
| Coincubation (4:1) | Cytotoxic | 36±1 | 59± 2 | 67 ± 3 |
| | N= | (9) | (9) | (9) |
| | P= | **0.030** | **0.001** | **0.001** |
| Effector control / alone | Spontaneous | 2±1 | 3 ± 1 | 6 ± 1 |
| Target (**Raji**) control / alone | Spontaneous | 3±1 | 4 ± 1 | 8 ± 3 |
| Coincubation (1:1) | Cytotoxic | 13±1 | 16 ± 1 | 47± 3 |
| | N= | (9) | (9) | (9) |
| | P= | **0.049** | **0.046** | **0.008** |
| Effector alone | Spontaneous | 5±1 | 3 ± 1 | 4 ± 1 |
| Target (Raji) alone | Spontaneous | 7±1 | 5 ± 1 | 9 ± 3 |
| Coincubation (2:1) | Cytotoxic | 19±1 | 26 ± 1 | 67± 3 |
| | N= | (3) | (9) | (9) |
| | P= | **0.044** | **0.016** | **0.001** |
| Effector alone | Spontaneous | 4±1 | 6 ± 1 | 5 ± 1 |
| Target (Raji) alone | Spontaneous | 3±1 | 7 ± 1 | 8 ± 3 |
| Coincubation (4:1) | Cytotoxic | 19±1 | 30 ± 1 | 69± 3 |
| | N= | (9) | (9) | (9) |
| | P= | **0.040** | **0.014** | **0.001** |

The death/killings (percentage based cytotoxicity) in this table reflect the death at 1:1, 2:1, 4:1 ratios in this study. Spontaneous kill reflects the death in target or effector alone tubes. Cytotoxic death shows the target cell death by only mast cell-mediated cytotoxicity in the coincubation sample. The percentage based cytotoxicity was calculated according to the given formula in the methods. All values are given as mean±SEM. P values reflect the significance of differences between spontaneous and mast cell mediated cytotoxic killing. N denotes the number of experiments were repeated in each series. NS means not significant.

Table 2B. In vitro human mast cell-mediated cytotoxicity % (percentage based killing) measured by FCM-MCMCA against human LAK-sensitive tumor cells at different ratios and time periods (2h- 24h) are shown.

| Percentage Based Human Mast Cell- Mediated Cytotoxicity (%, PC) | | | | | | |
|---|---|---|---|---|---|---|
| **Cell characteristics** | | **%, PC on Coincubation Times** | | | | |
| **LAK-sensitive** | **Death Type** | **2h** | **12h** | **18h** | **24h** | **48h** |
| Effector (**Mast**) control/alone | Spontaneous | 2±1 | 4±1 | 3±1 | 5±1 | 7±1 |
| Target (**K562**) control | Spontaneous | 3±1 | 4±1 | 5±1 | 6±1 | 5±1 |
| Coincubation (2:1) | Cytotoxic | 0±1 | 6±1 | 6±1 | 14±1 | 16±2 |
| | N= | (3) | (9) | (9) | (9) | (9) |
| | P= | NS | NS | NS | NS | NS |
| Effector control | Spontaneous | 4±1 | 3 ± 2 | 3 ± 2 | 4 ± 2 | 4 ± 2 |
| Target **(Daudi**) control | Spontaneous | 4±1 | 3 ± 1 | 4 ± 1 | 5 ± 2 | 8 ± 2 |
| Coincubation (2:1) | Cytotoxic | 30±1 | 57± 2 | 59± 2 | 63 ± 3 | 65 ± 3 |
| | N= | (3) | (9) | (9) | (9) | (9) |
| | P= | **0.030** | **0.001** | **0.001** | **0.001** | **0.001** |
| Effector control | Spontaneous | 5±1 | 2 ± 1 | 2 ± 1 | 4 ± 1 | 4 ± 1 |
| Target (**Raji**) control | Spontaneous | 7±1 | 5 ± 1 | 7 ± 1 | 9 ± 3 | 10 ± 3 |
| Coincubation (2:1) | Cytotoxic | 19±1 | 26 ± 1 | 46 ± 1 | 67± 3 | 75± 3 |
| | N= | (3) | (9) | (9) | (9) | (9) |
| | P= | **0.044** | **0.016** | **0.006** | **0.001** | **0.001** |
| **LAK-resistant** | **Death Type** | **2h** | **12h** | **18h** | **24h** | **48h** |
| Effector (**Mast**) control/alone | Spontaneous | 5±1 | 3±1 | 4±1 | 6±1 | 8±1 |
| Target (**DAMI**) control/alone | Spontaneous | 2±1 | 5±1 | 5±1 | 7±1 | 7±1 |
| Coincubation (2:1) | Cytotoxic | 6±1 | 15±2 | 17±2 | 20±2 | 22±2 |
| | N= | (3) | (6) | (6) | (6) | (6) |
| | P= | NS | NS | NS | NS | NS |
| Effector control | Spontaneous | 3±1 | 5±1 | 4±1 | 6±1 | 6±1 |
| Target (**Meg-01**) control | Spontaneous | 1±0 | 6±1 | 5±1 | 8±1 | 8±1 |
| Coincubation (2:1) | Cytotoxic | 4±1 | 14±2 | 18±2 | 22±4 | 25±4 |
| | N= | (3) | (5) | (5) | (5) | (5) |
| | P= | NS | NS | NS | NS | **0.039** |
| Effector control | Spontaneous | 3±1 | 6±1 | 3±1 | 5±1 | 5±1 |
| Target (**HL-60**) control | Spontaneous | 5±1 | 7±1 | 8±1 | 9±2 | 11±2 |
| Coincubation (2:1) | Cytotoxic | 5±1 | 13±1 | 16±1 | 28±3 | 36±3 |
| | N= | (3) | (6) | (6) | (6) | (6) |
| | P= | NS | NS | NS | **0.034** | **0.019** |
| Effector control | Spontaneous | 3±1 | 2±1 | 4±1 | 6±1 | 6±1 |
| Target (**Patients`**) control | Spontaneous | 2±1 | 6±1 | 8±1 | 10±1 | 13±1 |
| Coincubation (2:1) | Cytotoxic | 5±1 | 15±1 | 18±1 | 20±2 | 21±2 |
| | N= | (6) | (6) | (6) | (6) | (6) |
| | P= | NS | NS | NS | NS | NS |

The death/killings (percentage based cytotoxicity) in this table reflect the death at a 2:1 ratio in this study. Spontaneous kill reflects the death in target or effector alone tubes. Cytotoxic death shows the target cell death by only mast cell-mediated cytotoxicity in the coincubation sample. The percentage based cytotoxicity was calculated should be given formula. All values are given as mean±SEM. P values reflect the significance of differences between spontaneous and mast cell mediated cytotoxic killing. N denotes the number of experiments were repeated in each series. NS means not significant.

Table 2C. In vitro human mast cell -mediated cytotoxicity (%, PC) against different human tumor cells measured by both cytotoxicity assays is shown at various periods.

| Cell Types | Percentage Based Human Mast Cell- Mediated Cytotoxicity (%) | | | | | |
|---|---|---|---|---|---|---|
| | 12h | | | 24h | | |
| | **Early Apoptotic** | **Late Apoptotic** | **Total Killing** | **Early Apoptotic** | **Late Apoptotic** | **Total Killing** |
| **Daudi** | 7% | 50% | 57 % | 23% | 40% | 63 % |
| **Raji** | 8 % | 18% | 26 % | 27% | 40% | 67 % |

Table 2D. The distribution of mean killing (%, PC) measured by FCM-MCMCA in human LAK-sensitive tumor cells at 2:1 ratio on different coincubation times in a representative sample.

In the literature, MCC did not seem to be very effective against some types of LAK-sensitive tumor cells, such as K562 and YAC-1 (Henderson, 1981; Ghiara, 1985; Richards 1988).Consistently, there was not significant killing (18% killing at most) in NK-/LAK-sensitive K562 cells even with 5:1 ratio at 48h (Table 2A,C). These findings supported well-known resistance to MCC by some LAK-sensitive cells. However, human MCC for first time was found to be very effective against different type of LAK-sensitive cells, such as Daudi and Raji, in this study. As shown in these studies, most of the total killing of both human target cells was necrotic kill and it increased over time. Interestingly, Raji killing, especially necrotic, apparently maximized at 24h, even though Daudi cell killing stayed almost stable and peaked at 12h. Both LAK-sensitive Daudi and Raji cell death were statistically significant between 2h-48h, compared to spontaneous killing. In vitro human MCC against LAK-sensitive cells at different ratios/times was shown in table 2B-C.

Moreover, in this study the FCM-MCMCA method allowed us to separate cytotoxic killing into different stages, early and late apoptotic (necrotic) kill. And distribution of apoptotic type killing according to the cell lines at 12h and 24h was shown at 2:1 ratio (Table 2D). Early apoptotic cell death up to 46% was also detected in the representative samples (Fig.1H2,I2), indicating the role of pro-apoptotic components of MC granules in human MCC.

Although at 2h/12h/18h there was some killing, statistically significant killing in LAK-resistant cells such as Meg-01 and HL-60 cells was demonstrated with both 2:1 and 5:1 ratios at 48h (Table 2A,C). In HL-60 cells, there was a statistically significant degree of kill at 18h (ratio 5:1) and 24h (ratio 2:1) as well. Moreover, the AML patient samples seemed to be very resistant to MCC. In patient cells, there was a fair amount of killing (≤25 %) but was not statistically significant (Table 2A,C). Insignificant killing in patient samples and LAK-resistant cells, probably due to small number of sample, but it was noticeably important. This is the first study demonstrating human MCC against some human LAK-resistant cells too.

After 2h/12h coincubations, neither at 2:1 nor at 5:1 ratios was there significant killing in any experiments except for Daudi and Raji cells. In LAK-sensitive Daudi/Raji cells, statistically significant death at different rates was demonstrated and remained significant from 2h-48h coincubation (Table 2B-C). Concurrently, short term MCC (≤18h) was observed in patient samples as well as DAMI/HL-60/Meg-01 cells in this study, although MCC in the long term is well-known. We even observed some degree of cytotoxicity in very short-term incubation (2h) in DAMI/Meg-01 cells, although there was not statistically significant killing. The killing detected between 2h-48h in all LAK-resistant cells including patients' was close to statistical significance, partly due to an inadequate number of experiments (Table 2A,C). In overall; Daudi/Raji/Meg-01 and HL-60 cell deaths were found to be statistically significant at different periods in long term, compared to spontaneous (control) killing (Table 2A-C). Thus, these findings reveal human MC`s cytotoxic capacity against human LAK-resistant/-sensitive cells.

Briefly, interestingly, MCs did not seem to be very effective against some type of human NK-/LAK-sensitive cells such as K562; but LAK-resistant cells including Meg-01/HL-60/DAMI/patients' were killed somewhat effectively by MCC.

The ability to study MCC in longer coincubation times (≤48h), in addition to shorter coincubation times (2h-18h), is another advantage of our established FCM methods in this study. This appears to be a drawback for CRA as well as other methods utilizing dyes such as fluorochromes (PKH-26) due to increased risk in release of $^{51}$Cr or dye leakage, which results in staining of other populations. Nevertheless, our applications are potentially important for studying certain apoptotic pathways that take longer to become operational, such as membranous TNF-α-induced apoptosis, which is believed to be one of most important components of MCC. Membranous TNF-α has been shown to kill WEHI-164/L929/Raji cells in 24h assays (Henderson, 1981; Ghiara, 1985; Richards 1988; Heikkilä, 2008; Özdemir, 2003, 2006).

In this study, our results were found to be reproducible and reliable when experiments repeated (mean coefficients of variation (CV) of 1.1%). Incremental increase in MCC detected at different ratios/times shows reproducibility and reliability of our methods (Table 2A-C). When our flow cytometric data compared with CRA results, there was a significant correlation ($n=104$, $r=0.82$, $p<0.001$), similar to our earlier studies (Özdemir, 2003, 2007, 2011).

In addition, Wright-Giemsa slides showed conjugate formations between MC and some tumor cells (MC-target cell doublets), indicating possible initial steps of human MCC, perhaps via cell-to-cell contact thru their membranous components such as membranous TNF-α/Fas Ligand (Fig.1A1-4).

## 4. Discussion

This study first of all demonstrated human MCC against human tumor targets by two different approaches that were very comparable to CRA. These are established and reliable methods elucidating MCC by a two- and three-color FCM assays using DIOC18 and mAb target-cell marking, respectively. Our research experiences with these methods have been recently published (Özdemir, 2003, 2007, 2011).

As mentioned above, murine MCC against lysis-sensitive murine tumor cell lines (WEHI-164/L929) in long term was previously well demonstrated (Henderson, 1981; Ghiara, 1985; Richards 1988). Nevertheless, to the best of our knowledge, this is the first study using human BM-derived effector MCs against human tumor cells to show and verify short- and long-term human MCC in vitro. Even significant kill in different LAK-sensitive/-resistant cells was also demonstrated for the first time. MCC was shown to be effective against different types of NK-/LAK-sensitive Daudi/Raji cells, but not to K562 cells or LAK-resistant cells. These findings are consistent with earlier murine studies demonstrating murine MCC against lysis-sensitive cells. Like murine cells, Daudi/Raji are also known to be somewhat lysis (TNF-α)-sensitive, and this explains statistically significant and mostly necrotic killing in Daudi/Raji, which probably reflects pro-necrolytic characteristics of MCC.

Early cell death of LAK-sensitive/-resistant cells in our experiments detected from 2h indicated human MCC occurring in short-term coincubation. These results strongly suggest a possible contribution of a fast-acting secretory pathway via the exocytosis of pro-apoptotic granules of MCs to the human MCC. Accordingly, these findings verify the recent literature suggestive of MC-induced apoptosis in smooth muscle cell, cardiomyocytes and endothelial cells (Leskinen, 2003; Heikkilä, 2008).

The killing at various coincubation times in all LAK-resistant cells including patient cells was close to statistical significance partly due to an inadequate number of experiments. However, it was still noticeably important since these cells are known to be resistant to even LAK cells, and they are not essentially TNF-α sensitive cell. Thus our results also indicate a role for MC as a contributory effector cell in cellular immune surveillance of human innate immunity, resembling recently reported studies (Marshall, 2004; Özdemir, 2006).

Contrary to the findings of this in vitro study, MC availability in tissues and tumor stroma has still been controversial. The important point is here: increased tissue MCD could be primary and/or secondary since MCD is also found to be increased physiologically around healing tissue (Özdemir, 2006). MCs might be just as a reflection of generalized inflammatory reaction as well. For instance; the infiltration of MCs was thought to be a reflection of the host inflammatory response and is favorable prognostic factor in diffuse large B-cell lymphoma (Hedström, 2007). Similarly, MCs were believed to represent reactive cell types involve in the pathophysiology of the host reaction in lymphoma (Sharma, 1992). MCs also accumulate at sites of tumor growth in response to numerous chemoattractants or mediators. For example, CCL5/CXCR3 chemokines in lymphoma and tumor-derived stem cell factor and CD30 expressions lead to tumor growth and MCD in tumor tissues (Fischer, 2003). While evaluating the tumor-MC relationship, not only the MCD, but several other factors, such as the relationship of MCs with other stromal (fibroblasts, endothelial) and inflammatory cells should also be considered (Aldinucci, 2010). Hence it is important to find an answer to the following question: can the increased MCD be a result of tumor progression or a cause of tumor progression and a poor prognosis? Then the next question becomes, is the MC really an active player or an innocent passerby in a tumor stroma?

Increased MCD in the tumor stroma was assumed to be a stimulator of tumor progression through angiogenesis. As with other tumors; there are also conflicting results about the role of MCD and its relation to microvessel density (MVD) in lymphoma/leukemia (Özdemir, 2006). In addition, lymphoma progression is recently considered to be potentiated by at least two distinct angiogenic mechanisms. Autocrine stimulation of tumor cells via expression of vascular endothelial growth factor (VEGF) and VEGF receptors by lymphoma cells, as well as paracrine influences of proangiogenic tumor stroma on both local neovascularization and recruitment of circulating BM-derived progenitors (Ruan, 2009). Similarly, isolated AML blasts were shown to overexpress the VEGF/VEGFR-2 pathway, which can promote the growth of leukemic blasts in an autocrine and paracrine manner (Mesters, 2001). Yet, in some literature the following are hematological tumors in which MCD correlates with MVD: B-cell non-Hodgkin lymphoma, HL, follicular/angioimmunoblastic T-cell lymphoma, and B-cell chronic lymphocytic leukemia (Ribatti, 1998; Fukushima, 2001; Ribatti, 2009; Tripodo, 2010; Taskinen, 2010). And human tumors in which MCD is supposed to correlate with a poor prognosis include HL, diffuse large B-cell lymphoma, follicular and angioimmunoblastic T-cell lymphoma (Molin, 2002; Gratzinger, 2007; Ribatti, 2009;

Taskinen, 2010;). Amazingly, in some studies, human tumors in which MCD is supposed to correlate with a good prognosis include HL, diffuse large B-cell lymphoma, and follicular lymphoma (Koster, 2005; Hedström, 2007; Rygoł, 2007;Ribatti, 2009;). Although it is hard to explain these conflicting results above and in the literature, they may be associated with different methodologies used in studies such as timing of biopsy (e.g. doing in early instead of late stage of tumor), the tumor type, as well as environmental factors surrounding that tumor (Özdemir, 2006). Only observing increased MCD in various tumors with good or bad prognosis on pathological specimens seems to be far behind to explain the real role of MCs. The net effect of MCs on tumor growth, therefore, is likely to be the result of multiple interactions between MC, tumor, and associated inflammatory cells with their signaling pathways, and adjacent stromal cells such as vascular endothelium and fibroblasts (Ribatti, 1998; Özdemir, 2006; Ribatti, 2009; Aldinucci, 2010).

Consequently, antiangiogenic strategies have recently become an important therapeutic modality for solid tumors. And MCs have been thought of as a new target for the adjuvant treatment of tumors through the selective inhibition of angiogenesis, tissue remodeling and tumor promoting molecules. Preliminary studies with cromolyn in mice mammary adenocarinoma and pancreatic cancer therapy was ineffective. Although some therapeutics like alemtuzumab were also given as an example of antiangiogenic treatment success, it is known as an anti-myeloid cell antiangiogenic agent used for the treatment of ovarian cancer, not an anti-MC agent (Ruan, 2009). Beside MCs and myeloid cells, Tie2-expressing monocytes and vascular leukocytes have recently been shown as new targets in the regulation of tumor associated angiogenesis (De Palma, 2007). In the age of targeted therapy, studies of the targeting MCs` role in cancer might have direct clinical consequences and should be further elucidated via the use of histopathological and complex biological models.

Since the aim of this study was basically to show MCC using human effector/target cells, the mechanisms and specificity of human MCC were not evaluated in this study. Our studies still continue studying MC-tumor cell relations and the characteristics of MCC on human pathological biopsy specimens. We hypothesize that human MCC may happen thru non-secretory pathway (cell-to-cell contact) of membranous TNF-α/Fas L, and secretory pathway via released mediators like soluble TNF-α, granzymes and chymase. Simply, MCC happens via pro-apoptotic/-necrolytic granules of MCs in the short term, as well as through its membranous components (non-secretory pathway of MCC) in the long term as shown in this study. Consistently, observing effector-target doublets on Wright-Giemsa slides of this study might suggest the importance of cell-to-cell contact in this process. The mechanisms with characteristics of human MCC against human tumor cells, as well as the role of MC mediators, are discussed by us in detail somewhere (Özdemir, 2006).

## 5. Conclusion

Our findings in this study verify possible anti-tumor role of MC as a contributory effector cell to NK and other cytotoxic cells in immunosurveillance within human innate immunity. As current literature is still very confusing regarding MC`s role in and around the tumor tissue, this in vitro study may help enlighten its interactions with tumor cells and trigger new explanatory in vitro/in vivo studies like, for example, delineating the killing mechanisms of MCC.

These conflicting reports might indicate that there seem to be other factors determining the relationship between MCD and tumor progression. The conflicting results may also depend on wide variations in timing, tumor types/stages, methodologies, and the chemotherapy application as well. Importantly, some studies are not able to reflect the direct effects of MCs on tumor biology because many patients receive adjuvant chemotherapy in the time of sampling. So, some of the effects can be accounted for by the therapeutic response to chemotherapy. Nonetheless, by only observing increased MCD in and around a tumor, making a correlation between good or bad prognosis and specimens seems inadequate to explain their real role.

## 6. Acknowledgment

Development of this method was initiated by the author in Wayne State University in Detroit, MI and later completed during his tenure at Louisiana State University—HSC, New Orleans, LA in USA. The author thanks to Liqiao Ma for editing English in the chapter.

## 7. References

Prior, C. & Sesenna, R. (1953). Mast cells and their relation to the tumors of the bladder. *Rivista di Anatomia Patologica e di Oncologia,* Vol.7, No.8, pp. 809- 838.

Henderson, W.R.; Chi, E.Y.; Jong, E.C. & Klebanoff, S.J. (1981). Mast cell-mediated tumor-cell cytotoxicity. Role of the peroxidase system. *The Journal of Experimental Medicine,* Vol.153, No.3, (1981 Mar), pp. 520-533. Print ISSN: 0022-1007

Ghiara, P.; Boraschi, D.; Villa, L.; Scapigliati, G.; Taddei C. &Tagliabue A. (1985). In vitro generated mast cells express natural cytotoxicity against tumour cells. *Immunology,* Vol.55, No.2, (1985 June), pp. 317-324. Online ISSN: 1365-2567

Richards, A.L.; Okuno, T.; Takagaki, Y. & Djeu, J.Y. (1988). Natural cytotoxic cell-specific cytotoxic factor produced by IL-3-dependent basophilic/mast cells. Relationship to TNF. *The Journal of Immunology,* Vol.141, No.9, (1988 November), pp.3061-3066. Print ISSN: 0022-1767

Marshall, J.S. & Jawdat, D.M. (2004). Mast cells in innate immunity. *The Journal of Allergy and Clinical Immunology,* Vol.114, No.1, (2004 July), pp. 21-27. ISSN: 0091-6749

Özdemir, Ö. (2007). Evaluation of human mast cell-mediated cytotoxicity by DIOC18 target cell labeling in flow cytometry. *Journal of Immunological Methods,* Vol.319, No.1-2, (2007 January), pp. 98-103. ISSN: 0022-1759.

Özdemir, Ö. (2011). Flow cytometric mast cell-mediated cytotoxicity assay: a three-color flow cytometric approach using monoclonal antibody staining with annexin V/propidium iodide co-labeling to assess human mast cell-mediated cytotoxicity by fluorosphere-adjusted counts. *Journal of Immunological Methods.* Vol.365, No.1-2, (2011 February), pp. 166-173. ISSN: 0022-1759.

Della Rovere, F.; Granata, A.; Monaco, M. & Basile G. (2009). Phagocytosis of cancer cells by mast cells in breast cancer. *Anticancer Research.* Vol.29, No.8, (2009 August), pp. 3157-3161. ISSN: 0250-7005.

Leskinen, M.J.; Lindstedt, K.A.; Wang, Y. & Kovanen, P.T. (2003). Mast cell chymase induces smooth muscle cell apoptosis by a mechanism involving fibronectin degradation and disruption of focal adhesions. *Arteriosclerosis, Thrombosis, and Vascular Biology.* Vol.23, No.2, (2003 February), pp. 238-243. Print ISSN:1079-5642

Heikkilä, H.M.; Lätti, S.; Leskinen, M.J.; et al. (2008 ). Activated mast cells induce endothelial cell apoptosis by a combined action of chymase and tumor necrosis factor-alpha. *Arteriosclerosis, Thrombosis, and Vascular Biology*. Vol.28, No.2, (2008 February), pp. 309-314. Print ISSN:1079-5642

Wagelie-Steffen, A.L.; Hartmann, K.; Vliagoftis, H. & Metcalfe, D.D. (1998). Fas ligand (FasL, CD95L, APO-1L) expression in murine mast cells. *Immunology*. Vol.94, No.4, (1998 August), pp. 569-574. Online ISSN: 1365-2567

Pardo, J.; Wallich, R.; Ebnet, K.; et al. (2007). Granzyme B is expressed in mouse mast cells in vivo and in vitro and causes delayed cell death independent of perforin. *Cell death and Differentiation*. Vol.14, No.10, (2007 October), pp. 1768-1779. ISSN : 1350-9047

Kataoka, T.R.; Morii, E.; Oboki, K. & Kitamura Y. (2004). Strain-dependent inhibitory effect of mutant mi-MITF on cytotoxic activities of cultured mast cells and natural killer cells of mice. *Laboratory Investigation*. Vol.84, No.3, (2004 March), pp. 376-384. ISSN: 0023-6837

Özdemir, Ö. (2006). Mast cells and the tumor-associated neoangiogenesis. *Medical Science Monitor*. Vol.12, No.6, (2006 June), pp. LE9-11. Print ISSN: 1234-1010

Ribatti, D.; Vacca, A.; Marzullo, A.; et al. (2000). Angiogenesis and mast cell density with tryptase activity increase simultaneously with pathological progression in B-cell non-Hodgkin's lymphomas. *International Journal of Cancer*. Vol.85, No.2, (2000 January), pp. 171-175. Print ISSN: 0020-7136

Ribatti, D. & Crivellato, E. (2009). The controversial role of mast cells in tumor growth. *International Review of Cell and Molecular Biology*. Vol.275, pp. 89-131.

Molin, D.; Edström, A.; Glimelius, I.; et al. (2002). Mast cell infiltration correlates with poor prognosis in Hodgkin's lymphoma. *British Journal of Haematology*. Vol.119, No.1, (2002 October), pp. 122-124. Online ISSN : 1365-2141

Özdemir, Ö.; Ravindranath, Y. & Savaşan, S. (2003). Cell-mediated cytotoxicity evaluation using monoclonal antibody staining for target or effector cells with AnnexinV/Propidium Iodide co-labeling by fluorosphere-adjusted counts on three-color flow cytometry. *Cytometry*. Vol.56A, No.1, (2003 November), pp. 53-60.;56 : ISSN (electronic):1552-4930

Hedström, G.; Berglund, M.; Molin, D.; Fischer, M.; Nilsson, G. & Thunberg, U. (2007). Mast cell infiltration is a favourable prognostic factor in diffuse large B-cell lymphoma. *British Journal of Haematology*. 2007; Vol.138, No.1, (2007 July), pp. 68-71. Online ISSN: 1365-2141

Sharma, V.K.; Agrawal, A.; Pratap, V.K.; Nagar, A.M. & Mehrotra, M.L. (1992). Mast cell reactivity in lymphoma: a preliminary communication. *Indian Journal of Cancer*. Vol.29, No.2, (1992 June), pp. 61-65. ISSN 0019-509X

Fischer, M.; Juremalm, M.; Olsson, N.; et al. (2003). Expression of CCL5/RANTES by Hodgkin and Reed-Sternberg cells and its possible role in the recruitment of mast cells into lymphomatous tissue. *International Journal of Cancer*. Vol.107, No.2, (2003 November), pp. 197-201. Print ISSN: 0020-7136

Aldinucci, D.; Gloghini, A.; Pinto, A.; De Filippi, R. & Carbone, A. (2010). The classical Hodgkin's lymphoma microenvironment and its role in promoting tumour growth and immune escape. *The Journal of Pathology*. Vol.221, No.3, (2010 July), pp. 248-263. ISSN 1096-9896

Ruan, J.; Hajjar, K.; Rafii, S. & Leonard J.P. (2009). Angiogenesis and antiangiogenic therapy in non-Hodgkin's lymphoma. *Annals of Oncology*. Vol.20, No.3, (2009 March), pp. 413-424. Print ISSN 0923-7534

Mesters, R.M.; Padró, T.; Steins, M.; et al. (2001). Angiogenesis in patients with hematologic malignancies. *Onkologie*. Vol.24, No. Suppl 5, (2001 September), pp. 75-80. ISSN (electronic): 1423-0240

Fukushima, N.; Satoh, T.; Sano, M. & Tokunaga, O. (2001). Angiogenesis and mast cells in non-Hodgkin's lymphoma: a strong correlation in angioimmunoblastic T-cell lymphoma. *Leukemia and Lymphoma*. Vol.42, No.4, (2001 August), pp. 709-720. Print ISSN: 1042-8194

Tripodo, C.; Gri, G.; Piccaluga, P.P.; et al. (2010). Mast cells and Th17 cells contribute to the lymphoma-associated pro-inflammatory microenvironment of angioimmunoblastic T-cell lymphoma. *American Journal of Pathology*. Vol.177, No.2, (2010 August), pp. 792-802. Print ISSN: 0002-9440

Ribatti, D.; Nico, B.; Vacca, A.; et al. (1998). Do mast cells help to induce angiogenesis in B-cell non-Hodgkin's lymphomas? *British Journal of Cancer*. Vol.77, No.11, (1998 June), pp. 1900-1906. ISSN: 0007 0920

Taskinen, M.; Jantunen, E.; Kosma, V.M.; Bono, P.; Karjalainen-Lindsberg, M.L. & Leppä, S. (2010). Prognostic impact of CD31-positive microvessel density in follicular lymphoma patients treated with immunochemotherapy. *European Journal of Cancer*. Vol.46, No.13, (2010 September), pp. 2506-2512. ISSN 1359-6349

Gratzinger, D.; Zhao, S.; Marinelli, R.J.; et al. (2007). Microvessel density and expression of vascular endothelial growth factor and its receptors in diffuse large B-cell lymphoma subtypes. *American Journal of Pathology*. Vol.170, No.4, (2007 April), pp. 1362-1369. Print ISSN: 0002-9440

Rygoł, B.; Kyrcz-Krzemień, S.; Pajiak, J.; Konicki, P.; Kowai E. & Gasińska, T. (2007). Tryptase- and chymase-positive mast cells as possible prognostic factor in patients with Hodgkin's lymphoma. *Polskie Archiwum Medycyny Wewnętrznej*. Vol.117, No.1-2, (2007 January-February), pp. 27-32.

Koster, A.; van Krieken, J.H.; Mackenzie, M.A.; et al. (2005). Increased vascularization predicts favorable outcome in follicular lymphoma. *Clinical Cancer Research*. Vol.11, No.1, (2005 January), pp. 154-161. ISSN: 1078-0432

De Palma, M.; Murdoch, C.; Venneri, M.A.; et al. (2007). Tie2-expressing monocytes: regulation of tumor angiogenesis and therapeutic implications. *Trends in Immunology*. Vol.28, No. 12, (2007 December), pp. 519-524. ISSN: 1471-4906

Özdemir, Ö. (2006). Mast cell density, angiogenesis and their significance in tumor development. *Gynecologic Oncology*. Vol.100, No.3, (2006 March), pp. 628–629. Print ISSN: 0090-8258

2

# The Application of Membrane Vesicles for Cancer Therapy

Khan Salma, Jutzy Jessica M.S., Aspe Jonathan R., Valenzuela Malyn May A., Park Joon S., Turay David and Wall Nathan R.
*Loma Linda University, Dept. of Biochemistry, Ctr. for Health Disparities & Mol. Med.Loma Linda, California, United States of America*

## 1. Introduction

Cancer, a leading cause of death globally, is projected to become more prevalent in coming years due to increasing life expectancy. Among possible treatment options, the use of biomarkers especially has shown great potential as a gateway to personalized medicine, and in turn, great promise for improved diagnosis, prognosis and treatment of cancer and other diseases. However, the use of biomarkers in cancer therapeutics has thus far exhibited mild success, at best. The most common tool used for biomarker discovery is plasma proteomics due to the accessibility of blood samples and the rapid development of highly sensitive proteomics technologies. However, other body fluids such as urine may also be a reservoir for important marker proteins.

Extracellular membrane vesicles ranging in diameter of 30-1000 nm and originating from various cellular origins have been increasingly recognized for their participation in a variety of both normal and pathological cellular processes. Regardless of their cell type of origin these membrane bound vesicles or exosomes provide a protected and controlled internal microenvironment outside the cell for metabolic objectives of the host cell to be carried out at a distance from the host cell. They are also believed to be instrumental in cell-cell and cell-extracellular communication. Moreover, while knowledge of exosome biogenesis and physiological relevance remains limited, accumulating evidence suggests that their bioactivity may be clinically applicable in cancer therapeutics. One recent work suggests that the use of exosomes in immunotherapy may prime the immune system to recognize and kill cancer cells and thus could form a viable basis for the development of novel cancer vaccines.

This chapter will review current knowledge pertaining to exosomes, describe possible uses of exosomes in immunotherapy, and address challenges and future directions in bringing exosome-based cancer vaccines or immunotherapies closer to clinical reality.

## 2. Exosome biogenesis, secretion and physiologic considerations

Since their description in the process of reticulocyte maturation almost a quarter century ago (Johnstone *et al.*, 1987), exosomes; the intralumenal vesicles (ILV's) of multivesicular bodies (MVB's), have gained significant notoriety as evidenced by the nearly 10-15 fold rise in the amount of publications devoted to the subject just within the past decade (Raimondo *et al.*, 2011).

Many types of vesicles have been described in the literature having quite heterogeneous size, protein content, RNA content and origin. As a result there have been many names given to these different vesicle types (**Table 1**) (Ronquist & Brody, 1985; Ronquist & Frithz, 1986; Rooney *et al.*, 1993; Arienti *et al.*, 1997; Thery *et al.*, 2006; Lehmann *et al.*, 2008; Schiller *et al.*, 2008; Simpson *et al.*, 2008; Skog *et al.*, 2008; Dashevsky *et al.*, 2009; Di Vizio *et al.*, 2009; Haubold *et al.*, 2009; Jansen *et al.*, 2009; Nilsson *et al.*, 2009; Duijvesz *et al.*, 2010). Unfortunately, the different names given to these vesicles lead to much confusion and it is still unclear if all of the different vesicles are unique in biological function or if they represent a sliding scale of one entity (Duijvesz *et al.*, 2010). Exosomes are nanometer sized lipid bound vesicles derived from late endosomes contained in MVB's. They are characterized by their size 40-100nm, density ranging from 1.13g/ml to 1.19g/ml on a sucrose gradient (Record *et al.*, 2011) and their specific protein content (heat shock proteins, tetraspanins, Rab proteins, etc) **Figure 1**. Exosomes are secreted by both hematopoietic (eg dendritic cells, lymphocytes, mast cells) and non-hematopoietic cells such as fibroblasts, intestinal epithelium, neurons and various tumor cells. Exosomes have been isolated from serum and other biological fluids such as urine, ascitic fluid, amniotic fluid and even cerebrospinal fluid (Vella *et al.*, 2008). Exosome biogenesis involves an inward budding of the limiting membrane of late endosomes, also known as multivesicular bodies (MVBs) **(Figure 2)**, concurrent protein sorting into these budding exosomes, and subsequent splitting (scission) of these microvesicles (Keller et al., 2006). As a consequence, the nascent exosome contains the inner leaflet of the limiting membrane, membrane associated proteins, both native and recruited, and some amount of cytosol and cytosolic proteins.

| Vesicle | Size (nm) | Marker Proteins | Function | Reference |
|---|---|---|---|---|
| Exosomes | 50-150 | CD9, CD63, CD81, CD82, annexins, and RAB proteins | Antigen presentation, immune regulation, metastatic activity | Jansen FH, et al., 2009; Nilsson J, et al., 2009; Simpson RJ, et al., 2008; Thery C, et al., 2006 |
| Prostasomes | 50-500 | CD13, CD46, CD55, CD59, annexins, and RAB proteins | Immunosuppressive and sperm cell motility improving | Ronquist G, et al., 1985; Arienti G, et al., 1997; Ronquist G, et al., 1986; Rooney IA, et al., 1993 |
| Oncosomes | 50-500 | Signal transduction proteins | Function unknown | Di Vizio D, et al., 2009 |
| Microvessicles | 100-1000 | Integrins, selectins, CD40 ligands | Procoagulation and anticoagulation | Skog J, et al., 2008; Lehmann BD, et al., 2008 |
| Ectosomes (microparticles) | 50-1000 | CR1 and proteolytic enzymes, no CD63 | Procoagulation and anticoagulation | Haubold K, et al., 2009; Dashevsky O, et al., 2009; Duijvesz D, et al., 2011 |
| Membrane Particles | P4: 50-80<br>P2: 600 | CD133, no CD63 | Stem cell marker, possible role in tissue development and maintenance | Marzesco AM, et al., 2005 |
| Exosome-like Vesicles | 20-50 | TNFR1 | Constitutive production of soluble cytokine receptors may be regulated | Hawari FI, et al., 2004 |
| Apoptotic Vesicles | 50-500 | Histones H1, H2A, H2B, H3 and H4 as well as DNA & RNA, no cytochrome c, p53 or Hsp70 | Autoantigen seclusion/ isolation | Thery C, et al., 2001; Schiller M et al., 2008 |

Table 1. Characteristics of different types of microvessicles.

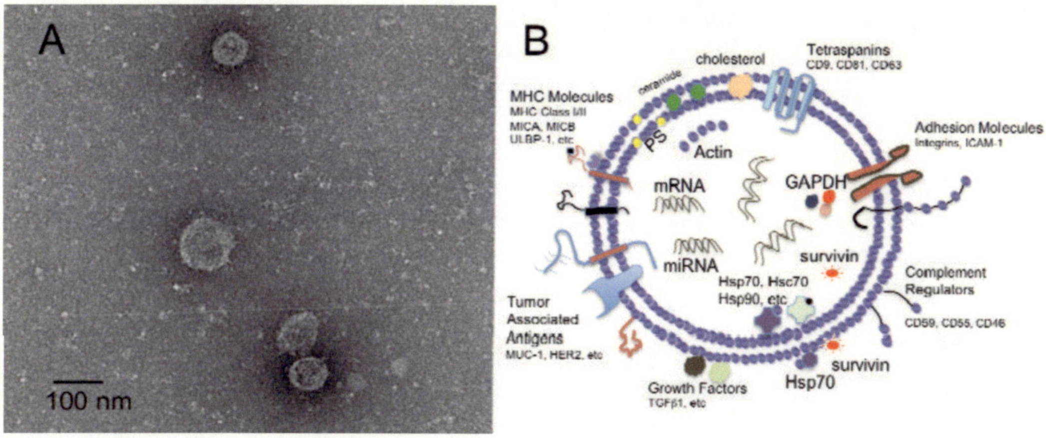


Fig. 1. Tumor derived exosomes (TEX). A. Electron microscopy revealed 50-100 nm sized microvesicles (Khan et al., 2011). B. Diagram depicting a typical TEX (modified from JP Mitchel, exosomes in cancer immunology).

The presence of specific proteins within and on the vesicle suggest the existence of a protein sorting mechanism during its formation. Some of these proteins are shared by exosomes derived from different sources and used to identify these vesicles during proteomic analysis. In our laboratory, we have consistently used the lysosomal associated membrane protein LAMP1 (common to exosomes from a wide variety of cells) as a positive control for exosome presence in western blot analysis (Khan *et al.*, 2011).

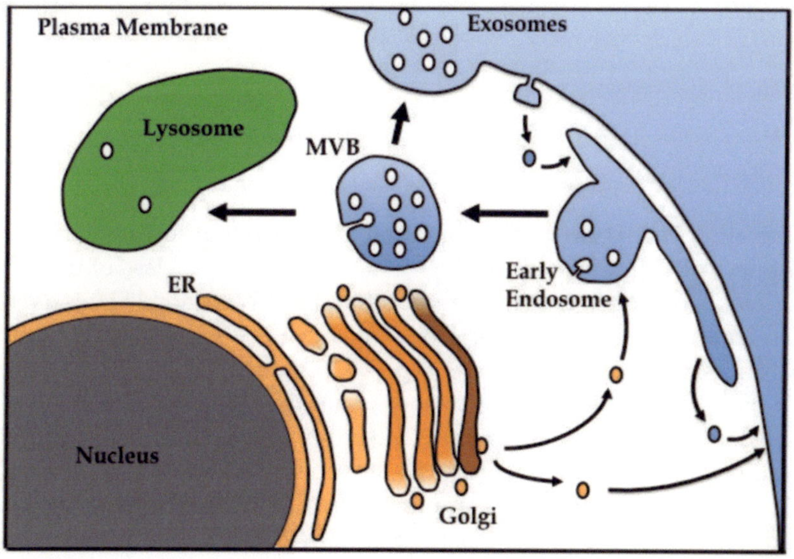


Fig. 2. Protein loading and release by exosomes. Endocytosed surface proteins as well as a subset of cytosolic proteins are taken by the endosomal system. Those destined for release as exosomes or for lysosomal degradation are sorted into lumenal vesicles called multivesicular bodies (MVB).

### 2.1 ESCRT-dependent protein sorting

The specific protein content of exosomes can be exploited to identify these exosomes and the cell-types from which they are derived via proteomic analysis. The fact that the exosome's protein content can be used as an identifier suggests the existence of a protein sorting mechanism during its formation. Endosomal Sorting Complex Required for Transport (ESCRT), comprised of a series of three protein complexes: ESCRT I, ESCRT II, and ESCRT III **(Figure 3)**, is suspected to play a critical role in sorting proteins into exosomes at the endosomal limiting membrane.

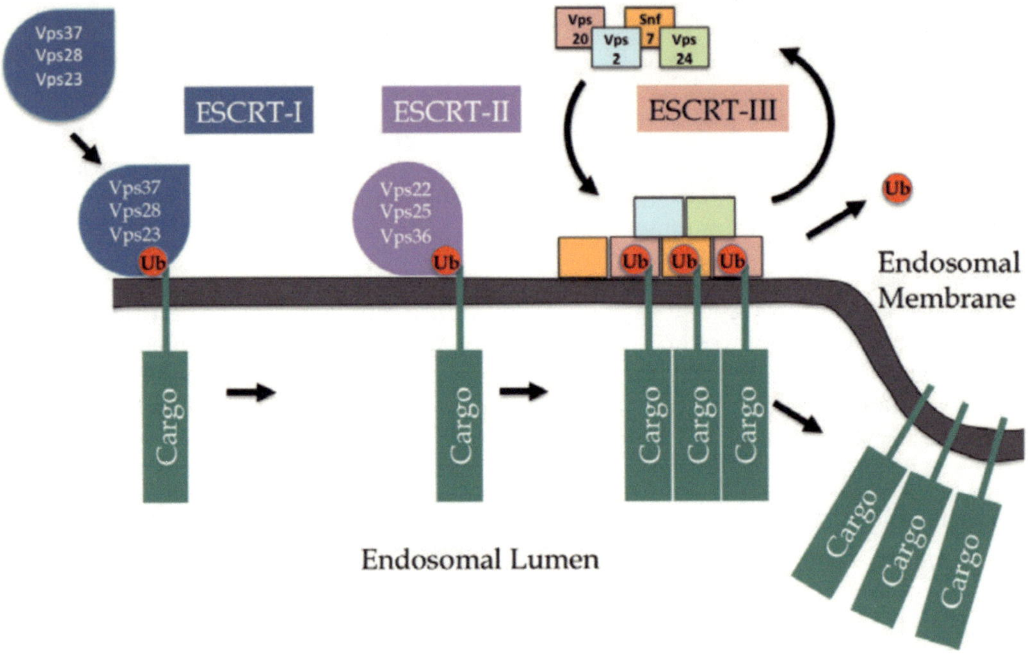


Fig. 3. Ubiquitin marks cargo proteins for endosomal sorting.

Monoubiquitination appears to mark cargo proteins for protein sorting within the MVBs. In yeast, recruitment of ubiquitinated cargo proteins depends on a class of proteins known as class E Vps (Vacuolar Protein Sorting) proteins that have been highly conserved from yeast to mammals—at least one mammalian homolog has been identified for each yeast class member (Babst, 2005). In the yeast model, Vps 27, is thought to complex on the endosomal membrane's outer leaflet with clathrin and ubiquitin-binding proteins, such as Golgi-associated, γ-adaptin homologs, Arf-binding (GGA) proteins, to form an endosomal clathrin coat that recruits monoubiquitinated cargo to the inner leaflet of the endosomal membrane. This complex recruits the ESCRT I complex from the cytoplasm and transfers to it the ubiquitinated cargo. ESCRT I then activates ESCRT II, which in turn occasions the oligomerization of Vps 2, Vps 20, Vps 24, and Snf 7 to form the ESCRT III complex and transfers to ESCRT III the ubiquitinated cargo. ESCRT III continues to accumulate and concentrates the cargo into still-budding exosomes of the MVB (Babst, 2005). The deubiquitinating protein Doa4 is then recruited into the complex where it functions to remove the ubiquitin from the cargo protein (Luhtala & Odorizzi, 2004). The ESCRT III complex subsequently dissociates from the cargo when the ATPase Vps 4 binds, thus releasing the cargo protein into the budding exosome.

### 2.2 Other modes of protein sorting

Other exosomal proteins, for which no ESCRT mechanisms have been described, may be incorporated into the exosome via varying levels of co-sorting. For example, tetraspanins may sort into exosomes due to their affinity for exosomal membrane components like sphingolipids and ceramides and may follow these phospholipids to further aggregate into lipid raft domains (de Gassart *et al.*, 2003). Protein-protein associations also contribute to co-sorting. MHC Class II molecules can associate with tetraspanins and be co-sorted into exosomal membranes (Blanc & Vidal, 2010). Some evidence also suggests lipid co-sorting into exosomes. The exosomal lipid LBPA (Lysobisphosphatidic Acid) can sort into exosomal membranes by interaction with the exosomal protein Alix. When present in media, LBPA was also shown to assist with the formation of vesicles in the MVBs (Matsuo *et al.*, 2004).

Hematopoietic cells including dendritic cells, lymphocytes and mast cells, and non-hematopoietic cells such as fibroblasts, intestinal epithelial cells, neurons and various tumor cells secrete exosomes. Exosome release from cells may follow a constitutive versus an inducible mode of secretion. The constitutive pathway utilizes the trans-golgi network, after which the vesicles travel through the cytoplasm via an intricate tubular network and eventually are released into the extracellular space (Ponnambalam & Baldwin, 2003). The inducible mode involves the release of preformed vesicles contained in MVBs. Such release may be dependent on known cellular triggers of vesicle release, such as increased intracellular calcium levels (Savina *et al.*, 2003). Other triggers, such as cellular depolarization, have also been described. These events culminate in the fusion of MVB membrane with the cell membrane and subsequent exosome release into the extracellular space.

Exosomes interact with target cells via specific receptors present on these target cells (Losche *et al.*, 2004). The exosome thus exerts its effect either via receptor-receptor interaction or internalization of the exosome with subsequent interaction of the exosome content with the recipient cellular machinery (Record *et al.*, 2011).

As will be described in other sections of this chapter, exosomes influence immune cells both in normal and abnormal states such as cancer. Furthermore RNA contained in exosomes could be translated within the recipient cell and as a result exert an epigenetic influence (Baj-Krzyworzeka *et al.*, 2006). In this regard, exosomes mimic viral particles by directing host cellular processes to its advantage. The role of exosomes in inflammatory conditions has recently been questioned after platelets and macrophage derived microparticles/exosomes were found in the lipid core of artherosclerotic plaques (Leroyer *et al.*, 2008). It is of interest to better understand the precise pro-inflammatory and thrombotic roles of exosomes and potentially use them as therapeutic targets in these conditions. Finally, the discovery of exosomes in urine has opened up the possibility of exosomal proteins being used as biomarkers for disease. It was recently shown that decreased levels of exosomal aquaporin-1 correlates with renal ischemia-reperfusion injury (Sonoda *et al.*, 2009). What makes this prospect exciting is the relative abundance of urine that can be obtained without an invasive procedure.

### 2.3 Summary

Exosomes are small membrane bound vesicles of endocytic origin that are released by most cells. The purpose for release seemed at first to be to discard membrane proteins and those believed to be resistant to lysosomal degradation. Now, it is believed that they mediate intercellular communication without the need for direct cell-to-cell interaction.

## 3. Existence of secreted membrane vesicles in cancers

Tumors are known to shed membrane vesicles (Taylor & Gercel-Taylor, 2005). In particular, human and mouse tumor cells have been shown to secrete tumor cell-derived exosomes (TEX), constitutively into the extracellular space (Wolfers *et al.*, 2001). The morphology, density and certain membrane markers expressed, such as LAMP1, MHC class I, HSP70 and HSP80, on the released TEX are similar to the dendritic cell-derived exosomes (DEX) (Andre *et al.*, 2002b) which will be discussed later. Despite similarities to DEX, there are differences in the molecular profiles and biological roles of TEXs, both of which give an indication of the cell of origin (Wieckowski & Whiteside, 2006). The specific protein content found on and within exosomes not only reflects their origin, but in addition, establishes their functional role (Zitvogel *et al.*, 1998) **(Table 2)**. TEX secreted from neoplastic cells express diverse tumor antigens, which signifies the type of tumor cells from where TEXs were released (Iero *et al.*, 2008). *In-vitro,* it has been shown that TEX released from breast carcinoma cells contain HER2, while carcinoembryonic antigen (CEA) was found in the exosomes secreted from colon carcinoma cells, and proteins MelanA/Mart-1 and gp100 that are expressed in melanoma cells are found on the released TEX (Andre *et al.*, 2002b; Andreola *et al.*, 2002). This phenomenon is also evident *in-vivo,* where plasma from cancer patients contain membrane vesicles that are characterized by the expression of tumor antigens which reflect the tumor of origin (Hegmans *et al.*, 2004; Mears *et al.*, 2004).

When immunocompetent and nude mice were pre-treated with murine mammary TEX, an accelerated growth of the tumor was observed (Liu *et al.*, 2006). This observation led to various studies to try to elucidate the role of secreted membrane vesicles in cancer. TEX can be described as "multi-purpose carriers" which have important roles in the communication, protection, as well as the exchange of genetic information with neighboring cells (Nieuwland & Sturk, 2010). The production and secretion of TEX is important for the tumor. They serve a protective function, have a supportive role in the survival and growth of the tumor cells, are involved in the promotion of host tissue invasion and subsequent metastasis, and facilitate evasion from the immune response (Valenti *et al.*, 2007; Anderson *et al.*, 2010). Acting in a paracrine fashion, the diverse function of TEX is speculated to be due to the various bioactive molecules found within and on the vesicles having a strong influence on the surrounding environment (Hegmans *et al.*, 2004; Mears *et al.*, 2004; van Niel *et al.*, 2006; Iero *et al.*, 2008).

The promotion of angiogenesis is due in part to the upregulation of vascular endothelial growth factor (VEGF) (Skog *et al.*, 2008) and release of matrix metalloproteinases (MMPs) in neighboring, even distant endothelial cells, which are brought by TEX containing tetraspanin family members (Gesierich *et al.*, 2006), epithelial growth factor receptor (EGFR) (Al-Nedawi *et al.*, 2009), platelet-derived tissue factor (TF) (Osterud, 2003) or developmental endothelial locus-1 protein (Hegmans *et al.*, 2004). TEX has also been implicated in the further growth of tumor by the exchange of genetic material. mRNA was detected within exosomes released from glioblastoma cells. Neighboring microvascular endothelial cells that take up the exosomes and translate the mRNA become liable for further tumor growth leading to the stimulation of angiogenesis (Skog *et al.*, 2008). In addition, tissue invasion and stromal remodeling can be facilitated by proteases and MMP transport and release via exosomes (Ginestra *et al.*, 1998; Graves *et al.*, 2004).

| Cancer Type | Protein | References |
|---|---|---|
| **Breast adenocarcinoma** (BT-474 MDA-MB-231, TS/A, H-2, P815) | ERBB2*/HER2* | (Andre *et al.*, 2002b; Koga *et al.*, 2005) |
| **Cervical Cancer** (heLa) | Survivin, HSP 70, HSP 90 | (Khan *et al.*, 2011) |
| **Colorectal Cancer** (LIM1215, HT29, SW403, 1869COL, AND CRC28462, LIM1215) | GPA 33*, CEACAM5*, EFNB1* annexins, ARFs*, Rabs*, ADAM10*, CD44*, NG2 ephrin-B1, MIF*, b-catenin, junction plakoglobin galectin-4, RACK1*, and tetraspanin-8, FASL* AND TRAIL* FASLG* TNFSF10* | (Andreola *et al.*, 2002; Abusamra *et al.*, 2005b; Huber *et al.*, 2005; Taylor & Gercel-Taylor, 2005; Choi *et al.*, 2007; Simpson *et al.*, 2009) |
| **Glioma** Cancer | EGFR* | (Al-Nedawi *et al.*, 2009) |
| **Melanoma** (Fon and Mel-888) | TRP*GP100*MART-1* Mel-CAM*FASLG*TNFSF10* A33*, CEA, EGFR*, ADAM10*, dipeptidase 1 ephrin-B1, hsc70, tetraspanins, ESCRT proteins (integrins, annexins, Rabs, and GTPases) | (Andre *et al.*, 2002b; Mears *et al.*, 2004; Abusamra *et al.*, 2005b) |
| **Mesothelioma** | PLVAP* | (Hegmans *et al.*, 2004) |
| **Ovarian** | ERBB2* | (Andre *et al.*, 2002b; Andreola *et al.*, 2002; Koga *et al.*, 2005) |
| **Prostate** | FASLG* TNFSF10* | (Huber *et al.*, 2005; Kim *et al.*, 2005) |
| **Squamous cell cancer** | FASLG TNFSF10 | (Taylor *et al.*, 2006; Martinez-Lostao *et al.*, 2010) |

Table 2. Protein content on and within exosomes reflects their origin and establishes their functional role. Cell surface A33 antigen precursor (GPA 33); Carcinoembryonic antigen-related cell Adhesion molecule 5 (CEACAM5); Ephrin-B1 (EFNB1); ADP-ribolysing factor (ARF), Ras-Gprotein superfamily (Rabs), A disintegrin and metaloprotease (ADAM10), Macrophage Migration inhibitory factor (MIF), Receptor for activated C-kinase (RACK1), 5,6-Dihydroxyyindole-2 carboxylic acid oxidase (TRP); Epidermal-growth factor receptor (EGFR); Receptor tyrosine-protein kinase erbB-2 (ERBB2); Plasmalemma vesicle associated protein (PLVAP); Melanocyte Protein Pmel 17 (GP100); Melanoma Antigen Recognized by T cells 1 (MART-1), Mel-CAM, TNF-ligand superfamily member 10 (TRAIL) TNF-ligand superfamily member 6 (FasL).

Recent studies have shown that TEX provide a protective role to the cancer cells, which can be manifested in different ways. Survivin, a member of the inhibitor of apoptosis (IAP) protein family, was found to be released from tumor cells via exosomes (Khan *et al.*, 2011). The protective role of TEX can be attained by the accumulation and packaging of chemotherapeutic drugs or its metabolites into the vesicles, thus decreasing cellular levels of the drug, a factor leading to drug resistance (Shedden *et al.*, 2003; Safaei *et al.*, 2005). This phenomenon has been observed in various cancer cells. Cisplatin enhanced the shedding of the vesicle from melanoma cells (Chen *et al.*, 2006a), while doxorubicin was found in the exosomes released from ovarian carcinoma cells (Shedden *et al.*, 2003).
Despite the beneficial roles of TEX for the tumor cells and the tumor microenvironment, TEX can be a useful tool for detecting the malignant condition. Serum levels of exosomes taken from cancer patients are significantly increased. These vesicles taken from serum (Ginestra *et al.*, 1999), as well as from malignant tumor fluids, such as ascites fluids (Adams *et al.*, 2005), pleural effusions (Andre *et al.*, 2002b) and urine (Nilsson *et al.*, 2009), positively correlate with the tumor progression.

### 3.1 Constitutive and inducible vesicle secretion in cancer and cancer therapy

In the tumor microenvironment, various changes are taking place, which could have an effect on the release of vesicles, such as exosomes. Environmental changes, such as stress induced by chemo- and radio-therapy, can modulate TEX release and the biome they contain. This phenomenon may induce the tissues to adapt to changes taking place in the microenvironment (Thery *et al.*, 2009). Tumor cells that have undergone radiation or chemotherapy treatment have been shown to increase the release of TEX (Yu *et al.*, 2006; Lehmann *et al.*, 2008). Interestingly, when treated with chemotherapeutic agents, there is a significantly enhanced membrane vesicle secretion in chemoresistant cells compared to chemosensitive cells. This activity may be a factor leading to drug resistance (Shedden *et al.*, 2003; Safaei *et al.*, 2005).
Chemotherapy and radiation (Chen *et al.*, 2006b) treatment lead to DNA-damaging conditions. In this state, the p53 pathway is activated, leading, among various other changes physiologically, to an induced expression of the transmembrane protein tumor suppressor-activated pathway 6 (TSAP6). TSAP6 is an important cellular component as it regulates the secretion of protein via the non-classical pathway or the ER/Golgi-independent protein secretion pathway needed for the enhanced release of exosomes (Nickel, 2003; Yu *et al.*, 2006; Lespagnol *et al.*, 2008). Normally, the secretion of exosomes in various cell types happens at a low rate. However, when p53 is activated, endosomal compartment activities are activated. Simultaneously, there is an increased expression of TSAP6, inducing the release of exosomes at a higher rate (Yu *et al.*, 2009) (**Figure 4**). It is suggested that following p53 activation, exosomal release may act as a 'detoxifier' to expel unwanted chemotherapeutic agents (Shedden *et al.*, 2003; Safaei *et al.*, 2005; Chen *et al.*, 2006b; Lespagnol *et al.*, 2008). Communication to the microenvironment is the other proposed role of TSAP6 and exosomal release after p53 activation, which may act as a warning signal to the neighboring cells, the immune system, and the extracellular matrix, that there are abnormal intracellular events happening (Lespagnol *et al.*, 2008; Yu *et al.*, 2009).

### 3.2 Summary

TEX can be used as an important biomarker for the disease, which will give information not only on the disease progression, but on the tumor type. As previously mentioned, TEX express specific tumor antigens which reflect the protein content of the tumor, giving an indication of the tumor type. The content of these vesicles can also be useful as markers for the aggressiveness of the disease.

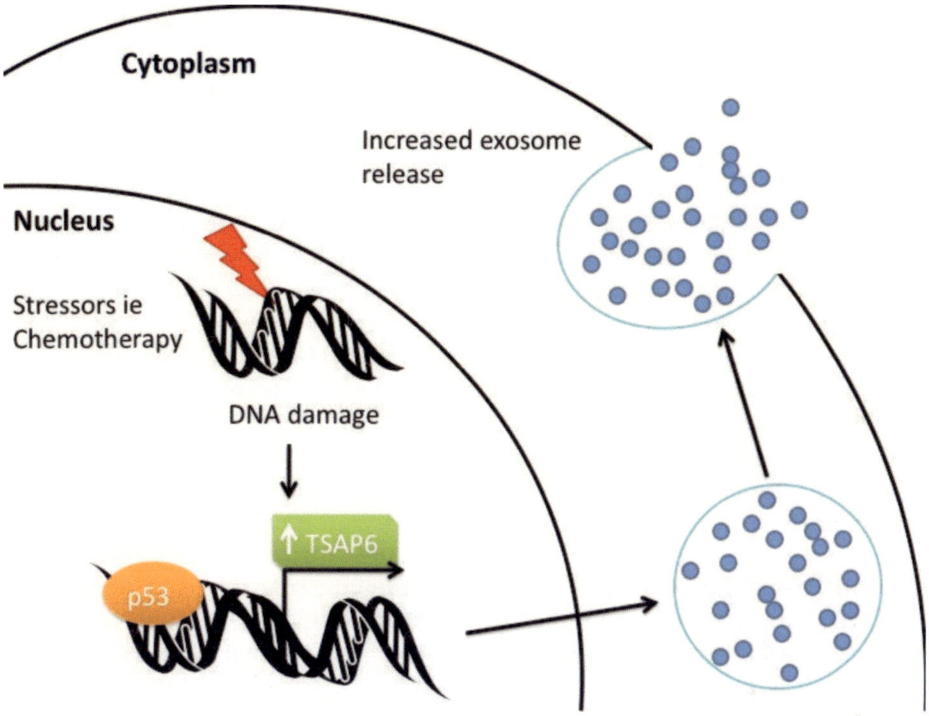


Fig. 4. Activation of p53 by DNA damage induces the expression of TSAP6 which enhances exosome-mediated secretion.

## 4. Proteome of cancer membrane vesicles

Mass spectrometry-based proteomic tools coupled with advanced purification methods for exosomes, has allowed more in-depth proteome analyses, contributing immensely to our understanding of the molecular composition of exosomes. Proteomic analysis of exosomes from diverse cell types, including cancers has revealed a common set of membrane and cytosolic proteins, suggesting the evolutionary importance of these membrane particles. In addition, exosomes express an array of proteins that reflect the originating host cell. The excessive release of exosomes in tumor cells, as evidenced by their increased levels in body fluids during the late stage of a disease and their overexpression of certain tumor cell biomarkers, suggests an important role of exosomes in diagnosis and biomarker studies (Simpson *et al.*, 2009).

By proteomic analysis we can enrich low abundance membrane proteins from underrepresented conventional cell lysates and unfractionated biological fluids. Identification of a conserved set of common proteins that are essential for vesicle biogenesis, structure and trafficking mechanisms can be explored. We can also detect cell-specific biomarkers. These concepts suggest that analyzing the composition and abundance of such proteins in exosomes may be useful to reveal different cell behaviors.

### 4.1 Proteomics of cell-type dependent exosomes

Exosomes have a unique protein composition that varies depending on cellular origin **(Table 2)**. Analysis of exosomes from a wide variety of cells and body fluids have been identified. Exosomes from various cancer cells expose Fas ligand (FasL, CD95L), a ligand of the death receptor Fas (CD95), which induces T-cell apoptosis and diminishes the function of adaptive immune cells (Andreola *et al.*, 2002; Huber *et al.*, 2005). It was shown that a modest correlation exists between lymph node infiltration and tumor burden and the numbers of circulating FasL-exposing exosomes in blood from patients with oral squamous cell cancers (Kim *et al.*, 2005). Exosomes from lymphoblastoma cells exposed latent membrane protein-1 (LMP-1), another immune suppressing transmembrane protein, thereby inhibiting leukocyte proliferation. In addition, low numbers of circulating exosomes, in cancer patients, stained positive for MUC1, a cancer cell antigen, and glycoprotein IIIa (integrin β3), which is mainly present on platelets and platelet-derived exosomes. Exosomes are released after fusion of exosomes from malignant epithelial cells with platelets (Tesselaar *et al.*, 2007). Alternatively, platelet-derived exosomes were shown to transfer integrins to breast and lung cancer cells (Janowska-Wieczorek *et al.*, 2001; Janowska-Wieczorek *et al.*, 2005). Thus, cancer cells can fuse with non-cancer cell-derived exosomes, thereby receiving lipids and membrane specific proteins which may help them escape from immune surveillance.

Degradation of the extracellular matrix (ECM) is essential for tumor growth (Hotary *et al.*, 2003). Exosomes expose and contain proteases, including matrix metalloproteinase 2 (MMP-2) and MMP-9 and its zymogens, and urokinase-type plasminogen activator (uPA). Neovascularization is also responsible for the increased entry of tumor cells into the circulation and metastasis. It is believed that tumor and stromal cells secrete angiogenic factors such as VEGF and basic fibroblast growth factor (bFGF) and that tumor-associated angiogenesis occurs by the action of these factors (Carmeliet, 2005). Furthermore, growing evidence suggests that exosomes derived from tumor cells and platelets also possess angiogenic activities. Vesicular components such as sphingomyelin, CD147, tetraspanin-8, VEGF, and bFGF are likely involved in exosome-mediated neovascularization (Kim *et al.*, 2002; Brill *et al.*, 2004; Gesierich *et al.*, 2006; Millimaggi *et al.*, 2007).

In a colorectal cancer cell line study, several exosomal proteins have been identified that are believed to be involved in tumor-associated angiogenesis: ADAM 10, CD44, NG2, ephrin-B1, macrophage migration inhibitory factor (MIF), RACK1, and tetraspanin-8 (Dong-Sic *et al.*, 2007). Clinical exosome analysis may also prove useful for solid cancers (Mathivanan *et al.*, 2010). Using exosomes from ovarian carcinoma cell lines, malignant ascites and sera from ovarian carcinoma patients, it was found that malignant ascites-derived exosomes cargo tumor progression related proteins (L1CAM, CD24, ADAM10 and EMMPRIN). It was also observed that exosomes move systemically via the blood stream (Keller *et al.*, 2009). Therefore, if some membrane proteins are typically and specifically expressed by a certain tumor, their detection on circulating exosomes, (which could be isolated from only 1mL of blood), may be exploited for diagnostic purposes as an early signal of cancer presence. Proteomic analysis of exosomes was also performed on human mesothelioma cell lines and malignant pleural effusions. Bard and colleagues, described exosomes which contained antigen presenting molecules, cytoskeletal proteins, and signal tranduction-involved proteins were in mesothelioma, lung, breast, and ovarian cancers. In addition, SNx25, BTG1, PEDF, and Thrombospondin were also identified (Bard *et al.*, 2004).

Characterization of urinary exosomal composition may be proposed as a potential source of diagnostic markers in bladder cancer. Two different approaches (Smalley *et al.*, 2008; Welton *et al.*, 2010) were taken to characterize these exosomes. In the first, urine exosomes were isolated from a limited number of individuals with bladder cancer and their protein composition compared to that of healthy controls. Eight proteins were found elevated, among which five have been linked to the EGF receptor pathway (Smalley *et al.*, 2008). In the second study, extensive steps were taken to produce high purity and quality-assured exosome preparations prior to beginning proteomics workflows. Working with conditioned media from cultured bladder cancer cell lines, 350 proteins were identified. Eighteen were proven to be present in exosomes isolated from the urine of three bladder cancer patients (Welton *et al.*, 2010). This suggests that conditioned media from cultured cell lines could represent an interesting starting model to detect exosomal proteomic alterations, which must then be confirmed *in vivo*, using biological fluids from a wide cohort of patients, in order to supply a non-invasive source for biomarker discovery.
Exosomes prepared from urine of prostate cancer patients contain typical markers of such a tumor (PSA and PCA3) (Mitchell *et al.*, 2009; Nilsson *et al.*, 2009). Moreover, δ-catenin immunoreactivity was identified in vesicles prepared from culture media of PC3 cells and found significantly increased in prostasomes of the urine of prostate cancer patients (Lu *et al.*, 2009).

### 4.2 Summary

Studies confirm that urinary exosome protein profiling is an important topic and may be a valuable tool for biomarker discovery in the field of urinary tract pathology. Proteomic approaches to investigate membranous vesicles and exosomes are still immature. However, they show a great potential for future developments in the diagnostic and prognostic applications.

## 5. Targeting interactions of membrane vesicles with neighboring tumor microenvironment

Tumor cells release large quantities of exosomes containing procoagulant, growth regulatory, and oncogenic cargo, which can be transferred throughout the cancer cell population and to transformed stromal cells, endothelial cells and possibly to the inflammatory infiltrates. These events likely impact tumor invasion, angiogenesis, metastasis, drug resistance, and cancer stem cells. Instead of physical contact, the influence of exosomes on the target cell may also involve pericellular discharge/activation of the bioactive cargo (Dolo *et al.*, 2005; Hendrix *et al.*, 2010; Muralidharan-Chari *et al.*, 2010). For instance, this may involve proteolytic remodelling of the extracellular microenvironment, modulation of ligand-receptor interactions, and a variety of other effects that could change the behaviour of target cells and properties of their surroundings (Hendrix *et al.*, 2010) **(Figure 5)**. In some instances, such interactions could be rather complex and multifactorial. The recently described Rab27B-regulated exosomal release of MMPs and HSP90a from metastatic cancer cells is believed to control invasive cellular behaviour by inducing changes in the extracellular matrix (ECM) as well as through modification of growth factor responses (Hendrix *et al.*, 2010). Likewise, procoagulant exosomes may facilitate tumor initiation, invasion, and dissemination by activating the clotting cascade extracellularly and coagulation-dependent signalling intracellularly (Milsom *et al.*, 2007). Exosome-mediated emission of various factors including tetraspanins, chemoattractants, adhesion molecules and proteases from cancer cells, platelets, and other cellular sources contributes to metastatic regulation in several experimental systems (Janowska-Wieczorek *et al.*, 2005; Jung *et al.*, 2009). As mentioned earlier, exosomes may also act as important reservoirs of cytokines and mediators of inflammatory and immune responses (Bianco *et al.*, 2009; Thery *et al.*, 2009).

### 5.1 Mediators of intercellular communication

Contact with the cell death ligand (FasL) exposed on certain tumor cell-derived exosomes is lethal for Fas-expressing lymphoid cytotoxic effector cells, a process implicated in the induction of immunotolerance in colorectal cancer and possibly other malignancies (Albanese *et al.*, 1998). These influences may affect recipient cells via a random distribution of exosomes in tissue and body fluids, or more directional exosome homing/uptake mechanisms. For instance, an acidic pH commonly present in hypo-perfused areas of solid tumors may lead to localized disruption of exosomes and consequent discharge of their proangiogenic and pro-inflammatory cargo such as VEGF and other factors (Taraboletti *et al.*, 2006). Exosomes may also be directed to specific sites due to the molecular addresses they carry on their surfaces (Celi *et al.*, 2004; Zhou *et al.*, 2008; Xiao *et al.*, 2009). The nature, directionality, and efficiency of this molecular exchange depends on several factors. For instance, the physical properties of vesicular plasma membranes affect the fusion rate between exosomes and target cells, which may increase their exosome uptake under acidic pH (Parolini *et al.*, 2009). In some instances, exosome transfer could also be directed by specific molecular addresses, for example, a high concentration of phosphatydyl serines (PS) on the surface of certain exosomes (e.g. ectosomes or procoagulant microparticles) may enable their recognition by PS receptors (PSRs) on the surface of specific types of target cells. Many of such PSRs have been described within the context of phagocytosis of apoptotic cells by mononuclear cells; examples of such PSRs include Tim1, Tim4, stabilin 2 and BAI1 (Park *et al.*, 2007; Zhao *et al.*, 2010), at least some of which could be expressed more widely and may be involved in the uptake of exosomes. Indeed, blocking PSRs often obliterates exosome incorporation by endothelial cells, platelets and cancer cells (Del Conde *et al.*, 2005; Al-Nedawi *et al.*, 2008; Al-Nedawi *et al.*, 2009). A corollary to this point would be that phagocytes could be particularly susceptible to molecular influences of PS-positive exosomes, beyond their simple destruction. It has also been proposed that Tim1/4 receptors on two adjacent cells could allow formation of exosome bridges, thereby promoting additional indirect intercellular interactions (Xiao *et al.*, 2009). Similarly, the presence of PSGL-1 (P-selectin ligand) on the surface of procoagulant exosomes directs them to P-selectin-expressing platelets and endothelial cells (Thomas *et al.*, 2009).

### 5.2 Oncosomes: Oncogene-driven vesiculation

During malignant transformation, the action of mutant oncogenes, such as K-ras, EGFR, or its constitutively active mutant EGFR (variant III) (EGFRvIII), as well as several others, appear to stimulate the formation and release of exosomes (Yu *et al.*, 2005; Al-Nedawi *et al.*, 2008). Similarly, the activation or loss of specific tumor suppressor proteins appears to impact cellular vesiculation either positively or negatively (Yu *et al.*, 2005; Yu *et al.*, 2006). While the exact nature of the signalling pathways involved in oncogene-driven exosome biogenesis remains largely unknown, recent studies have begun to shed more light on the underlying processes. For instance, in cultures of prostate cancer cells, elevated exosome production was detected in association with increased oncogenic activity of protein kinase B (PKB/Akt), or upon stimulation with growth factors (EGF), and depending on the status of the actin regulating protein known as diaphanous related formin 3 (DRF3) (Di Vizio *et al.*, 2009). In this case, inhibition of DRF3 expression through RNA interference enhanced the rate of exosome formation, and membrane blebbing activity, suggesting that DRF3 may be an inhibitor of ectosome release (Di Vizio *et al.*, 2009). Interestingly, DRF3 expression is lost during the progression of prostate cancer to metastatic disease, which suggests an intriguing link between oncogenesis, vesiculation and metastasis (Di Vizio *et al.*, 2009).

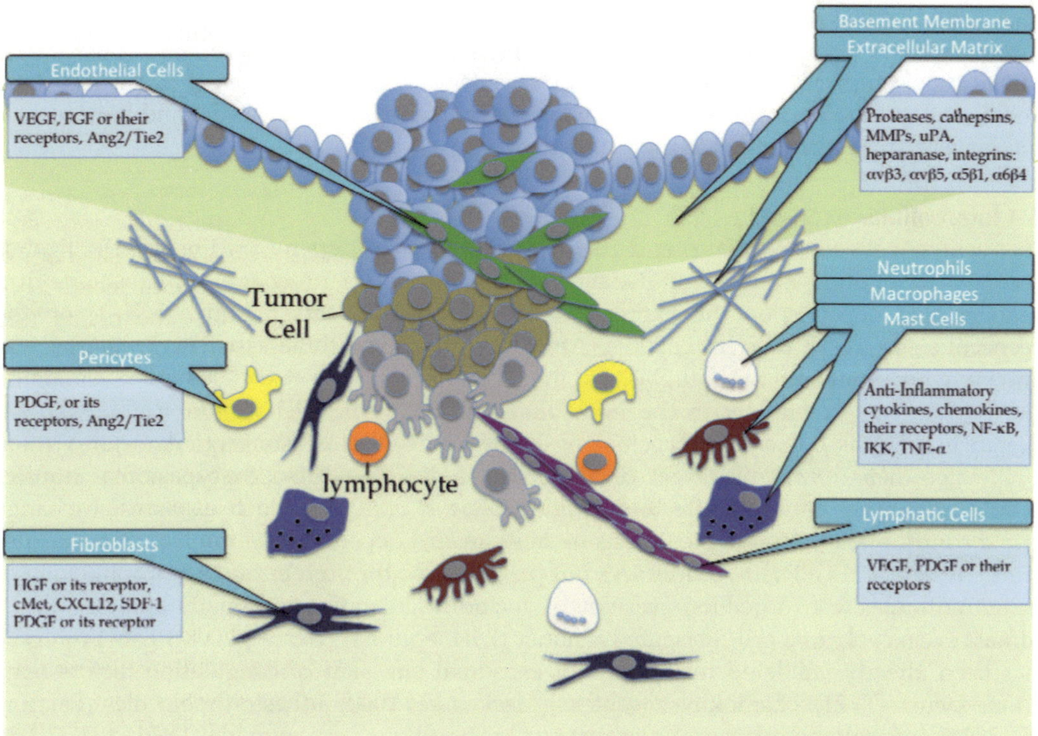


Fig. 5. Tumor microenvironment. The heterotypic interactions within the tumor microenvironment and their give and take of exosomes and their contents provide many targets for possible therapy. The goal of targetting these interactions will interrupt the heterotypic signaling that would thus deprive the cancer cells of the support they have within the tumor microenvironment.

### 5.3 Effect of TEX on tumor microenvironment

Exosome release by colorectal cancer cells is a function of K-ras and p53 status (Yu *et al.*, 2005). It is noteworthy that oncoproteins not only stimulate exosome formation but also become incorporated into their cargo (Al-Nedawi *et al.*, 2008; Al-Nedawi *et al.*, 2009). As a result, oncogene-containing exosomes (sometimes refered to as *oncosomes*) may serve as vehicles that carry oncogenic cargo and mediate its transfer between cells (Al-Nedawi *et al.*, 2009). At least four different modes of such oncogenic transfer have been described: (a) intercellular passage of active oncoproteins (Al-Nedawi *et al.*, 2008), (b) transfer of oncogenic mRNA transcripts

(Skog *et al.*, 2008), (c) exchange of oncogenic miR and/or (d) passage of genomic sequences containing oncogenic DNA (Bergsmedh *et al.*, 2001). In many instances, this horizontal transfer may have marked biological (transforming) consequences. Thus, oncosomes containing EGFRvIII may emanate from malignant tumor cells and be taken up by their indolent counterparts inducing their growth, survival, and clonogenic and angiogenic capacity (Al-Nedawi *et al.*, 2008). These exosomes may also act on endothelial cells and reprogram their responses such that they exhibit an increase in angiogenic activity (Skog *et al.*, 2008) or switch to an autocrine mode of secretory pathway, e.g. by turning on VEGF production (Al-Nedawi *et al.*, 2008). Indeed, blocking exosome uptake using the Annexin V analogue (Diannexin) is associated with a measurable anti-angiogenic effect *in vivo* (Al-Nedawi *et al.*, 2008). In chronic lymphoblastic leukaemia (CLL), exosomes containing AXL kinase conditioned the bone marrow stroma to support disease progression (Ghosh *et al.*, 2010). These and similar effects identify exosomes as possible effectors of oncogenic and proangiogenic *field effects*, long postulated to exist in cancer (Slaughter *et al.*, 1953; Al-Nedawi *et al.*, 2009) and viewed as a mechanism of cell recruitment to the malignant process.

### 5.4 Intercellular exchange

Interactions between exosomes and their target cells may depend on the specific ligand-receptor recognition events. For instance, platelets take up procoagulant exosomes in a manner that depends on the expression of P-selectin and its ligand (PSGL-1) on the respective surfaces (Falati *et al.*, 2003). After the uptake, exosome-associated material was shown to penetrate into the cytoplasm of the acceptor cell (Skog *et al.*, 2008) or to remain on the cell surface, potentially in the immediately active form (Del Conde *et al.*, 2005; Al-Nedawi *et al.*, 2008). Interestingly, cloaking PS by exposure of exosomes to Annexin V often obliterates their uptake by target cells. Recent studies suggested that exosomal transfer would encompass multiple effectors at once (Skog *et al.*, 2008). Such exosomal exchange could contribute to tumor angiogenesis by mechanisms dependent on transfer of oncogenes (Rak, 2010) (e.g., EGFRvIII4 or mRNA), but possibly also through bidirectional trafficking of other molecules (e.g., VEGFRs, Tie, Notch), including ligands traditionally assumed to act almost exclusively in a cell-associated manner (Dll4, ephrins) (Kerbel, 2008). This prototype has been already validated in the case of exosomal emission of coagulation factors (e.g., tissue factor—TF21), chemokine receptors (Mack *et al.*, 2000) adhesion molecules (Falati *et al.*, 2003), immunomodulators (Valenti *et al.*, 2007), cell surface antigens (Dolo *et al.*, 2005), intact RNA species (Ratajczak *et al.*, 2006; Valadi *et al.*, 2007), and oncogenic proteins (Koga *et al.*, 2005; Al-Nedawi *et al.*, 2008; Sanderson *et al.*, 2008).

### 5.5 Summary

So far in the literature, exosomal cargo associated proteins and their importance in angiogenesis, inflammation, proteolysis regulators, membrane receptors, soluble factors, oncoproteins and tumor suppressors, lipids, nucleic acids are described briefly. Therefore, exosomes represent an integral part of both physiological regulation and disease pathogenesis, which may influence new therapeutic and diagnostic modalities.

## 6. Membrane vesicles and antigen presentation

As described earlier in this chapter, various cell types release exosomes, which contain a proteomic sampling from the cell of origin. Proteins within exosomes can be presented as antigens to the immune system and, when derived from certain cell types, are capable of presenting antigens to immune cells directly. Antigen presentation by antigen presenting cells (APCs) requires several important steps to elicit an immune response: 1. the APC internalizes and processes the antigen, 2. the processed antigen is inserted into Major Histocompatibility Complex (MHC) molecules and displayed on the cell surface, 3. MHC molecules interact with T cell receptors to start a signaling cascade to activate the T cell (Kim *et al.*, 2004). Dendritic cells are the primary APC type that stimulates T cells *in vivo*, which requires MHC molecules on the dendritic cell, as well as expression of co-stimulatory molecules that enhance T cell activation, such as CD40, CD80 and CD86 (Kim *et al.*, 2004). Like many other cell types, dendritic cells release membrane vesicles, particularly exosomes, which help modulate the immune response (Chaput *et al.*, 2006; Schorey & Bhatnagar, 2008; Thery *et al.*, 2009).

### 6.1 Antigen presentation by immune cell exosomes

Antigen presenting cells, such as dendritic cells and B cells, release exosomes equipped with MHC class I and class II molecules that allow direct presentation of antigens to cytotoxic and helper T cells, respectively (Kim *et al.*, 2004; Chaput *et al.*, 2006). Antigens processed by APCs are loaded into MHC molecules and the MHC-antigen complex is released into the extracellular space within exosomes. These exosomes then travel throughout the body and induce an immune response by stimulating antigen-specific T cells. In addition to MHC molecules, APC exosomes express surface co-stimulatory molecules CD40, CD80 and CD86 to enhance T cell activation (Raposo *et al.*, 1996). The ability of exosomes to induce a T cell response is dependent on the expression of these molecules, as introduction of antibodies against CD40, CD80 and CD86 inhibit antigen presentation and T cell activation by APC exosomes. Additionally, the tetraspanin molecule CD54 (ICAM1) plays a crucial role in this process by enhancing exosome-T cell contact through its interaction with CD11a (LFA-1) on the T cell (Kim *et al.*, 2004). This interaction allows MHC and co-stimulatory molecules to bind to their receptors on the T cells long enough to provide sufficient signaling. As observed with inhibition of the co-stimulatory molecules, antibody blockade of CD54 on exosomes dramatically reduces T cell activation by APC exosomes (Kim *et al.*, 2004).

### 6.2 Transfer of antigens by exosomes

In addition to their ability to present processed antigens, exosomes can also transfer antigens from one cell to another. Exosomes containing cellular antigens are taken up by APCs, where the antigens are processed and inserted into MHC molecules for presentation (Obregon *et al.*, 2006). This is a very important mechanism in disease states, where infected or malignant cells release exosomes into the bloodstream that can be processed and presented by APCs throughout the body to induce an immune response (Bhatnagar & Schorey, 2007). In cancer, TEXs are taken up by APCs and activate tumor-specific T cells (Andre *et al.*, 2002a). *In vitro* studies have shown that when T cells are incubated with TEX in the presence of naïve dendritic cells, both helper and cytotoxic T cells are activated in an antigen-specific manner (Thery *et al.*, 2009). Additionally, *in vivo* vaccination studies comparing TEX and irradiated tumor cells showed a stronger immune response in animals vaccinated with TEXs. These studies have led to two clinical trials, which will be discussed in detail later.

### 6.3 Summary

Antigen presentation to T cells is the first and most critical step in the adaptive immune response. The ability of exosomes to supply antigens to dendritic cells for presentation as well as present antigens directly via exosomal MHC molecules is an important mechanism for detection of infection and malignancy. Induction of anti-cancer responses via tumor-released exosome antigens is likely a key mechanism in immune surveillance to prevent tumor progression. Whether this can be utilized in tumor immunotherapies is under investigation and could prove useful in combination therapies.

## 7. Antigen-independent roles of membrane vesicles in immune responses

Antigen presentation by exosomes is primarily an immunostimulatory process, however exosomes have many antigen-independent functions that can both stimulate and inhibit the immune system (Schorey & Bhatnagar, 2008; Thery *et al.*, 2009). These roles are dependent on the type of cell the exosomes originate from and the molecules they express (Andre *et al.*, 2002a; Abusamra *et al.*, 2005a; Xiang *et al.*, 2009; Chalmin *et al.*, 2010; Szajnik *et al.*, 2010; Zhang *et al.*, 2011). In this way exosomes are important for proper immune function and immune regulation, but can also be hijacked by malignant cells to prevent detection by the immune system.

### 7.1 Immune cell exosomes induce immune responses

Dendritic cell exosomes (DEXs) are vital for stimulation of the adaptive immune response by their presentation of antigen to T cells (**Figure 6**), but induction of the humoral immune response is as important a function (Chaput *et al.*, 2006). DEXs have been shown to stimulate Natural Killer (NK) cell responses critical to the clearance of infection and malignancy (Viaud *et al.*, 2009). This function is mediated by the expression of interleukin-15 receptor alpha (IL-15Rα) and Natural Killer Group 2D (NKG2D) ligands on dendritic cell exosomes. Interleukin-15 (IL-15) is a cytokine that stimulates NK cell activation and proliferation. Exosomal IL-15Rα can bind IL-15 in the extracellular space and deliver it to NK cells by exosomal binding to NKG2D on the surface of the NK cells (Viaud *et al.*, 2009). Delivery of IL-15 in this manner significantly increases NK cell responses *in vitro* and in mice injected with autologous DEXs (Thery *et al.*, 2009; Viaud *et al.*, 2009). Because of their critical importance to tumor clearance, NK cell stimulation by DEXs could provide therapeutic benefits by increasing NK cell numbers in cancer patients.

### 7.2 Tumor cell exosomes and the immune response

The role of TEX in the progression of cancer is multifaceted, as they can affect tumor growth, invasion and metastasis, and therapy resistance. In addition to influencing other malignant cells, TEXs have significant effects on the immune response, both positive and negative.

#### 7.2.1 Exosomes from heat-shocked tumor cells induce immune activation

The release of exosomes from normal and malignant cells is increased by heat shock and stress, with amplified proportions of Hsps within the exosome (Schorey & Bhatnagar, 2008). Culture of dendritic cells with exosomes from heat-shocked tumors resulted in higher expression of CD40, CD80 and CD86 than in dendritic cells cultured with control immune cell exosomes or non-heat shocked tumor exosomes (Chen *et al.*, 2006c). Additionally, the dendritic cells treated with heat shocked TEXs exhibited increased production of pro-inflammatory cytokines tumor necrosis factor alpha (TNFα), IL-1β, and IL-12 (Chen *et al.*, 2006c). This is thought to be mediated by the increased amount of Hsps in the heat-shocked TEXs, though the exact mechanism is still under investigation.

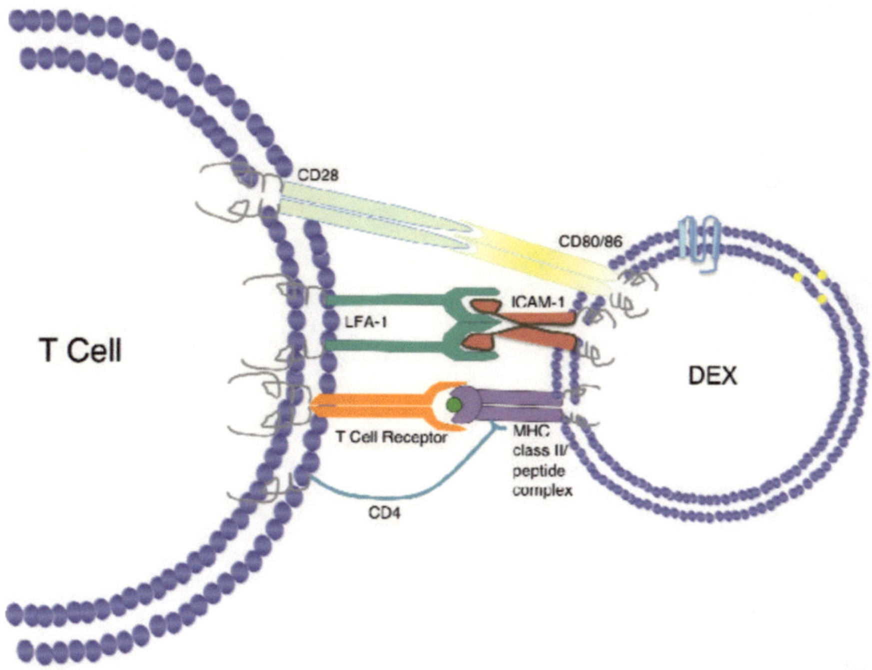


Fig. 6. Dendritic cell-derived exosomes interact with T cells through MHC class I, II, tetraspanins such as CD9, CD63, CD81 and through co-stimulatory molecules such as CD86.

### 7.2.2 Tumor cell exosomes inhibit natural killer cells via NKG2D

NK cells kill cancer cells by release of granules and perforins (**Figure 7**). NK cell activity is often lost in cancer patients, resulting in a reduced ability of the immune system to eliminate malignant cells (Clayton *et al.*, 2008; Viaud *et al.*, 2009; Ahiru *et al.*, 2010). The NK cell receptor NKG2D is important in regulation of NK cell function, with some ligands stimulating and others inhibiting cytotoxic function (Clayton *et al.*, 2008). As discussed earlier, DEXs expressing activating NKG2D ligands can enhance NK cell function and promote tumor clearance (Viaud *et al.*, 2009). Other NKG2D ligands, such as MHC class I-related chain A (MICA) can reduce NK cell function. Tumor cells abuse this normal ligand by upregulating MICA on the cell surface as well as on TEXs (Ahiru *et al.*, 2010). Ovarian cancer exosomes expressing high levels of MICA were shown to decrease NK cell function *in vitro* by reducing their NKG2D receptor expression and their responsiveness to activating NKG2D ligands (Ahiru *et al.*, 2010). This reduction in NK cell function is highly detrimental to the anti-tumor response and is one of many mechanisms by which tumors escape immune detection (Thery *et al.*, 2009).

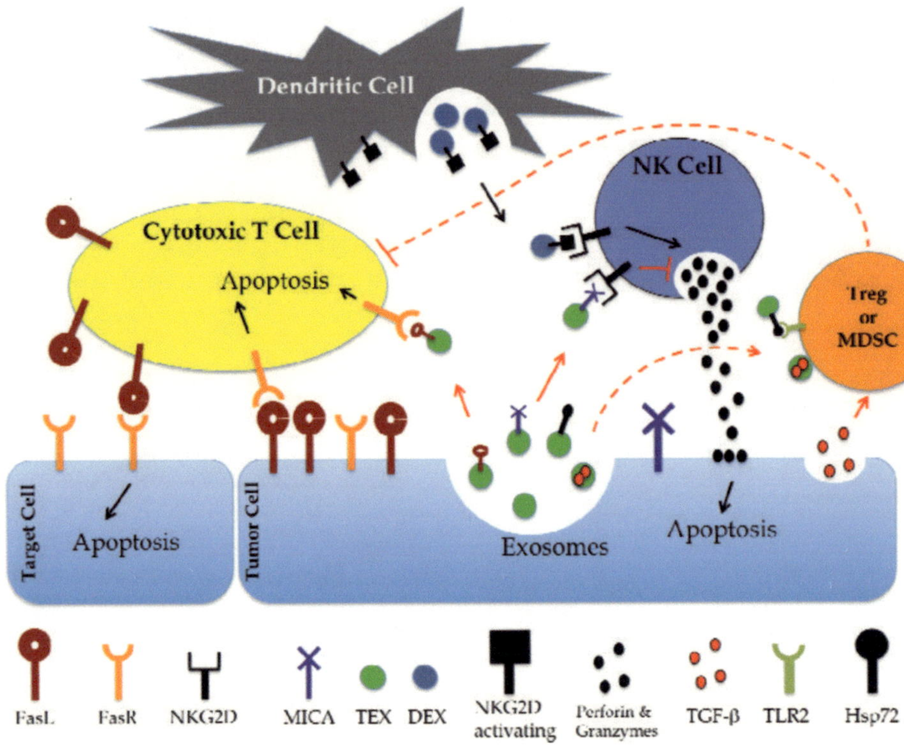


Fig. 7. DEX and TEX play opposing roles with regard to immune cell activation and prohibition.

### 7.2.3 Fas ligand expression on tumor cell exosomes induce immune cell apoptosis

Cytotoxic immune cells like cytotoxic T cells express Fas Receptor (FasR; CD95) and Fas ligand (FasL; CD95L) that allow them to induce apoptosis in target cells. Several cancer types including colon and ovarian carcinoma and melanoma cells express FasL to induce death of the very immune cells that attempt to kill them (Koyama *et al.*, 2001). This is a primary mechanism of tumor-immune escape that prevents the immune system from eliminating transformed cells, resulting in disease progression. To further prevent cytotoxic killing by T cells, TEXs have been found to express high levels of surface-bound FasL (Abusamra *et al.*, 2005a). Release of FasL via exosomes allows the tumor to kill FasR-expressing immune cells at distant sites, as well as in the tumor microenvironment, further preventing tumor clearance. Interestingly, although both helper and cytotoxic T cells express FasR, exosomes containing FasL preferentially induce apoptosis in cytotoxic T cells and not in helper T cells (Abusamra *et al.*, 2005a). The mechanism behind this is not fully understood, but may be due to favored interactions between exosomes and cytotoxic T cells due to other exosomal surface molecules (**Figure 7**).

### 7.2.4 Tumor exosomes induce suppressive immune cell phenotypes

Immune suppression within the tumor microenvironment prevents cytotoxic attack and promotes tumor progression. Like FasL and NKG2D inhibition, increasing immunosuppressive cell types can reduce cytotoxic immune responses. Two primary inhibitory cell types have been implicated in cancer progression: regulatory T cells (Tregs) (Szajnik *et al.*, 2010) and myeloid derived suppressor cells (MDSCs) (Xiang *et al.*, 2009). These cell types inhibit both helper and cytotoxic T cell responses and reduces their production of inflammatory cytokines like interferon gamma (IFN-γ). Large numbers of immune cells are found within the tumor microenvironment, but Tregs and MDSCs are far more prominent in cancer patients than in healthy patients, leading to the hypothesis that immune suppression can be induced by the tumors (Xiang *et al.*, 2009; Szajnik *et al.*, 2010). Tumor cells can directly induce regulatory populations by secreting transforming growth factor beta (TGF-β), which promotes differentiation of naïve T cells and myeloid precursor cells into their respective suppressive phenotypes. A similar mechanism is utilized by tumors to induce Tregs and MDSCs within the tumor microenvironment and the periphery by secretion of TGF-β in exosomes (Xiang *et al.*, 2009; Chalmin *et al.*, 2010; Szajnik *et al.*, 2010). Ovarian carcinoma derived exosomes were found to induce $CD4^+CD25^+Foxp3^+$ Tregs from $CD4^+CD25^-$ naïve T cells *in vitro (Szajnik et al., 2010)*. This was found to be dependent on the presence of TGF-β and IL-10 in the exosomes and was inhibited by addition of neutralizing antibodies to both cytokines. In a similar study, mouse bone marrow myeloid precursor cells were shown to take up TEXs, inducing their differentiation into $CD11b^+Gr\text{-}1^+$ myeloid derived suppressor cells. Exosomal expression of TGF-β and prostaglandin E2 (PGE2) was shown to induce this differentiation, which was inhibited by antibody neutralization (Xiang *et al.*, 2009). The suppressive function of existing MDSCs is also increased by TEXs. Interaction of Hsp72 on the exosome with Toll-like receptor 2 (TLR2) on the MDSC induces Stat3 signaling to induce their immunosuppressive functions (Chalmin *et al.*, 2010). By increasing immunosuppressive cell types, TEXs can prevent attack by cytotoxic cells (**Figure 7**).

### 7.3 Summary

Exosomes can have important antigen-independent effects on immune cells that vary with the cell type they are derived from as well as the state of the cells upon release. DEXs and TEXs can stimulate immune responses, which could provide therapeutic benefits. In contrast, tumor derived exosomes from several cancer types have been shown to prevent cytotoxic attack on the tumor by FasL-induced T cell death, NKG2D ligand-mediated suppression of NK cells and through induction of immune suppressor cells like Tregs and MDSCs. How TEXs can be utilized or inhibited therapeutically remains to be seen, but currently is an active area of research.

## 8. Immune responses induced by *in vitro* purified membrane vesicles *in vivo*

Many studies described in the Sections 6 and 7 were performed using membrane vesicles and exosomes isolated and introduced to immune cell cultures *in vitro*. Before these findings can be utilized therapeutically, they must be confirmed in *in vivo* animal models. Results from these animal studies have demonstrated the importance of exosomes in immune modulation and are currently being implemented in clinical trials.

### 8.1 Vaccination with tumor exosomes prevent tumor growth in mice

Early studies in tumor vaccination utilized irradiation-killed tumor cells with limited success. With the discovery of TEXs, mouse vaccination studies with TEXs were shown to be more effective at generating tumor-specific T cell responses than irradiated tumor cells.

Additionally, vaccination of mice with exosomes containing ovalbumin resulted in delayed growth of ovalbumin-expressing tumors and induced pro-inflammatory Th1 T cell responses. As described in Section 7.2, exosomes isolated from heat-shocked cancer cells are more immunogenic *in vitro*. Using heat-shocked TEXs for immunization in mice showed similar immunogenicity, with 80% of mice remaining tumor free after challenge. While these studies have provided the groundwork for cancer vaccines, the immunosuppressive functions of cancer exosomes have caused many to be skeptical of their use as vaccine.

### 8.2 Dendritic cell exosomes containing tumor antigens induce anti-tumor immune responses

The use of DEXs as artificial antigen presenting cells can elicit strong antigen-specific T cell responses (Kim *et al.*, 2004). Mouse studies using DEXs pulsed with tumor peptides resulted in the activation of tumor-specific T cells, proliferation of NK cells and tumor regression (Kim *et al.*, 2004; Chaput *et al.*, 2006). Utilization of this technology with great success in murine studies has led to the development of several clinical trials using autologous DEXs as a treatment in cancer patients (**Figure 8**).

#### 8.2.1 Melanoma phase I trial

A Phase I trial using dendritic cell exosomes to induce tumor regression was evaluated in 15 patients with metastatic melanoma (Escudier *et al.*, 2005). Autologous monocytes were isolated from patients by leukapheresis and differentiated *in vitro* to dendritic cells. These dendritic cells were cultured, exosomes isolated from the culture medium and pulsed with peptides from the tumor antigen MAGE3 (Escudier *et al.*, 2005). Patients received escalating doses of cryopreserved exosomes and their tumor progression and immune responses monitored. All 15 patients completed therapy but only 1 had specific T cell responses. Skin and lymph node mass reduction was observed in 5 of 15 patients and 7 of 15 patients showed increased NK cell activity (Escudier *et al.*, 2005; Thery *et al.*, 2009).

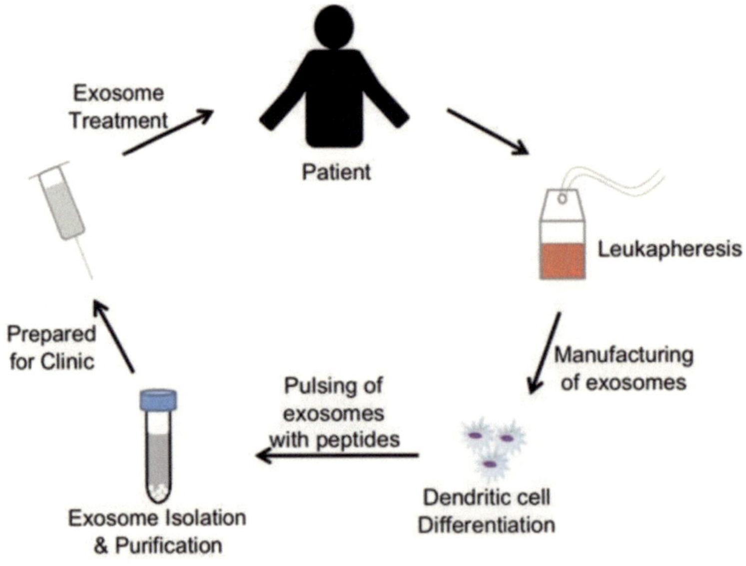


Fig. 8. Dendritic cell exosomes can be harvested and used in immunotherapy.

### 8.2.2 Non-small cell lung cancer phase I and II trials

A similar trial to the melanoma study was performed in Stage III and IV non-small cell lung cancer (NSCLC) (Morse *et al.*, 2005). Of the 13 patients enlisted in the trial, 9 finished the treatments and no toxicity was observed. Immune responses to MAGE3 was observed in 3 of 9 patients, with MAGE3-specific T cells only detected in 1 patient and while an increase in Treg cells was observed in 2 patients (Morse *et al.*, 2005). This trial concluded that dendritic cell exosomes are safe for use therapeutically, but that better responses may result from including Treg inhibitors in the treatment. A Phase II trial has begun adding IL-15R and NKG2D to the exosomes as well as Treg inhibitor therapy in NSCLC patients whose disease has been stabilized by chemotherapy (Thery *et al.*, 2009).

### 8.3 Summary

The use of exosomes as a cancer therapeutic has been demonstrated to be effective in murine studies and safe by Phase I clinical trials. Although some benefit was seen in patient trials, making these exosomal therapies more effective will likely require combination immunotherapies, chemotherapies and radiation. The use of exosomes to induce anti-cancer responses presents an exciting new field in cancer immunotherapy.

## 9. Membrane vesicles as therapeutic agents

Secreted microvesicles, known as exosomes, provide a form of cell to cell signaling in which the recipient cell can be modified by the contents of the delivered exosomes. The contents (cytosolic proteins, lipids, siRNA, miRNA, DNA, etc) (Tan *et al.*, 2010; Khan *et al.*, 2011) are protected and stably delivered unlike those secreted into the extracellular matrix (Pap *et al.*, 2010); thus securing the bioactivity of the delivered contents. Exosomes could be an attractive tool as an immunotherapeutic as they maintain much of the anti-tumor activity of a dendritic cell with the advantage of a cell free vehicle. Understanding that exosomes are involved in many levels of tumorigenesis, and potential strategies against this form of cellular communication has led to the creation of potential therapeutics against exosomes.

TEXs are a protective measure for tumor cells that aids in survival, growth, invasion, metastasis, and evasion of the immune system (Clayton *et al.*, 2007; Valenti *et al.*, 2007; Anderson *et al.*, 2010; Khan *et al.*, 2011). Taxol and vinca alkaloids are well known chemotherapeutic agents, but they also limit exosome release via the microtubule formation. Exosome formation has also been shown to be blocked by decreasing acidity of the microcellular environment (Iero *et al.*, 2008; Pap *et al.*, 2010). Prevention of exosome formation involves a broad variety of proteins and is essential for life in all cells. Therefore any inhibition of exosomes within the body could lead to unwarranted side effects (Pap *et al.*, 2010). It was thought that inhibition or treatment focused against TEXs and its ability to aid tumor cells could bear significant benefit to patients, but that was overshadowed by the realization that exosomes could potentially be employed as biomarkers and diagnostic tools of malignancy in blood (Anderson *et al.*, 2010) and urine (Nilsson *et al.*, 2009). One such study analyzed the correlation between serum PSA and urinary-exosomes, but none was observed. However, the data suggests that healthy donor urinary-exosomes were negative for PSA, PSMA, and 5T4 (Mitchell *et al.*, 2009).

Realizing that exosomes are secreted/released by a wide variety of cell types (Skokos *et al.*, 2001; Wolfers *et al.*, 2001; Chaput *et al.*, 2004b; Tan *et al.*, 2010; Khan *et al.*, 2011) including immune cells and tumor cells, many studies set out to manipulate exosomes for cancer therapy, specifically immunotherapy. Ever since B lymphocytes were described to contain MHC class II molecules and stimulate CD4+ T cells (Raposo *et al.*, 1996), studies have suggested exosomes may have an immunogenic role. Currently, DEXs from pulsed dendritic cells are under investigation for their ability to enhance and prime the immune system against tumor cells. Dendritic cells activate T cell responses through direct dendritic to T cell contacts. However, exosomes secreted by dendritic cells are also able to stimulate T cells (Zitvogel *et al.*, 1998).

### 9.1 Anti-cancer therapy

The importance of exosomes in cell to cell communication can be seen in their antigen presenting ability. Seminal work during the late 1990's showed DC's pulsed/loaded with cancer antigens or tumor peptides could yield DEXs which elicited better immune responses towards tumor cells (Zitvogel *et al.*, 1998; Wolfers *et al.*, 2001; Couzin, 2005; Chaput *et al.*, 2006; Tan *et al.*, 2010). The immune response was due to DEXs displaying the appropriate MHC class I molecules and tumor peptides. In fact, DC can be pulsed with both MHC class I and II, therefore effectively priming T cells against tumors (Thery *et al.*, 2002; Andre *et al.*, 2004; Chaput *et al.*, 2004a; Mignot *et al.*, 2006) as well as stimulating the activation and proliferation of NK cells (Clayton *et al.*, 2007; Viaud *et al.*, 2009). Current literature suggests that MHC class I and II containing exosomes are potential cell-free cancer vaccines (Zitvogel *et al.*, 1998; Andre *et al.*, 2004; Chaput *et al.*, 2004a; Tan *et al.*, 2010). Unlike current clinical cancer vaccines, exosomes are not technically vaccines as they are preventative and not therapeutic. The prophylactic vaccines are only effective against oncogenic viruses and do not treat the cancer directly, not to mention too expensive for the average patient (Tan *et al.*, 2010). Treatment of tumors with DEXs has had beneficial results such as initiation of immune response (Couzin, 2005), tumor growth suppression (Zitvogel *et al.*, 1998), tumor shrinking (Viaud *et al.*, 2009), and tumor rejection (Wolfers *et al.*, 2001; Mignot *et al.*, 2006). Exosomes are a better alternative than DC in terms of therapy because its composition can be identified, measured, is stable for storage, and has predictable behavior after administration (Thery *et al.*, 2002; Chaput *et al.*, 2004b).

The utilization of exosomes for cancer immunotherapy is a very new but very rapidly growing field. Most studies were conducted *in vitro*, but it is still unclear how oncologists will be able to translate the literature's data into the realm that will be most beneficial for the patient. One such complication is how the DEXs will be collected and implemented for patient treatment, and will the collected DEXs be sufficient enough? One potential strategy involves isolating DEXs through filtration of the patient's blood which will then be returned and employed to stimulate the immune system (Couzin, 2005). This would certainly allow for personalized therapy, but the question still remains: would there be enough DEXs and if not could adjuvant augmentation increase their numbers. Although the mode of exosome action in vivo is not clear yet, DEXs are a very interesting and potential substitute for dendritic cells in tumor vaccination therapy.

## 10. Conclusion

Various secreted extracellular vesicles have been found in blood, saliva, breast milk, bronchoalveolar lavage fluid, urine and amniotic fluid. Cellular uptake mechanisms have been shown to range from ligand/receptor interactions, integrin/cell adhesion molecule attachment and fusion, or through transcytosis. Physiologically, these extracellular vesicles have been shown to play a role in inter-cellular communication, disposal of defective or weakened proteins, formation of morphogen gradients for tissue patterning during development and for antigen presentation to T cells. Pathologically, these vesicles have been shown to aid in the transmission of viruses, prions, β-amyloid in Alzheimer's disease, and specifically to this chapter, tumor pathogenesis. Although additional investigation is still needed to fully exploit these extracellular vesicles for therapy, there is increasing evidence that in better understanding them and the molecules that they transport, determinations of diagnosis and prognosis and the prediction of response to treatment may be possible. However, it is also the hope that these vesicles may also act at therapeutic targets and perhaps even replacement therapies.

Conventional treatments for cancer include the use of chemotherapeutic drugs, radiation therapy and interventional surgery if the tumors are operable. Recent data suggests that the application of dendritic cell-derived, tumor cell-derived and even ascitic cell-derived exosomes could be developed as novel treatments for cancer. In fact, is has already been established that exosomes can be safely administered to patients, though the number of patients in these trials have been small and thus argue for larger studies. Furthermore, the goal of exosome therapy is to increase the biological magnitude of the immune response and as such exosomal immunotherapy is heavily reliant on the immune system. It will therefore be important to address issues such as patient immunosuppression due to therapeutic treatment, as the efficacy of the immunotherapy will be reliant upon the capability of the immune system. In order to increase the biological magnitude of the immune response researchers are artificially coating and engineering exosomes with tumor antigens to make them more recognizable to the immune system. The affects of heat shocking exosomes is also being investigated as heat shocked tumor exosomes are more effective than those not receiving heat treatment. Heating of the exosome confers a greater immunogenicity and thus elicits a greater immune response. Another possible application for exosomes is in vaccine delivery as exosome-producing cells could be engineered to produce a miRNA or specific genetic component or toxin that could be loaded into a exosome with the proper surface molecules for a cell specific uptake and response. Finally, the application of exosomes as immunotherapeutics represents a new chapter in cancer treatment development. However, much more research must go into elucidation of mechanism and targeting in order to improve potency.

## 11. Acknowledgment

The authors would like to thank the sponsors of their work on exosomes over the past few years: NCMHD Project EXPORT Program 5P20MD001632/Project 3 (NRW), also a generous start up package by Loma Linda University (NRW) and a National Merit Test Bed (NMTB) award sponsored by the Department of the Army under cooperative agreement number DAMD17-97-2-7016 (NRW).

## 12. References

Abusamra, A.J., Zhong, Z., Zheng, X., Li, M., Ichim, T.E., Chin, J.L. & Min, W.P. (2005a) Tumor exosomes expressing Fas ligand mediate CD8+ T-cell apoptosis. *Blood Cells, Molecules & Diseases*, 35, 169-173.

Abusamra, A.J., Zhong, Z., Zheng, X., Li, M., Ichim, T.E., Chin, J.L. & Min, W.P. (2005b) Tumor exosomes expressing Fas ligand mediate CD8+ T-cell apoptosis. *Blood Cells Mol Dis*, 35, 169-173.

Adams, M., Navabi, H., Croston, D., Coleman, S., Tabi, Z., Clayton, A., Jasani, B. & Mason, M.D. (2005) The rationale for combined chemo/immunotherapy using a Toll-like receptor 3 (TLR3) agonist and tumour-derived exosomes in advanced ovarian cancer. *Vaccine*, 23, 2374-2378.

Ahiru, O., Boutet, P., Fernandez-Messina, L., Aguera-Gonzalez, S., Skepper, J.N., Vales-Gomez, M. & Reyburn, H.T. (2010) Natural killer cell cytotoxicity is suppressed by exposure to the human NKG2D ligand MICA*008 that is shed by tumor cells in exosomes. *Cancer Research*, 70, 481-489.

Al-Nedawi, K., Meehan, B., Micallef, J., Lhotak, V., May, L., Guha, A. & Rak, J. (2008) Intercellular transfer of the oncogenic receptor EGFRvIII by microvesicles derived from tumour cells. *Nat Cell Biol*, 10, 619-624.

Al-Nedawi, K., Meehan, B. & Rak, J. (2009) Microvesicles: messengers and mediators of tumor progression. *Cell Cycle*, 8, 2014-2018.

Albanese, J., Meterissian, S., Kontogiannea, M., Dubreuil, C., Hand, A., Sorba, S. & Dainiak, N. (1998) Biologically active Fas antigen and its cognate ligand are expressed on plasma membrane-derived extracellular vesicles. *Blood*, 91, 3862-3874.

Anderson, H.C., Mulhall, D. & Garimella, R. (2010) Role of extracellular membrane vesicles in the pathogenesis of various diseases, including cancer, renal diseases, atherosclerosis, and arthritis. *Lab Invest*, 90, 1549-1557.

Andre, F., Chaput, N., Schartz, N.E., Flament, C., Aubert, N., Bernard, J., Lemonnier, F., Raposo, G., Escudier, B., Hsu, D.H., Tursz, T., Amigorena, S., Angevin, E. & Zitvogel, L. (2004) Exosomes as potent cell-free peptide-based vaccine. I. Dendritic cell-derived exosomes transfer functional MHC class I/peptide complexes to dendritic cells. *J Immunol*, 172, 2126-2136.

Andre, F., Schartz, N.E., Chaput, N., Flament, C., Raposo, G., Amigorena, S., Angevin, E. & Zitvogel, L. (2002a) Tumor-derived exosomes: a new source of tumor rejection antigens. *Vaccine*, 20, A28-A31.

Andre, F., Schartz, N.E., Movassagh, M., Flament, C., Pautier, P., Morice, P., Pomel, C., Lhomme, C., Escudier, B., Le Chevalier, T., Tursz, T., Amigorena, S., Raposo, G., Angevin, E. & Zitvogel, L. (2002b) Malignant effusions and immunogenic tumour-derived exosomes. *Lancet*, 360, 295-305.

Andreola, G., Rivoltini, L., Castelli, C., Huber, V., Perego, P., Deho, P., Squarcina, P., Accornero, P., Lozupone, F., Lugini, L., Stringaro, A., Molinari, A., Arancia, G., Gentile, M., Parmiani, G. & Fais, S. (2002) Induction of lymphocyte apoptosis by tumor cell secretion of FasL-bearing microvesicles. *J Exp Med*, 195, 1303-1316.

Arienti, G., Carlini, E., Verdacchi, R., Cosmi, E.V. & Palmerini, C.A. (1997) Prostasome to sperm transfer of CD13/aminopeptidase N (EC 3.4.11.2). *Biochim Biophys Acta*, 1336, 533-538.

Babst, M. (2005) A protein's final ESCRT. *Traffic*, 6, 2-9.

Baj-Krzyworzeka, M., Szatanek, R., Weglarczyk, K., Baran, J., Urbanowicz, B., Branski, P., Ratajczak, M.Z. & Zembala, M. (2006) Tumour-derived microvesicles carry several surface determinants and mRNA of tumour cells and transfer some of these determinants to monocytes. *Cancer Immunol Immunother*, 55, 808-818.

Bard, M.P., Hegmans, J.P., Hemmes, A., Luider, T.M., Willemsen, R., Severijnen, L.A., van Meerbeeck, J.P., Burgers, S.A., Hoogsteden, H.C. & Lambrecht, B.N. (2004)

Proteomic analysis of exosomes isolated from human malignant pleural effusions. *Am J Respir Cell Mol Biol*, 31, 114-121.

Bergsmedh, A., Szeles, A., Henriksson, M., Bratt, A., Folkman, M.J., Spetz, A.L. & Holmgren, L. (2001) Horizontal transfer of oncogenes by uptake of apoptotic bodies. *Proc Natl Acad Sci U S A*, 98, 6407-6411.

Bhatnagar, S. & Schorey, J.S. (2007) Exosomes released from infected macrophages contain Mycobacterium avium glycopeptidolipids and are proinflammatory. *Journal of Biological Chemistry*, 282, 25779-25789.

Bianco, N.R., Kim, S.H., Ruffner, M.A. & Robbins, P.D. (2009) Therapeutic effect of exosomes from indoleamine 2,3-dioxygenase-positive dendritic cells in collagen-induced arthritis and delayed-type hypersensitivity disease models. *Arthritis Rheum*, 60, 380-389.

Blanc, L. & Vidal, M. (2010) Reticulocyte membrane remodeling: contribution of the exosome pathway. *Curr Opin Hematol*, 17, 177-183.

Carmeliet, P. (2005) VEGF as a key mediator of angiogenesis in cancer. *Oncology*, 69 Suppl 3, 4-10.

Celi, A., Lorenzet, R., Furie, B.C. & Furie, B. (2004) Microparticles and a P-selectin-mediated pathway of blood coagulation. *Dis Markers*, 20, 347-352.

Chalmin, F., Ladoire, S., Mignot, G., Vincent, J., Bruchard, M., Remy-Martin, J.P., Boireau, W., Rouleau, A., Simon, B., Lanneau, D., De Thonel, A., Multhoff, G., Hamman, A., Martin, F., Chauffert, B., Solary, E., Zitvogel, L., Garrido, C., Ryffel, B., Borg, C., Apetoh, L., Rebe, C. & Ghiringhelli, F. (2010) Membrane-associated Hsp72 from tumor-derived exosomes mediates STAT3-dependent immunosuppressive function of mouse and human myeloid-derived suppressor cells. *The Journal of Clinical Investigation*, 120, 457-471.

Chaput, N., Flament, C., Viaud, S., Taieb, J., Roux, S., Spatz, A., Andre, F., LePecq, J.B., Boussac, M., Garin, J., Amigorena, S., Thery, C. & Zitvogel, L. (2006) Dendritic cell derived-exosomes: biology and clinical implementations. *J Leukoc Biol*, 80, 471-478.

Chaput, N., Schartz, N.E., Andre, F., Taieb, J., Novault, S., Bonnaventure, P., Aubert, N., Bernard, J., Lemonnier, F., Merad, M., Adema, G., Adams, M., Ferrantini, M., Carpentier, A.F., Escudier, B., Tursz, T., Angevin, E. & Zitvogel, L. (2004a) Exosomes as potent cell-free peptide-based vaccine. II. Exosomes in CpG adjuvants efficiently prime naive Tc1 lymphocytes leading to tumor rejection. *J Immunol*, 172, 2137-2146.

Chaput, N., Taieb, J., Schartz, N.E., Andre, F., Angevin, E. & Zitvogel, L. (2004b) Exosome-based immunotherapy. *Cancer Immunol Immunother*, 53, 234-239.

Chen, K.G., Valencia, J.C., Lai, B., Zhang, G., Paterson, J.K., Rouzaud, F., Berens, W., Wincovitch, S.M., Garfield, S.H., Leapman, R.D., Hearing, V.J. & Gottesman, M.M. (2006a) Melanosomal sequestration of cytotoxic drugs contributes to the intractability of malignant melanomas. *Proc Natl Acad Sci U S A*, 103, 9903-9907.

Chen, S.Q., Du, Y., Wang, X., Gu, Q.L., Huang, Y.M. & Dong, Z.M. (2006b) [Production of specific CTL induced by exosomes derived from K562 cells]. *Zhongguo Shi Yan Xue Ye Xue Za Zhi*, 14, 1168-1171.

Chen, W., Wang, J., Shao, C., Liu, S., Yu, Y., Wang, Q. & Cao, X. (2006c) Efficient induction of antitumor T cell immunity by exosomes derived from heat-shocked lymphoma cells. *European Journal of Immunology*, 36, 1598-1607.

Choi, D.S., Lee, J.M., Park, G.W., Lim, H.W., Bang, J.Y., Kim, Y.K., Kwon, K.H., Kwon, H.J., Kim, K.P. & Gho, Y.S. (2007) Proteomic analysis of microvesicles derived from human colorectal cancer cells. *J Proteome Res*, 6, 4646-4655.

Clayton, A., Mitchell, J.P., Court, J., Linnane, S., Mason, M.D. & Tabi, Z. (2008) Human tumor-derived exosomes down-modulate NKG2D expression. *Journal of Immunology*, 180, 7249-7258.

Clayton, A., Mitchell, J.P., Court, J., Mason, M.D. & Tabi, Z. (2007) Human tumor-derived exosomes selectively impair lymphocyte responses to interleukin-2. *Cancer Res*, 67, 7458-7466.

Couzin, J. (2005) Cell biology: The ins and outs of exosomes. *Science*, 308, 1862-1863.

Dashevsky, O., Varon, D. & Brill, A. (2009) Platelet-derived microparticles promote invasiveness of prostate cancer cells via upregulation of MMP-2 production. *Int J Cancer*, 124, 1773-1777.

de Gassart, A., Geminard, C., Fevrier, B., Raposo, G. & Vidal, M. (2003) Lipid raft-associated protein sorting in exosomes. *Blood*, 102, 4336-4344.

Del Conde, I., Shrimpton, C.N., Thiagarajan, P. & Lopez, J.A. (2005) Tissue-factor-bearing microvesicles arise from lipid rafts and fuse with activated platelets to initiate coagulation. *Blood*, 106, 1604-1611.

Di Vizio, D., Kim, J., Hager, M.H., Morello, M., Yang, W., Lafargue, C.J., True, L.D., Rubin, M.A., Adam, R.M., Beroukhim, R., Demichelis, F. & Freeman, M.R. (2009) Oncosome formation in prostate cancer: association with a region of frequent chromosomal deletion in metastatic disease. *Cancer Res*, 69, 5601-5609.

Dolo, V., D'Ascenzo, S., Giusti, I., Millimaggi, D., Taraboletti, G. & Pavan, A. (2005) Shedding of membrane vesicles by tumor and endothelial cells. *Ital J Anat Embryol*, 110, 127-133.

Dong-Sic, C., Jae-Min, L., Wook, P., Hyeon-Woo, L., Young, B., Yoon-Keun, K., Kyung-Hoon, K., Jeong, K., Pyo, K. & Song, Y. (2007) Proteomic analysis of microvesicles derived from human colorectal cancer cells. *J Proteo Res*, 6, 10.

Duijvesz, D., Luider, T., Bangma, C.H. & Jenster, G. (2010) Exosomes as Biomarker Treasure Chests for Prostate Cancer. *Eur Urol*.

Escudier, B., Dorval, T., Chaput, N., Andre, F., Caby, M.P., Novault, S., Flament, C., Leboulaire, C., Borg, C., Amigorena, S., Baccaccio, C., Bonnerot, C., Dhellin, O., Movassagh, M., Piperno, S., Robert, C., Serra, V., Valente, N., LePecq, J.B., Spatz, A., Lantz, O., Tursz, T., Angevin, E. & Zitvogel, L. (2005) Vaccination of metastatic melanoma patients with autologous dendritic cell (DC) derived-exosomes: results of the first phase I clinical trial. *Journal of Translational Medicine*, 3.

Falati, S., Liu, Q., Gross, P., Merrill-Skoloff, G., Chou, J., Vandendries, E., Celi, A., Croce, K., Furie, B.C. & Furie, B. (2003) Accumulation of tissue factor into developing thrombi in vivo is dependent upon microparticle P-selectin glycoprotein ligand 1 and platelet P-selectin. *J Exp Med*, 197, 1585-1598.

Gesierich, S., Berezovskiy, I., Ryschich, E. & Zoller, M. (2006) Systemic induction of the angiogenesis switch by the tetraspanin D6.1A/CO-029. *Cancer Res*, 66, 7083-7094.

Ghosh, A.K., Secreto, C.R., Knox, T.R., Ding, W., Mukhopadhyay, D. & Kay, N.E. (2010) Circulating microvesicles in B-cell chronic lymphocytic leukemia can stimulate marrow stromal cells: implications for disease progression. *Blood*, 115, 1755-1764.

Ginestra, A., La Placa, M.D., Saladino, F., Cassara, D., Nagase, H. & Vittorelli, M.L. (1998) The amount and proteolytic content of vesicles shed by human cancer cell lines correlates with their in vitro invasiveness. *Anticancer Res*, 18, 3433-3437.

Ginestra, A., Miceli, D., Dolo, V., Romano, F.M. & Vittorelli, M.L. (1999) Membrane vesicles in ovarian cancer fluids: a new potential marker. *Anticancer Res,* 19, 3439-3445.

Graves, L.E., Ariztia, E.V., Navari, J.R., Matzel, H.J., Stack, M.S. & Fishman, D.A. (2004) Proinvasive properties of ovarian cancer ascites-derived membrane vesicles. *Cancer Res,* 64, 7045-7049.

Haubold, K., Rink, M., Spath, B., Friedrich, M., Chun, F.K., Marx, G., Amirkhosravi, A., Francis, J.L., Bokemeyer, C., Eifrig, B. & Langer, F. (2009) Tissue factor procoagulant activity of plasma microparticles is increased in patients with early-stage prostate cancer. *Thromb Haemost,* 101, 1147-1155.

Hegmans, J.P., Bard, M.P., Hemmes, A., Luider, T.M., Kleijmeer, M.J., Prins, J.B., Zitvogel, L., Burgers, S.A., Hoogsteden, H.C. & Lambrecht, B.N. (2004) Proteomic analysis of exosomes secreted by human mesothelioma cells. *Am J Pathol,* 164, 1807-1815.

Hendrix, A., Westbroek, W., Bracke, M. & De Wever, O. (2010) An ex(o)citing machinery for invasive tumor growth. *Cancer Res,* 70, 9533-9537.

Hotary, K.B., Allen, E.D., Brooks, P.C., Datta, N.S., Long, M.W. & Weiss, S.J. (2003) Membrane type I matrix metalloproteinase usurps tumor growth control imposed by the three-dimensional extracellular matrix. *Cell,* 114, 33-45.

Huber, V., Fais, S., Iero, M., Lugini, L., Canese, P., Squarcina, P., Zaccheddu, A., Colone, M., Arancia, G., Gentile, M., Seregni, E., Valenti, R., Ballabio, G., Belli, F., Leo, E., Parmiani, G. & Rivoltini, L. (2005) Human colorectal cancer cells induce T-cell death through release of proapoptotic microvesicles: role in immune escape. *Gastroenterology,* 128, 1796-1804.

Iero, M., Valenti, R., Huber, V., Filipazzi, P., Parmiani, G., Fais, S. & Rivoltini, L. (2008) Tumour-released exosomes and their implications in cancer immunity. *Cell Death Differ,* 15, 80-88.

Janowska-Wieczorek, A., Majka, M., Kijowski, J., Baj-Krzyworzeka, M., Reca, R., Turner, A.R., Ratajczak, J., Emerson, S.G., Kowalska, M.A. & Ratajczak, M.Z. (2001) Platelet-derived microparticles bind to hematopoietic stem/progenitor cells and enhance their engraftment. *Blood,* 98, 3143-3149.

Janowska-Wieczorek, A., Wysoczynski, M., Kijowski, J., Marquez-Curtis, L., Machalinski, B., Ratajczak, J. & Ratajczak, M.Z. (2005) Microvesicles derived from activated platelets induce metastasis and angiogenesis in lung cancer. *Int J Cancer,* 113, 752-760.

Jansen, F.H., Krijgsveld, J., van Rijswijk, A., van den Bemd, G.J., van den Berg, M.S., van Weerden, W.M., Willemsen, R., Dekker, L.J., Luider, T.M. & Jenster, G. (2009) Exosomal secretion of cytoplasmic prostate cancer xenograft-derived proteins. *Mol Cell Proteomics,* 8, 1192-1205.

Johnstone, R.M., Adam, M., Hammond, J.R., Orr, L. & Turbide, C. (1987) Vesicle formation during reticulocyte maturation. Association of plasma membrane activities with released vesicles (exosomes). *J Biol Chem,* 262, 9412-9420.

Jung, T., Castellana, D., Klingbeil, P., Cuesta Hernandez, I., Vitacolonna, M., Orlicky, D.J., Roffler, S.R., Brodt, P. & Zoller, M. (2009) CD44v6 dependence of premetastatic niche preparation by exosomes. *Neoplasia,* 11, 1093-1105.

Keller, S., Konig, A.K., Marme, F., Runz, S., Wolterink, S., Koensgen, D., Mustea, A., Sehouli, J. & Altevogt, P. (2009) Systemic presence and tumor-growth promoting effect of ovarian carcinoma released exosomes. *Cancer Lett,* 278, 73-81.

Keller, S., Sanderson, M.P., Stoeck, A. & Altevogt, P. (2006) Exosomes: from biogenesis and secretion to biological function. *Immunol Lett,* 107, 102-108.

Kerbel, R.S. (2008) Tumor angiogenesis. *N Engl J Med,* 358, 2039-2049.

Khan, S., Jutzy, J.M., Aspe, J.R., McGregor, D.W., Neidigh, J.W. & Wall, N.R. (2011) Survivin is released from cancer cells via exosomes. *Apoptosis*, 16, 1-12.

Kim, J.V., Latouche, J.B., Riviere, I. & Sadelain, M. (2004) The ABCs of artificial antigen presentation. *Nature Biotechnology*, 22, 403-410.

Kim, J.W., Wieckowski, E., Taylor, D.D., Reichert, T.E., Watkins, S. & Whiteside, T.L. (2005) Fas ligand-positive membranous vesicles isolated from sera of patients with oral cancer induce apoptosis of activated T lymphocytes. *Clin Cancer Res*, 11, 1010-1020.

Koga, K., Matsumoto, K., Akiyoshi, T., Kubo, M., Yamanaka, N., Tasaki, A., Nakashima, H., Nakamura, M., Kuroki, S., Tanaka, M. & Katano, M. (2005) Purification, characterization and biological significance of tumor-derived exosomes. *Anticancer Res*, 25, 3703-3707.

Koyama, S., Koike, N. & Adachi, S. (2001) Fas receptor counterattack against tumor-infiltrating lymphocytes in vivo as a mechanism of immune escape in gastric carcinoma. *Journal of Cancer Research and Clinical Oncology*, 127, 20-26.

Lehmann, B.D., Paine, M.S., Brooks, A.M., McCubrey, J.A., Renegar, R.H., Wang, R. & Terrian, D.M. (2008) Senescence-associated exosome release from human prostate cancer cells. *Cancer Res*, 68, 7864-7871.

Leroyer, A.S., Tedgui, A. & Boulanger, C.M. (2008) Role of microparticles in atherothrombosis. *J Intern Med*, 263, 528-537.

Lespagnol, A., Duflaut, D., Beekman, C., Blanc, L., Fiucci, G., Marine, J.C., Vidal, M., Amson, R. & Telerman, A. (2008) Exosome secretion, including the DNA damage-induced p53-dependent secretory pathway, is severely compromised in TSAP6/Steap3-null mice. *Cell Death Differ*, 15, 1723-1733.

Liu, C., Yu, S., Zinn, K., Wang, J., Zhang, L., Jia, Y., Kappes, J.C., Barnes, S., Kimberly, R.P., Grizzle, W.E. & Zhang, H.G. (2006) Murine mammary carcinoma exosomes promote tumor growth by suppression of NK cell function. *J Immunol*, 176, 1375-1385.

Losche, W., Scholz, T., Temmler, U., Oberle, V. & Claus, R.A. (2004) Platelet-derived microvesicles transfer tissue factor to monocytes but not to neutrophils. *Platelets*, 15, 109-115.

Lu, Q., Zhang, J., Allison, R., Gay, H., Yang, W.X., Bhowmick, N.A., Frelix, G., Shappell, S. & Chen, Y.H. (2009) Identification of extracellular delta-catenin accumulation for prostate cancer detection. *Prostate*, 69, 411-418.

Luhtala, N. & Odorizzi, G. (2004) Bro1 coordinates deubiquitination in the multivesicular body pathway by recruiting Doa4 to endosomes. *J Cell Biol*, 166, 717-729.

Mack, M., Kleinschmidt, A., Bruhl, H., Klier, C., Nelson, P.J., Cihak, J., Plachy, J., Stangassinger, M., Erfle, V. & Schlondorff, D. (2000) Transfer of the chemokine receptor CCR5 between cells by membrane-derived microparticles: a mechanism for cellular human immunodeficiency virus 1 infection. *Nat Med*, 6, 769-775.

Martinez-Lostao, L., Garcia-Alvarez, F., Basanez, G., Alegre-Aguaron, E., Desportes, P., Larrad, L., Naval, J., Martinez-Lorenzo, M.J. & Anel, A. (2010) Liposome-bound APO2L/TRAIL is an effective treatment in a rabbit model of rheumatoid arthritis. *Arthritis Rheum*, 62, 2272-2282.

Mathivanan, S., Lim, J.W., Tauro, B.J., Ji, H., Moritz, R.L. & Simpson, R.J. (2010) Proteomics analysis of A33 immunoaffinity-purified exosomes released from the human colon tumor cell line LIM1215 reveals a tissue-specific protein signature. *Mol Cell Proteomics*, 9, 197-208.

Matsuo, H., Chevallier, J., Mayran, N., Le Blanc, I., Ferguson, C., Faure, J., Blanc, N.S., Matile, S., Dubochet, J., Sadoul, R., Parton, R.G., Vilbois, F. & Gruenberg, J. (2004) Role of LBPA and Alix in multivesicular liposome formation and endosome organization. *Science*, 303, 531-534.

Mears, R., Craven, R.A., Hanrahan, S., Totty, N., Upton, C., Young, S.L., Patel, P., Selby, P.J. & Banks, R.E. (2004) Proteomic analysis of melanoma-derived exosomes by two-dimensional polyacrylamide gel electrophoresis and mass spectrometry. *Proteomics*, 4, 4019-4031.

Mignot, G., Roux, S., Thery, C., Segura, E. & Zitvogel, L. (2006) Prospects for exosomes in immunotherapy of cancer. *J Cell Mol Med*, 10, 376-388.

Milsom, C., Yu, J., May, L., Meehan, B., Magnus, N., Al-Nedawi, K., Luyendyk, J., Weitz, J., Klement, P., Broze, G., Mackman, N. & Rak, J. (2007) The role of tumor-and host-related tissue factor pools in oncogene-driven tumor progression. *Thromb Res*, 120 Suppl 2, S82-91.

Mitchell, P.J., Welton, J., Staffurth, J., Court, J., Mason, M.D., Tabi, Z. & Clayton, A. (2009) Can urinary exosomes act as treatment response markers in prostate cancer? *J Transl Med*, 7, 4.

Morse, M.A., Garst, J., Osada, T., Khan, S., Hobeika, A., Clay, T.M., Valente, N., Shreeniwas, R., Sutton, M.A., Delcayre, A., Hsu, D.H., LePecq, J.B. & Lyerly, H.K. (2005) A phase I study of dexosome immunotherapy in patients with advanced non-small cell lung cancer. *Journal of Translational Medicine*, 3.

Muralidharan-Chari, V., Clancy, J.W., Sedgwick, A. & D'Souza-Schorey, C. (2010) Microvesicles: mediators of extracellular communication during cancer progression. *J Cell Sci*, 123, 1603-1611.

Nickel, W. (2003) The mystery of nonclassical protein secretion. A current view on cargo proteins and potential export routes. *Eur J Biochem*, 270, 2109-2119.

Nieuwland, R. & Sturk, A. (2010) Why do cells release vesicles? *Thromb Res*, 125 Suppl 1, S49-51.

Nilsson, J., Skog, J., Nordstrand, A., Baranov, V., Mincheva-Nilsson, L., Breakefield, X.O. & Widmark, A. (2009) Prostate cancer-derived urine exosomes: a novel approach to biomarkers for prostate cancer. *Br J Cancer*, 100, 1603-1607.

Obregon, C., Rothen-Rutishauser, B., Gitahi, S.K., Gehr, P. & Nicod, L.P. (2006) Exovesicles from human activated dendritic cells fuse with resting dendritic cells, allowing them to present alloantigens. *American Journal of Pathology*, 169, 2127-2136.

Osterud, B. (2003) The role of platelets in decrypting monocyte tissue factor. *Dis Mon*, 49, 7-13.

Pap, E., Pallinger, E. & Falus, A. (2010) The role of membrane vesicles in tumorigenesis. *Crit Rev Oncol Hematol*.

Park, D., Tosello-Trampont, A.C., Elliott, M.R., Lu, M., Haney, L.B., Ma, Z., Klibanov, A.L., Mandell, J.W. & Ravichandran, K.S. (2007) BAI1 is an engulfment receptor for apoptotic cells upstream of the ELMO/Dock180/Rac module. *Nature*, 450, 430-434.

Parolini, I., Federici, C., Raggi, C., Lugini, L., Palleschi, S., De Milito, A., Coscia, C., Iessi, E., Logozzi, M., Molinari, A., Colone, M., Tatti, M., Sargiacomo, M. & Fais, S. (2009) Microenvironmental pH is a key factor for exosome traffic in tumor cells. *J Biol Chem*, 284, 34211-34222.

Ponnambalam, S. & Baldwin, S.A. (2003) Constitutive protein secretion from the trans-Golgi network to the plasma membrane. *Mol Membr Biol*, 20, 129-139.

Raimondo, F., Morosi, L., Chinello, C., Magni, F. & Pitto, M. (2011) Advances in membranous vesicle and exosome proteomics improving biological understanding and biomarker discovery. *Proteomics*, 11, 709-720.

Rak, J. (2010) Microparticles in cancer. *Semin Thromb Hemost*, 36, 888-906.

Raposo, G., Nijman, H.W., Stoorvogel, W., Liejendekker, R., Harding, C.V., Melief, C.J. & Geuze, H.J. (1996) B lymphocytes secrete antigen-presenting vesicles. *J Exp Med*, 183, 1161-1172.

Ratajczak, J., Wysoczynski, M., Hayek, F., Janowska-Wieczorek, A. & Ratajczak, M.Z. (2006) Membrane-derived microvesicles: important and underappreciated mediators of cell-to-cell communication. *Leukemia*, 20, 1487-1495.

Record, M., Subra, C., Silvente-Poirot, S. & Poirot, M. (2011) Exosomes as intercellular signalosomes and pharmacological effectors. *Biochem Pharmacol*.

Ronquist, G. & Brody, I. (1985) The prostasome: its secretion and function in man. *Biochim Biophys Acta*, 822, 203-218.

Ronquist, G. & Frithz, G.G. (1986) Prostasomes in human semen contain ADP and GDP. *Acta Eur Fertil*, 17, 273-276.

Rooney, I.A., Atkinson, J.P., Krul, E.S., Schonfeld, G., Polakoski, K., Saffitz, J.E. & Morgan, B.P. (1993) Physiologic relevance of the membrane attack complex inhibitory protein CD59 in human seminal plasma: CD59 is present on extracellular organelles (prostasomes), binds cell membranes, and inhibits complement-mediated lysis. *J Exp Med*, 177, 1409-1420.

Safaei, R., Larson, B.J., Cheng, T.C., Gibson, M.A., Otani, S., Naerdemann, W. & Howell, S.B. (2005) Abnormal lysosomal trafficking and enhanced exosomal export of cisplatin in drug-resistant human ovarian carcinoma cells. *Mol Cancer Ther*, 4, 1595-1604.

Sanderson, M.P., Keller, S., Alonso, A., Riedle, S., Dempsey, P.J. & Altevogt, P. (2008) Generation of novel, secreted epidermal growth factor receptor (EGFR/ErbB1) isoforms via metalloprotease-dependent ectodomain shedding and exosome secretion. *J Cell Biochem*, 103, 1783-1797.

Savina, A., Furlan, M., Vidal, M. & Colombo, M.I. (2003) Exosome release is regulated by a calcium-dependent mechanism in K562 cells. *J Biol Chem*, 278, 20083-20090.

Schiller, M., Bekeredjian-Ding, I., Heyder, P., Blank, N., Ho, A.D. & Lorenz, H.M. (2008) Autoantigens are translocated into small apoptotic bodies during early stages of apoptosis. *Cell Death Differ*, 15, 183-191.

Schorey, J.S. & Bhatnagar, S. (2008) Exosome function: from tumor immunology to pathogen biology. *Traffic*, 9, 871-881.

Shedden, K., Xie, X.T., Chandaroy, P., Chang, Y.T. & Rosania, G.R. (2003) Expulsion of small molecules in vesicles shed by cancer cells: association with gene expression and chemosensitivity profiles. *Cancer Res*, 63, 4331-4337.

Simpson, R.J., Jensen, S.S. & Lim, J.W. (2008) Proteomic profiling of exosomes: current perspectives. *Proteomics*, 8, 4083-4099.

Simpson, R.J., Lim, J.W., Moritz, R.L. & Mathivanan, S. (2009) Exosomes: proteomic insights and diagnostic potential. *Expert Rev Proteomics*, 6, 267-283.

Skog, J., Wurdinger, T., van Rijn, S., Meijer, D.H., Gainche, L., Sena-Esteves, M., Curry, W.T., Jr., Carter, B.S., Krichevsky, A.M. & Breakefield, X.O. (2008) Glioblastoma microvesicles transport RNA and proteins that promote tumour growth and provide diagnostic biomarkers. *Nat Cell Biol*, 10, 1470-1476.

Skokos, D., Le Panse, S., Villa, I., Rousselle, J.C., Peronet, R., David, B., Namane, A. & Mecheri, S. (2001) Mast cell-dependent B and T lymphocyte activation is mediated by the secretion of immunologically active exosomes. *J Immunol*, 166, 868-876.

Smalley, D.M., Sheman, N.E., Nelson, K. & Theodorescu, D. (2008) Isolation and identification of potential urinary microparticle biomarkers of bladder cancer. *J Proteome Res*, 7, 2088-2096.

Szajnik, M., Czystowska, M., Szczepanski, M.J., Mandapathil, M. & Whiteside, T.L. (2010) Tumor-derived microvesicles induce, expand and up-regulate biological activites of human regulatory T cells (Treg). *PLoS One*, 5, e11469.

Tan, A., De La Pena, H. & Seifalian, A.M. (2010) The application of exosomes as a nanoscale cancer vaccine. *Int J Nanomedicine*, 5, 889-900.

Taraboletti, G., D'Ascenzo, S., Giusti, I., Marchetti, D., Borsotti, P., Millimaggi, D., Giavazzi, R., Pavan, A. & Dolo, V. (2006) Bioavailability of VEGF in tumor-shed vesicles depends on vesicle burst induced by acidic pH. *Neoplasia*, 8, 96-103.

Taylor, D.D., Akyol, S. & Gercel-Taylor, C. (2006) Pregnancy-associated exosomes and their modulation of T cell signaling. *J Immunol*, 176, 1534-1542.

Taylor, D.D. & Gercel-Taylor, C. (2005) Tumour-derived exosomes and their role in cancer-associated T-cell signalling defects. *Br J Cancer*, 92, 305-311.

Tesselaar, M.E., Romijn, F.P., Van Der Linden, I.K., Prins, F.A., Bertina, R.M. & Osanto, S. (2007) Microparticle-associated tissue factor activity: a link between cancer and thrombosis? *J Thromb Haemost*, 5, 520-527.

Thery, C., Amigorena, S., Raposo, G. & Clayton, A. (2006) Isolation and characterization of exosomes from cell culture supernatants and biological fluids. *Curr Protoc Cell Biol*, Chapter 3, Unit 3 22.

Thery, C., Duban, L., Segura, E., Veron, P., Lantz, O. & Amigorena, S. (2002) Indirect activation of naive CD4+ T cells by dendritic cell-derived exosomes. *Nat Immunol*, 3, 1156-1162.

Thery, C., Ostrowski, M. & Segura, E. (2009) Membrane vesicles as conveyors of immune responses. *Nat Rev Immunol*, 9, 581-593.

Thomas, G.M., Panicot-Dubois, L., Lacroix, R., Dignat-George, F., Lombardo, D. & Dubois, C. (2009) Cancer cell-derived microparticles bearing P-selectin glycoprotein ligand 1 accelerate thrombus formation in vivo. *J Exp Med*, 206, 1913-1927.

Valadi, H., Ekstrom, K., Bossios, A., Sjostrand, M., Lee, J.J. & Lotvall, J.O. (2007) Exosome-mediated transfer of mRNAs and microRNAs is a novel mechanism of genetic exchange between cells. *Nat Cell Biol*, 9, 654-659.

Valenti, R., Huber, V., Iero, M., Filipazzi, P., Parmiani, G. & Rivoltini, L. (2007) Tumor-released microvesicles as vehicles of immunosuppression. *Cancer Res*, 67, 2912-2915.

van Niel, G., Porto-Carreiro, I., Simoes, S. & Raposo, G. (2006) Exosomes: a common pathway for a specialized function. *J Biochem*, 140, 13-21.

Vella, L.J., Greenwood, D.L., Cappai, R., Scheerlinck, J.P. & Hill, A.F. (2008) Enrichment of prion protein in exosomes derived from ovine cerebral spinal fluid. *Vet Immunol Immunopathol*, 124, 385-393.

Viaud, S., Terme, M., Flament, C., Taieb, J., Andre, F., Novault, S., Escudier, B., Robert, C., Caillat-Zucman, S., Tursz, T., Zitvogel, L. & Chaput, N. (2009) Dendritic cell-derived exosomes promote natural killer cell activation and proliferation: a role for NKG2D ligands and IL-15Ralpha. *PLoS One*, 4, e4942.

Welton, J.L., Khanna, S., Giles, P.J., Brennan, P., Brewis, I.A., Staffurth, J., Mason, M.D. & Clayton, A. (2010) Proteomics analysis of bladder cancer exosomes. *Mol Cell Proteomics*, 9, 1324-1338.

Wieckowski, E. & Whiteside, T.L. (2006) Human tumor-derived vs dendritic cell-derived exosomes have distinct biologic roles and molecular profiles. *Immunol Res*, 36, 247-254.

Wolfers, J., Lozier, A., Raposo, G., Regnault, A., Thery, C., Masurier, C., Flament, C., Pouzieux, S., Faure, F., Tursz, T., Angevin, E., Amigorena, S. & Zitvogel, L. (2001) Tumor-derived exosomes are a source of shared tumor rejection antigens for CTL cross-priming. *Nat Med*, 7, 297-303.

Xiang, X., Poliakov, A., Liu, C., Liu, Y., Deng, Z.B., Wang, J., Cheng, Z., Shah, S.V., Zhang, L., Grizzle, W.E., Mobley, J. & Zhange, H.G. (2009) Induction of myeloid-derived suppressor cells by tumor exosomes. *International Journal of Cancer*, 124, 2621-2633.

Xiao, Z., Blonder, J., Zhou, M. & Veenstra, T.D. (2009) Proteomic analysis of extracellular matrix and vesicles. *J Proteomics*, 72, 34-45.

Yu, J.L., May, L., Lhotak, V., Shahrzad, S., Shirasawa, S., Weitz, J.I., Coomber, B.L., Mackman, N. & Rak, J.W. (2005) Oncogenic events regulate tissue factor expression in colorectal cancer cells: implications for tumor progression and angiogenesis. *Blood*, 105, 1734-1741.

Yu, X., Harris, S.L. & Levine, A.J. (2006) The regulation of exosome secretion: a novel function of the p53 protein. *Cancer Res*, 66, 4795-4801.

Yu, X., Riley, T. & Levine, A.J. (2009) The regulation of the endosomal compartment by p53 the tumor suppressor gene. *FEBS J*, 276, 2201-2212.

Zhang, H., Xie, Y., Li, W., Chibbar, R., Xiong, S. & Xiang, J. (2011) CD4+ T cell-released exosomes inhibit CD8+ cytotoxic T-lymphocyte responses and antitumor immunity. *Cellular & Molecular Immunology*, 8, 23-30.

Zhao, C.Q., Li, T.L., He, S.H., Chen, X., An, Y.F., Wu, W.K., Zhou, X.H., Li, P. & Yang, P.C. (2010) Specific immunotherapy suppresses Th2 responses via modulating TIM1/TIM4 interaction on dendritic cells. *Allergy*, 65, 986-995.

Zhou, H., Cheruvanky, A., Hu, X., Matsumoto, T., Hiramatsu, N., Cho, M.E., Berger, A., Leelahavanichkul, A., Doi, K., Chawla, L.S., Illei, G.G., Kopp, J.B., Balow, J.E., Austin, H.A., 3rd, Yuen, P.S. & Star, R.A. (2008) Urinary exosomal transcription factors, a new class of biomarkers for renal disease. *Kidney Int*, 74, 613-621.

Zitvogel, L., Regnault, A., Lozier, A., Wolfers, J., Flament, C., Tenza, D., Ricciardi-Castagnoli, P., Raposo, G. & Amigorena, S. (1998) Eradication of established murine tumors using a novel cell-free vaccine: dendritic cell-derived exosomes. *Nat Med*, 4, 594-600.

# 3

# The Airways: A Promising Route for the Pulmonary Delivery of Anticancer Agents

Guilleminault L.[1,2], Hervé-Grépinet V.[1],
Lemarié E.[1,2] and Heuzé-Vourc'h N.[1]
[1]*INSERM U618, Université François Rabelais, Faculté de médecine, Tours*
[2]*Service de Pneumologie, CHRU Tours*
*France*

## 1. Introduction

The outcome of lung cancer has not changed dramatically in recent years, despite the availability of new therapeutic agents. Lung cancer is the most common cause of cancer-related death in all industrialised countries (28 % in the USA for 2009). It is usually treated by a combination of surgery, radiotherapy and chemotherapy; and anticancer drugs are generally given intravenously. But this delivery route leads to high drug concentrations in the systemic circulation, with some adverse side effects and low drug concentrations in the respiratory tract. Clearly, a new route for administering anti-cancer drugs is needed: the airways. Drugs for treating chronic respiratory diseases like asthma, chronic obstructive pulmonary disease (COPD) and cystic fibrosis are commonly delivered *via* the airways. The main advantage of this route is that the drug is delivered directly into the bronchi, bronchioles or deep lungs. Airway delivery should theoretically ensure longer exposure of the intended target to higher concentrations of the drug, while reducing adverse side effects. The patient should therefore benefit from a minimum drug concentration in the bloodstream and other body tissues. The airways therefore appear to be an attractive route for delivering anticancer agents in lung cancer, especially when other treatments have limited success, and in particular pathological situations, such as bronchioloalveolar carcinoma (BAC). This chapter provides an overview of the delivery of anticancer agents by aerosoltherapy for treating lung cancers and metastases, including the current status in the use of aerosoltherapy in oncology and future progress.

## 2. Challenge of aerosol drug delivery in lung cancer

### 2.1 Aerosol deposition

Effective drug delivery to the lungs *via* the airways requires a detailed knowledge of aerosols. The main parameters that should be considered are the particle size, the inspiratory flow rate, the volume of the inhalation and the calibre of the patient's airways. The model developed by Weibel divides the lungs into 23 serial branching generations. The first sixteen form the conducting bronchial airways and the last seven, the respiratory zone (or alveolar region) (Weibel et al., 1963). The lungs may also be divided in three parts, upper (apex), middle and lower (base). Thus the major challenge involved in delivering drugs into the lungs is provided by the complex structure of the respiratory tract.

Aerosols generally have a polydisperse particle size distribution, and particle size is one of the most important factors influencing aerosol deposition in the lungs. The mass median aerodynamic diameter (MMAD) is usually used to estimate the particle size distribution. The MMAD describes an aerosol in terms of its mass and size. It is defined as 50 % of the mass of the particles less than MMAD and 50 % greater than the MMAD (Soderlom, 1989). Analysis of lung depositions indicated that almost all particles with a MMAD >5 µm are deposited in the oropharynx. Most of those with a MMAD of 2 to 6 µm are deposited in the bronchi (conducting airways) and fine particles with a MMAD <2 µm are deposited in the alveolar region. Most of the particles smaller than 1 µm are presumably exhaled (Newman et al., 1983).

The depositing of particles in the lungs also depends on several other parameters. One is the inspiratory flow rate (IFR). The particles display high velocity and turbulence when the IFR increases, causing them to be deposited in the conducting airways (Dolovich et al., 2000). Thus drug deposition in the upper airways can be improved by increasing the IFR. In contrast, a low IFR and gas density help aerosols to penetrate into the lung periphery (Anderson et al., 1990). The penetration of particles into the alveolar region also depends on the inhaled volume. Particles are better deposited in the lung peripheries of patients with a high FEV1 (forced expiratory volume in one second) (Pavia et al. 1976). Similarly, rapid exhalation following a short breath hold can influence particle deposition in the large airway. The calibre of the airways also modulates particle deposition. There is excessive mucus secretion and accumulation in some respiratory diseases, such as cystic fibrosis and certain tumours, which leads to obstruction of the airways. This reduction in airway calibre has a negative influence on the deposition and distribution patterns of aerosols. Particle deposition is dramatically decreased in cystic fibrosis patients, even from aerosols with fine particles (<2µm), because of the secretions and reduced airway calibre (Dolovich, 2009).

The diameter of the airways of children is much smaller than those of adults. Hence, particles are deposited mainly in the oropharynx or upper airways because they impact rapidly on the bronchus barrier. The breathing patterns of children also differ from those of adults. Their tidal volume is smaller (volume of air displaced between normal inspiration and expiration) and their respiratory rate higher than those of adults, which prevents drugs from being deposited in the alveolar region. Co-operation and compliance complicate the administration of drug to children *via* the airways. Cries can be assimilated to a rapid exhalation, leading to deposition of drug almost exclusively on the surface of the oropharynx (Schüepp et al., 2004).

Few studies focused on the deposition of inhaled particles in the lungs of the elderly. They have shown that the particle deposition in old and younger patients with lung diseases were similar. However, some pulmonary delivery devices are unsuitable for patients suffering from memory loss and disorders of movement coordination (Allen et al., 2008).

### 2.2 Technology of delivery devices

Several devices have been developed to generate aerosol particles. They include nebulisers, pressurized-metered dose inhalers (pMDI) and dry powder inhalers (DPI). Nebulisers are widely used for drug inhalation, and there are three types of nebuliser: pneumatic (or jet), ultrasonic and vibrating-mesh. Pneumatic nebulisers use compressed air to aerosolise drug solutions. These solutions are carried into the gas stream and dispersed into droplets due to surface tension (Hess et al., 2008). A fill volume of 4-5 ml is optimal and normal saline is added when the volume is lower. Ultrasonic nebulisers use a high-frequency piezoelectric system to produce ultrasound, which then nebulises a drug solution. This system is not compatible with all molecules because the ultrasound can destroy certain drugs. In vibrating-mesh nebulisers, the drug solution is compressed by perforated membranes that are vibrating rapidly. All types of nebuliser are only half as efficient with nasal inhalation as with oral inhalation (Everard et al., 1993).

A pMDI is a handheld device that contains a drug in solution or suspension and a gas like hydrofluoroalkane to propel the solution/suspension. It must be shaken before use to mix gas with the drug solution/suspension. The most important component of the pMDI is the metering valve (Hess et al., 2008). This is because the pMDI canister is used inverted, and the valve prevents the drug from leaking due to gravity. The advantages of this system are its small size, ease of use, and its portability. However, good coordination between hand movements and inhalation is needed for efficient drug deposition. Devices with an automatic release have been developed for patients with coordination disorders. A valve holding chamber can also be placed between the MDI and the patient to ensure that aerosol is retained in the chamber and released when the patient breathes.

The drug used in the DPI system is formulated as a dry powder. The devise has a dosing principle and an inhaler (Pedersen, 1996). The powder is broken down into small particles by the force of the patient's inhalation. DPI is available in multi-dose and single-dose models. The single-dose model has a single drug capsule that must be manually inserted into the device by the patient. These drug capsules must not be ingested.

Education is essential for effective drug delivery *via* the airways. Nurses, physicians and pharmacists must all learn how to use inhalers so as to prevent their misuse or inadequate treatment. Mishandling of aerosol devices like the pMDI is associated with decreased asthma control (Giraud and Roche, 2002). Patients must be also educated to inhale properly in order to maximize drug deposition in the intended lung compartment. Most of the anticancer drugs presently being evaluated in clinical trials have been administered to the airways with nebulisers. Nebulisers and endotracheal sprays have generally been used to deliver anticancer drugs in preclinical studies to animals.

### 2.3 Recommendations for delivering anticancer drugs *via* the airways

Official sources, such as the European Respiratory Society, have not yet established procedures for using anticancer drugs to treat lung cancer. They have only discussed the lack of evidence for using opiates and bronchodilators in palliative care (Boe et al., 2001). Herein, we propose some advices based on official recommendations established for other respiratory diseases (such as COPD and asthma). Certain steps should be scrupulously respected if a drug is administered *via* the airways. The choice of the device is critical because they are not compatible for all drugs. Physicians may prefer not to use pMDI or DPI systems for patients with coordination disorders or memory deficiency. A mouthpiece is the most suitable means of improving lung deposition and is safer for the patient as it avoids injuring the eyes. The manufacturer's instructions (formulation, solution volume and type of driver gas) should be respected to ensure optimal drug deposition, and effective treatment. Nebulisers should be cleaned carefully to prevent bacterial contamination and subsequent lung infections. Maintenance procedures are available for all nebulisers and they should be communicated to the patient. Single-dose nebulisers may be most suitable for hospitalised patients, with replacement every 24 hours.

Great care should be taken when administering anticancer agent *via* the pulmonary route. Anticancer agents are potentially toxic for the lung and may impair the pulmonary function in some patients, but most of them are not very toxic when the inhalation procedure is standardized and the dose well defined. The safety of healthcare workers should be considered. Aerosolised chemotherapy should be delivered in a well-ventilated room with an efficient air filtering system (Gagnadoux et al., 2007). Wittgen et al demonstrated the advantages of combining a mobile HEPA (High Efficiency Particulate Air) filter air cleaning system with a demistifier tent to prevent aerosol propagation during inhalation of nebulised liposomal cisplatin (Wittgen et al., 2006).

## 3. Aerosolisation of anticancer agents

### 3.1 Formulation of anticancer drugs for aerosol delivery

Particle size is one of the most critical parameters for ensuring efficient drug deposition in the respiratory tract. Several parameters influence drug targeting to the desired lung area: these are the size, shape, density, electrical charge and hygroscopicity of the aerosol particles (Pilcer and Amighi, 2010). It is also essential that the aerosolised drug remains pharmacologically active. Formulations for nebulised drug traditionally include sodium chloride or other salts to adjust the osmolarity, HCl or NaOH to obtain a stabilised neutral pH and a surfactant such as polysorbates to avoid drug aggregates. But other methods have been developed to produce particles with controlled properties; these include jet milling, spray drying and supercritical fluid techniques. Excipients like lipids and polymers are also used to improve pulmonary deposition (Pilcer and Amighi, 2010).

Some drugs are encapsulated into liposome to increase their resident time into the lungs (Cryan, 2005). Liposomal formulations generally provide sustained drug release, prevent local irritation, and improve drug stability. For example, the resident time in the lungs of liposomal cyclosporine A is nearly 17 times longer than that of the standard compound (Arppe et al., 1998). The lipids most commonly used to produce liposome are lecithins (phosphatidylcholines), phosphatidylethanolamines, phosphatidylserines, and phosphatidylinositols. Formulations with microspheres have also been developed. Although, they are mostly used to deliver drugs whose intended actions are systemic, such as vaccines and insulin, more and more formulations of anticancer agents associated with microspheres are being developed. Microspheres are produced using natural or synthetic polymers. The two most commonly used synthetic polymers are polylactic acid (PLA) and polylacticco-glycolic acid (PLGA) (Cryan, 2005). The rate at which a drug is released from microparticles depends on its dissolution and diffusion.

New formulations are today developed for the controlled release of the drug and to enhance anticancer efficacy. Biotinylated-EGF-modified gelatine was tested as a carrier for cisplatin with better anticancer and less toxic effect than free cisplatin after aerosolisation *in vitro* and *in vivo* (Tseng et al., 2009). Encapsulation of anticancer agent in nanoparticles is also evaluated, in particular through airways delivery with some promising results (El-Gendy and Berckland, 2009, Hureaux et al., 2009, Tomoda et al., 2009).

### 3.2 Pharmacological properties of aerosolised anticancer agents

Most anticancer drugs resist the physical constraints of aerosolisation, retain their pharmacological properties, and produce particles with aerodynamic properties that are compatible with lung deposition. A study by Gagnadoux et al. showed that the cytotoxicity of a nebulised formulation of the nucleoside analog gemcitabine (GCB) was similar to that of the native drug when tested against NCI-H460 and A549 Non-Small Cell Lung Cancer (NSCLC) cells (Gagnadoux et al., 2006). Another study of the cytotoxicity of a nebulised farnesol formulation containing polysorbate 80 (Tween 80) in vitro for NSCLC lines (H460 and A549) showed that the anticancer properties of nebulised farnesol were essentially the same as those of the native drug (Wang et al., 2003). The cytotoxic effects of doxorubicin before and after encapsulation were compared *in vitro* using growth inhibition assays. Azarmi et al. (2006) studied doxorubicin (DOX)-loaded nanoparticles formulated as a dry powder by spray-freeze-drying. The cytotoxic effects of free DOX, carrier particles containing blank nanoparticles and DOX-loaded nanoparticles were assessed using H460 and A549 lung cancer cells. The DOX-nanoparticles were more cytotoxic for both cell lines a higher than were the blank nanoparticles and the free DOX. The aerosolisation of therapeutic proteins such as anticancer antibodies has also been tested. The results showed that some inhalers are suitable for limiting the formation of aggregates and preserving the pharmacological activity of the antibody *in vitro* (Maillet et al., 2008). Cetuximab, a chimeric IgG1 that targets the epidermal growth factor receptor (EGFR), was tested with three types of nebulisers: jet, mesh and ultrasonic. The immunological and pharmacological properties of nebulised cetuximab were evaluated using A431 cells. Flow cytometric analyses and assays of EGFR-phosphorylation and the inhibitions of A431 cell growth demonstrated that the mesh and jet nebulisers did not destroy the ability of cetuximab to bind to EGFR or its inhibitory activity.

## 4. Airways delivery in preclinical studies

### 4.1 Animal models for aerosol delivery in cancer

#### 4.1.1 Animal model for assessing lung deposition

The structure of the human nasal system is very different from that of all other animals except the non-human primates. The nasal anatomy of primates (human and non-human) is much simpler than that of the majority of animals (Gross et al., 1991.). Rodents cannot breathe through their mouths. Particles must be smaller than 3 µm if they are to reach the airways of rodents (Miller et al., 2000). One way to avoid nasal deposition is to introduce a catheter connected to a high pressure syringe into the trachea to deliver aerosols directly into the lungs. There are two types of tracheo-bronchial anatomy, dichotomous division and monopodial division (McBride et al. 1991). The human respiratory tract is considered to undergo dichotomous branching, while those of rats, mice and dogs are monopodial. This anatomical difference does not seem to influence aerosol deposition in the lungs, but further studies are needed to confirm this. The transition between bronchial airways and the alveolar region is gradual in humans; humans have respiratory bronchioles, while rodents do not (Tyler et al., 1993). Inhaled particles are cleared faster from the alveoli of rodents than from the alveoli of humans because rodents lack bronchioles. However, additional studies are required to determine whether this difference influences the deposition of aerosolised particles in the lungs (Phalen et al., 2008). Total aerosol deposition is better in nasal breathing humans than in oral breathing humans. Upper respiratory tract deposition is similar in nasal breathing humans and in dogs, hamsters, and rabbits. However, pulmonary deposition in nasal breathing humans is comparable to that of dogs and monkeys, but lower than in hamsters and rats. The peak particle size for pulmonary deposition is larger in humans than in dogs, guinea pigs, monkeys, and rats (Phalen et al., 2008)

### 4.1.2 Animal models for anticancer drug studies

#### 4.1.2.1 Chemically induced lung cancer

Several animal models of lung cancer have been developed and used to understand carcinogenesis and test anticancer agents. One of them is chemically-induced lung cancer. These animal models are usually used only to study carcinogenesis and cancer prevention because of the long time required for tumour development and the poor therapeutic response. Newborn A/J mice injected intraperitoneally with ethyl carbamate (urethane) begin to develop benign lung adenomas within few months, followed by degenerate adenocarcinomas similar to those of humans (Shimkin et al., 1975). Some of the many chemical agents that have been tested for their ability to induce lung tumours and study carcinogenesis are benzopyrene, metals, aflatoxin, and constituents of tobacco smoke such as polyaromatic hydrocarbons and nitrosamines (Liu et al., 2002). But chemical models have rarely been used in aerosol studies except for aerosolised chemopreventive treatment.

#### 4.1.2.2 Transgenic lung cancer

Transgenic mouse models of lung adenocarcinoma expressing a mutant active K-ras transgene are available. Jonhson et al. (2001) created a mouse strain (K-ras LA1) carrying an oncogenic allele of K-ras that had an activating codon 12 mutation (gly to asp) on exon 1, that can be activated only on a spontaneous recombination event in the whole animal (Jonhson et al., 2001). This mutation, probably in combination with other somatically acquired mutations, leads to the development of multifocal lung adenocarcinomas in 100% of the mice, skin papillomas in 23%, and thymic lymphomas in 35%. Lung tumours can first be detected microscopically when the mice are 2 weeks old, and the number and size of tumours increase continuously until they essentially fill the thoracic cavity, causing the mouse to die of respiratory failure (mean survival 300 days). Extrathoracic metastases are rare and occur only at a very late stage of the disease, as in humans with adenocarcinoma (Wislez et al., 2003; Jonhson et al., 2001). The radiological appearance is also very similar to the human disease with multifocal lesions such as nodules with ground glass attenuation (Cody et al., 2005). We are presently using this model to analyze the administration of anticancer drugs *via* the airways.

#### 4.1.2.3 Human lung tumour xenografts

Human lung tumour xenografts are widely used in cancer therapeutic studies. Nude mice or SCID immunosuppressed mice are injected intravenously or into the lungs with human tumour cells. Orthotopic models of lung cancer have also been evaluated for aerosol studies. Lung cancer cells, mainly H460 (large cell lung carcinoma) and A549 (bronchioloalveolar lung carcinoma) or disaggregated lung tumours are implanted endotracheally in immunocompromised mice. Orthotopic models are interesting because the tumours grow directly into the lungs, in an environment mimicking that of human lung neoplastic cells. Models of pulmonary metastases have also been used in aerosol studies. For example, LM7 and LM8 osteosarcoma cells were injected intravenously into immunosuppressed mice, leading to the development of lung metastases (Koshkina and Kleinerman, 2005). Lastly, tumours grow better in the lungs than in the subcutaneous compartment. The cell lines most frequently used in animal studies are H460 (large cell lung carcinoma) and A549 (lung carcinoma).

### 4.2 Pharmacokinetics of anticancer agents delivered *via* the airways in animals

#### 4.2.1 Lung deposition

The concentrations in the lungs of anticancer drugs delivered by the pulmonary route are higher than the concentrations delivered by any other route. Cisplatin, one of the major drugs used to treat lung cancers, is administered systemically. Delivery of cisplatin *via* a catheter placed in right caudal lung lobe in dogs provided a concentration in the right caudal lobe that was 44 times higher than in other pulmonary lobes (Selting et al., 2008). The pulmonary delivery of other anticancer drugs that are clinically injected intravenously, but are unconventional for treating non small cell lung cancer, was also tested. The deposition of aerosolised liposomal camptothecin, a quinoline alkaloid, in the lungs was assessed in nude mice with colon, breast or lung tumour xenografts. The concentration of the encapsulated camptothecin in the lung was 100 times higher following airways administration than after intramuscular injection (Koshkina et al., 1999). Similarly, the concentration of aeorosolised 5-Fluorouracile (5-FU) in the lung tissue was 1000 times higher than in the serum of hamsters (Hitzman et al., 2006). High concentrations of 5-FU were detected in the trachea and bronchi of dogs after airways delivery, whereas a lower concentration was measured in the peripheral lung (Tatsumura et al., 1993). We have used near infrared imaging to analyze the distribution of cetuximab, an anti-EGFR antibody, in a xenograft model of lung tumour following systemic and pulmonary delivery, (Maillet et al., in press). The antibody accumulated rapidly and durably in the lungs (Figure 1), and the lung concentration was higher following airways delivery (not shown) (Maillet et al., in press).

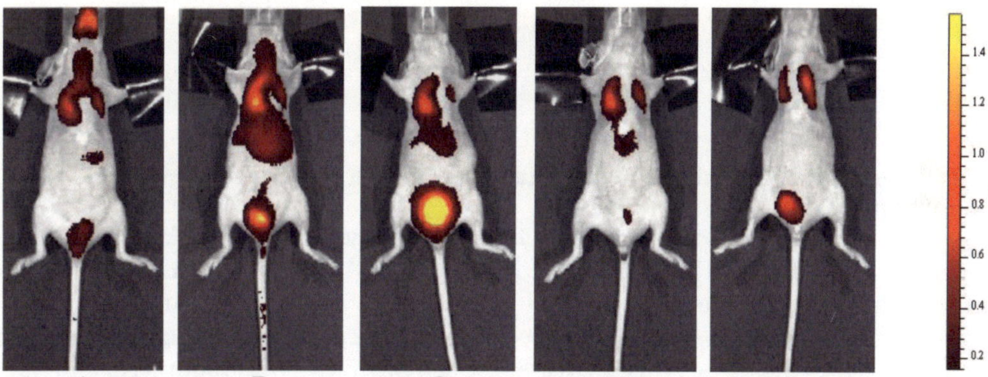


A B C D E

Fig. 1. Lung deposition of inhaled cetuximab at (A) 1h30 (B) 8h (C) 24h (D) 48h and (E) 72h.

#### 4.2.2 Blood passage

Most studies have shown that the concentration of an anticancer drug in the bloodstream is lower after airways delivery than after systemic injection. For example, the concentration of cisplatin in the serum was 15.6 times lower after pulmonary administration than after intravenous (i.v.) injection (Selting et al., 2008). Gemcitabine was given to 3 baboons *via* the airways and its concentration in the blood was 25 times lower than after its systemic delivery (Gagnadoux et al., 2006). Dogs with spontaneous pulmonary metastases were given aerosolized paclitaxel and doxorubicin and the drug concentrations in the bloodstream were measured 1 minute later (Hershey et al., 1999). The serum concentrations were lower than when the drugs were delivered intravenously. However a pharmacokinetic analysis is required to support this conclusion. We have recently determined the pharmacokinetics of cetuximab delivered systemically and *via* the lungs. Little cetuximab was found in the bloodstream after airways delivery (only 11% of the fraction delivered to the lungs) and its passage was slow with a peak around 48 hours (Maillet et al., in press).

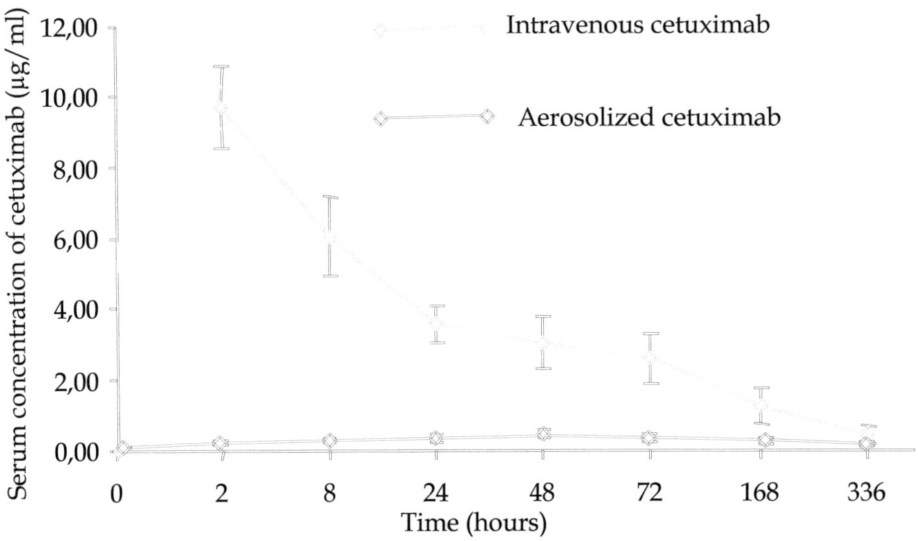


Fig. 2. Serum concentrations of cetuximab delivered systemically or *via* the pulmonary route.

### 4.3 Efficacy and safety of anticancer agents delivered *via* the airways in animals

#### 4.3.1 Cisplatin

Selting and co-workers aerosolised cisplatin directly into the right caudal lobes of healthy dogs (Selting et al., 2008). They found no haematological toxicity and this delivery of aerosolised cisplatin was generally very well tolerated. Radiological and histological analyses indicated that all the dogs developed mild to moderate pneumonitis in the right caudal lobe where the drug was delivered. Chemotherapy with both cisplatin and gemcitabine was also delivered through the pulmonary route in healthy dogs using the same method (Selting et al., 2011). As previously reported, the only adverse event observed was focal pneumonitis in the right caudal lung lobe. Overall, the local-regional delivery of cisplatin either alone or in combination was well tolerated, suggesting that aerosolised platin-based chemotherapy may be used safely to treat humans. However, this method may be difficult to administer to patients with chronic respiratory failure.

#### 4.3.2 Paclitaxel

Dogs with spontaneous primary or secondary lung tumours were given aerosolised paclitaxel using a jet nebuliser (Hershey et al., 1999). One of the 15 dogs had a partial response and one had a complete response with long term survival. The thirteen remaining had stabilised or progressive disease. In another study, mice with pulmonary metastases were given paclitaxel encapsulated in liposomes using a pneumatic nebuliser (Koshkina et al., 2001). There were significantly fewer tumours in the treated mice than in the mice given liposome alone. Survival was improved, with 40% of the mice treated with liposomal paclitaxel being alive after 45 days, whereas all the mice treated with liposome alone were dead. A recent study found that adding vitamin E to the aerosolised liposomal-encapsulated paclitaxel enhanced the anticancer response to paclitaxel in murine model of lung metastases from primary breast cancer (Latimer et al. 2009). Lastly, the feasibility of aerosolising paclitaxel encapsulated in lipid nanoparticles was tested *in vitro*. Preclinical studies in animal models of lung cancer are expected to evaluate whether encapsulation leads to the controlled release of the drug (Hureaux et al., 2009).

#### 4.3.3 Gemcitabine

Gagnadoux et al. evaluated the dose-limiting toxicity of gemcitabine delivered endotracheally to Wistar rats with a sprayer (Gagnadoux et al., 2005). The maximum tolerated dose was 4 mg/kg. They detected no toxicity, except for decreases in platelet and red blood cell counts, when gemcitabine had been inhaled once a week for 9 weeks. They also evaluated the antitumor efficacy of aerosolised gemcitabine in nude mice implanted intrabronchially with H460 cells (Gagnadoux et al., 2005). Of the 13 mice given aerosolised gemcitabine, 4 had no visible tumour at the end of the experiment. And those tumours remaining in the treated mice were smaller (2.05 mm) than those in the control group (5 mm). Aerosolised gemcitabine also significantly reduced tumour numbers in a pulmonary metastases murine model of osteosarcoma (Koshkina et al., 2005). Also, dogs with spontaneous lung metastases of osteosarcoma were treated in a preclinical study with aerosolised gemcitabine combined with a standard treatment regimen (Rodriguez et al., 2010). Almost half (46%) of the treated dogs showed over 50% tumour necrosis, but there was no necrosis in the untreated animals.

#### 4.3.4 Doxorubicine

Hershey et al. treated 18 dogs with spontaneous primary or secondary lung tumours with aerosolised doxorubicine using a jet nebuliser (Hershey et al., 1999). There were 4 partial responses and treatment was well tolerated except for some coughing by half of the subjects, cardiotoxicity in two animals, and mild to moderate pneumonitis in almost all the dogs.

#### 4.3.5 Camptothecin

Aerosolised liposomal 9-nitro-20(S)-camptothecin (L9-NC) was first assessed in mice with xenografts of breast, colon and lung tumours injected subcutaneously (Knight et al., 1999). Treatment started 1 to 4 weeks after tumour implantation and was given 5 days a week. The growth of subcutaneous tumours was 7- fold lower in treated animals with breast cancer than in the controls and 7 to 10-fold lower in the mice with colon cancers. The lung tumour xenografts were also smaller in the mice treated with aerosolised L9-NC than in the controls. The antitumor effect of L9-NC was better when it was delivered through the airways than orally in all the systems. L9-NC was also evaluated in nude mice with lung metastases produced by the i.v. injection of melanoma (B16) or osteosarcoma (LM6) cells (Koshkina et al., 2000). The mice were given aerosolized L9-NC 5 days a week for three weeks. The treated mice with lung metastases of melanoma had statistically smaller (mean diameter 32 mm) tumour foci than the control group (85 mm). Similarly, 10 of the 11 control mice with LM6 lung metastase, had visible tumours, whereas none of 11 treated mice had tumours, suggesting that these tumors were very sensitive to aerosolised L9-NC. Gilbert et al. evaluated the safety of aerosolised L9-NC in healthy dogs. They found no toxicity after treatment with this drug for 5 days a week for 8 weeks (Gilbert et al., 2002).

#### 4.3.6 Temozolomide

Wauthoz and co-workers evaluated aerosolised temozolomide, a recent alkylating agent, in mice with pulmonary metastases obtained by injecting B16 melanoma cells i.v. (Wauthoz et al., 2010). The treatment seemed to be very well tolerated because the maximum tolerated dose was not reached. The antitumor activity of temozolomide was similar whether it was delivered through the airways or intravenously and both routes gave significantly better results than the control group. And three of the mice were long-term survivors. These encouraging results might lead to clinical trials.

#### 4.3.7 Interleukin-2 (IL-2)

IL-2 is a cytokine that induces an antitumor immune response. Anderson et al. evaluated immunotherapy with aerosolised IL-2 using mice with pulmonary metastases of sarcoma (Anderson et al., 1990). The antitumor activity of IL-2 delivered *via* the airways appeared to be better than *via* the other routes tested. Aerosolisation of IL-2 encapsulated in liposomes gave better survival than free IL-2 or liposome alone delivered *via* the same route. Tumour size was reduced by 50% to 85% by aerosolised liposomal IL-2, which was better than the results with free IL-2. This suggested that liposomal IL-2 was better than free IL-2.

The efficacy of airways delivery of free IL-2 and liposomal IL-2 were also compared in healthy dogs (Khanna et al. 1996). There were increases in white cells and effector cells in the broncho-alveolar lavage fluid of dogs treated with liposomal IL-2 but no haematological or clinical toxicity. A preclinical study in which dogs were treated with aerosols of liposomal IL-2 gave spectacular results (Khanna et al., 1997). Aerosolised liposomal IL-2 was used to treat 9 dogs, 7 with pulmonary metastases of a primary osteosarcoma and 2 with primary lung carcinomas. The pulmonary nodules in 2 of the 4 dogs with metastatic pulmonary osteosarcomas were in complete regression. No relapse was observed over 12 and 20 months, respectively. The disease of one of the two dogs with a primary lung carcinoma was stabilized for up to 8 months. Aerosolised IL-2 was widely evaluated in clinical trials to treat pulmonary metastases of renal cell carcinoma but there are few published preclinical studies in animals with IL-2 delivered *via* the pulmonary route. Clinical trials were probably proposed based on results obtained with IL-2 administered i.v. (Rosenberg et al., 1994)

#### 4.3.8 Celecoxib

Celecoxib is a non-steroidal anti-inflammatory drug that inhibits cyclooxygenase 2. Treatment with aerosolised celecoxib was assessed in association with intravenous docetaxel in an orthotopic lung tumour model (A549) (Fulzele et al., 2006). Animals were given aerosolised celecoxib plus i.v docetaxel or oral celecoxib plus i.v. docetaxel, each of the drugs alone or a placebo. The aerosol was produced with a pneumatic nebuliser. Aerosolised celecoxib plus i.v. docetaxel reduced lung tumour volume by 61% compared to the placebo group while oral celecoxib plus i.v. docetaxel reduced it by 54%. Moreover, the combined treatments gave better results than the drugs alone.

#### 4.3.9 Monoclonal antibodies

We have recently evaluated the antitumor activity of aerosolised cetuximab in a xenograft model of lung tumours. Aerosolised cetuximab limited the growth of the lung tumours (Maillet et al., in press). This proof-of-concept study demonstrates that the airways can be suitable for delivering aerosolised monoclonal antibodies to treat lung cancer, but further studies are required to determine whether the pulmonary route really does increase the therapeutic benefit of monoclonal antibodies to patients with lung cancer.

## 5. Airways delivery of anticancer agents in clinical studies

### 5.1 Aerosolisation of anticancer drugs in primary lung cancer

#### 5.1.1 Cisplatin

Cisplatin is the standard drug for treating non small cell lung cancers. It is given combined with another chemotherapeutic agent. Aerosolised cisplatin was assessed in a phase I study on 17 patients with lung cancer, including 16 with non-small-cell-lung cancer and one with small cell lung cancer (Wittgen et al., 2007). The cancers were progressing despite all previous treatment. Increasing doses of cisplatin encapsulated in liposomes were given. Each aerosol treatment was for 20 minutes with a jet nebuliser. The particles produced had a MMAD of about 3 μm. Each patient was given cisplatin on 1 to 4 consecutive days over a period of 21 days. The initial dose was 24 mg/m$^2$, which was doubled to 48 mg/m$^2$ without toxicity. The cycle was then shortened from 3 to 2 weeks, and finally to 1 week. Nebulised cisplatin was administered 3 times a day instead of twice. No dose-limiting toxicity was observed and the maximum tolerated dose was not reached. Dyspnea was reported in 11 patients and a productive and irritating cough in 5. Eosinophilia was observed in 4 of these 11 (36.4%) patients. Cisplatin was detected in the blood of only 4 patients. The disease of 12 of the 17 patients became stable and it progressed in five of them, but the study was not constructed to assess the response to treatment. The dose-limiting toxicity was not reached, precluding a phase II study.

#### 5.1.2 Doxorubicin

##### 5.1.2.1 Safety and pharmacokinetic data

Anthracycline is usually administered intravenously to treat various cancers, including small cell lung cancer. The most severe adverse response is cardiac toxicity. Delivering the drug by inhalation is an interesting alternative route which may limit the cardiac toxicity. A phase I study was conducted by Otterson et al. to assess the safety of inhaled doxorubicin (Otterson et al., 2007). The 53 patients taking part included 16 patients with a primary lung tumour without histology details. The remaining 37 had pulmonary metastases of sarcoma (n=19), osteosarcoma (n=6), colorectal (n=4), thyroid (n=3) and other primary tumours (n=5). They were given doxorubicin with a pneumatic nebuliser fitted with a device that captured any fugitive aerosol to protect health worker. The starting dose was 0.4 mg/m$^2$. Inhalation was given every 3 weeks. The majority of adverse events were pulmonary with cough (n=27), dyspnea (n=9), chest pain (n=5), wheezing (n=4), hoarseness (n=3), hemoptysis (n=1), and bronchospasm (n = 1). While 5 patients suffered grade 3-4 pulmonary toxicity such as hypoxemia or decreased lung function tests, it was difficult to differentiate the adverse effects of treatment and the consequences of the pulmonary disease. Two patients suffered severe toxicity in response to a dose of 9.4 mg/m$^2$, with respiratory distress in 1 patient and bilateral ground glass infiltrates in the other. The lung function tests of the whole population were relatively stable and there was little non-pulmonary toxicity. There was no evidence of hematological toxicity. The authors concluded that the recommended dose for a phase II study is 7.5 mg/m². The maximal concentration ($C_{max}$) of doxorubicin in the blood was low when the dose was less than 3 mg/m². $C_{max}$ increased 1.6 times with doses of 3.8 - 7.5 mg/m². $C_{max}$ was more than doubled with doses of from 7.5 to 9.4 mg/m². The maximal doxorubicin peak in the blood occurred within 5 minutes. This was due to its rapid passage through the alveolar-capillary barrier because doxorubicin is small and lipophilic.

One patient with spindle cell sarcoma gave a partial response, while the diseases of 8 patients were stable after 5 courses: 2 with bronchoalveolar carcinoma, 2 with soft tissue sarcoma, 1 with endometrial carcinoma, and 3 with thyroid cancer. The diseases of 6 patients became stable after three courses. Two patients stopped treatment after first administration. The diseases of the remaining patients progressed.

Very little inhaled doxorubicin enters the blood and probably has little systemic toxicity. It is difficult to come to any conclusion about treatment efficacy because the study was not constructed to do so, and the histological subtypes of cancers varied greatly. However, the stabilized bronchioalveolar carcinoma cases suggest that this histological pattern might be suitable for inhalation treatment with doxorubicin.

#### 5.1.2.2 Efficacy data

Inhaled doxorubicin associated with systemic cisplatin and docetaxel at 75 mg/m² was tested in a phase I/II study on chemo-naive patients with advanced NSCLC (Otterson et al., 2010). Among the 36 patients included in the study, 28 were given dose 1 (6 mg/m²) and 8 were given dose 2 (7.5 mg/m²). The diffusing capacity of the lung for carbon monoxide (DLCO) of two of the patients given 7.5 mg/m² decreased and the recommended dose for the phase II study was 6 mg/m². The 34 patients in the phase II study, included 16 (47.1%) with adenocarcinoma, 5 (14.7%) with squamous cell carcinoma, 1 (2.9%), with large cell carcinoma, 11 (32.4%) with unspecified histology and 1 (2.9%) with a mixed tumour (squamous and adenocarcinoma). The patients were given 1 to 8 treatment cycles. Seven patients were given only one cycle and left the study because their disease progressed (n=3), adverse event (n=2), withdrawal of consent (n=1) or the physician's decision (n=1). There was little pulmonary toxicity except that the lung function of 5 patients decreased, but they did not stop their treatment. Among patients, 24 were evaluable, including 6 (25%) with a partial response and 1 (4%) with a complete response. The remaining 17 patients included 13 (54%) whose disease was stable and 4 (17%) whose disease progressed. Response rate was poorer than expected by the authors (at least 9 responding patients). The median overall survival time was 14.4 months for those given the level 1 dose and 19.5 months for those given the level 2 dose with no statistical difference. The median overall survival time was longer than is usually observed in clinical trials of lung cancer treatment. This discrepancy may be due to bias associated with the selection of the patients or because inhaled doxorubicin plus platinum chemotherapy really had some effect. A phase III study is expected to determine which of these hypotheses is correct.

### 5.1.3 Campthotecin

Vershraegen et al. examined the feasibility of using aerosolised liposomal 9-nitro-20(S)-camptothecin (L9-NC) (Verschraegen et al., 2000). They treated 6 patients with primary or secondary lung tumours who had not responded to previous treatment with L9-NC for 5

days a week every 3 weeks. The histology of the lung tumours was not specified, neither were any details about the nebulisation procedure given, except that an air flow of 10 liters per minute was used to generate the aerosol. No toxicity up to grade 2 was observed. The maximum drug concentration was seen 2 hours at the end of the aerosolisation, which rapidly decreased. The disease of two patients stabilized.
The same group then carried out a phase I study with nebulised L9-NC to determine the dose-limiting toxicity (Verschraegen et al., 2004). L9-NC was aerosolised with a pneumatic nebuliser with an air flow of 10 liters per minute and a mouth breathing-only face mask. Patients were treated for 5 days a week as above. The dose was increased by reducing the interval between treatments or increasing the concentration of L9-NC. The patients were premedicated with an inhaled bronchodilatator and steroids after one of them developed a grade 2 bronchial irritation. The starting dose was 6.7 µg/kg. All 25 patients completed the protocol except one who could not undergo nebulisation because of claustrophobia. The 26.6 µg/kg dose was poorly tolerated, with pharyngeal mucositis. The 20.0 µg/kg dose 2 patients to develop grade 3 asthenia but the 13.3 µg/kg treatment was well tolerated. There were mild side effects, such as a cough in 67% of patients, bronchial irritation in 46%, sore throat in 33%, nausea in 62%, vomiting in 33%, fatigue in 50%, anemia and neutropenia in 29%, and skin rash around the face mask in 21%. There was a 20% decrease in FEV1 during treatment which rapidly returned to baseline. Other lung function parameters were stable. The blood plasma L9-NC concentration peaked 2 hours after nebulisation, which was followed by a sustained decrease. The blood concentrations were similar to those obtained after oral administration, without any haematological toxicity. The responses to treatment were reported, but a phase I study is not designed to do so. Two patients had a partial remission, with endometrial carcinoma metastatic to the lungs only, but they suffered a relapse within 8 and 3 years respectively. One of these patients had a partial response of hepatic metastasis. The disease of the patients with lung tumours (3 of 6) was stabilized. Thus, nebulised L9-NC seems to be promising for treating pulmonary metastases rather than primary lung tumours. The recommended phase II study dose was 13.3 µg/kg 5 days a week every week.

#### 5.1.4 5-Fluorouracile

Tastumura et al. were the first to report chemotherapeutic nebulisation for cancer patients (Tatsumura et al., 1983). They treated six patients with lung cancer with 5-FU aerosolised with an ultrasonic nebuliser. Two of them had complete responses and two others partial responses. Only traces of 5-FU were detected in the blood. These encouraging results led to another clinical trial to assess nebulised 5-FU for treating primary lung tumour patients (Tatsumura et al., 1993). A first group of 19 patients with resectable lung cancer was given nebulised 5-FU, 2 hours before surgery to determine the 5-FU concentrations in excised lung tissue. The 5-FU concentration in the tumour tissue was 5-15 times higher than in the normal lung tissue ($p<0.05$). The 5-FU concentrations were higher in proximal tissue and regional lymph nodes than in the remaining tissue. No drug was detected in blood samples. A second group of ten patients with unresectable lung cancer (6 squamous cell carcinomas and 4 adenocarcinomas) were given inhaled 5-FU twice a day for 3 days per week to evaluate their response to treatment. Of these, 6 had objective responses, including two complete responses and four partial responses. The disease of the remaining four patients was unchanged and 3 of them died of their disease. No toxicity was detected. Despite these promising results, no clinical trial to assess the efficacy of inhaled 5-FU has been published, probably because i.v. injected 5-FU is not indicated for treating lung cancer.

### 5.1.5 Non-steroidal anti-inflammatory drugs

To the best of our knowledge, no clinical trial has assessed the efficacy of inhaled non-steroidal anti-inflammatory drugs for treating cancer patients, although aerosolised celecoxib plus i.v. chemotherapeutic agents showed good results in preclinical studies.

## 5.2 Aerosolisation of anticancer drugs in pulmonary metastases

### 5.2.1 Interleukin-2

The characteristics of clinical trials of inhaled interleukin-2 are summarized in Table 1.
Interleukin-2 (Il-2) was initially administered intravenously to treat patients with melanomas and renal cell carcinoma with some good results (Rosenberg et al., 1994). However, severe toxicity limits its intravenous administration (Mitani et al., 1992). It was logical, therefore, to evaluate IL-2 delivered *via* the airways. It was the first drug delivered *via* this route to be tested in a clinical trial for treating lung metastases (Huland et al., 1994). Patients with pulmonary metastases of renal-cell carcinoma were given IL-2 together with low doses of IL-2 injected subcutaneously (10% of total IL-2 dose) and systemic subcutaneous interferon alpha (IFN alpha). Toxicity was low, grade II toxicity occurred in only one patient who suffered bronchospasms. The pulmonary metastases did not increase during treatment. One of the 15 patients treated showed a complete response, 8 had partial responses, and the lung disease of 6 was stable. Surprisingly, 3 of 7 patients had partial responses of non-pulmonary metastases and one was stabilized. The mean survival time was 19.1 months, whereas the mean survival time of patients with renal carcinoma metastases is usually 9.9 months.
Inhaled natural IL-2 alone was also assessed in a phase I study on 16 patients, including 14 with pulmonary metastases of renal cell carcinomas and 2 non small cell lung cancers (Lorenz et al., 1996). Treatment was initially delivered once a day and progressively increased to reach 5 times a day over 43 days. Aerosol particles had an MMAD of about 2.3 μm. Treatment was relatively safe. Coughs were one of the most common adverse side effects and one patient fractured a rib, but no systemic toxicity was reported. The effect on lung function was mild to moderate. IL-2 was not detected in the blood with the low dose, but increased within 2 to 6 hours with the high dose. The pulmonary metastases of 3 patients went into complete regression, but 2 of them died from non-pulmonary metastases.
The safety and efficacy of inhaled IL-2 was evaluated in a study on 7 patients with pulmonary metastases of renal carcinomas (Nakamoto et al., 1997). The drug was aerosolised with an ultrasonic nebuliser and delivered over 10 minutes for 5 days a week. Treatment was associated with subcutaneous injections of interferon alpha. One patient stopped the treatment before three months because his overall health deteriorated. The disease of two of the remaining 6 became stable, 3 had partial responses and the disease of one patient with cystic renal disease progressed. One patient developed severe toxicity, pulmonary fibrosis appearing within 4 months and treatment was stopped. His metastases grew dramatically and he died 6 months after treatment cessation.
The safety of inhaled IL-2 led Huland et al. to perform a clinical trial on a large cohort (Huland et al., 1999a). The 116 patients with pulmonary metastases of renal carcinoma included this 6-year study were given high doses of aerosolised IL-2, either alone (11%),

with a low dose given subcutaneously IL-2 (33%), or with low-dose systemic IL-2 and interferon-alpha (56%). The overall response rate was 16% for IL-2 alone, 49% for IL-2 plus subcutaneous (s.c.) IL-2, and 35% for IL-2 plus s.c. IL-2 and interferon. The median overall response was 9.6 months. The pulmonary metastases of 15% of patients progressed and those of 55% were stabilized. The authors identified risk factors of poor response in patients treated with inhaled IL-2 (Huland et al., 1999b). Of the 116 patients given inhaled IL-2 (natural or recombinant), 86 had a poor response and at least one of the following risk factors: 1 metastatic location (86%), interval between diagnosis and treatment of <12 months (62%), weight loss prior to therapy (41%), and ECOG (Eastern Cooperative Oncology Group) performance status ≥2 (13%). However, the response rate, including long-term stabilization, was 27 to 57% in patients with these risk factors. Inhaled IL-2 should be proposed for all renal cancer patients with pulmonary metastases. However, patient with multiple nodules and who are tired may have reduced lung deposition of inhaled treatment. Another clinical trial was conducted on 40 patients with progressive pulmonary metastases of a renal cell carcinoma. They were treated with inhaled IL-2 3 times a day for a total dose of 18 million units (MU) plus a low dose of systemic IL-2 (Merimsky et al., 2004). The dose was reduced for one patient because of a cough and dyspnea. The dose was increased to 36 MU for seven patients whose disease progressed. The response rate was poorer than in previous studies supervised by Huland et al. Only one of the 40 patients had a partial response, but the disease of 22 patients was stabilized. The median time to progression was 8.7 months. Toxicity was low including cough, weakness, dyspnea, fever and abdominal pain. The efficacy and safety of inhaled IL-2 were also assessed in a retrospective study on 51 patients with pulmonary metastases of renal cell carcinoma (Esteban-González et al., 2007). The patients were given 3 cycles of 36 MU per day for 5 days per week for 12 weeks. Toxicity was low, always grade 1 or 2. Cough and fatigue were the most common problems. The overall objective response rate was 13.7%. The median progression-free survival time was 8.6 months and the overall survival time was 23 months. Inhaled IL-2 seemed to have an effect but it was not compared to a control group. A retrospective study compared 94 patients with metastases of renal carcinoma treated with inhaled IL-2 to 103 patients treated with systemic IL-2 (Huland et al., 2003). The toxicity in the two groups was radically different. Cough was observed in the inhaled IL-2 group and fever, fatigue, skin lesion in systemic IL-2 group. The 1-, 2- and 3-year survival rates were estimated to be 47%, 28% and 23% for inhaled IL-2 and 26%, 10% and 1% for the systemic IL-2 group. The hazard ratio for inhaled IL-2 was 0.435. The death risk of patients treated with inhaled IL-2 was decreased by 44%.

The largest clinical trial with a drug delivered *via* the pulmonary route to treat lung cancer was the study conducting by Atzpodien et al. (Atzpodien et al., 2006). The 379 patients with metastases of renal cell carcinoma were randomly assigned to group I (143 patients) or group II (236 patients). The group I patients in arm A were given subcutaneous IL-2, subcutaneous interferon-α plus 13-cis-retinoic acid; those in arm B were given the same treatment as arm A plus inhaled IL-2. The patients in group II were assigned to arm C (arm A plus intraveinous 5-FU) or arm D (arm A plus oral capecitabine). The 13-cis-retinoic acid used in this study is a regulator of cell differentiation that has been reported to enhance the antitumor effect of IL-2/IFN-α on renal cell carcinoma metastases (Atzpodien et al, 1995). Patients with pulmonary metastases were preferentially assigned to group I. Arm B patients were given systemic IL-2 and IFN-α plus inhaled IL-2 on days 1 to 5 of weeks 2 and 3 and

| | Drugs | Patients | Toxicity | Response rate | Outcome |
|---|---|---|---|---|---|
| **Huland et al. 1994** | Inhaled IL2 + low dose systemic IL-2 + systemic IFN | 15 patients with RCC | Grade 2 (7%)<br>Bronchospasm in 1 patient | 1 CR<br>8 PR<br>6 SD | OS= 19,1 months |
| **Lorenz et al. 1996** | Inhaled IL-2 alone | 14 patients with RCC<br>2 patients with NSCLC | Cough<br>Mild to moderate decrement of lung function | 1 CR<br>1 PR<br>6 SD | NA |
| **Nakamoto et al. 1997** | Inhaled IL-2 and s.c. IFN | 7 patients with RCC | 1 patient with pulmonary fibrosis | 3 PR<br>2 SD | NA |
| **Huland et al. 1999** | Inhaled IL-2 either alone or with low dose s.c. IL-2 or with low-dose s.c. IL-2 and IFN | 116 patients with RCC | Grade 3 (16%) | CR/PR/SD:<br>-16% IL-2<br>-49% with inhaled and s.c. IL-2<br>-35% with tritherapy | PFS= 9.6 months<br><br>OS= 11.8 months |
| **Huland et al. 2003** | Inhaled IL-2 vs systemic IL-2 | 94 patients with inhaled IL-2 and 103 patients with systemic IL-2 | cough | CR/PR/SD:<br>-45% inhaled IL-2<br>-35% systemic IL-2 | Inhaled IL-2<br>1-year survival : 47%<br>2- year survival: 28%<br>3-year survival: 23%<br>Systemic IL-2<br>1-year survival : 26%<br>2- year survival: 10%<br>3-year survival: 1% |
| **Merimsky et al. 2003** | Inhaled IL-2 and low dose systemic IL-2 | 40 patients with RCC | cough, weakness, dyspnea, fever and abdominal pain | 1 PR<br>22 SD | PFS=8.7 months |
| **Atzpodien et al. 2006** | Arm A : and systemic IL-2 and 13-cis-retinoic acid<br>Arm B: Arm A and Inhaled IL-2 | 379 patients with RCC | Equal toxicity for each arm (more than 5% of grade III/IV toxicity). No respiratory toxicity was reported in arm B | Arm A:<br>12% CR<br>19% PR<br>26% SD<br>Arm B:<br>10% CR<br>19% PR<br>36% SD | Arm A : PFS=5 months<br>OS= 22 months<br>Arm B : PFS= 4 months<br>OS= 18 months |
| **Esteban-González et al. 2007** | Inhaled IL-2 | 51 patients with RCC | Grade 1 and 2 exclusively | CR/PR/SD:<br>13.7% | PFS=8.6 months<br>OS=23 months |

Table 1. Main characteristics of clinical trials assessing inhaled interleukin-2. PFS: progression-free survival, OS: overall survival, CR: complete response, PR: partial response, SD: stable disease.

weeks 5 to 8 with a pneumatic nebuliser producing 3 µm particles. A cycle was considered to be 8 weeks and patients were given 3 courses. Sixty patients (15.8%) (arm A: 14%; arm B: 9.2%; arm C: 21.6%; arm D: 15%) did not complete treatment due to disease progression before the first evaluation (2.9%), intolerance (8.7%), death during therapy (1.6%), patients' wish (2.1%), and non-compliance (0.5%). The endpoints were overall survival, progression-free survival and objective response to treatment. In arm A, 8 patients (10%) had a complete response and 15 patients (19%) had a partial response, 28 (36%) had stable disease and the disease of 27 (35%) progressed despite treatment. The overall objective response rate was 29% (95% CI 19, 40). In arm B, 8 patients (12%) had a complete response, 12 (19%) a partial response, 17 (26%) had stable disease, and the disease of 28 (43%) progressed. The overall objective response rate was 31% (95% CI 20, 44). The patients in arms C and D had similar results. Progression-free survival was 5 months in arm A, 4 months in arm B, 0 month in arm C and 4 months in arm D with no statistical difference between them. The overall survival time was 22 months in arm A, 18 months in arm B, 18 months in arm C, and 16 months in arm D with no statistical difference. All four treatments were moderately well tolerated with equal toxicity for each arm (more than 5% of grade III/IV toxicity). No respiratory toxicity was reported in arm B with inhaled IL-2. The treatment based on s.c. IL-2, s.c. IFN and oral 13-cis-retinoic acid was probably too toxic for the advantages of inhaled IL-2 to be detected. Clinical trials associating an oral tyrosine kinase inhibitor like sorafenib with inhaled IL-2 might be interesting. A study on 10 patients reported asthma in response to inhaled IL-2 (Loppow et al., 2007), but only one patient had to stop treatment.

Skubitz et al. demonstrated that interleukin-2 encapsulated in liposomes could be delivered by aerosol to patients with pulmonary metastases (Skubitz et al., 2000). They gave 9 patients liposomes containing IL-2 or placebo with a jet nebuliser and a standard compressor. The IL-2 treatment was inhaled for about 20 minutes 3 times a day. No significant toxicity was observed and inhalation was well tolerated. Further studies are expected. However, it is hard to see the clinical advantage of inhaled liposomal IL-2 considering the impressive results of the free form, unless it could improve IL-2 resident time in the airways, so reducing the number of treatments.

### 5.2.2 Monoclonal antibodies and tyrosine kinase inhibitor

To the best of our knowledge, no clinical trials have tested inhaled antibodies or tyrosine kinase inhibitors for treating lung cancer patients.

### 5.2.3 Granulocyte Macrophage Colony Stimulating Factor (GM-CSF)

GM-CSF was first assessed in a dose escalation study on 7 patients with pulmonary metastases (2 patients with osteosarcoma, 2 with melanoma, 1 with leiomyosarcoma, 1 with renal cell carcinoma and 1 with Ewing's sarcoma) (Anderson et al., 1999). They were given GM-CSF aerosolised with a pneumatic nebuliser. One was not treated due to rapid disease progression. The remaining 6 patients were given the drug twice a day for one week, and treatment was stopped for one week. The starting dose was 60 µg. The dose was increased to determine dose-limiting toxicity. Those given the high dose showed a minor increase in their white blood cell count that was not statistically different from their white blood cell count before treatment. Lung function was stable except in one patient with osteosarcoma whose FVC increased. No toxicity was described. Although it was a dose escalation study, treatment response was reported. Of the six patients who completed study, the disease of 4 stabilized for 9 months, 1 had a partial response and 1 had a complete response (patient with Ewing's sarcoma). The authors suggest that the low GM-CSF concentration into the bloodstream after airways delivery may be attributed to GM-CSF sequestration into the lungs by immune effectors. This therapy was given to 45 other patients (40 with pulmonary metastases) to better evaluate the toxicity of inhaled GM-CSF (Rao et al., 2003). They were given nebulised GM-CSF (250 µg) twice a day for 1 week followed by a 1 week rest. Moderate toxicity was observed in 18 patients. The disease of 24 patients was stabilized or partially responded (8 of 13 with a sarcoma, 6 of 14 with melanoma, and 5 of 12 with renal cell carcinoma). The efficacy of aerosolised GM-CSF might be due to stimulation of an antitumor immune response because one patient with pulmonary metastases of melanoma had a 10-fold increase in specific cytotoxic T lymphocytes resulting in a partial response. The authors suggested that there was a dose-dependent response to the treatment and conducted a third dose escalation study with doses higher than in previous trials (Markovic et al., 2008). Only patients with pulmonary metastases of melanomas were included because the authors postulated that there could be an antitumor auto-immunization against the melanoma, as suggested by increase in melanoma-specific lymphocyte T in previous study. Aerosolised GM-CSF was delivered with a pneumatic nebuliser twice daily on days 1 to 7 and 15 to 21 in a 28-day cycle. Doses ranged from 500 to 2000 µg. The author considered aerosolised GM-CSF to be well tolerated.because only 3 of the 40 patients had severe toxicity, including grade 4 dyspnea in 1 patient given 2000 µg and 1 patient given 1750 µg, and grade 3 fatigue in 1 patient given 1000 µg. There were increases in melanoma-specific cytotoxic T lymphocytes in 9 patients (1 given 500 µg, 1 given 750 µg, 2 given 1500 µg, 1 given 1750 µg, and 4 given 2000 µg). Although the data are descriptive, the authors reported that one patient on 2000 µg had a partial response and the disease of 6 became stable. None of the GM-CSF doses used induced antitumor immunity in the majority of patients. Further studies are needed to determine the extent of the antitumor immunity induced by aersosolised GM-CSF in melanoma. A recent clinical trial treated 43 adults and children with lung relapses of osteosarcoma with inhaled GM-CSF. They were given 2 cycles of inhaled GM-CSF, then the tumour nodules were surgically removed. The patients were then given 12 cycles of inhaled GM-CSF (Arndt et al., 2010). Treatment was given 5 days per week every 2 weeks and the dose range was from 250 µg to 1750 µg. The Fas and Fas ligand were assayed in the removed nodules to assess the immunomodulatory effect of GM-CSF. Nine patients had grade 3 respiratory toxicity, including 5 patients on 1750 µg. Thirty seven patients suffered relapses. The median free survival time was 4.3 months and the overall survival rates were 63.1% at 2 years and 35.4% at 3 years. GM-CSF was found to have no immunomodulatory effect, and this potential property of GM-CSF remains controversial.

### 5.3 Aerosols in palliative cancer care

Breathlessness is a serious problem for cancer patients in palliative care because of the discomfort it causes. Drugs are usually given systemically to relieve this discomfort, but this is invasive and often requires hospitalization.

#### 5.3.1 Morphine and other opiod analgesics

The opiate analgesic morphine is widely used and is given orally, intravenously or subcutaneously to cancer patients to relieve pain. The effect of morphine on breathlessness was suggested more than 20 years ago (Bruera et al. 1990) and reported in a systematic review in 2002 (Jennings et al., 2002). Delivering morphine *via* the pulmonary route might decrease breathlessness because there are morphine receptors in the lungs. The safety and pharmacology of aerosolised-morphine have been evaluated in cancer patients with dyspnea.

#### 5.3.1.1 Safety

A safety trial conducted on 50 cancer patients with dyspnea revealed no major adverse reactions, such as respiratory distress or vomiting (Tanaka et al., 1999). The 20 mg dose of morphine was delivered with an ultrasonic nebuliser. Dyspnea was measured using a visual analog scale based on the subjective quantification of breathlessness by the patient. Nebulised morphine produced a significant 10% decrease in dyspnea.

#### 5.3.1.2 Pharmacokinetics

Morphine 6 glycuronide (M6G) is an active metabolite of morphine. The pharmacokinetics of inhaled M6G were analysed on 10 healthy volunteers (Penson et al., 2002). M6G was delivered as an intravenous bolus (2 mg), subcutaneously (2 mg) or by inhalation (4 mg). The bioavailability of M6G was 102% after s.c. delivery and 6% after airways delivery compared to intravenous route. The peak of M6G in the blood appeared from 30 minutes to 2 h after s.c. delivery and from 1.2 to 8 hours after airways delivery. A previous study found that the bioavailability of nebulised morphine was 17%, suggesting that little passed into the blood (Chrubasik et al., 1988). A recent study by Krajnik et al. compared two methods of morphine nebulisation (Krajnik et al, 2009). Morphine, at a dose of 5 mg, was given to 10 breathless cancer patients with a nebuliser producing 2-5 μm or 0.5-2 μm particle droplets. The nebuliser producing the larger particles resulted in more metabolite being released into the blood, but a longer procedure was needed to deliver the 5 mg dose and the maximum plasma concentration of the metabolite occurred later. No toxicity was observed. A clinical trial comparing the efficacy of the two devices is required.
The published pharmacokinetic studies on morphine and its metabolite suggest that little passes into the blood.

#### 5.3.1.3 Efficacy

5.3.1.3.1 Uncontrolled trials

The safety profile and poor passage into the blood led to clinical trials to analyse the efficacy of inhaled morphine. Quigley el al. treated 9 cancer patients suffering from breathlessness with M6G in a phase I/II study (Quigley et al., 2002). They were given a single dose of 5 mg, 10 mg, or 20 mg M6G. Treatment was well tolerated. Pharmacokinetic analysis showed a blood peak at 2 hours for all doses with a blood concentration proportional to the dose. The patient status based on visual analog scale of breathlessness and dyspnea (Borg score) was significantly improved, with no difference between doses. The inhalation of a derivative of morphine, hydromorphone, was also evaluated in cancer patients (Coyne et al., 2002). These 32 breathless patients inhaled hydromorphone and were assessed at baseline, 5 minutes and 60 minutes after nebulisation. The patients assessed their change as the same, worse, or improved. Most of them (26; 81%) reported improved breathing and 6 (9%) found no change. Oxygen saturation was improved from 94.6% at baseline to 96.8% at 5 minutes and 96.7% at 60 minutes.

5.3.1.3.2 Controlled trials

The above results should be interpreted with caution because there was no control group (aerosolised placebo or i.v. opioids). A few years ago we performed a trial with inhaled

morphine (20 mg) or normal saline in 10 cancer patients (Grimbert et al., 2004). The patients were given both treatments over 48 hours, separated by a wash-out period. Dyspnea, respiratory rate and oxygen saturation were assessed on a visual analog scale before and after treatment. The scores improved after both treatments, but respiratory rate and oxygen saturation did not change, indicating no specific drug response. We postulated that the improved comfort was due to a nebulisation-dependent humidification of the airways or a placebo response. Our results differ from those of Coyne et al., who described an improved perception of breathing, respiratory rate and oxygen saturation following treatment with nebulised fentanyl citrate (Coyne et al., 2002). This difference may be due to a great variation in the oxygen saturation measured and the subjective dyspnea measurement.
Bruera et al. compared the effects of nebulised morphine and subcutaneous morphine on 11 cancer patients suffering from breathlessness (Bruera et al., 2005). On day 1 they were given nebulised morphine plus a subcutaneous placebo, or nebulised placebo plus subcutaneous morphine. The treatments were reversed on day 2. Both treatments were very well tolerated. The score of the group given morphine subcutaneously decreased significantly from 5 to 3 on a visual analog scale, and that of the nebulised drug group decreased from 4 to 2. However, only 11 patients were studied and the visual analog scale fluctuated during the subcutaneous morphine treatment. A more recent study compared the effects of nebulised hydromorphone, intravenous hydromorphone, and nebulised normal saline on twenty patients (Charles et al., 2008). Patients needing treatment for breathlessness were randomly given 5 mg of nebulised hydromorphone, a systemic breakthrough dose of hydromorphone, or 3 ml of nebulised saline on three different occasions. A placebo given by another route was administrated. The primary goal of a decrease in the visual analog scale within 10 minutes was not reached. There were significant decreases over a longer period but no difference between treatments.
Thus, these studies with a placebo control group have not demonstrated any difference between nebulised opioid and placebo. However both treatments seemed to significantly improve the patients' perception of breathing, which may be attributed to a placebo effect or improved airway humidity.

### 5.3.2 Furosemide

Inhaled furosemide was used with some success to treat breathlessness asthma patients and healthy volunteers whose breathlessness was induced (Bianco et al., 1989, Nishino et al., 2000).
This finding led to inhaled furosemide being evaluated in cancer patients. A group of three cancer patients reported improved dyspnea when given nebulised furosemide (20 mg) (Shimoyama et al., 2002). Nebulisation of a bronchodilator before giving inhaled furosemide had no effect and the authors excluded a placebo effect. A study on 15 cancer patients suffering from breathlessness assessed the effect of ultrasonically nebulised furosemide (20 mg) (Kohara et al., 2003). Cancer dyspnea was measured with a brief self-rating scale of 12 items. Most patients (n=12; 80%) reported significant improvements in their cancer dyspnea and anxiety. Their heart rates, respiratory rates and oxygen saturation were not improved. The improved dyspnea might have been due to a placebo effect or improved airway humidity, as observed in inhaled morphine studies. A controlled trial on 7 cancer patients treated with inhaled normal saline or furosemide (20 mg) found that the scores of the visual analog scale were better after saline than after furosemide, but without statistical

significance (Stone et al., 2002). Another study that included placebo group confirmed that inhaled furosemide had little effect on the breathlessness of 15 cancer patients (Wilcock et al., 2008). They assessed the patients' perception of breathing before and 60 minutes after treatment; they found no improvement in either group. There were small decreases in FEV1 and vital capacity after nebulised normal saline but not after nebulised furosemide.

### 5.4 Chemoprevention of lung cancer by aerosolisation

The chemoprevention of lung cancer with aerosolised drugs was first tested in animals. Budesonide, an inhaled steroid, inhibited the formation of lung tumour by over 80% (Wattenberg et al., 1997). Squamous cell carcinoma in hamsters was reduced by 50% with inhaled difluoromethylornitine and 60% with and inhaled 5-FU (Wattenberg et al., 2004).

The results of clinical trials of the chemopreventive effects of inhaled steroid have been equivocal. Lam et al. suggested that budesonide had no effect on bronchial dysplastic lesions and did not prevent new lesions forming in 112 smokers (Lam et al., 2004). In contrast, fluticasone delivered by aerosol gave promising results, with significantly fewer treated patients with increasing numbers of nodules than in the placebo group (Van den Berg et al., 2008). A clinical trial in which 11 subjects with lung metaplasia or dysplasia were given aerosolized vitamin A found complete or partial responses in 56% of cases (Kohlhäufl et al., 2002)

Further studies are needed to determine whether inhaled steroid and vitamin A really do have chemopreventive effects.

Others aerosolised agents such as pioglitazone (an antidiabetic agent), polyphenons E (a mixture of polyphenons) and bexarotene (a retinoid X receptor (RXR) agonist) had promising results in animal studies (Fu et al. 2009, 2011, Yan et al., 2007, Zhang et al. 2011).

## 6. Perspectives and conclusion

Most of the preclinical studies have shown that aerosolisation preserves anti-cancer properties of a large amount of agents. Administration through the pulmonary route of anticancer drugs is well tolerated in animal models. Lung deposition is better following airways than systemic delivery. Moreover, blood passage is often lower when anti-cancer agents are administered through the airways. To date, the clinical studies of inhaled anticancer agents such as cisplatin, campthotecin, 5-fluoro-uracile, have demonstrated the safety and the pharmacokinetic advantages of airways administration in cancer patients. Moreover, antitumor responses have been observed including complete remission with inhaled interleukin-2 in renal cell carcinoma patients or with inhaled doxorubicin in lung cancer patients. However, studies were constructed with a small number of patients, the histological patterns were mostly heterogeneous with primary and secondary lung tumour mixed in the same trial and different devices or dosage were used to evaluate response to the same agent. Thus, it is difficult to bring conclusions on the real efficacy of anti-cancer agents administered through the airways, but significant effects are obvious. Despite promising results of inhaled anticancer drugs, the aerosol delivery of opioid or furosemide in palliative cancer patients was not convincing. Chemoprevention of lung cancer with inhaled agents is interesting, but further studies are needed to validate this approach.

It would be valuable to systematically integrate aerosol metrology and pharmacokinetic analysis with preclinical studies in order to improve drug deposition at the target site in the respiratory tract, and define the formulation that enables drugs to be retained in the lungs.

Standardisation of administration procedures should be considered to enhance homogeneity of clinical studies. Data on drug deposition is essential to make comparison between patients and drug pharmacokinetics and would be informative in future clinical trials. As reported, combined administration of an inhaled anti-cancer agent with drugs administered intravenously may be relevant to enhance the anticancer effect. It may also be interesting to consider the association of several anticancer agents delivered through the pulmonary route. Selting et al. simultaneously delivered in healthy dogs, aerosolised cisplatin and gemcitabine *via* a catheter in right caudal lung lobe without clinical toxicity (Selting et al., 2011). Along with conventional agent, biotherapeutics such as IL-2 and GM-CSF were assessed with promising preclinical and clinical results. Airways may also be suited for the local delivery of other biologics, such as monoclonal antibodies (Maillet et al. in press). But, researchers now need to evaluate the relative benefits of drug delivery by the airways and the systemic route before aerosolised anticancer agents can become a clinical reality in oncology.

## 7. Acknowledgements

The English text was edited by Dr Owen Parkes.

## 8. References

Allen, S. (2008). Are inhaled systemic therapies a viable option for the treatment of the elderly patient? *Drugs Aging,* Vol. 25, No. 2, pp. 89-94, ISSN 1170-229X

Anderson, M., Svartengren, M., Bylin, G., Philipson, K. & Camner, P. (1993). Deposition in asthmatics of particles inhaled in air or in helium-oxygen. *Am Rev Respir Dis,* Vol. 147, No. 3, (Mar), pp. 524-8, ISSN 0003-0805

Anderson, P.M., Katsanis, E., Leonard, A.S., Schow, D., Loeffler, C.M., Goldstein, M.B. & Ochoa, A.C. (1990). Increased local antitumor effects of interleukin 2 liposomes in mice with MCA-106 sarcoma pulmonary metastases. *Cancer Res,* Vol. 50, No. 6, (Mar 15), pp. 1853-6, ISSN 0008-5472

Anderson, P.M., Markovic, S.N., Sloan, J.A., Clawson, M.L., Wylam, M., Arndt, C.A., Smithson, W.A., Burch, P., Gornet, M. & Rahman, E. (1999). Aerosol granulocyte macrophage-colony stimulating factor: a low toxicity, lung-specific biological therapy in patients with lung metastases. *Clin Cancer Res,* Vol. 5, No. 9, (Sep), pp. 2316-23, ISSN 1078-0432

Arndt, C.A., Koshkina, N.V., Inwards, C.Y., Hawkins, D.S., Krailo, M.D., Villaluna, D., Anderson, P.M., Goorin, A.M., Blakely, M.L., Bernstein, M., Bell, S.A., Ray, K., Grendahl, D.C., Marina, N. & Kleinerman, E.S. (2010). Inhaled granulocyte-macrophage colony stimulating factor for first pulmonary recurrence of osteosarcoma: effects on disease-free survival and immunomodulation. a report from the Children's Oncology Group. *Clin Cancer Res,* Vol. 16, No. 15, (Aug 1), pp. 4024-30, ISSN 1078-0432

Arppe, J., Vidgren, M. & Waldrep, J.C. (1998). Pulmonary pharmacokinetics of cyclosporin A liposomes. *International Journal of Pharmaceutics,* Vol. 161, No. 2, (23 February 1998), pp. 205-214, ISSN 0378-5173.

Atzpodien, J., Kirchner, H., Duensing, S., Lopez Hanninen, E., Franzke, A., Buer, J., Probst, M., Anton, P. & Poliwoda, H. (1995). Biochemotherapy of advanced metastatic renal-cell carcinoma: results of the combination of interleukin-2, alpha-interferon, 5-fluorouracil, vinblastine, and 13-cis-retinoic acid. *World J Urol,* Vol. 13, No. 3, pp. 174-7, ISSN 0724-4983

Atzpodien, J., Kirchner, H., Rebmann, U., Soder, M., Gertenbach, U., Siebels, M., Roigas, J., Raschke, R., Salm, S., Schwindl, B., Muller, S.C., Hauser, S., Leiber, C., Huland, E., Heinzer, H., Siemer, S., Metzner, B., Heynemann, H., Fornara, P. & Reitz, M. (2006). Interleukin-2/interferon-alpha2a/13-retinoic acid-based chemoimmunotherapy in advanced renal cell carcinoma: results of a prospectively randomised trial of the German Cooperative Renal Carcinoma Chemoimmunotherapy Group (DGCIN). *Br J Cancer,* Vol. 95, No. 4, (Aug 21), pp. 463-9, ISSN 0007-0920

Azarmi, S., Tao, X., Chen, H., Wang, Z., Finlay, W.H., Lobenberg, R. & Roa, W.H. (2006). Formulation and cytotoxicity of doxorubicin nanoparticles carried by dry powder aerosol particles. *Int J Pharm,* Vol. 319, No. 1-2, (Aug 17), pp. 155-61, ISSN 0378-5173

Bianco, S., Pieroni, M.G., Refini, R.M., Rottoli, L. & Sestini, P. (1989). Protective effect of inhaled furosemide on allergen-induced early and late asthmatic reactions. *N Engl J Med,* Vol. 321, No. 16, (Oct 19), pp. 1069-73, ISSN 0028-4793

Boe, J., Dennis, J.H., O'Driscoll, B.R., Bauer, T.T., Carone, M., Dautzenberg, B., Diot, P., Heslop, K. & Lannefors, L. (2001). European Respiratory Society Guidelines on the use of nebulizers. *Eur Respir J,* Vol. 18, No. 1, (Jul), pp. 228-42, ISSN 0903-1936

Bruera, E., Macmillan, K., Pither, J. & MacDonald, R.N. (1990). Effects of morphine on the dyspnea of terminal cancer patients. *J Pain Symptom Manage,* Vol. 5, No. 6, (Dec), pp. 341-4, ISSN 0885-3924

Bruera, E., Sala, R., Spruyt, O., Palmer, J.L., Zhang, T. & Willey, J. (2005). Nebulized versus subcutaneous morphine for patients with cancer dyspnea: a preliminary study. *J Pain Symptom Manage,* Vol. 29, No. 6, (Jun), pp. 613-8, ISSN 0885-3924

Charles, M.A., Reymond, L. & Israel, F. (2008). Relief of incident dyspnea in palliative cancer patients: a pilot, randomized, controlled trial comparing nebulized hydromorphone, systemic hydromorphone, and nebulized saline. *J Pain Symptom Manage,* Vol. 36, No. 1, (Jul), pp. 29-38, ISSN 1873-6513

Chrubasik, J., Wust, H., Friedrich, G. & Geller, E. (1988). Absorption and bioavailability of nebulized morphine. *Br J Anaesth,* Vol. 61, No. 2, (Aug), pp. 228-30, ISSN 0007-0912

Cody, D.D., Nelson, C.L., Bradley, W.M., Wislez, M., Juroske, D., Price, R.E., Zhou, X., Bekele, B.N. & Kurie, J.M. (2005). Murine lung tumor measurement using respiratory-gated micro-computed tomography. *Invest Radiol,* Vol. 40, No. 5, (May), pp. 263-9, ISSN 0020-9996

Coyne, P.J., Viswanathan, R. & Smith, T.J. (2002). Nebulized fentanyl citrate improves patients' perception of breathing, respiratory rate, and oxygen saturation in dyspnea. *J Pain Symptom Manage,* Vol. 23, No. 2, (Feb), pp. 157-60, ISSN 0885-3924

Cryan, S.A. (2005). Carrier-based strategies for targeting protein and peptide drugs to the lungs. *AAPS J,* Vol. 7, No. 1, pp. E20-41, ISSN 1550-7416

Dolovich, M.A. (2000). Influence of inspiratory flow rate, particle size, and airway caliber on aerosolized drug delivery to the lung. *Respir Care,* Vol. 45, No. 6, (Jun), pp. 597-608, ISSN 0020-1324

Dolovich, M.B. (2009). 18F-fluorodeoxyglucose positron emission tomographic imaging of pulmonary functions, pathology, and drug delivery. *Proc Am Thorac Soc,* Vol. 6, No. 5, (Aug 15), pp. 477-85, ISSN 1943-5665

El-Gendy, N. & Berkland, C. (2009). Combination chemotherapeutic dry powder aerosols via controlled nanoparticle agglomeration. *Pharm Res,* Vol. 26, No. 7, (Jul), pp. 1752-63, ISSN 1573-904X

Esteban-Gonzalez, E., Carballido, J., Navas, V., Torregrosa, Z., Munoz, A. & de Mon, M.A. (2007). Retrospective review in patients with pulmonary metastases of renal cell carcinoma receiving inhaled recombinant interleukin-2. *Anticancer Drugs,* Vol. 18, No. 3, (Mar), pp. 291-6, ISSN 0959-4973

Everard, M.L., Hardy, J.G. & Milner, A.D. (1993). Comparison of nebulised aerosol deposition in the lungs of healthy adults following oral and nasal inhalation. *Thorax,* Vol. 48, No. 10, (Oct), pp. 1045-6, ISSN 0040-6376

Fu, H., He, J., Mei, F., Zhang, Q., Hara, Y., Ryota, S., Lubet, R.A., Chen, R., Chen, D.R. & You, M. (2009). Lung cancer inhibitory effect of epigallocatechin-3-gallate is dependent on its presence in a complex mixture (polyphenon E). *Cancer Prev Res (Phila),* Vol. 2, No. 6, (Jun), pp. 531-7, ISSN 1940-6215

Fu, H., Zhang, J., Pan, J., Zhang, Q., Lu, Y., Wen, W., Lubet, R.A., Szabo, E., Chen, R., Wang, Y., Chen, D.R. & You, M. Chemoprevention of lung carcinogenesis by the combination of aerosolized budesonide and oral pioglitazone in A/J mice. *Mol Carcinog,* (Mar 3), ISSN 1098-2744

Fulzele, S.V., Chatterjee, A., Shaik, M.S., Jackson, T. & Singh, M. (2006). Inhalation delivery and anti-tumor activity of celecoxib in human orthotopic non-small cell lung cancer xenograft model. *Pharm Res,* Vol. 23, No. 9, (Sep), pp. 2094-106, ISSN 0724-8741

Gagnadoux, F., Hureaux, J., Vecellio, L., Urban, T., Le Pape, A., Valo, I., Montharu, J., Leblond, V., Boisdron-Celle, M., Lerondel, S., Majoral, C., Diot, P., Racineux, J.L. & Lemarie, E. (2008). Aerosolized chemotherapy. *J Aerosol Med Pulm Drug Deliv,* Vol. 21, No. 1, (Mar), pp. 61-70, ISSN 1941-2711

Gagnadoux, F., Le Pape, A., Urban, T., Montharu, J., Vecellio, L., Dubus, J.C., Leblond, V., Diot, P., Grimbert, D., Racineux, J.L. & Lemarie, E. (2005a). Safety of pulmonary administration of gemcitabine in rats. *J Aerosol Med,* Vol. 18, No. 2, (Summer), pp. 198-206, ISSN 0894-2684

Gagnadoux, F., Leblond, V., Vecellio, L., Hureaux, J., Le Pape, A., Boisdron-Celle, M., Montharu, J., Majoral, C., Fournier, J., Urban, T., Diot, P., Racineux, J.L. & Lemarie, E. (2006). Gemcitabine aerosol: in vitro antitumor activity and deposition imaging for preclinical safety assessment in baboons. *Cancer Chemother Pharmacol,* Vol. 58, No. 2, (Aug), pp. 237-44, ISSN 0344-5704

Gagnadoux, F., Pape, A.L., Lemarie, E., Lerondel, S., Valo, I., Leblond, V., Racineux, J.L. & Urban, T. (2005b). Aerosol delivery of chemotherapy in an orthotopic model of lung cancer. *Eur Respir J,* Vol. 26, No. 4, (Oct), pp. 657-61, ISSN 0903-1936

Gilbert, B.E., Seryshev, A., Knight, V. & Brayton, C. (2002). 9-nitrocamptothecin liposome aerosol: lack of subacute toxicity in dogs. *Inhal Toxicol,* Vol. 14, No. 2, (Feb), pp. 185-97, ISSN 0895-8378

Giraud, V. & Roche, N. (2002). Misuse of corticosteroid metered-dose inhaler is associated with decreased asthma stability. *Eur Respir J,* Vol. 19, No. 2, (Feb), pp. 246-51, ISSN 0903-1936

Grimbert, D., Lubin, O., de Monte, M., Vecellio None, L., Perrier, M., Carre, P., Lemarie, E., Boissinot, E. & Diot, P. (2004). [Dyspnea and morphine aerosols in the palliative care of lung cancer]. *Rev Mal Respir,* Vol. 21, No. 6 Pt 1, (Dec), pp. 1091-7, ISSN 0761-8425

Gross, E.A. & Morgan, K.T. (1991). Architecture of nasal passages and larynx. In: *Comparative Biology of the Normal Lung.* Parent, R.A. (Ed.). pp. 7-25, Boca Raton, FL: CRC Press.

Hershey, A.E., Kurzman, I.D., Forrest, L.J., Bohling, C.A., Stonerook, M., Placke, M.E., Imondi, A.R. & Vail, D.M. (1999). Inhalation chemotherapy for macroscopic primary or metastatic lung tumors: proof of principle using dogs with spontaneously occurring tumors as a model. *Clin Cancer Res,* Vol. 5, No. 9, (Sep), pp. 2653-9, ISSN 1078-0432

Hess, D.R. (2008). Aerosol delivery devices in the treatment of asthma. *Respir Care,* Vol. 53, No. 6, (Jun), pp. 699-723; discussion 723-5, ISSN 0020-1324

Hitzman, C.J., Wattenberg, L.W. & Wiedmann, T.S. (2006). Pharmacokinetics of 5-fluorouracil in the hamster following inhalation delivery of lipid-coated nanoparticles. *J Pharm Sci,* Vol. 95, No. 6, (Jun), pp. 1196-211, ISSN 0022-3549

Huland, E., Burger, A., Fleischer, J., Fornara, P., Hatzmann, E., Heidenreich, A., Heinzer, H., Heynemann, H., Hoffmann, L., Hofmann, R., Huland, H., Kampfer, I., Kindler, M., Kirchner, H., Mehlhorn, G., Moniak, T.H., Rebmann, U., Roigas, J., Schneider, T.H., Schnorr, D., Schmitz, H.J., Wenisch, R., Varga, Z. & Vinke, J. (2003). Efficacy and safety of inhaled recombinant interleukin-2 in high-risk renal cell cancer patients compared with systemic interleukin-2: an outcome study. *Folia Biol (Praha),* Vol. 49, No. 5, pp. 183-90, ISSN 0015-5500

Huland, E., Heinzer, H. & Huland, H. (1994). Inhaled interleukin-2 in combination with low-dose systemic interleukin-2 and interferon alpha in patients with pulmonary metastatic renal-cell carcinoma: effectiveness and toxicity of mainly local treatment. *J Cancer Res Clin Oncol,* Vol. 120, No. 4, pp. 221-8, ISSN 0171-5216

Huland, E., Heinzer, H. & Huland, H. (1999a). Immunotherapy of pulmonary metastatic renal cell carcinoma: success dependant on risk factors? *Hepatogastroenterology,* Vol. 46 Suppl 1, (May), pp. 1257-62, ISSN 0172-6390

Huland, E., Heinzer, H. & Huland, H. (1999b). Treatment of pulmonary metastatic renal-cell carcinoma in 116 patients using inhaled interleukin-2 (IL-2). *Anticancer Res,* Vol. 19, No. 4A, (Jul-Aug), pp. 2679-83, ISSN 0250-7005

Hureaux, J., Lagarce, F., Gagnadoux, F., Vecellio, L., Clavreul, A., Roger, E., Kempf, M., Racineux, J.L., Diot, P., Benoit, J.P. & Urban, T. (2009). Lipid nanocapsules: ready-to-use nanovectors for the aerosol delivery of paclitaxel. *Eur J Pharm Biopharm,* Vol. 73, No. 2, (Oct), pp. 239-46, ISSN 1873-3441

Jennings, A.L., Davies, A.N., Higgins, J.P., Gibbs, J.S. & Broadley, K.E. (2002). A systematic review of the use of opioids in the management of dyspnoea. *Thorax,* Vol. 57, No. 11, (Nov), pp. 939-44, ISSN 0040-6376

Johnson, L., Mercer, K., Greenbaum, D., Bronson, R.T., Crowley, D., Tuveson, D.A. & Jacks, T. (2001). Somatic activation of the K-ras oncogene causes early onset lung cancer in mice. *Nature,* Vol. 410, No. 6832, (Apr 26), pp. 1111-6, ISSN 0028-0836

Khanna, C., Anderson, P.M., Hasz, D.E., Katsanis, E., Neville, M. & Klausner, J.S. (1997). Interleukin-2 liposome inhalation therapy is safe and effective for dogs with spontaneous pulmonary metastases. *Cancer,* Vol. 79, No. 7, (Apr 1), pp. 1409-21, ISSN 0008-543X

Khanna, C., Hasz, D.E., Klausner, J.S. & Anderson, P.M. (1996). Aerosol delivery of interleukin 2 liposomes is nontoxic and biologically effective: canine studies. *Clin Cancer Res,* Vol. 2, No. 4, (Apr), pp. 721-34, ISSN 1078-0432

Knight, V., Koshkina, N.V., Waldrep, J.C., Giovanella, B.C. & Gilbert, B.E. (1999). Anticancer effect of 9-nitrocamptothecin liposome aerosol on human cancer xenografts in nude mice. *Cancer Chemother Pharmacol,* Vol. 44, No. 3, pp. 177-86, ISSN 0344-5704

Kohara, H., Ueoka, H., Aoe, K., Maeda, T., Takeyama, H., Saito, R., Shima, Y. & Uchitomi, Y. (2003). Effect of nebulized furosemide in terminally ill cancer patients with dyspnea. *J Pain Symptom Manage,* Vol. 26, No. 4, (Oct), pp. 962-7, ISSN 0885-3924

Koshkina, N.V., Gilbert, B.E., Waldrep, J.C., Seryshev, A. & Knight, V. (1999). Distribution of camptothecin after delivery as a liposome aerosol or following intramuscular injection in mice. *Cancer Chemother Pharmacol,* Vol. 44, No. 3, pp. 187-92, ISSN 0344-5704

Koshkina, N.V. & Kleinerman, E.S. (2005). Aerosol gemcitabine inhibits the growth of primary osteosarcoma and osteosarcoma lung metastases. *Int J Cancer,* Vol. 116, No. 3, (Sep 1), pp. 458-63, ISSN 0020-7136

Koshkina, N.V., Kleinerman, E.S., Waidrep, C., Jia, S.F., Worth, L.L., Gilbert, B.E. & Knight, V. (2000). 9-Nitrocamptothecin liposome aerosol treatment of melanoma and osteosarcoma lung metastases in mice. *Clin Cancer Res,* Vol. 6, No. 7, (Jul), pp. 2876-80, ISSN 1078-0432

Koshkina, N.V., Waldrep, J.C., Roberts, L.E., Golunski, E., Melton, S. & Knight, V. (2001). Paclitaxel liposome aerosol treatment induces inhibition of pulmonary metastases in murine renal carcinoma model. *Clin Cancer Res,* Vol. 7, No. 10, (Oct), pp. 3258-62, ISSN 1078-0432

Latimer, P., Menchaca, M., Snyder, R.M., Yu, W., Gilbert, B.E., Sanders, B.G. & Kline, K. (2009). Aerosol delivery of liposomal formulated paclitaxel and vitamin E analog reduces murine mammary tumor burden and metastases. *Exp Biol Med (Maywood),* Vol. 234, No. 10, (Oct), pp. 1244-52, ISSN 1535-3699

Liu, J. & Johnston, M.R. (2002). Animal models for studying lung cancer and evaluating novel intervention strategies. *Surg Oncol,* Vol. 11, No. 4, (Dec), pp. 217-27, ISSN 0960-7404

Loppow, D., Huland, E., Heinzer, H., Gronke, L., Magnussen, H., Holz, O. & Jorres, R.A. (2007). Interleukin-2 inhalation therapy temporarily induces asthma-like airway inflammation. *Eur J Med Res,* Vol. 12, No. 11, (Nov 5), pp. 556-62, ISSN 0949-2321

Lorenz, J., Wilhelm, K., Kessler, M., Peschel, C., Schwulera, U., Lissner, R., Struff, W.G., Huland, E., Huber, C. & Aulitzky, W.E. (1996). Phase I trial of inhaled natural interleukin 2 for treatment of pulmonary malignancy: toxicity, pharmacokinetics, and biological effects. *Clin Cancer Res,* Vol. 2, No. 7, (Jul), pp. 1115-22, ISSN 1078-0432

Maillet, A., Congy-Jolivet, N., Le Guellec, S., Vecellio, L., Hamard, S., Courty, Y., Courtois, A., Gauthier, F., Diot, P., Thibault, G., Lemarie, E. & Heuze-Vourc'h, N. (2008). Aerodynamical, immunological and pharmacological properties of the anticancer antibody cetuximab following nebulization. *Pharm Res,* Vol. 25, No. 6, (Jun), pp. 1318-26, ISSN 0724-8741

Maillet, A., Guilleminault, L., Lemarié, E., Lerondel, S., Azzopardi, N., Montharu, J., Congy-Jolivet, N., Reverdiau, P., Legrain, B., Parent, C., Douvin, D., Hureaux, J., Courty, Y., De Monte, M., Diot, P., Paintaud, G., Le Pape, A., Watier, H. & Heuzé-Vourc'h, N. (In press). Aerosolized Immunotherapy in lung cancer: proof-of-principle study with cetuximab in a mouse model of lung tumor. *Pharm Res*. In Press.

Markovic, S.N., Suman, V.J., Nevala, W.K., Geeraerts, L., Creagan, E.T., Erickson, L.A., Rowland, K.M., Jr., Morton, R.F., Horvath, W.L. & Pittelkow, M.R. (2008). A dose-escalation study of aerosolized sargramostim in the treatment of metastatic melanoma: an NCCTG Study. *Am J Clin Oncol,* Vol. 31, No. 6, (Dec), pp. 573-9, ISSN 1537-453X

McBride, J.T. (1991). Architecture of the tracheobronchial tree. In: *Comparative Biology of the Normal Lung*. Parent, R. (Ed.). pp. 49–61, CRC, Press, Boca Raton, FL.

Merimsky, O., Gez, E., Weitzen, R., Nehushtan, H., Rubinov, R., Hayat, H., Peretz, T., Ben-Shahar, M., Biran, H., Katsenelson, R., Mermershtein, V., Loven, D., Karminsky, N., Neumann, A., Matcejevsky, D. & Inbar, M. (2004). Targeting pulmonary metastases of renal cell carcinoma by inhalation of interleukin-2. *Ann Oncol,* Vol. 15, No. 4, (Apr), pp. 610-2, ISSN 0923-7534

Miller, F.J. (2000). Dosimetry of particles in laboratory animals and humans in relationship to issues surrounding lung overload and human health risk assessment: a critical review. *Inhal Toxicol,* Vol. 12, No. 1-2, (Jan-Feb), pp. 19-57, ISSN 0895-8378

Mitani, S., Nakamoto, T., Usui, A. & Usui, T. (1992). Interleukin-2 immunotherapy for advanced renal cell carcinoma. *Biotherapy (Jpn),* Vol. 6, pp. 452-453.

Nakamoto, T., Kasaoka, Y., Mitani, S. & Usui, T. (1997). Inhalation of interleukin-2 combined with subcutaneous administration of interferon for the treatment of pulmonary metastases from renal cell carcinoma. *Int J Urol,* Vol. 4, No. 4, (Jul), pp. 343-8, ISSN 0919-8172

Newman, S.P. (1983). Therapeutic aerosols 1—Physical and practical considerations. *Thorax,* Vol. 38, pp. 881s-886s.

Nishino, T., Ide, T., Sudo, T. & Sato, J. (2000). Inhaled furosemide greatly alleviates the sensation of experimentally induced dyspnea. *Am J Respir Crit Care Med,* Vol. 161, No. 6, (Jun), pp. 1963-7, ISSN 1073-449X

Otterson, G.A., Villalona-Calero, M.A., Hicks, W., Pan, X., Ellerton, J.A., Gettinger, S.N. & Murren, J.R. (2010). Phase I/II study of inhaled doxorubicin combined with platinum-based therapy for advanced non-small cell lung cancer. *Clin Cancer Res,* Vol. 16, No. 8, (Apr 15), pp. 2466-73, ISSN 1078-0432

Otterson, G.A., Villalona-Calero, M.A., Sharma, S., Kris, M.G., Imondi, A., Gerber, M., White, D.A., Ratain, M.J., Schiller, J.H., Sandler, A., Kraut, M., Mani, S. & Murren, J.R. (2007). Phase I study of inhaled Doxorubicin for patients with metastatic tumors to the lungs. *Clin Cancer Res,* Vol. 13, No. 4, (Feb 15), pp. 1246-52, ISSN 1078-0432

Pavia, D. & Thomson, M.L. (1976). The fractional deposition of inhaled 2 and 5 mum particles in the alveolar and tracheobronchial regions of the healthy human lung. *Ann Occup Hyg,* Vol. 19, No. 2, (Nov), pp. 109-14, ISSN 0003-4878

Pedersen, S. (1996). Inhalers and nebulizers: which to choose and why. *Respir Med,* Vol. 90, No. 2, (Feb), pp. 69-77, ISSN 0954-6111

Penson, R.T., Joel, S.P., Roberts, M., Gloyne, A., Beckwith, S. & Slevin, M.L. (2002). The bioavailability and pharmacokinetics of subcutaneous, nebulized and oral morphine-6-glucuronide. *Br J Clin Pharmacol,* Vol. 53, No. 4, (Apr), pp. 347-54, ISSN 0306-5251

Phalen, R.F., Oldham, M.J. & Wolff, R.K. (2008). The relevance of animal models for aerosol studies. *J Aerosol Med Pulm Drug Deliv,* Vol. 21, No. 1, (Mar), pp. 113-24, ISSN 1941-2711

Pilcer, G. & Amighi, K. (2010). Formulation strategy and use of excipients in pulmonary drug delivery. *Int J Pharm,* Vol. 392, No. 1-2, (Jun 15), pp. 1-19, ISSN 1873-3476

Quigley, C., Joel, S., Patel, N., Baksh, A. & Slevin, M. (2002). A phase I/II study of nebulized morphine-6-glucuronide in patients with cancer-related breathlessness. *J Pain Symptom Manage,* Vol. 23, No. 1, (Jan), pp. 7-9, ISSN 0885-3924

Rao, R.D., Anderson, P.M., Arndt, C.A., Wettstein, P.J. & Markovic, S.N. (2003). Aerosolized granulocyte macrophage colony-stimulating factor (GM-CSF) therapy in metastatic cancer. *Am J Clin Oncol,* Vol. 26, No. 5, (Oct), pp. 493-8, ISSN 1537-453X

Rodriguez, C.O., Jr., Crabbs, T.A., Wilson, D.W., Cannan, V.A., Skorupski, K.A., Gordon, N., Koshkina, N., Kleinerman, E. & Anderson, P.M. (2010). Aerosol gemcitabine: preclinical safety and in vivo antitumor activity in osteosarcoma-bearing dogs. *J Aerosol Med Pulm Drug Deliv,* Vol. 23, No. 4, (Aug), pp. 197-206, ISSN 1941-2703

Rosenberg, S.A., Yang, J.C., Topalian, S.L., Schwartzentruber, D.J., Weber, J.S., Parkinson, D.R., Seipp, C.A., Einhorn, J.H. & White, D.E. (1994). Treatment of 283 consecutive patients with metastatic melanoma or renal cell cancer using high-dose bolus interleukin 2. *JAMA,* Vol. 271, No. 12, (Mar 23-30), pp. 907-13, ISSN 0098-7484

Schuepp, K.G., Straub, D., Moller, A. & Wildhaber, J.H. (2004). Deposition of aerosols in infants and children. *J Aerosol Med,* Vol. 17, No. 2, (Summer), pp. 153-6, ISSN 0894-2684

Selting, K., Waldrep, J.C., Reinero, C., Branson, K., Gustafson, D., Kim, D.Y., Henry, C., Owen, N., Madsen, R. & Dhand, R. (2008). Feasibility and safety of targeted cisplatin delivery to a select lung lobe in dogs via the AeroProbe intracorporeal nebulization catheter. *J Aerosol Med Pulm Drug Deliv,* Vol. 21, No. 3, (Sep), pp. 255-68, ISSN 1941-2711

Selting, K., Essman, S., Reinero, C., Branson, K.R., Henry, C.J., Owen, N., Guntur, V.P., Waldrep, J.C., Kim, D.Y. & Dhand, R. (2011). Targeted combined aerosol chemotherapy in dogs and radiologic toxicity grading. *J Aerosol Med Pulm Drug Deliv,* Vol. 24, No. 1, (Feb), pp. 43-8, ISSN 1941-2703

Shimkin, M.B. & Stoner, G.D. (1975). Lung tumors in mice: application to carcinogenesis bioassay. *Adv Cancer Res,* Vol. 21, pp. 1-58, ISSN 0065-230X

Shimoyama, N. & Shimoyama, M. (2002). Nebulized furosemide as a novel treatment for dyspnea in terminal cancer patients. *J Pain Symptom Manage,* Vol. 23, No. 1, (Jan), pp. 73-6, ISSN 0885-3924

Skubitz, K.M. & Anderson, P.M. (2000). Inhalational interleukin-2 liposomes for pulmonary metastases: a phase I clinical trial. *Anticancer Drugs,* Vol. 11, No. 7, (Aug), pp. 555-63, ISSN 0959-4973

Soderholm, S.C. (1989). Proposed international conventions for particle size-selective sampling. *Ann Occup Hyg,* Vol. 33, No. 3, pp. 301-20, ISSN 0003-4878

Stone, P., Rix, Kurowska, A. & Tookman (2002). Re: nebulized furosemide for dyspnea in terminal cancer patients. *J Pain Symptom Manage,* Vol. 24, No. 3, (Sep), pp. 274-5; author reply 275-6, ISSN 0885-3924

Tanaka, K., Shima, Y., Kakinuma, R., Kubota, K., Ohe, Y., Hojo, F., Matsumoto, T., Ohmatsu, H., Goto, K., Nagai, K. & Nishiwaki, Y. (1999). Effect of nebulized morphine in cancer patients with dyspnea: a pilot study. *Jpn J Clin Oncol,* Vol. 29, No. 12, (Dec), pp. 600-3, ISSN 0368-2811

Tatsumura, T., Koyama, S., Tsujimoto, M., Kitagawa, M. & Kagamimori, S. (1993). Further study of nebulisation chemotherapy, a new chemotherapeutic method in the treatment of lung carcinomas: fundamental and clinical. *Br J Cancer,* Vol. 68, No. 6, (Dec), pp. 1146-9, ISSN 0007-0920

Tatsumura, T., Yamamoto, K., Murakami, A., Tsuda, M. & Sugiyama, S. (1983). [New chemotherapeutic method for the treatment of tracheal and bronchial cancers--nebulization chemotherapy]. *Gan No Rinsho,* Vol. 29, No. 7, (Jun), pp. 765-70, ISSN 0021-4949

Tomoda, K., Ohkoshi, T., Hirota, K., Sonavane, G.S., Nakajima, T., Terada, H., Komuro, M., Kitazato, K. & Makino, K. (2009). Preparation and properties of inhalable nanocomposite particles for treatment of lung cancer. *Colloids Surf B Biointerfaces,* Vol. 71, No. 2, (Jul 1), pp. 177-82, ISSN 1873-4367

Tseng, C.L., Su, W.Y., Yen, K.C., Yang, K.C. & Lin, F.H. (2009). The use of biotinylated-EGF-modified gelatin nanoparticle carrier to enhance cisplatin accumulation in cancerous lungs via inhalation. *Biomaterials,* Vol. 30, No. 20, (Jul), pp. 3476-85, ISSN 1878-5905

Tyler, W.S. (1983). Comparative subgross anatomy of lungs. Pleuras, interlobular septa, and distal airways. *Am Rev Respir Dis,* Vol. 128, No. 2 Pt 2, (Aug), pp. S32-6, ISSN 0003-0805

Verschraegen, C.F., Gilbert, B.E., Huaringa, A.J., Newman, R., Harris, N., Leyva, F.J., Keus, L., Campbell, K., Nelson-Taylor, T. & Knight, V. (2000). Feasibility, phase I, and pharmacological study of aerosolized liposomal 9-nitro-20(S)-camptothecin in patients with advanced malignancies in the lungs. *Ann N Y Acad Sci,* Vol. 922, pp. 352-4, ISSN 0077-8923

Verschraegen, C.F., Gilbert, B.E., Loyer, E., Huaringa, A., Walsh, G., Newman, R.A. & Knight, V. (2004). Clinical evaluation of the delivery and safety of aerosolized liposomal 9-nitro-20(s)-camptothecin in patients with advanced pulmonary malignancies. *Clin Cancer Res,* Vol. 10, No. 7, (Apr 1), pp. 2319-26, ISSN 1078-0432

Wang, Z., Chen, H.T., Roa, W. & Finlay, W. (2003). Farnesol for aerosol inhalation: nebulization and activity against human lung cancer cells. *J Pharm Pharm Sci,* Vol. 6, No. 1, (Jan-Apr), pp. 95-100, ISSN 1482-1826

Wattenberg, L.W., Wiedmann, T.S., Estensen, R.D. (2004). Chemoprevention of cancer of the upper respiratory tract of the Syrian golden hamster by aerosol administration of difluoromethylornithine and 5-fluorouracil. *Cancer Res,* Vol. 64, No. 7, (Apr 1), pp. 2347-9, ISSN 0008-5472

Wattenberg, L.W., Wiedmann, T.S., Estensen, R.D., Zimmerman, C.L., Steele, V.E., Kelloff, G.J. (1997). Chemoprevention of pulmonary carcinogenesis by aerosolized budesonide in female A/J mice. *Cancer Res,* Vol. 57, No. 24, (Dec 15), pp. 5489-92. ISSN 0008-5472

Wauthoz, N., Deleuze, P., Hecq, J., Roland, I., Saussez, S., Adanja, I., Debeir, O., Decaestecker, C., Mathieu, V., Kiss, R. & Amighi, K. (2010). In vivo assessment of temozolomide local delivery for lung cancer inhalation therapy. *Eur J Pharm Sci,* Vol. 39, No. 5, (Mar 18), pp. 402-11, ISSN 1879-0720

Weibel, E.R. (1963). Principles and methods for the morphometric study of the lung and other organs. *Lab Invest,* Vol. 12, (Feb), pp. 131-55, ISSN 0023-6837

Wilcock, A., Walton, A., Manderson, C., Feathers, L., El Khoury, B., Lewis, M., Chauhan, A., Howard, P., Bell, S., Frisby, J. & Tattersfield, A. (2008). Randomised, placebo controlled trial of nebulised furosemide for breathlessness in patients with cancer. *Thorax,* Vol. 63, No. 10, (Oct), pp. 872-5, ISSN 1468-3296

Wislez, M., Massiani, M.A., Milleron, B., Souidi, A., Carette, M.F., Antoine, M. & Cadranel, J. (2003). Clinical characteristics of pneumonic-type adenocarcinoma of the lung. *Chest,* Vol. 123, No. 6, (Jun), pp. 1868-77, ISSN 0012-3692

Wittgen, B.P., Kunst, P.W., Perkins, W.R., Lee, J.K. & Postmus, P.E. (2006). Assessing a system to capture stray aerosol during inhalation of nebulized liposomal cisplatin. *J Aerosol Med,* Vol. 19, No. 3, (Fall), pp. 385-91, ISSN 0894-2684

Wittgen, B.P., Kunst, P.W., van der Born, K., van Wijk, A.W., Perkins, W., Pilkiewicz, F.G., Perez-Soler, R., Nicholson, S., Peters, G.J. & Postmus, P.E. (2007). Phase I study of aerosolized SLIT cisplatin in the treatment of patients with carcinoma of the lung. *Clin Cancer Res,* Vol. 13, No. 8, (Apr 15), pp. 2414-21, ISSN 1078-0432

Yan, Y., Cook, J., McQuillan, J., Zhang, G., Hitzman, C.J., Wang, Y., Wiedmann, T.S. & You, M. (2007). Chemopreventive effect of aerosolized polyphenon E on lung tumorigenesis in A/J mice. *Neoplasia,* Vol. 9, No. 5, (May), pp. 401-5, ISSN 1476-5586

Zhang, Q., Pan, J., Zhang, J., Liu, P., Chen, R., Chen, D.R., Lubet, R., Wang, Y. & You, M. Aerosolized bexarotene inhibits lung tumorigenesis without increasing plasma triglyceride and cholesterol levels in mice. *Cancer Prev Res (Phila),* Vol. 4, No. 2, (Feb), pp. 270-6, ISSN 1940-6215

4

# Cell Division Gene from Bacteria in Minicell Production for Therapy

Nguyen Tu H.K.
*International University, Hochiminh City National University*
*Vietnam*

## 1. Introduction

Drug resistance is one of our biggest problems in terms of cancer therapy. Chemotherapeutic drug therapy in cancer is seriously hampered by severe toxicity primarily due to indiscriminate drug distribution and consequent collateral damage to normal cells. Therefore, the cancer treatment requires the combination with pharmaceutical science, cell biology, chemistry, electronics, materials, science and technology to improve the cancer therapy development. The results of genome sequencing and studies of biological–genetic function (functional genomics) are combined with chemical, microelectronic and micro system technologies to produce medical devices, known as diagnostic 'Biochips'. The multitude of biologically active molecules is expanded by additional novel structures created with newly arranged 'gene clusters' and (bio-) catalytic chemical processes. With the nanotechnology involving the ability to arrange molecules and atoms into molecular structures, the drug development in cancer treatment is also limitted. The application of micro-machining techniques is growing rapidly and has applications in microfluidics (for labs-on-a-chip), in sensors as well as in fiber optics and displays. Nowsaday, direct-write technologies are of increasing importance in materials processing. Building the structures are made directly without the use of masks, allowing rapid prototyping. The techniques comprise plasma spray, laser particle guidance, matrix-assisted pulsed-laser evaporation, laser chemical vapor deposition, micro-pen, ink jet, e-beam, focused ion beam and several droplet micro-dispensing methods. Micrometer-scale patterns of viable cells are required for the next generation of tissue engineering, fabrication of cell-based microfluidicbiosensor arrays, and selective separation and culturing of microorganisms. The patterns of viable *Escherichia coli* bacteria have been transferred onto various substrates with laser-based forward transfer technique. These tools can be used to create three-dimensional mesoscopically engineered structures of living cells, proteins, DNA strands and antibodies and two co- fabricate electronic devices on the same substrate to generate cell-based biosensors and bioelectronic interfaces and implants. Discrete nanoparticles with controlled chemical composition and size distribution are readily synthesized using reverse micelles and microemulsions as confined reaction media, but their assembly into well-defined superstructures amenable to practical use remains a difficult and demanding task. This usually requires the initial synthesis of spherical nanoparticles, followed by further processing such as solvent evaporation, molecular crosslinking or template patterning. The interfacial activity of reverse micelles and microemulsions can be exploited to couple nanoparticle synthesis and self-assembly over a range of length scales to produce materials with complex organization arising from the interdigitation of surfactant molecules attached to specific nanoparticle crystal faces. The construction and the evolutionary improvement of micro- and nanodevices may be carried out using evolving populations of artificial creatures. The biological life is in the control of its own means of reproduction, which generally involves in the complex, auto-catalyzing chemical reactions. However, this autonomy of the design and manufacture has not yet been realized artificially. Therefore, the requirements for cancer treatment are essential and developed rapidly with the involvement in numerous physical and chemical methodologies.

Gene therapy and tissue engineering are new concepts in the treatment of cancer disease. The oligonucleotides used in gene therapy with the potential to alter cell function for an extended period of time in relation to more established therapeutic agents. Tissue engineering aims to regrow tissue structure lost as a result of trauma or cancer through the application of engineered materials. Both fields can demonstrate initial success, such as the replacement of adenosine deaminase genes in children with severe immunodeficiency and the use of synthetic materials to accelerate healing of burns and skin ulcers. Major limitations are the low level of expression in gene therapy and the tissue engineers have not yet learned to reproduce complex architecture, such as vascular networks, which are essential for normal tissue function. A combination of both methods has been used as a new strategy to overcome problems remaining. DNA delivery has been described in situ from polymer coatings, microspheres and synthetic matrices. DNA material hybrid systems promise to enable forms of gene therapy not possible with other gene delivery systems, e.g., polymeric microspheres facilitate the expression of orally administered genes.

Besides, an F1-ATPase biomolecular motor and fabricated nanopropellers was constructed. The molecular dynamics of the F1-ATPase at the molecular level were described and the suitability of biomolecular devices as nanomolecular machines comprehensively reviewed. This chapter aims to present an integrated view of the developments on the discovery of new therapy for cancer disease.

The chapter will drive why cell division gene from bacteria may play a role in drug delivery to treat the cancer diseases. The topics will deal with the affects of hyaluronan in cell morphology of *Lactobacillus acidophilus* in minicell producing study and the role of the cell division gene from bacteria in minicell production for therapy. In order to study the minicell production from bacteria, the function of cell division genes in bacteria as well as minicells in cancer treatment. The role of *min* gene from *Streptomyces lavendulae* in minicell formation for therapy will be studied as the first contribution to cancer therapy.

## 2. Minicell production for therapy

Up to now, the major factor limiting cancer chemotherapeutics is toxicity to the host cells. The efforts to the develop the targeted drug delivery systems as nanoparticles, polymer therapeutics to cancer cell via cell-surface receptors are also not perfect in leakage in vivo or production scale up. Remarkably, bacterial minicells are anucleate nanoparticles produced as a result of inactivating the genes controlling the normal bacterial cell division (de Boer et al., 1989) due to depressing the polar sites of cell division, may provide the better way for cytotoxic drug delivery. The minicells are also prepared from genetically defined *minCED(-)*

chromosomal deletion bacteria and then the subsequent minicells were purified. The deletion of *minCED(-)* out of the bacteria cell may affect on their growth under their control so far. Therefore, to find out many methods in the minicell formation without the above mentioned discussion is essential. This chapter will point the difficulties in minicell production in the hyaluronic acid combination and then suggest the role of minicell production in drug resistance that may be the better way for cancer treatment.

### 2.1 Affects of hyaluronic acid in cell morphology in *Lactobacillus acidophilus*

In order to study the role of minicell formation, this chapter had also used probiotic named *Lactobacillus acidphilus* having a positive impact to the host by helping balance the intestinal flora. Relying on the benefit properties of *Lactobacillus acidphilus*, the new application of this probiotic in minicell formation is discussed in this chapter.

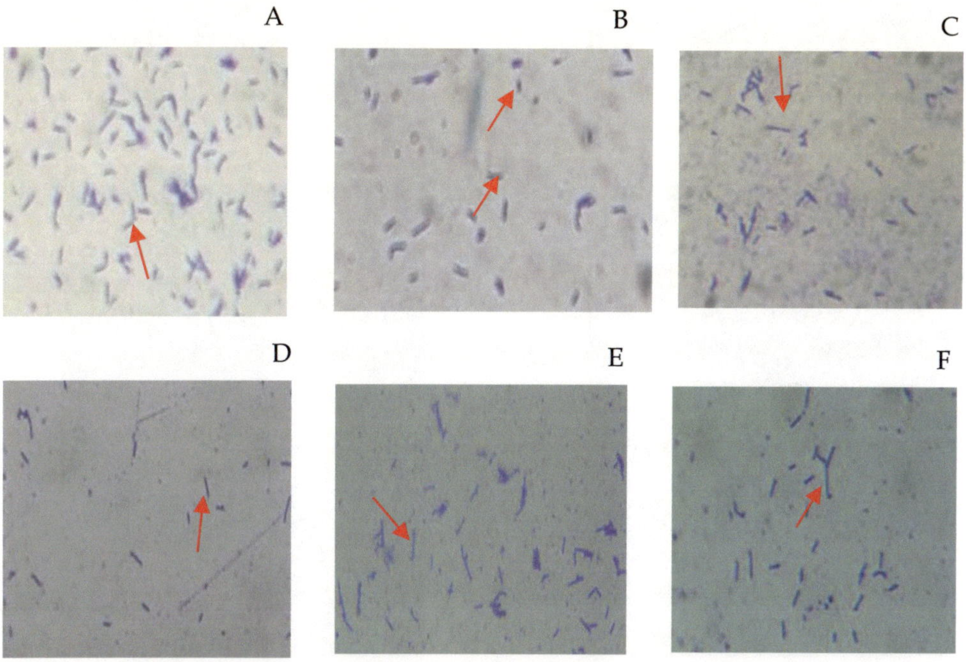


Fig. 1. The gram stainning of *L. acidophilus* with different HA concentration A: 0% ; B: 0.02%; C: 0.03% ; D: 0.05%; E: 0.08% ; F: 0.1%. The arrows showed the shape differentiation in medium with different concentration of hyaluronic acid.

The hypothesis was to apply a polymer named hyaluronic acid (HA) commonly used in foods, cosmetics, pharmaceutical field to form minicell. Besides, HA was also used to study in drug delivery. The delivery system prepared from *Lactobacillus acidophilus* and probiotic was thought to prevent many side effects in cancer treatment. *Lactobacillus acidophilus* was used and maintained in MRS agar and MRS broth. The incubation was performed at 25 - 30°C in anaerobic condition for 3-4 days. The HA was added into the MRS broth in 5 tubes to obtain the final concentrations as 0, 0.03%, 0.05%, 0.08% and 0.1%, respectively. *Lactobacillus acidophilus* in medium with 0.03%, 0.05% of HA was shorter than in the medium without HA (Fig.1C).

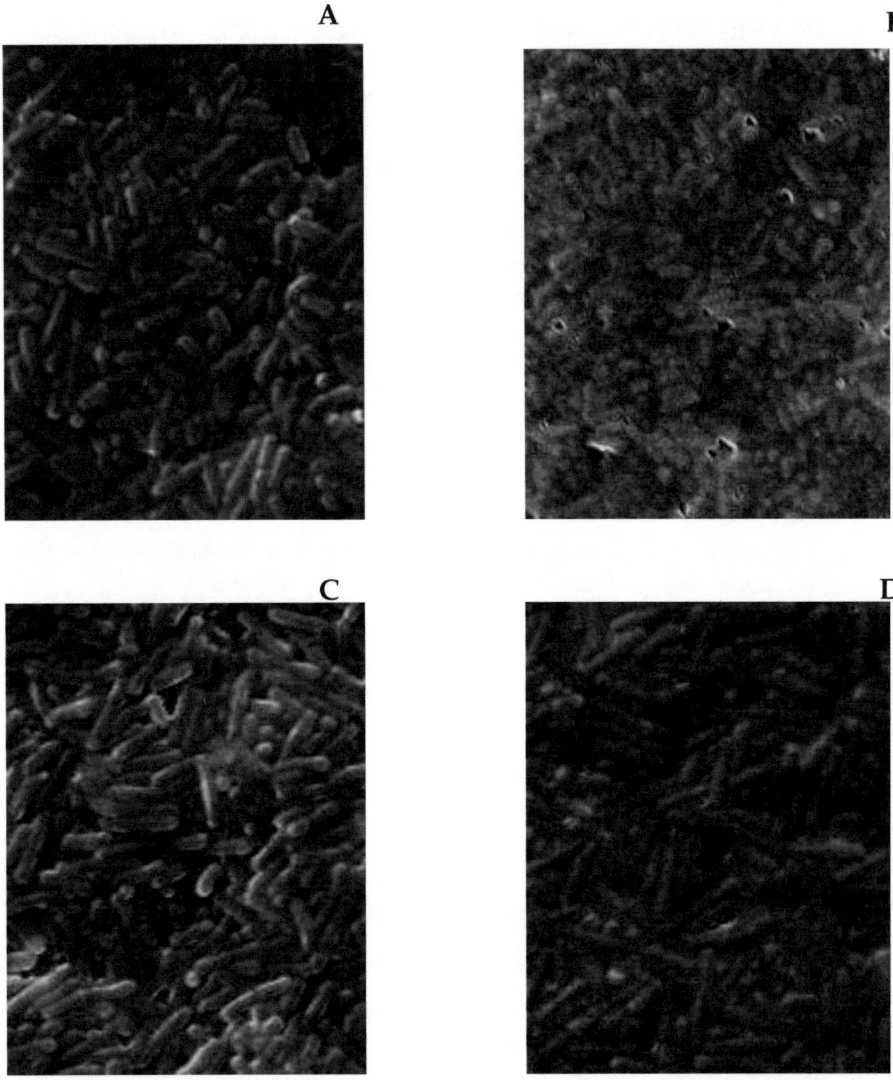


Fig. 2. *L. acidophilus* with HA concentration at A: 0%; B: 0.03%; C: 0.08%; D: 0.1% with the zoom out of 1.300 times of scanning electron microscope. Photographs of scanning electron microscope with the scale bar is 10μm.

The cell was shortest in the medium with 0.03% HA and become longer in the medium with 0.08% and 0.1% than in the medium without HA (Fig.1E and F). To confirm the morpholgical differentiation of *L. acidophilus* with HA, the scanning electron microscope was used to observe the cells and the results were showed (Fig.2 A, B, C, D).

The differentiation of cell caused by HA depends on the different HA concentration . This results showed that the minicell phenotype produced by HA were the simple way. Maybe HA participate in the gene expression in *Lactobacillus acidophilus* that will be studied so far. Therefore, looking for the new tools to form minicell is neccesary. The chapter suggested the way to produce minicell obviously for healthcare.

### 2.2 Cell division gene from bacteria in minicell production for therapy

#### 2.2.1 Min gene in cell division function

In *E. coli*, a number of proteins involved in cell division were identified by Hirota and co-workers who isolated thermo-sensitive mutants that failed to divide at elevated temperatures (Hirota et al., 1968). Since these mutants form long filaments, fts (filamentous temperature sensitive) was designated. Additional cell division proteins have been identified. For example, 10 proteins such as FtsZ, A, K, Q, L, B, W, I, N and ZipA, which are required for cell division, are known until now (Addinall & Holland, 2002; Buddelmeijer & Beckwith, 2002; Errington et al., 2003; Margolin, 2000; Rothfield et al., 1999). These 10 proteins assemble at the site of division into a multi-protein complex called the septal ring. Formation of this complex is thought to initiate with the assembly of FtsZ into a ring-like structure, the Z-ring, which requires the activity of at least one of the two essential FtsZ binding proteins, ZipA or FtsA (Pichoff & Lutkenhaus, 2002). Following addition of both ZipA and FtsA to the Z-ring, the remaining division proteins are recruited to mature the septal ring (Addinall & Holland, 2002; Buddelmeijer and Beckwith, 2002; Errington et al., 2003; Hale & de Boer, 2002; Mangolin, 2000; Pichoff & Lutkenhaus, 2002; Rothfield et al., 1999). After the assembly is completed, the proteins for the formation of the septal ring function in concert to mediate the coordinated invagination of three cell envelope layers such as the inner membrane, the peptidoglycan layer, and the outer membrane. Unfortunately, very little is known about the roles of many of the division proteins in this process. Spatital regulation of Z-ring assembly by the Min system is independent of nucleoid occlusion, which is evident in anucleate cells produced by chromosome segregation mutants. In the cells, the Z-rings assemble at or near mid-cell, suggesting that the Min system alone is sufficient to regulate the proper placement of the Z-ring (Sun et al., 1998). In contrast, in cells lacking a functional Min system, nucleoid occlusion is not sufficient to direct Z-ring assembly, and the division occurs consequently at any one of the three potential division sites dictated by the nucleoid occlusion. If the cell division occurs at a polar potential division site, a chromosomeless-minicell and a multinucleate filament are produced (Adler et al., 1967; de Boer et al., 1989). The first minicell mutant in *E. coli* has been isolated in 1967 (Adler et al., 1967). The mutations responsible for the minicell phenotype were mapped to the *minB* locus (Adler et al., 1967), which was later cloned and characterized (de Boer et al., 1989). The *minB* locus encodes three proteins, designated MinC, MinD, and MinE, all of which are required for proper the Min system function. In *B. subtilis*, the Min system includes MinC, MinD and DivIVA.

#### 2.2.2 MinC

MinC comprised of two domains of roughly equal size (de Boer et al., 1989; Hu & Lutkemhaus, 2001). The *N*-terminal domain interacts with FtsZ and is required and sufficient to inhibit FtsZ polymerization in vitro and Z-ring formation in vivo (Hu & Lutkenhaus, 2003). The mechanistic basis of this inhibition is unknown. The C-terminal domain is required for homodimerization of the protein and for interaction with activators of Min function, MinD and DicB (Hu & Lutkenhaus, 2003; Johnson et al., 2002; Szeto et al., 2001b). The DicB protein is encoded on the cryptic prophage Kim, and under normal conditions, expression of DicB is actively repressed (Cam et al., 1988). In the absence of these activators, MinC blocks cell division only when present at a level at least 25-fold greater than normal. In the presence of either activator, physiological levels of MinC are sufficient to inhibit division (de Boer et al., 1990; 1992b).

### 2.2.3 MinD

MinD is a part of the ParA superfamily of ATPase and is the most highly conserved of the Min proteins (Szeto et al., 2003). It generally associates with the inner membrane and is required for the binding and activation of MinC (Zhou et al., 2004). It contains five distinct domains. Three of which (P-loop, Switch I and Switch II) are thought to be important for ATP-binding (Gérard et al., 1998). The P-loop and switch II sites are deviant Walker A and B-type ATP binding motifs. Mutations in the P-loop, Switch I and Switch II domains are effective to ATP-binding causing the mislocalization of MinD and a concurrent mislocalization of MinC (Karoui et al., 2001). This suggests that ATP-binding is essential for membrane binding and activation of MinC. The ATPase domain is also required for an appropriate MinE-dependent localization to the cell poles (Maston et al., 1999b). Mutations in the ATPase domain of *B. subtilis* MinD are no longer restricted to the cell poles (Karoui et al., 2001). Instead, they diffuse throughout the inner membrane, suggesting a loss of interaction with DivIVA. However, MinD can localize to the division sites, in the presence or absence of DivIVA (Lee & Price, 1993). Mutations of the Switch I and Switch II in *E. coli* disrupt MinC activation, but not MinD localization (Zhou et al., 2004). Initial attempts for *B. subtilis* MinD with GFP (green fluorescence protein) at the C-terminal end have suggested that the protein does not function (Marston et al., 1998). Sequence analysis revealed a conserved C-terminal amphipathic helix (Hu et al., 2003; Szeto et al., 2002), that was likely disrupted by the addition of GFP. Even though structure prediction algorithms and the crystal structure failed to predict any membrane or membrane binding domains (Hayashi et al., 2001), deletion analysis has shown that the last 10 amino acids are required for membrane binding in *E. coli* (Zhou et al., 2003). *B. subtilis* also contains a C-terminal amphipathic helix required for membrane binding (Szeto et al., 2002). Truncations or mutations in this region disrupt MinD's ability to bind the membrane. Mutations that allow MinC activation but disrupt DivIVA interaction have also been identified (Karoui et al., 2001). *E. coli* MinD binds the membrane in an ATP-dependent manner in vitro (Lackner et al., 2003). MinD will associates with the phospholipids vesicles in the presence of ATP and $Mg^{2+}$, while the ADP-bound form will not. MinE stimulates the ATPase activity of MinD to release it from the membrane. Substitution with non hydrolysable forms of ATP cause MinD to remain associated with the membrane even in the presence of MinE. The ability of MinE to release MinD, and thus MinC, from the membrane is thought to be the driving force behind the oscillations in *E. coli* (Howard et al., 2001).

### 2.2.4 MinE

MinE is an 88 amino acid protein with two known functional domains. The *N*-terminal domain ( $^{D}$MinE, amino acids 1-33) is required and sufficient to interact with MinD and to counteract MinCD-mediated division inhibition (Huang et al., 1996). The C-terminal topological specificity domain ($^{TS}$MinE, amino acids 34-88) is required to suppress the inhibitory activities of MinCD specifically at mid-cell. Additionally, this domain mediates homodimerization of the protein (King et al., 1999; 2000; Pichoff et al., 2002). The structure of the C-terminal domain has been solved (King et al., 2000), revealing that the protein dimerizes in an anti-parallel fashion. The *N*-terminal domain is not shown in the structure, but is predicted to be a nascent helix (King et al., 1999).

### 2.2.5 DivIVA

A major difference between *E. coli* and *B. subtilis* is that *B. subtilis* uses DivIVA to sequester MinCD to the cell poles. Unlike the MinCD oscillations caused by MinE in *E. coli*, the localization of *B. subtilis* MinCD is static (Edwards et al., 1997). Furthermore, *E. coli* does not contain a DivIVA homologue, nor does *B. subtilis* have a MinE homologue (Lee & Price, 1993). DivIVA in *B. subtilis* is a 19.5 kDa protein, but soluble DivIVA exists as a 145 kDa oligomer *in vivo* (Muchova et al., 2002). The structure of membrane associated DivVIA (~40%) remains unknown. Transmissible electron microscope images of DivIVA (Glu162Lys), a functional point mutant, reveals a 'doggy-bone' like structure capable of further assembly into two dimensional structures (Stahler et al., 2004). DivIVA localizes to the poles and midcell division sites, sometime, during the assembly of the cell division machinery. The timing and mechanism of localization is still unclear. After division, DivIVA remaining at the division sites is not essential, however. DivIVA must then have some function beyond that of localizing MinCD. DivIVA$_{SC}$ from the *S. coelicolor*, which is homologues to DivIVA from *Bacillus subtilis*, is essential and directly involved in hyphal tip growth and morphogenesis. A DivIVA$_{SC}$-EGFP hybrid was distinctively localized to hyphal tips and lateral branches. DivIVA$_{SC}$ is a novel bacterial morphogenesis, and it is closely localized at the apical sites of peptidoglycan assembly in *Streptomyces* hyphae.

### 2.2.6 Min system dynamics regulate the activity of MinC

The cell division is determined by the cellular distribution of MinC, which is regulated by both MinD and MinE. In addition, MinD and MinE influence the other cellular distribution. MinD, MinC and MinE are cytoplasmic, and MinC is unable to efficiently inhabit Z-ring assembly (Hu & Lutkenhaus, 2001). As a result, cells show a minicelling division phenotype (Min cells), where the cells frequently divide close to either cell pole (de Boer et al., 1989). In MinE cells, MinC and MinD are assembled along the entire membrane. This static, uniform distribution of MinC blocks the Z-ring assembly at all sites, resulting in the formation of long, non-septate filamentous cell (Sep-cells) (de Boer et al., 1989; Hu & Lutkenhaus, 2001; Rowland et al., 2000). In cells expressing three Min proteins (MinC, D and E), a wild-type scenario, MinC undergoes a rapid and dynamic localization cycle in which the protein oscillates from one cell pole to other every 20-30 seconds (Hu and Lutkenhaus, 2001). As the result of this pole-to-pole oscillation, the time-averaged concentration of the division inhibitor is greatest as the cell poles and lowest at mid-cell, and this concentration differential is proposed to direct Z-ring assembly to mid-cell (Hale et al., 2001; Howard et al., 2001; Huang et al., 2003; Kruse, 2002; Meinhardt and de Boer, 2001). This dynamic distribution of MinC is driven by MinD and MinE, which themselves undergo a coupled oscillatory localization cycle (Hale et al., 2001, Shih et al., 2002). At the start of this cycle, MinD and a portion of MinE assemble on the membrane along one half of the cell in a pattern resembling a test tube (MinD/E tube), while another portion of MinE assembles at the rim of this tube forming a ring (E-ring). The MinD/E tube undergoes a continuous cycle of disassembly from the membrane at one cell end and concurrent reassembly on the membrane at the opposite cell end. The E-ring closely follows the location of the MinD/E tube, always appearing to be associated with its rim. MinC plays no role in the mechanism of oscillation, and the cellular location of MinC follows that of MinD (Hale et al., 2001; Rowland et al., 2000). While the MinD/E tube and E-ring do not appear to have an underlying structure in live cells analyzed by conventional 2-dimensional fluorescence microscopy, spiral-like accumulations of the proteins in what would represent the MinD/E tube and E-ring have been observed in fixed cells analyzed by 3-dimensional deconvolution microscopy. This observation suggests that the bulk of Min protein dynamics occurs along spiral tracks within the cell (Shih et al., 2003).

### 2.2.7 MinCD during sporulation

Deletions in the MinCD locus cause a decrease in sporulation of nearly ten fold (Barak et al., 1998) although the relative sporulation efficiency is nearly identical to wild-type. The cause of the decrease is unclear as MinCD's role in sporulation has not been well examined. *B. subtilis* with null mutations in MinCD form thin, sporulation like septa at the midcell, suggesting that MinCD is helpful to inhibit sporulation septa from forming at the midcell. Since its role during vegetative growth is to prevent FtsZ ring formation at the poles, MinCD may also trigger the switch from midcell division to polar division in conjunction with spo0A. It's also been suggested that MinCD confers polarity to SpoIIIE dependent chromosome translocation by inhibiting the assembly of forespore expressed SpoIIIE (Sharp et al., 2002). In the absence of MinCD, SpoIIIE can assemble on the forespore side of the septum and can reverse translocate DNA into the mother cell leading to anucleate forespores.

### 2.2.8 Conservation of Min proteins

MinD is well conserved among many bacteria and archaea and is also found in number of eukaryotic chloroplasts (Gérard et al., 1998). Interestingly, this high degree of conservation is not shared with MinC and/or MinE suggesting that the mechanism by which MinD homologues lack MinC and/or MinE regulates division site placement is not conserved in all organisms (Margolin, 2000; Rothfield et al., 1999). For example, *B. subtilis* has both MinC and MinD but lacks MinE. In *B. subtilis*, DivIVA imparts topological specificity to MinCD-mediated division inhibition in a manner very different from that of MinE (Cha & Stewart, 1997). DivIVA, which stably associates with cell poles, recruits MinCD to the poles and thereby, spatially restricts the inhibitory activity of the complex to the polar potential division sites (Marston & Errington, 1999b; Marston et al., 1998). Therefore, the Min protein oscillation is not required to spatially regulate the Z-ring assembly in all organisms.

### 2.2.9 Minicells in cancer treatment

Molecularly targeted drugs such as cell cycle inhibitors are being developed to achieve a higher degree of tumor cell specificity and reduce toxic side effects. Unfortunately, relative to the cytotoxics, many of the molecularly targeted drugs are less potent and the target protein is expressed only at certain stages of the cell cycle thus necessitating regimens like continuous infusion therapy to arrest a significant number of tumor cells in a heterogeneous tumor mass (Jennifer et al., 2007). Therefore, trend to produce minicells or nanocells from non-pathogen bacteria is essential. The minicells were made from bacteria and contained pieces of genetic material, known as short interference RNA (siRNA), which knockout or "silence" the drug-resistant genes of tumours. Bacterial membranes might be quite different because they have protein channels (in their membrane) through which siRNAs can enter (Jennifer et al., 2009). By means of the receptors in the tumor surface, the minicell will specify and deliver the drugs to the tumors. Minicells are produce by minicell producing parent cells. These parent cells undergo cell division in an abnormal manner that produces a chromosomal-containing cell and a minicell lacking a copy of the parental chromosome. Minicells are often smaller than their parent cells. For example, minicells produced from E. coli are generally spherical in shape and are about 0.1 to about 0.3 μm, whereas whole E. coli cells are about 2 to about 10μm in length. The minicell can be tagged with siRNA that is also play a role in disease prevention and drug resistant reduce. It was discovered that an unprecedented concentration of one million to ten million drug molecules can be packaged within a minicell. In contrast, other nanovectors such as liposomes have been shown to package ~10,000 molecules of drug within each liposome. Similarly, armed antibodies can conjugate only four to ten drug molecules per antibody. The potency of observed anti-tumor effects may depend on the concentration of a drug that is delivered intracellularly within cancer cells. At present, the cancer treatment is the big pressure in the world because of the high cost for treatment such as the high price of monoclonal antibodies. This is the difficulties of the pharmaceutical companies which did not supply enough demands wheras minicell will made the cost reduce and delivers the small amounts of many drugs intracellularly and then decrease the drug resistance of the cell (Jennifer et al., 2007). To get improvement of minicells, the research of *min* gene encoding for cell division will be done to understand about the new approach for drug treatment. The *min* gene was cloned and studied for the function. The generated minicells or nanocells during gene expression will be used to study as the drug delivery to cancer cell.

### 2.2.10 Role of *min* gene from *Streptomyces lavendulae* in minicell formation for therapy

There are many cell division genes in bacteria summarized as above. However, only one *minD* gene exists in the human chromosome. To understand the role of minicell in drug delivery in human, the study tried to find the diversity of *minD* gene in the bacteria which have the linear structure as human chromosome that belong to *Streptomyces. Streptomyces* have a complex morphological differentiation and are well-known for their ability to produce an enormous variety of bioactive secondary metabolites, such as antibiotics and immunosuppressant drugs (Wright et al., 1976b).The *minD* gene *Streptomyces coelicolor* and *Streptomyces avernitilis* genome have been sequenced completely (Ikeda et al., 2003; Betley et al., 2002). In *Streptomyces*, there are *minD1*, *minD2* or *minD3* depending on the these strains. Clearly, the *min* gene cluster has also tried to obtain in *Streptomyces lavendulae*. Because *Streptomyces coelicolor* and *Streptomyces avernitilis* are well studied, the aim of the *minD* gene study focused on *Streptomyces lavendulae*. The cloned *min* gene was expressed in many way to analyze the functional regulations of cell division. The goal is to develop the effects of Min homolog harbored by *Streptomyces* in morphological change, especially the minicell and filamentous morphology in *Escherichia coli*. The minicells generated by *min* gene expression gave many hopes for cancer- targeted drug delivery in cancer therapy while the chemotherapeutic therapy used nowadays are not specific but also toxic to cancer cell.

The introduction of *min* gene with the sequence containing 49 nucleotides at upstream of *min* gene gave the apparent morphological alteration into minicells when using the pET 28a(+) as expression vector while the introduction of *min* gene gave the filamentous under the pET 21a(+). To construct *E. coli* expressing the *S. lavendulae min* gene, a PCR with primers as 5′- CAC*CATATG*ACCACTCGAATCCTCCCCGC- 3′ and 5′- CAC*CTCGAG*GCC CTCCCGGCCGCGC- 3′ was performed. The product was treated with *NdeI* and *XhoI* (italic sites), and inserted into pET 21a(+) to create pET 21a(+)/*min*. To amplify upregulated-*min* gene (*min* containing 49-bp upstream of *min*), PCR primers (5′-GGA*ATTC*CAGTCCCACCGACCGCACGTAC-3′and 5′-CCG*CTCGAG*CGGGCCACGAGC AGCAGGATC-3) were designed. The resulting amplified product was digested with *EcoRI* and *XhoI* (italic sites) and inserted into pET 28a(+) to create pET 28a(+)/upregulated-*minDSL*.

Transformation the constructed plasmids in *E. coli* were performed. *E. coli* BL21(DE3) harboring pET 21a(+)/*min* and pET 28a(+)/upregulated-*min* was grown at 37°C in 1L of an LB medium to OD600=0.5, whereupon isopropyl-D-thiogalacto-pyranoside (IPTG) was added to culture at the final concentration of 0.5 mM to induce the expression of Min. The *E. coli* cells were grown for 5.5 h at 28°C and observed by microscope. Introduction of pET 21a(+)/*min* into *E. coli* BL21(DE3) cell caused a filamentous shape, as observed by a light microscope (Fig. 3B) and scanning electron microscope (Fig. 3D). The investigation of

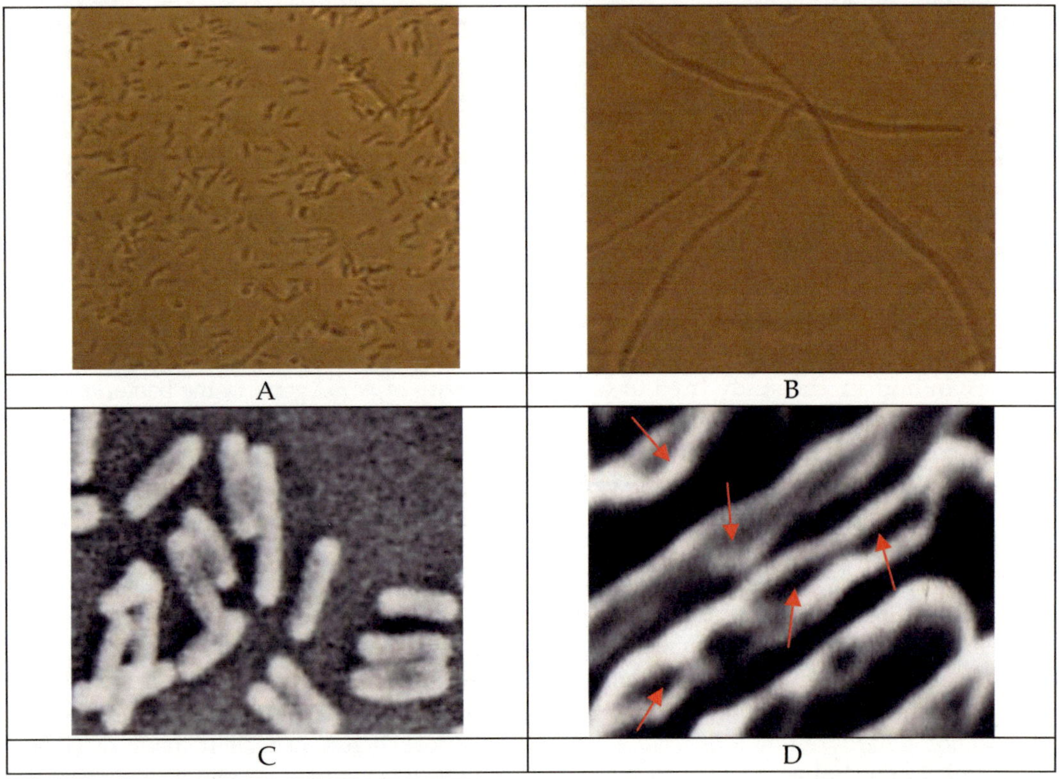


Fig. 3. The cell shapes of *E. coli* BL21 (DE3) carrying *min* gene when using pET 21a(+) as an expression vector. (A) and (B) are the pictures filmed by light microscope, but (C) and (D) are the picture filmed by scanning electron microscope. *E. coli* BL21 (DE3) transformed with pET 21a(+) is a typical rod shape, as shown in (A) and (C). The same host transformed with pET 21a(+)/*min* exhibits a filamentous phenotype, as shown in (B) and (D). Red arrows show the indentations along the cells.Photographs of light microscope with the scale bar is 5 m, and both figures are at the same magnification. Photographs of scanning electron microscope with the scale bar is 1 m.

minicell production indicates that the production of minicells is blocked when maltose was added in the culture. By the microscopic analysis, the indentations in the cell wall of *E. coli* reflect the *min* gene may be play a role in cellular mechanism. The relationship between phenotype differentiation and drug resistance was not clear. However, in the *E. coli* system with the overexpression of MinCDE, the function of *min* gene from *Streptomyces* was activated by means of the putative primary promoter upstream of *min* gene along with the

selective conditions of environment. The interaction between Min proteins in *E. coli* in the different cultured conditions maybe also affected on the cells. This hypothesis should be studied before the minicells formed by this way will be applied in treatment.
To facilitate further study the function of Min protein, the *E. coli* BL21(DE3) carrying the pET 28a(+)/upregulated-*min* gene carrying plasmid was overexpressed. Under the presence of IPTG, the transformant took a minicell phenotype (Fig. 4B), whereas the same cell transformed with pET 28a(+) exhibited a normal rod-shaped morphology (Fig. 4A). The minicells are produced by a process that is similar to the normal cell division except that it occurs near one or both poles of the cell. The division process, that generates the minicells,

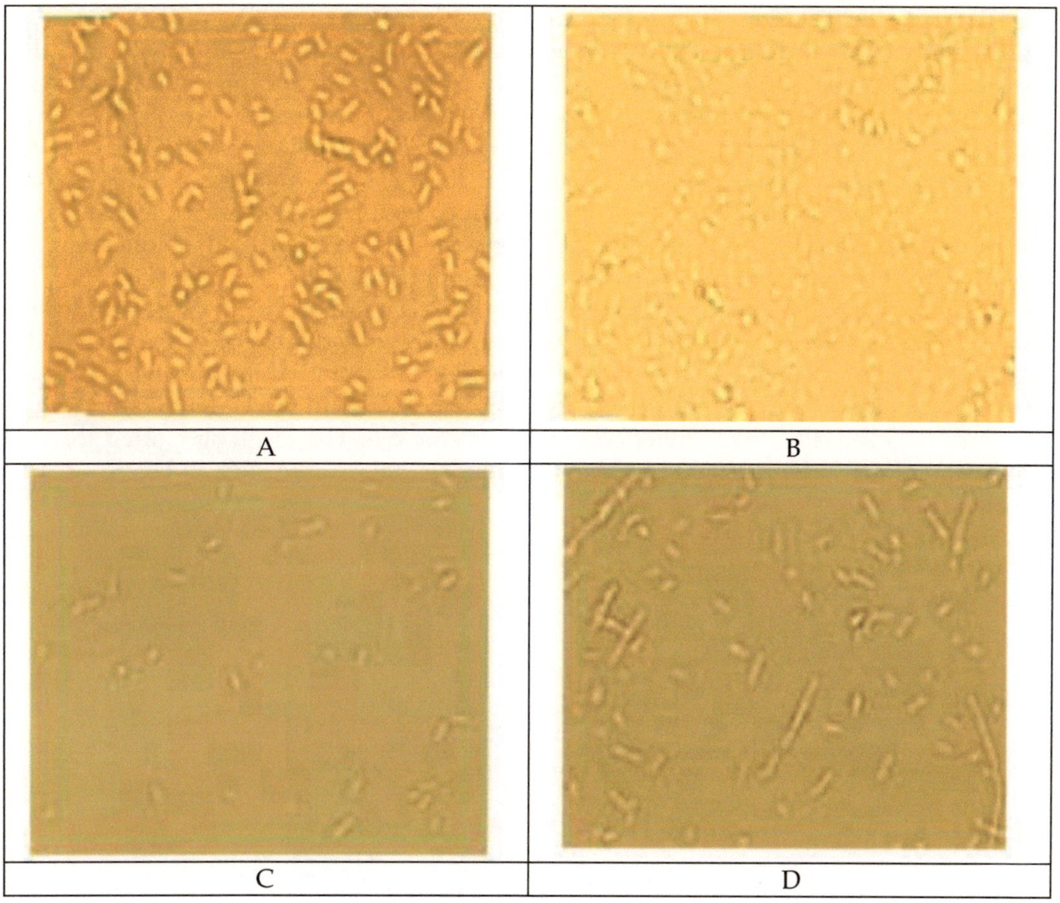


Fig. 4. The cell shapes of *E. coli* BL21 (DE3) carrying *min* gene when using pET 28a(+) as an expression vector.(A) *E.coli* BL21(DE3) cells were transformed with pET 28a(+). (B) *E. coli* BL21(DE3) cells were transformed pET 28a(+)/upregulated-*min*. (C) Phenotype of *E.coli* BL21 (DE3) cells were transformed with pET 28a(+) in LB medium supplemented with maltose (1%). (D) *E. coli* BL21(DE3) cells were transformed pET 28a(+)/ upregulated-*min* in LB medium supplemented with maltose (1%). Photographs of light microscope with the scale bar is 5m, and both figures are at the same magnification.

seems to be "normal" in many ways. In this case, DNA is not distributed to both sides of the division plane. The production of minicells is a consequence of the unusual genetic constitution and does not require any unusual manipulation of the environment. They has anticipated that the minicell phenotype will be valuable in a variety of genetic and biochemical studies. During morphological change in bacteria, the Min expression caused different solubility (Nguyen et al., 2008; Nguyen, 2010). Because the morphological change, the physiological differentiation concerning to drug resistant may also be effected. That is the why min gene is essential for cell division and viability in *E. coli*. The *E. coli* BL21(DE3) carrying the pET 28a(+)/upregulated-*min* carrying plasmid was overexpressed under the presence of maltose, the cell are longer than the *E. coli* BL21(DE3) carrying the pET 28a(+) (Fig. 4C, D). In a conclusion, the overexpression of *S. lavendulae minDSL* in *E. coli* causes the cellular shape change. That is the consequence of the *min* gene in fused construction that results in the filamentous shape, whereas the native Min corrects the minicell phenotype in *E. coli* (Fig. 4B). Since the minicell phenotype will be valuable in a variety of genetic and biochemical studies, a native Min protein was purified. After *E. coli* BL21 (DE3) carrying *min* was grown, the cell mass was collected in the inclusion body from the cell-free extract. Washing the inclusion body with 1% n-decyl-D-glucopyranoside was useful to reduce the contaminated proteins. The washed inclusion body was dissolved in a buffer containing 1% n-decyl-D-maltopyranoside. The Min protein was purified from the inclusion body, as described in the experimental procedures section. The Min protein was purified to homogeneity, as shown in Fig. 5. This procedure showed the difference of the native Min protein properties from the tagged one. The experiment pointed out the morphological differentiation as well as the different expressing ways caused by *min* gene. Probably the *min* gene of *Streptomyces* had any effects on *Escherichia coli*. The result supported that the application of minicells obtained by this procedure should be studied well before used as drug delivery.

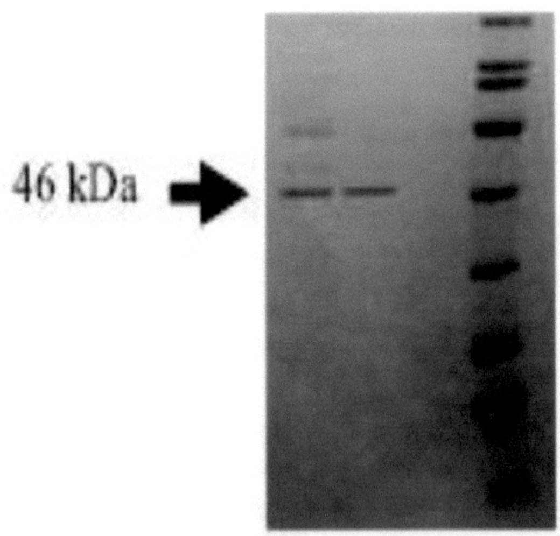


Fig. 5. Purification of Min protein was analyzed by Tricine-SDS-PAGE. The arrow showed the purified 46 kDa of Min protein after it was dissolved in a buffer containing 1% n-decyl-D-maltopyranoside.

Because there were the shape changes in *E. coli* transformed by these constructions as pET 21a(+), pET 28a(+), pET 21a(+)/ *min*, pET 28a(+)/upregulated-*min*, the drug resistance assay of minicells was also performed curiously. Interestingly, there was also drug resistance. The test was measured the turbidity after the *E. coli* were cultured with D-cycloserine at the interval time. To investigate the role of *min* gene in antibiotic resistance, the D-cycloserine resistant assay was performed. The results were in fig. 6. Remarkably, the resistance in minicells carrying pET 28a(+)/upregulated-*min* was the highest than the filament cells pET 21a(+)/ *min* and other controls. As the result, the minicell formation will give a mission in drug delivery and drug resistance in tuberculosis but in cancer diseases. More studies will be done so far to explain the mechanisms and to give more design for drug delivery in cancer therapy.

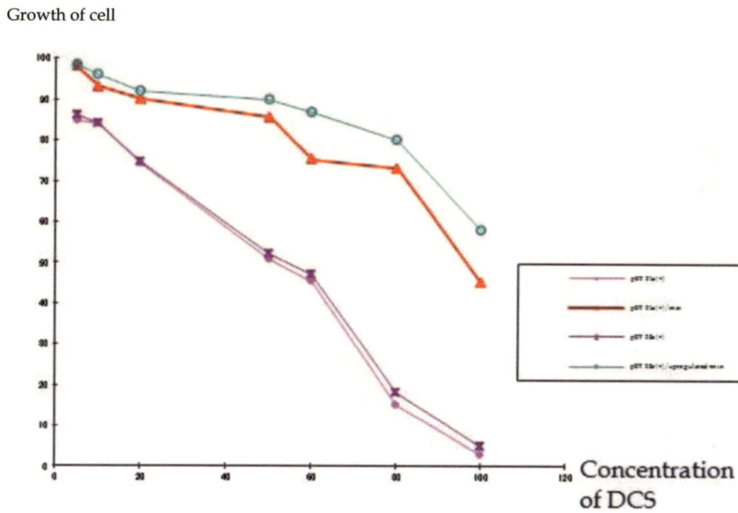


Fig. 6. D-cycloserine resistance assay in *E. coli*. the resistance in minicells carrying pET 28a(+)/upregulated-*min* was the highest than the filament cells pET 21a(+)/ *min* and the controls.

## 3. Conclusion

The phenotype differentiation and drug resistance in *Escherichia coli* were not clear. However, by the microscopic analysis, the indentations in the cell wall reflect that *min* may play a role in cellular mechanism. Our experiment suggests the considerations that bacterial shapes are not accidental but are biologically important. In the *E. coli* system with the overexpression of MinCDE, the function of Min protein from *S. lavendulae* was activated by means of the putative primary promoter upstream of *min* gene along with the selective conditions of environment. The chapter showed the effects of *min* gene of *Streptomyces* in *E. coli* in the formation of minicell phenotype which may participate in drug resistance that is interested in cancer treatment and vaccine preparation. The minicells produced by the expression of *min* gene with the upstream gave the high resistance of D-cycloserine, an antibiotic for tuberculosis treatment. This chapter provided the benefit of bacterial minicells which play in drug delivery and resistant to the drug used in cancer treatment. In the other hands, the *min* gene in human containing F1-ATPase is also similar to *min* genes bacteria. The purified Min protein (Fig. 5) showed the activity of an ATPase (data not shown). The molecular dynamics of the F1-ATPase at the molecular level will be studied to develop the biomolecular devices as nanomolecular machines for therapy.

## 4. References


Addinall, S.G., and Holland, B. (2002). The tubulin ancestor, FtsZ, draughtsman, designer and driving force for bacterial cytokinesis. *J. Mol. Biol.* 318, 219-236.

Adler, H.I., Fisher, W.D., Cohen, A., and Hardigree, A.A. (1967) Miniature *Escherichia coli* cells deficient in DNA. *Proc. Natl. Acad. Sci. USA* 57, 321-326.

Barak, I., Prepiak, P., Schmeisser, F. (1998) MinCD proteins control the septation process during sporulation of *Bacillus subtilis*. *J. Bacteriol. 180(20)*, 5327-5333.

Bentley SD, Chater KF, Cerdeno-Tarraga AM, Challis GL, Thomson NR, James KD, Harris DE, Quail MA, Kieser H, Harper D et al. (2002) Complete genome sequence of the model actinomycete *Streptomyces coelicolor* A3(2). *Nature* 417: 141–147

Buddelmeijer, N., and Beckwith, J. (2002) Assembly of cell division proteins at the *E. coli* cell center. *Curr. Opin. Microbiol.* 5, 553-557.

Cam, K., Béjar, S., Gil, D., and Bouché, J.P. (1988) Identification and sequence of division inhibitor gene dicB suggests expression from an internal in-frame translation start. *Nucleic Acids Res.* 16, 6327-6338.

Cha, J.H., and Stewart, G.C. (1997) The divIVA minicell locus of *Bacillus subtilis*. *J. Bacteriol.* 179, 1671-1683.

de Boer, P.A.J., Crossley, R.E., and Rothfield, L.I. (1989) A division inhibitor and a topological specificity factor coded for by the minicell locus determine proper placement of the division septum in *E. coli*. *Cell* 56, 641-649.

de Boer, P.A.J., Crossley, R.E., and Rothfield, L.I. (1990) Central role for the *Escherichia coli* minC gene product in two different cell division-inhibition systems. *Proc. Natl. Acad. Sci.USA* 87, 1129-1133.

de Boer, P.A.J., Crossley, R.E., and Rothfield, L.I. (1992b) Roles of MinC and MinD in the site-specific septation block mediated by the MinCDE system of *Escherichia coli*. *J. Bacteriol.* 174, 63-70.

Edwards, D.H., and Errington, J. (1997) The *Bacillus subtilis* DivIVA protein targets to the division septum and controls the site specificity of cell division. *Mol. Microbiol.* 24(5), 905-915.

Errington, J., Daniel, R.A., and Scheffers, D.J. (2003) Cytokinesis in bacteria. *Microbiol. Mol. Biol. Rev.* 67, 52-65.

Gérard, E., Labedan, B., and Forterre, P. (1998) Isolation of a minD-like gene in the hyperthermophilic archaeon *Pyrococcus* AL585, and phylogenetic characterization of related proteins in the three domains of life. *Gene* 222, 99-106.

Hale, C.A., and de Boer, P.A.J. (2002) ZipA is required for recruitment of FtsK, FtsQ, FtsL, and FtsN to the septal ring in *Escherichia coli*. *J. Bacteriol.* 184, 2552-2556.

Hale, C.A., Meinhardt, H., and de Boer, P.A.J. (2001) Dynamic localization cycle of the cell division regulator MinE in *E. coli*. *EMBO J.* 20, 1563-1572.

Hayashi, I., Oyama, T., and Morikawa, K. (2001) Structural and functional studies of MinD ATPase: implications for the molecular recognition of the bacterial cell division apparatus. *EMBO J.* 20, 1819-1828.

Hirota, Y., Ryter, A., and Jacob, F. (1968) Thermosensitive mutants of *E. coli* affected in the process of DNA synthesis and cellular division. *Cold Spring Harbor Symp Quant. Biol.* 33, 677-693.

Howard, M., Rutenberg, A.D., and de Vet, S. (2001) Dynamic compartmentalization of bacteria: Accurate division in *E. coli*. *Phys. Rev. Lett.* 87, 278102.

Hu, Z., and Lutkenhaus, J. (2001) Topological Regulation of Cell Division in *E. coli*. Spatiotemporal Oscillation of MinD Requires Stimulation of its ATPase by MinE and Phospholipid. *Mol. Cell* 7, 1337-1343.

Hu, Z., Saez, C., and Lutkenhaus, J. (2003) Recruitment of MinC, an inhibitor of Z-Ring formation, to the membrane in Escherichia coli: Role of MinD and MinE. *J. Bacteriol.* 185, 196-203.

Huang, J., Cao, C., and Lutkenhaus, J. (1996) Interaction between FtsZ and inhibitors of cell division. *J. Bacteriol.* 178, 5080-5085.

Ikeda H, Ishikawa J, Hanamoto A, Shinose M et al. (2003) Complete genome sequence and comparative analysis of the industrial microorganism *Streptomyces avernitilis*. *Nat Biotechnol* 21: 526-531.

Jennifer AM, Nancy BA et al. (2007) Sequential treatment of drugresistant tumors with targeted minicells containing siRNA of a cytotoxic drug. *Nat Biotech* 27: 643-654

Jennifer AM, Nancy BA, Jocelyn M, Ilya S, Stefanie W, Kartini K, Vatsala NB, Leo P, Scott TP, Carlotta P (2009) Sequential treatment of drug-resistant tumors with targeted minicells containing siRNA or a cytotoxic drug. *Nat Biotechnology* 27: 643-651

Johnson, J.E., Lackner, L.L., and de Boer, P.A.J. (2002) Targeting of DMinC/MinD and DMinC/DicB complexes to septal rings in *Escherichia coli* suggests a multistep mechanism for MinC-mediated destruction of nascent FtsZ-rings. *J. Bacteriol.* 184, 2951-2962.

Karoui, M.E., and Errington, J. (2001) Isolation and characterization of topological specificity mutants of minD in *Bacillus subtilis*. *Mol. Microbiol.* 42, 1211-1221.

King, G.F., Rowland, S.L., Pan, B., Mackay, J.P., Mullen, G.P., and Rothfield, L.I. (1999) The dimerization and topological specificity functions of MinE reside in a structurally autonomous C-terminal domain. *Mol. Microbiol.* 31, 1161-1169.

King, G.F., Shih, Y.L., Maciejewski, M.W., Bains, N.P., Pan, B., Rowland, S.L., Mullen, G.P., and Rothfield, L.I. (2000) Structural basis for the topological specificity function of MinE. *Nat. Struct. Biol.* 7, 1013-1017.

Kruse, K. (2002) A dynamic model for determining the middle of *Escherichia coli*. *Biophys. J.* 82, 618-627.

Lackner, L.L., Raskin, D.M., and de Boer, P.A. (2003) ATP-dependent interactions between *Escherichia coli* Min proteins and the phospholipid membrane in vitro. *J. Bacteriol.* 185, 735-749.

Lee, S., Price, C.W. (1993) The minCD locus of *Bacillus subtilis* lacks the minE determinant that provides topological specificity to cell division. *Mol. Microbiol.* 7, 601-610.

Margolin, W. (2000). Themes and variations in prokaryotic cell division. *FEMS Microbiol. Rev.* 24, 531-548.

Marston, A.L., and Errington, J. (1999b) Selection of the midcell division site in *Bacillus subtilis* through MinD-dependent polar localization and activation of MinC. *Mol. Microbiol.* 33, 84-96.

Marston, A.L., Thomaides, H.B., Edwards, D.H., Sharpe, M.E., and Errington, J. (1998) Polar localization of the MinD protein of *Bacillus subtilis* and its role in selection of the mid-cell division site. *Genes & Dev.* 12, 3419-3430.

Meinhardt, H., and de Boer, P.A.J. (2001) Pattern formation in *Escherichia coli*: A model for the pole-to-pole oscillations of Min proteins and the localization of the division site. *Proc. Natl. Acad. Sci. U S A* 98, 14202-14207.

Muchova, K., Kutejova, E., Scott, D., Brannigan, J.A., Lewis, R.J., Wilkenson, A.J., Barak, I. (2002) Oligomerization of the *Bacillus subtilis* division protein DivIVA. *Microbiology* 148, 807-813.

Nguyen HKT, Kumagai T, Matoba Y, Sugiyama M (2008) Molecular cloning and functional analysis of minD gene from *Streptomyces lavendulae* ATCC 25233. *J Bioscience Bioeng* 106(3): 303-305

Nguyen HKT (2010) Regulations of cell division from Streptomyces that may play an important role in drug resistance. *Proceedings of the 3rd International Conference on the Development of BME in Vietnam*, 11-14th, Jan 2010: 170-173.

Pichoff, S., and Lutkenhaus, J. (2002) Unique and overlapping roles for ZipA and FtsA in septal ring assembly in *Escherichia coli*. *EMBO J* 21, 685-693.

Rothfield, L., Justice, S., and García-Lara, J. (1999) Bacterial cell division. *Annu. Rev. Genet.* 33, 423-448.

Rowland, S.L., Fu, X., Sayed, M.A., Zhang, Y., Cook, W.R., and Rothfield, L.I. (2000) Membrane redistribution of the *Escherichia coli* MinD protein induced by MinE. *J. Bacteriol.* 182, 613-619.

Sharp, MD., Pogliano, K. (2002) MinCD-dependent regulation of the polarity of SpoIIIE assembly and DNA transfer. *EMBO J.* 21(22), 6267-74.

Shih, Y.L., Fu, X., King, G.F., Le, T., and Rothfield, L. (2002) Division site placement in *E. coli*: mutations that prevent formation of the MinE ring lead to loss of the normal midcell arrest of growth of polar MinD membrane domains. *EMBO J.* 21, 3347-3357.

Shih, Y. L., Le, T., and Rothfield, L. (2003) Division site selection in *Escherichia coli* involves dynamic redistribution of Min proteins within coiled structures that extend between the two cell poles. *Proc. Natl. Acad. Sci. USA* 100, 7865-7870.

Stahler, H., Kutejova, E., Muchova, K., Gregorini, M., Lustig, A., Muller, SA., Olivieri, V., Engel, A., Wilkinson, AJ., Barak, I. (2004) Oligomeric structure of *Bacillus subtilis* cell division protein DivIVA determined by transmission electron microscopy. *Mol. Microbiol.* 52(5), 1281-1290.

Sun, Q., and Margolin, W. (1998) FtsZ dynamics during the division cycle of live *Escherichia coli* cells. *J. Bacteriol.* 180, 2050-2056.

Szeto, T.H., Rowland, S.L., and King, G.F. (2001b) The dimerization function of MinC resides in a structurally autonomous C-terminal domain. *J. Bacteriol.* 183, 6684-6687.

Szeto, T.H., Rowland, S.L., Habrukowich, C.L., and King, G.F. (2003) The MinD membrane targeting sequence is a transplantable lipid-binding helix. *J. Biol. Chem.* 278, 40050-40056.

Wright, L.F., Howood, D.A. (1976b) Actinorhdin is a chromosomally determined antibiotic in *Streptomyces coelicolor* A3(2). J. Gen. Microbiol. 96, 289-297.

Zhou, H., and Lutkenhaus, J. (2004) The switch I and II regions of MinD are required for binding and activating MinC. *J. Bacteriol.* 186, 1546-1555.

# 5

# Vascular-Targeted Photodynamic Therapy (VTP)

Ezatul Ezleen Kamarulzaman[1,4], Hamanou Benachour[2], Muriel Barberi-Heyob[2,5], Céline Frochot[3,5], Habibah A Wahab[4], François Guillemin[2,5] and Régis Vanderesse[1,5]

*[1]Laboratoire de Chimie Physique Macromoléculaire (LCPM)*
*Nancy-University, CNRS, Nancy*
*[2]Centre de Recherche en Automatique de Nancy, Nancy-University, CNRS, Centre Alexis Vautrin, Vandœuvre-lès-Nancy*
*[3]Laboratoire Réactions et Génie des Procédés (LRGP), Nancy-University, CNRS, Nancy*
*[4]School of Pharmaceutical Sciences, Universiti Sains Malaysia, Penang*
*[5]GDR CNRS 3049 "Médicaments Photoactivables – Photochimiothérapie(PHOTOMED)"*
*[1, 2, 3, 5]France*
*[4]Malaysia*

## 1. Introduction

Despite recent advances in surgery, chemotherapy, and radiation treatment, survival of patients with advanced malignancy remains suboptimal. Photodynamic therapy (PDT) is now established as a clinical treatment modality for various diseases including cancer (Dougherty et al., 1998). PDT involves the combined action of a photosensitizer, visible light of an appropriate wavelength and molecular oxygen to produce reactive oxygen species (ROS) like singlet oxygen, a short-lived species with highly cytotoxic effect (Dougherty et al., 1998, Solban et al., 2005). In biological system, the generated ROS trigger a cascade of biochemical effects that result in cell death. Singlet oxygen is thought to be the main mediator of cellular death, involving apoptotic and necrotic responses within treated tumours and produces microvascular injury leading to inflammation and hypoxia. PDT effects are mediated not only through direct killing of tumour cells but also through indirect effects, which involve both the initiation of an immune response against tumour cells and the destruction of tumour neovasculature. Indeed, the vascular effect plays a critical role in the eradication of tumour by PDT as it may cause deprivation of life-sustaining nutrients and oxygen supply from the existing blood vessels of the surrounding tissue. This present chapter will focus on recent and significant advances and developments in targeting strategies in PDT with the emphasis on vascular target specificity.

## 2. Targeted photodynamic therapy

In cancer treatment, PDT is a locoregional treatment used to reduce the volume of a tumour mass and obtain a radical cure of a small superficial tumour. PDT has been developed for the treatment of various cancers, e.g. esophagus (Radu et al., 2000), bronchi (Metz & Friedberg 2001, Savary et al., 1997), and bladder (Guillemin et al., 2001, Jichlinski &

Leisinger 2001), as well as for other non-oncological applications, such as for the treatment of age-related macular degeneration (AMD) (Brown et al., 2004). Moreover, PDT has also been used as a successful non-invasive therapeutic modality for treating cutaneous neoplasm (Fritsch et al., 1998, Karrer et al., 2001).

PDT can enhance the quality of life and lengthen survival. It has minimal side effects, selective and curative targeting therapy, no drug resistance and reduced toxicity that allows for repeated treatment (Dolmans et al., 2003). Thus, the successful of PDT will widely depend on the nature of the photosensitizer, which upon absorption of light, induces a chemical or physical alteration of another chemical entity. Early studies of photosensitizers for PDT were focused on a complex mixture of porphyrins named haematoporphyrin derivative (HpD), the first generation of photosensitizer.

One of the most clinically used photosensitizer is porfimer sodium (Photofrin®), a purified product from the HpD derivative. Photofrin® is the first drug approved by the Food and Drug Administration (FDA) (Konan et al., 2002). It has also been indicated for the treatment of superficial bladder cancer in Canada and early lung and advanced esophageal cancers in Netherlands and Japan. It has been used in thousands of patients for more than 20 years and no long-term safety issues have emerged. Despite its continuing effectiveness, Photofrin® has several disadvantages. The main disadvantages are the drug induces protracted skin photosensitivity and the initial selectivity for the tumour tissue remains low (Gilson et al., 1988, Moriwaki et al., 2001). These limitations led to the development of the second generation of photosensitizers.

One of the well known second generation photosensitizer is temoporfin (*meta*-tetra(hydroxyphenyl)chlorin, also known as *m*-THPC or Foscan®). It has been effectively used for the palliative treatment of head and neck cancers and it has received an approval in Europe for this indication in 2001. Nonetheless, like Photofrin®, temoporfin is also correlated with a pronounced skin photosensitivity, slow elimination from the blood compartment and weak selectivity between tumour and healthy tissue (Sharman et al., 1999). The disadvantages of temoporfin are contrast to Pd-bacteriopheophorbide (Tookad® or WST09) and its derivative WST11 which are believed to be purely vascular mediated (Woodhams et al., 2006). Moreover, Tookad® exhibits rapid elimination from the circulation and its plasma half-life is less than a few hours. Another second generation photosensitizer is benzoporphyrin derivative, verteporfin (Visudyne®), which was also recently approved, but it was only developed for the treatment of age-related macular degeneration, and not indicated for cancer treatment (Kertes 2006). Protoporphyrin IX (PpIX) is the one example of photosensitizers used for topical application to treat skin lesions. It can be produced in nucleated cells after topical application of either aminolevulinic acid (ALA) or methyl aminolevulinate (mALA) to the site of skin cancer or precancerous lesion (Vihinen et al., 2005 ). This discovery has resulted in the approval of ALA in the USA and mALA in Europe (Brown et al., 2004).

Thousands of patients have already been treated with PDT using the first and second generation of photosensitizers for a variety of advanced neoplasms, and have shown a great improvement in their quality of life and lengthened their survival. In spite of PDT advantages, it has a limitation in the cancer treatment due to the low of selectivity of photosensitizers; the ideal drug delivery system in PDT should be selectively accumulated in the tumour tissues and the delivery of therapeutic concentrations of photosensitizer to the target site with little or no uptake by non-target cells. However, the majority of photosensitizers are taken up non-selectively by all cell types, hence, they are found accumulated not only in tumour cells but also in normal cells.

This situation led to the development of the third generation of photosensitizers, a derivative of the second generation of photosensitizer attached to or introduced into chemical devices. The chemical devices inquiring some biological specificity to deliver or to target such drug for selective accumulation of photosensitizer or vectors with photosensitizer such as nanoparticles, liposomes and miscellaneous (Bechet et al., 2008). Indeed, the new generation of photosensitizers are being designed and developed to enhance selectivity and efficacy of PDT. This could be done by improving the existing photosensitizers, adding specific moieties and using delivery vehicles to specifically target these compounds (Sharman et al., 2004). Thus, targeted-PDT employing the improved photosensitizers could offer better advantage in delivering the photosensitizers across the cellular plasma membrane and resulting in intracellular accumulation of the photosensitizer. For example the use of nanoparticles or peptides as carriers of photosensitizers offer very promising approach for an ideal PDT targeting agent (Bechet et al., 2008). The advantages of targeting strategy include the selective targeted delivery of the photosensitizer to the tumour site that induces low toxicity and minimal damage to the normal tissues. This strategy contributes in the mechanism of PDT in cancer treatment through direct killing of tumour cells but also through indirect effects, which involves both the initiation of an immune response against tumour cells and the destruction of the neovasculature.

## 3. PDT - Tumour vascular targeting

The targeting of tumour vasculature has become a very promising area of focus for the development of new cancer therapeutics (Tozer et al., 2005). It is well known that solid tumours cannot grow larger than 1 $mm^3$ without developing a vascular network (Siemann et al., 2004). This is due to the fact that when a tumour grows, its need for nutrients and oxygen increases, as well as the removal of metabolic waste, and consequently the number and size of blood vessels increase proportionately. In addition, to sustain the tumour growth, tumour tissues need to depend upon existing blood vessels as well as development of new blood vessels from the pre-existing vasculature (angiogenesis) for maintaining the blood supply. Tumour vasculature is also responsible for the progression of cancer from small, localized neoplasm to larger, growing and potentially spread cancer to other parts of the body.

The vessels that nourish tumours possess structural and functional properties different from those of normal vessels (Fig. 1). Normal vasculature is characterized by dichotomous branching, but tumour vasculature is unorganized and exhibits significant abnormalities in vessel architectures (tortuousity, dilatation, irregular branching, and lack of pericyte and basement membrane coverage) and functions (stagnant blood flow and increased vascular permeability) (Fukumura & Jain 2007). Moreover, tumour vasculature can present trifurcations and branches with uneven diameters. Perivascular cells in tumour vessels have abnormal morphology and heterogeneous association with vessels (McDonald & Choyke 2003).

The process of angiogenesis involves the initiation, progression and metastasis of smooth muscle and endothelial cells to invade, proliferate, migrate and survive in response to angiogenic stimuli, leading to the formation of new microvessels. This process is facilitated by a variety of proangiogenic factors that basically consist of four groups of proteins, which are the angiogenic factors, the integrins, the matrix metalloproteinases (MMP) and the plasminogen activator system. The first class of angiogenic factors group is composed of molecules that promote endothelial cells survival and proliferation, including VEGFs, angiopoietins, epithelial growth factor (EGF), fibroblast growth factors (FGFs), platelet-derived growth factor (PDGF), placenta growth factor (PlGF), insulin-like growth factor (IGF), angiogenic cytokines such as interelukin-8 (IL-8) and their endothelial receptors. Among them, VEGF plays a critical role in vascular formation and it is the most potent angiogenic cytokines. It has been first characterized for its ability to induce vascular leakage and permeability and to promote vascular endothelial cell proliferation (Dvorak et al., 1999, Ferrara & Davis-Smyth 1997). Another group of proangiogenic factors is the molecules that related with the cell-cell and cell-matrix interactions, which provide signals for endothelial survival, adhesion and vascular integrity. This group consists of integrins and other adherent molecules. A selective expression of adhesion receptor, $\alpha_v\beta_3$ integrin, has been detected during tumour angiogenesis (Brooks et al., 1994a, Brooks et al., 1994b). The survival of new endothelial cells is increased by a specific signal following the recognition of $\alpha_v\beta_3$ integrin from its receptor. The other group of proangiogenic factors is matrix metalloproteinases which comprise a group of proteolytic enzymes that facilitate the propagation of tumour and break down the extracellular matrix (ECM), thereby facilitating cell motility and thus allow the migration of endothelial cells to form new vessels (Ahmad et al., 2010). The last group is a cascade of proteases called the plasminogen activator system which plays an important role during the process of angiogenesis.

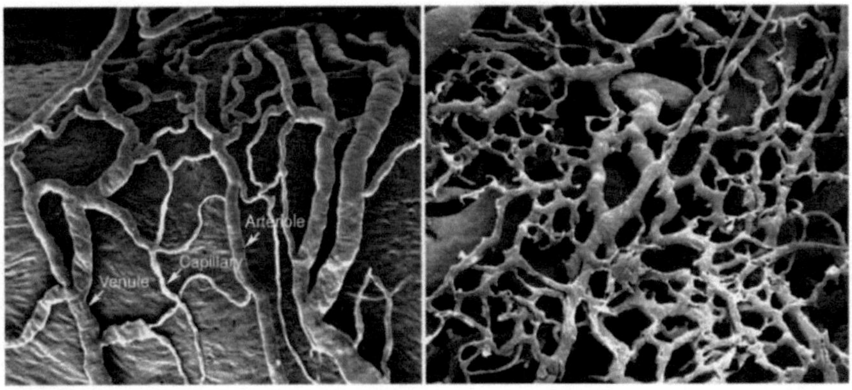


Fig. 1. Structural differentiation of normal blood vessels (*vasa vasorum* of carotid sinus rat, *left*) and tumour vasculature (human tumour xenograft in nude mice, *right*) using SEM microscopy (Konerding et al., 2001, McDonald & Choyke 2003).

On the basis of angiogenesis and vasculogenesis studies, Judah Folkman had proposed a hypothesis that "solid tumours are angiogenesis-dependent" and "anti-angiogenesis could be a potential therapeutic approach" (Folkman 1971). In his pioneer work, he found cancer cells implanted in vascular sites of animal grew rapidly and formed large tumours. In contrast, cells implanted in avascular sites were unable to form tumour masses more than 1 to 2 mm in size. Therefore, he proposed to inhibit the new blood vessels formation to prevent the tumour growth and thus kill cancer cells. Since then, it becomes a relevant target for tumour therapy. It gives some hopes that tumour growth can be interrupted or stopped by inhibiting the progression of angiogenesis and therefore destroys the tumour metastasis. In addition, the malignant tissue would be starved of its oxygen and nutrients supply and also unable to eliminate metabolic wastes (Denekamp 1999). This also implies the destroying of tumour neovasculature, which can be an effective approach to control the tumour growth and provide the basis for selective tumour vasculature targeting.

Tumour vascular targeting can be divided into two general categories, anti-angiogenic therapy, referring to interfere with new blood vessel development and vascular targeted therapy, associating with the damage of the established tumour vasculature (Bloemendal et al., 1999, Ellis et al., 2001, Siemann et al., 2005, Siemann et al., 2004, Thorpe 2004). The inhibitors of anti-angiogenic therapy seek to inhibit or interrupt the tumour-initiated angiogenesis process by disrupting essential aspects of angiogenesis, particularly signaling between the tumour and endothelial cells, and between the tumour and stromal cells. In addition, anti-angiogenic therapy can disrupt endothelial function in order to prevent new blood vessel formation. Nevertheless, anti-angiogenic therapy is the other subject that can be discussed in another topic interest and will therefore not be discussed further in the present chapter.

Vascular targeted photodynamic therapy (VTP) is related to the destruction of functional vasculature which is necessary for efficient tumour eradication by PDT. The strategy aims to destroy neovasculature of tumours. Thereby, vascular damage is considered to be a major phenomenon occurring during PDT of tumours, which largely contributes to its efficacy. Vascular targeting in PDT is considered active when the photosensitizing compounds selectively accumulate in the targeted neovascular components, thus bringing out a preferential vascular response (B. Chen et al., 2006a). Vascular targeting can be passive when the injected photosensitizer is mainly confined in the blood vessels and reaches peak plasma concentration and will further provide a therapeutic window for vascular treatment. Recently, a combination of vascular targeted strategy and photodynamic therapy named vascular targeted photodynamic therapy (VTP) has become a promising subject to be explored and developed. VTP is being developed either by changing PDT schedule, for example, decrease the period between the photosensitizer's injection and irradiation of the tumour site (drug-light interval, DLI) or by designing photosensitizers localizing primarily in the vascular compartment (Star et al., 1986, Fingar et al., 1996, Kurohane et al., 2001).

VTP has several advantages, which are:

i. the tumour endothelial cells are directly accessible to intravenously administered photosensitizer thus permitting a rapid localization of a high percentage of the injected dose
ii. the molecular oxygen required for photochemical reaction is also more readily available
iii. since each capillary provides oxygen and nutrients and also removes the metabolic wastes for thousands of tumour cells, occlusion of the vessel has an amplified effect on tumour cells
iv. the outgrowth of mutant endothelial cells lacking the target antigen is unlikely because they are a normal, genetically stable cells population
v. finally, since tumour vessels share common morphological and biochemical properties, this strategy should be applicable to different tumour types (Veikkola et al., 2000).

For example, the use of hematoporphyrin in the tumour cell death after photoirradiation by PDT is caused by vasoconstriction and complete stasis that occurs secondary to demolish the microvasculature (Star et al., 1986). It changes the morphological of neovasculature which led to the absence of the capillary layer and mitochondrial degeneration, thus supporting tumour demolition (Chaudhuri et al., 1987). By using vertoporfin in VTP, it resulted to cause a dose- and time-dependent increase in vascular permeability, but decrease in blood perfusion. Vertoporfin in VTP is known to permeabilize blood vessels through the formation of endothelial intercellular gaps, hence, triggering the loss of endothelial barrier function that enhance the tumour vascular shutdown (Chen et al., 2008, Chen et al., 2006b). Another example is Photofrin® which induces changes in vessel constriction, vessel leakage and thrombus formation (Fingar et al., 1992), while higher dosage of Photofrin® during PDT causes vessel constriction and changes in permeability (Fingar et al., 1997).

With these several advantages, tumour targeting has become a promising strategy for the development of active photosensitizer delivery systems that able to enhance selectivity and efficiency of vascular PDT for cancer treatment. The next subtopic will focus on the main molecular targets explored in the vascular-targeting PDT for cancer, including the vascular endothelial growth factor receptors (VEGFRs such as neuropilin-1 (NRP-1)), $\alpha_v\beta_3$ integrin, matrix metalloproteinase (MMPs) and receptor tissue factor (TF) activities.

### 3.1 Vascular Endothelial Growth Factor (VEGF) receptors

Vascular endothelial growth factor (VEGF) is an endothelial cell -specific mitogen for vascular endothelial cells which is an important regulator of normal and pathological angiogenesis including cells survival and proliferation (Ferrara 2002, Ferrara & Davis-Smyth 1997). VEGF is upregulated in the bulky neoplastic cells, generally as a response to hypoxia and many oncogenes, and its overproduction is correlated with high microvascular density and poor prognosis (Ishigami et al., 1998). VEGF encourages the growth of vascular endothelial cells derived from arteries, veins, and lymphatics. VEGF induces a strong angiogenic response in a variety of both *in vivo* (Leung et al., 1989, Plouet et al., 1989) and *in vitro* models (Pepper et al., 1994) and also inducing confluent microvascular endothelial cells to invade collagen gels and form capillary-like-structures (Pepper et al., 1992).

The overexpression of VEGF results in the upregulation of VEGF receptors namely VEGFR-1 (also known as fms-like tyrosine kinase, flt-1), VEGFR-2 (fetal liver kinase-1, flk-1 or kinase domain region, KDR) and VEGFR-3 (KDR/flt-1) (Bando et al., 2005, Kremer et al., 1997, Plate et al., 1992). VEGFR-1 and VEGFR-3 are expressed in distinct vascular beds, whereas VEGFR-2 is selectively expressed on almost all endothelial cells (Ferrara 2004). VEGFR-1 and VEGFR-2 are associated with angiogenesis, while VEGFR-3 is affiliated with lymphangiogenesis (Ferrara 2004).

Among of the three primary receptors of VEGF, VEGFR-2 becomes an interest for most active targeting strategies and this receptor is believed to be the main receptor that mediates VEGF biological activities and also plays a major role in tumour-associated angiogenesis. VEGF/VEGFR-2 signaling pathway is critical for tumour angiogenesis and for solid tumour growth. Expression of VEGFR-2 in various cell types results in the ability to respond ligands by the transduction of a mitogenic signal. VEGFR-2 is highly expressed in both vascular endothelial cells and lymphatic endothelial cells in tumour neovasculature, as well as other cell types such as megakaryocytes (Katoh et al., 1995), hematopoietic stem cells (Katoh et al., 1995), and chronic myelogenous leukemia (CML) (Grosskreutz et al., 1999, Ishida et al., 2001). Therefore, VEGFR-2 is seen as promising molecular target for anti-angiogenic drug delivery, and that specific targeting of VEGFR-2 could provide an interesting approach for selective and efficient photosensitizer delivery to tumour neovasculature.

Although VEGFR-2 has been widely known as a promising target for the selective delivery of therapeutic drugs for conventional therapies, the number of photoactivatable drugs targeting VEGFR-2 remains limited. Targeted verteporfin (Visudyne®) has been reported as the first research works that investigated the potential of VEGFR-2 as a molecular target for vascular PDT. In a recent study Renno *et al.* conjugated the verteporfin, first to polyvinyl alcohol (PVA) polymer, then to a peptidic motif ATWLPPR which was reported to bind VEGFR-2. The use of the conjugated drug efficiently caused choroidal neovascularization (CNV) closure and exhibited more selective than nonconjugated verteporfin (Renno et al., 2004). Although these results showed the targeting VEGFR-2 can be an effective strategy to the tumour neovasculature, more recent studies demonstrated a contrast finding that ATWLPPR does not recognize KDR but bind to NRP-1 (Perret et al., 2004, Tirand et al., 2006). These results have then attracted a great interest on the potential of NRP-1 as promising target for targeted vascular PDT.

The neuropilins were originally reported as a mediator of axon guidance and later serve as a receptor that involved in normal blood vessel development, tumour angiogenesis and tumour progression (Ellis 2006, Favier et al., 2006, Gu et al., 2002, Neufeld et al., 2002). Therefore, neuropilins appear to serve as a co-receptor or a 'hub' receptor due to its ability to bind with high affinity into two structurally unrelated classes of ligands with distinct biological functions, the class 3 semaphorins and various members of the VEGF family. As co-receptors of VEGF, the neuropilins have been identified to modulate binding to other receptors without being active in signaling (Soker et al., 1998) and though to increase the binding affinity of the various VEGF ligands to the primary receptors. Neuropilins are described in two family members, neuropilin-1 (NRP-1) and neuropilin-2 (NRP-2). NRP-1 was identified at first as high-affinity cell surface receptors for secreted class 3 semaphorins, but more recently, it was reported as a co-receptor for VEGF. NRP-2 was recognized by sequence analysis and it was reported to share the same domain arrangement as NRP-1 and also share with 44% identity with NRP-1 (Chen et al., 1997, Kolodkin et al., 1997).

Neuropilins are expressed specifically in tumour angiogenic vessels and some tumour cells, and also promote tumour angiogenesis and progression (Miao et al., 2000). When co-expressed with VEGFR-2, NRP-1 enhanced the binding of $VEGF_{165}$ to VEGFR-2. This situation can be explained when the NRP-1 serve as a receptor for the $VEGF_{165}$ isoform through the exon 7-encoded region of VEGF (Soker et al., 1998). $VEGF_{165}$ has also been shown to bind with the receptors VEGFR-1 and VEGFR-2 via the exons 3-and 4-encoded peptides, respectively (Keyt et al., 1996). This situation leads the $VEGF_{165}$ to form a bridge between VEGFR-2 and NRP-1 (Soker et al., 1998), and thus mediate the formation of a ternary complex between $VEGF_{165}$, VEGFR-2 and NRP-1 (Fuh et al., 2000, Soker et al., 2002, Staton et al., 2007). It may explain the possible reason why NRP-1 enhances VEGF binding and activity by bringing these receptors into closer proximity (Soker et al., 2002, Soker et al., 1998). Besides that, NRP-1 co-expression with VEGFR-2 enhanced VEGF-induced chemotaxis in comparison with cells expressing VEGFR-2 alone, and also enhanced the VEGF binding to VEGFR-2, VEGFR-2 phosphorylation and VEGF-induced signaling and migration (Bernatchez et al., 2002, Rollin et al., 2004). Therefore, NRP-1 has become a promising target for selective vascular localization of photosensitizers, and thus enhances the vascular photodynamic effects.

In conjunction with that, our group introduced the conjugation of a photosensitizer (5-(4-carboxyphenyl)-10,15,20-triphenyl-chlorin, TPC) to a VEGF receptor-specific heptapeptide, H-Ala-Thr-Trp-Leu-Pro-Pro-Arg-OH (ATWLPPR), via a spacer (6-aminohexanoic acid, Ahx), noticed TPC-Ahx-ATWLPPR (Fig. 2) (Tirand et al., 2006). We showed that ATWLPPR and TPC-Ahx-ATWLPPR bound exclusively to NRP-1 but were devoid of affinity for VEGFR-2 or KDR, to which ATWLPPR was originally thought to bind. This peptide conjugation ATWLPPR has proved to be very efficient in endothelial cells compared to its nonconjugated counterpart. Our study demonstrated that TPC-Ahx-ATWLPPR accumulated up to 25-fold more in human umbilical vein endothelial cells (HUVEC) than free TPC over a 24 hours period. The accumulation of the conjugated photosensitizer was related to NRP-1-dependent mechanisms but also to non-specific mechanisms (Thomas et al., 2008, Tirand et al., 2007). *In vivo* biodistribution studies in nude mice xenografted with U87 human malignant glioma cells revealed significant tumour level to normal ratios as early as 1 hour after intravenous injection of TPC-Ahx-ATWLPPR. We also studied the *in vivo* vascular effect by measuring the tumour blood flow during PDT using both conjugated and nonconjugated photosensitizer (Fig. 3). Only the conjugate-mediated VTP produced a selective vascular effect, leading to vascular shutdown and tumour growth delay (Bechet et al., 2010).

From the biological mechanism point of view, the conjugate-mediated vascular effect implies the induction of tissue factor (TF) expression leading to the thrombogenic effect within the vessel lumen (Fig. 4) (Bechet et al., 2010).

These findings shed some light that the targeting strategy using a peptide competing with $VEGF_{165}$ binding on NRP-1 could have a better accumulation of photosensitizer in endothelial cells lining tumour vessels. Nonetheless, using this strategy, the affinity of conjugated photosensitizer for NRP-1 remains low compared to the peptide alone. The possible reason may include, *(i)* intramolecular interactions between chlorin and peptide, and steric hindrance due to the TPC moiety, (Ishigami et al., 1998) *(ii)* aggregation of the photosensitizer molecules, and *(iii)* low stability of the peptide moiety that, may be due to sensitivity to circulating peptidases action. In order to overcome these drawbacks, a linker can be used as a spacer to couple the photoactivable compound to the peptides, in order to individualize these two moieties. The bioavailability of the peptide can also be enhanced by the introduction of a non-amidic moiety at the cleavage site (Pernot et al, 2011).

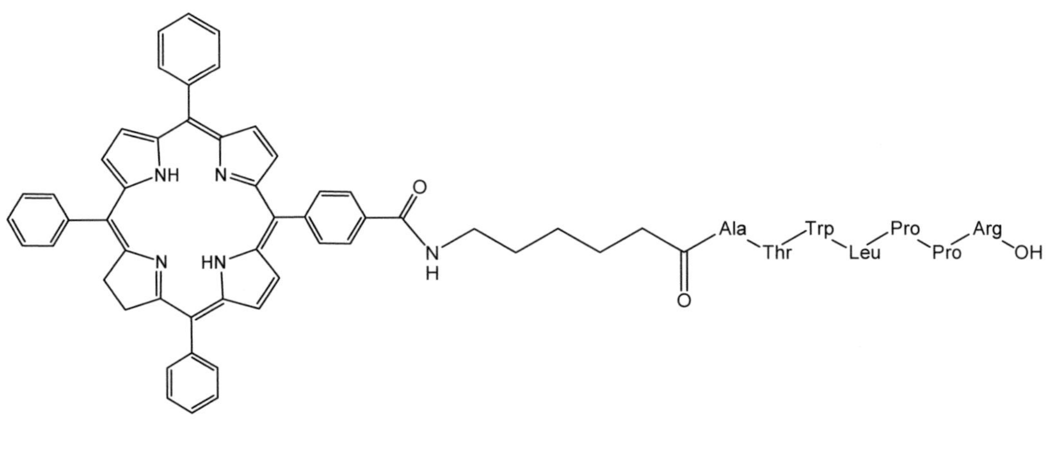


Fig. 2. ATWLPPR peptide conjugated with a chlorin (Tirand *et al.*, 2006)

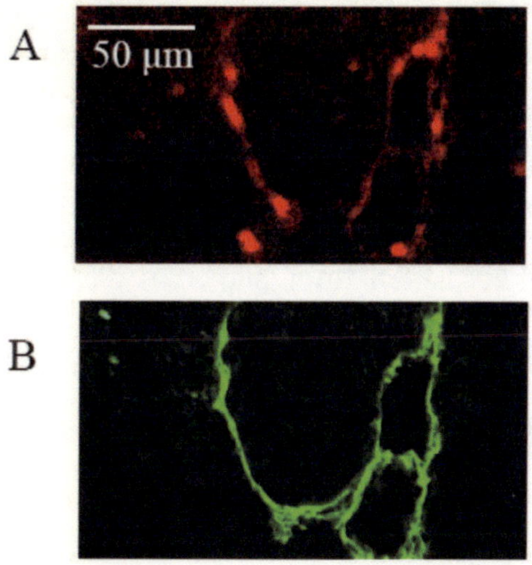


Fig. 3. Localization of the photosensitizers 4 hours after intravenous injection. (A) Color composite image of TPC-Ahx-ATWLPPR fluorescence (red). (B) Color composite image of CD31-staining (green) in the same region as (A). Analysis of the tumour sections 4 hours after TPC-Ahx-ATWLPPR administration showed that the photosensitizer was mainly colocalized inside the vascular endothelium (Thomas et al., 2008).

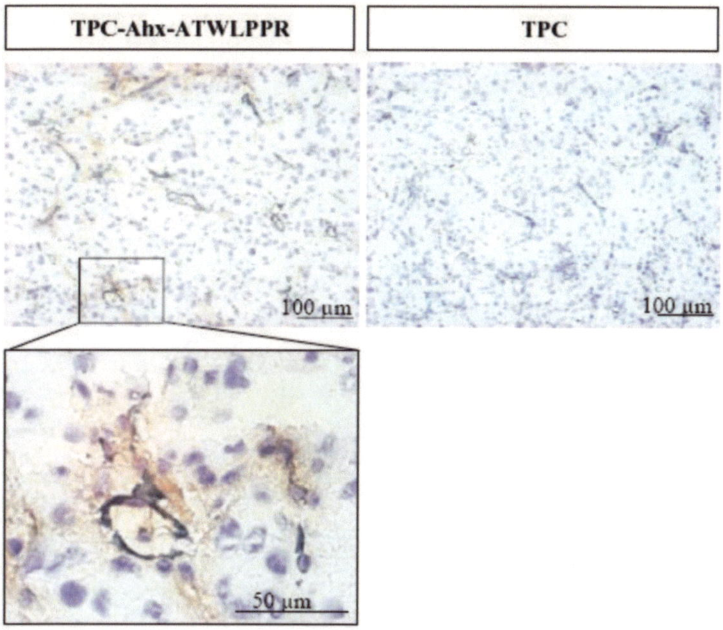


Fig. 4. Immediately after PDT, TPC-Ahx-ATWLPPR-induced (*upper left*) photodynamic activity induced TF expression (brown staining) compared to the nonconjugated photosensitizer (TPC) (*upper right*). Tissue factor staining appeared to be non-uniform and was not limited to vessel *lumen* areas but also present in tumour tissues. *Bottom* is the enlarged view of the corresponding specimen (Bechet et al., 2010).

### 3.2 $\alpha_v\beta_3$ Integrin

The $\alpha_v\beta_3$ integrin, a heterodimeric transmembrane glycoprotein receptor is highly expressed in many tumour cells including osteocarcinomas, neuroblastomas and lung carcinomas. The $\alpha_v\beta_3$ integrin is upregulated in both tumour cells and angiogenic endothelial cells (Desgrosellier & Cheresh 2010) but poorly expressed in resting endothelial cells and most normal organs. This integrin serves as an endothelial cell receptor for extracellular matrix proteins which includes fibrinogen (fibrin), vibronectin, thrombospondin, osteopondin and fibronectin (Desgrosellier & Cheresh 2010), and plays an important role in the calcium-dependent signaling pathway leading to endothelial cell migration (Byrne et al., 2008). Linear and cyclic derivatives of RGD peptidic motif (H-Arg-Gly-Asp-OH) are the well characterized oligopeptides known to bind to endothelial $\alpha_v\beta_3$ integrin. Therefore, $\alpha_v\beta_3$ integrin is believed as an attractive molecular target for antivascular therapies. In this sense, several studies have been done to explore the potential of $\alpha_v\beta_3$ integrin in vascular-targeted PDT.

Solid phase synthesis of four porphyrin derivatives bearing the $\alpha_v\beta_3$ integrin ligand RGD peptide was reported by Chaleix *et al.* (Chaleix et al., 2004). Three of these porphyrin derivatives exhibited photodynamic activity on K562 leukemia cells to a degree comparable to that of Photofrin®. The same authors later described the synthesis of a cyclic dithiopentapeptide CRGDC, containing the RGD sequence which has been found to adopt conformations showing an increased affinity for integrins (Fig. 5) (Chaleix et al., 2004, Haubner et al., 2001). The replacement of the disulfide bonds of the cyclic peptide by carbon-carbon bond increases it stability and plasmatic residence time (Haubner et al., 2001). Carboxy-glucosylporphyrins coupled to this cyclic peptide *via* a spacer arm showed the same efficiency for singlet oxygen production as hematoporphyrin under the same experimental conditions.

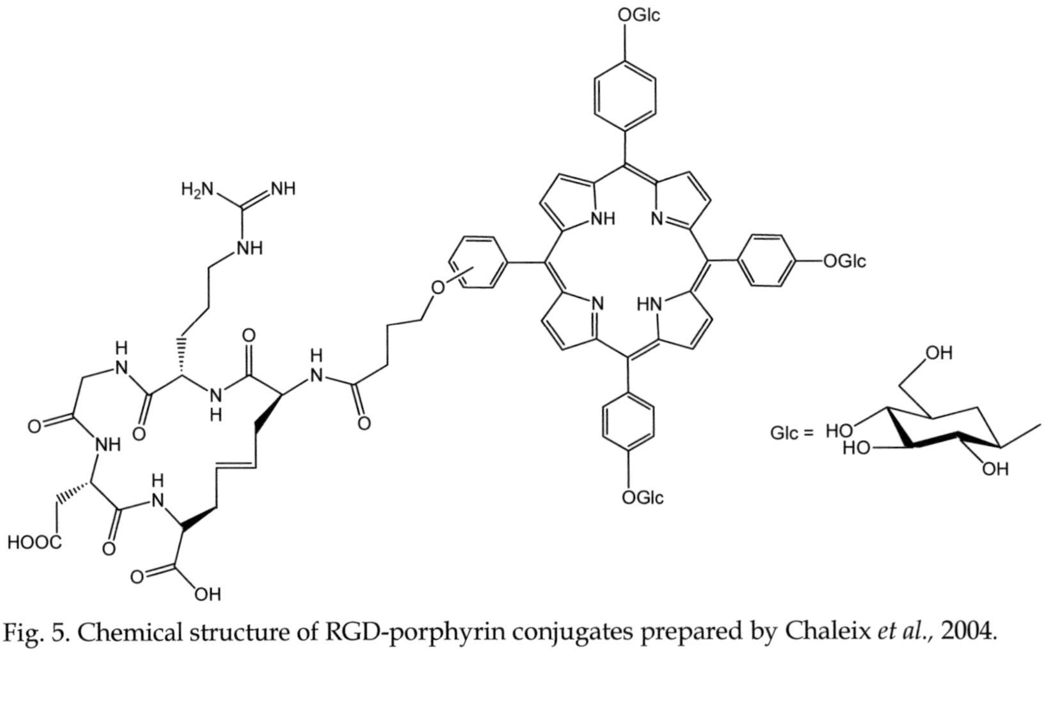


Fig. 5. Chemical structure of RGD-porphyrin conjugates prepared by Chaleix *et al.*, 2004.

In another study, Allen *et al.* tested the use of viral proteins as delivery vehicles for photosensitizer to enhance their target selectivity (Allen et al., 1999). Adenoviruses most commonly caused illness of the respiratory system but they may also cause various other illnesses such as gastroenteritis, conjunctivitis, cystitis and rash illness. Adenoviruses received a great deal of attention as gene therapy vectors, due to ease and safe to manipulate and to store. Haddada *et al.* have shown that adenoviruses can infect several cell and tissue types including fully differentiated tissues and nonreplacing cells, and gain access into a cell *via* receptor-mediated endocytosis. This requires two separate receptors; one mediating attachment and the other mediating internalization. The first receptor allows the attachment of adenoviruses to cells *via* the fiber capsid protein/receptor interaction, while the second receptor, known as $\alpha_v$ integrin, is required for virus internalization. The binding of adenoviruses to $\alpha_v$ integrin is mediated by adenoviruses penton base proteins containing RGD peptide motif. Tetrasulfonated aluminum phthalocyanines ($AlPcS_4$) was covalently coupled to the various adenoviruses capsid proteins including the hexon, penton bases and fiber antigen *via* one or two caproic acid spacer chains, and these derivatives were tested both *in vitro* and *in vivo*. It was shown that the penton base conjugate was the most efficient *in vitro,* as measured in two positive cell lines (A549, Hep2) expressing integrins (Allen et al., 1999). These findings suggested that adenoviral proteins can be used as delivery vehicles for photosensitizers to target tumour cells. However, vehicles may promote inflammation and anti-protein cellular immunity, which could limit their usefulness.

Some years ago, our group described a new family of peptidic photosensitizer by the conjugation of 5-(4-carboxyphenyl)-10,15,20-triphenylchlorin or porphyrin to the linear RGD or cyclic [RGDfK] motif (Frochot et al., 2007). The results showed that RGD-containing linear or cyclic peptide targeted tetraphenylchlorin were incorporated up to 98- and 80-fold more, respectively, than the nonconjugated photosensitizer over a 24 hour exposure in HUVEC overexpressing $\alpha_v\beta_3$ integrin. However, we found a non-specific increased cellular uptake by murine mammary carcinoma cells (EMT-6), lacking $\alpha_v\beta_3$ integrin receptor. Survival measurements clearly demonstrated that HUVEC were more sensitive to peptide conjugate-mediated photodynamic therapy than the nonconjugated photosensitizer, demonstrating that the higher photodynamic efficiency was related to the high cellular uptake of the conjugate (Frochot et al., 2007). Moreover, study showed that the peptide moiety also introduces a balance between hydrophilicity and hydrophobicity providing excellent water solubility and weak tendency to form aggregates, which is a required feature for an efficient photodynamic activity. More recently, our team has described the synthesis, characterization, fluorescence, and singlet oxygen quantum yields of tetraphenylporphyrin and tetraphenylchlorin coupled to RGD peptides and they found that some of these compounds are very promising for potential photodynamic therapy applications (Boisbrun et al., 2008).

### 3.3 Matrix metalloproteinases

The matrix metalloproteinases (MMPs) are a family of extracellular proteinases (Fig. 6) that have an essential role in tumour metastasis and angiogenesis, more particularly in endothelial cell growth, invasion and migration, in the formation of capillary tubes and in the recruitment of accessory cells, due to its ability to degrade components of the extracellular matrix (ECM) (van Kempen et al., 2006, Vihinen et al., 2005). ECM is a complex network of macromolecules secreted by the cells, including carbohydrates and proteins such as fibronectin, vitronectin, laminin, tenascin and collagen. While components of the ECM are involved in the regulation of different cell functions such as motility, morphogenesis, differentiation and proliferation, proteolytic degradation of the ECM is considered as an important mechanism favouring cancer development, invasion and metastasis, which is associated with increased expression of several proteases. Indeed, several studies have reported increased expression of proteases such as MMPs in many human malignant tissue types often correlating with poor prognosis (Egeblad & Werb 2002).

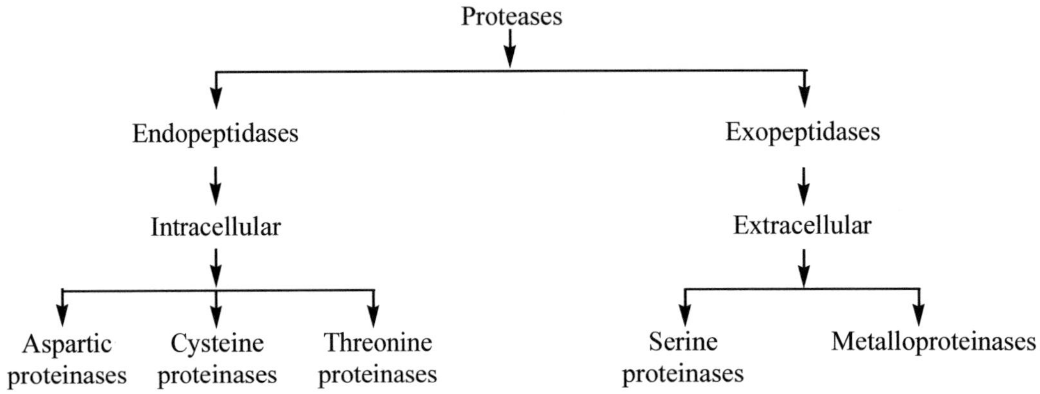


Fig. 6. Overview of different proteases.

MMPs-induced extracellular matrix proteolysis is also involved in the angiogenesis necessary for the continued growth of solid tumors. Indeed, MMPs are involved in different steps of angiogenesis (Chetty et al., 2010, Sharwani et al., 2006), thus become potential interesting targets in PDT for cancer treatment. MMPs facilitate endothelial cell migration by releasing them from their basement membranes, degrading perivascular ECM, and generating ECM degradation products that are chemotactic for endothelial cells. Fiore *et al.* demonstrated that MMPs have an ability to cleave not only components of the ECM, but also other proteinases, latent growth factors and growth factor binding proteins, chemotactic molecules, cell surface receptors and cell-cell adhesion molecules (Fiore et al., 2002). These findings came out with at least five main groups of MMPs; collagenases, gelatinases, stromelysins, the matrilysins and membrane-type MMPs, which differ according to their substrate specificity, primary structure and cellular localization.

MMPs are thought to play an important role at different stages of tumour development. Many studies offer strong evidence that MMP-2 (gelatinase A) and MMP-9 (gelatinase B) play a major role in the tumour growth and angiogenesis processes. These gelatinases can degrade the type IV collagen of basal laminae and other nonhelical collagen domains such as laminin (Chambers & Matrisian 1997, Xu et al., 2005). There is increasing evidence supporting the theory that MMP-2 and MMP-9 expression is associated with disease outcomes in different cancers such as ovarian and breast tumours (Davidson et al., 1999, Yoneda et al., 1997). Therefore, protease-sensitive macromolecular prodrugs have attracted interest for bio-responsive drug delivery to sites with up-regulated proteolytic activities.

Another interesting target is MMP-7, which is associated with many cancers. The MMPs regulate normal development but also play a role in the pathogenesis of cancers. MMP-7 in particular is found upregulated in several cancers including pancreatic, colon, breast, and non small-cell lung cancer (Leinonen et al., 2006, Shiomi & Okada 2003). Pham and co-workers designed a peptide-based near-infrared (NIR) fluorescence probe consisting of a NIR fluorescence emitter linked *via* a MMP-7 substrate peptide linker to a NIR fluorescence absorber for sensing tumour-associated MMP-7 activity (Pham et al., 2004). They applied the Forster resonance energy transfer (FRET) principle for controlling fluorescence emission between the donor and the acceptor. The absence of proteases results in the quenched fluorescence for the donor; however, in the presence of proteases, the substrate peptide linker is cleaved, releasing the FRET interaction between the donor-acceptor fluorophore, which result in a four-fold increase in the fluorescence signal for an initially quenched molecular dye (Verma et al., 2007).

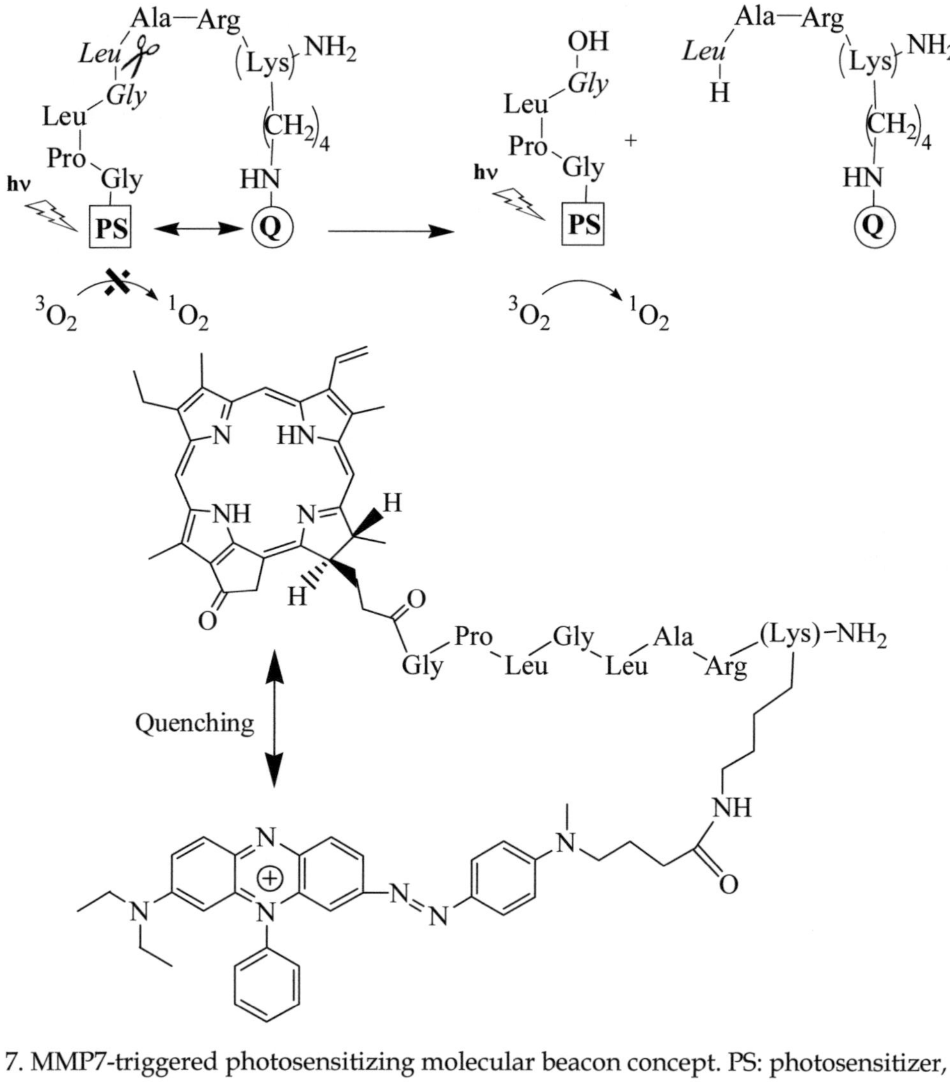


Fig. 7. MMP7-triggered photosensitizing molecular beacon concept. PS: photosensitizer, Q: quencher.

Considering this, photodynamic molecular beacons (PMB) provide an additional mechanism of selectivity in PDT over and above the targeting afforded by current photosensitizers and specific light delivery (Zheng et al., 2007). Photodynamic molecular beacons consist of a disease-specific linker, a photosensitizer, and a fluorescence singlet oxygen quencher (Q). The photodynamic molecular beacons are noncytotoxic because of the energy transfer from the excited photosensitizer to quencher. Upon activation by the target enzyme, the linker will be cleaved, which allows the separation between the photosensitizer and the quencher. Upon irradiation, this leads to fluorescence emission restoration and singlet oxygen generation. Therefore, photodynamic molecular beacons offer a control of fluorescence emission and singlet oxygen generation of photosensitizer in response to specific cancer target activation. Thus, molecular beacons are FRET-based target-activatable probes.

Zheng *et al.* have combined the two principles of FRET and PDT and introduced a concept of photodynamic molecular beacons for controlling the photosensitizer's ability to generate singlet oxygen, and thus for controlling its PDT activity (Zheng et al., 2007). They reported the synthesis and characterization of a MMP-7-triggered photodynamic molecular beacon, using: (i) pyropheophorbide as the photosensitizer, because of its excellent singlet oxygen quantum yield, NIR fluorescence emission and high tumour affinity; (ii) black hole quencher 3 (BHQ3) as a dual fluorescence and singlet oxygen quencher; and (iii) a short peptide sequence, G*PL*GLARK, as the MMP-7 cleavable linker, with the cleavage site, as indicated by italics in Fig. 7 (Ishigami et al., 1998). This figure shows that the pyropheophorbide and the quencher are linked to the opposite ends of the MMP-7-specific cleavable peptide linker to keep them in close proximity, permitting FRET and singlet oxygen quenching to form inactive prodrug; silent and photodynamically inactive, until the linker interacts with the target tumour-associated MMP-7. After characterizing the MMP-7-triggered production of singlet oxygen in solution, the authors also demonstrated the MMP-7-mediated photodynamic cytotoxicity in cancer cells. *In vivo* studies revealed the MMP-7-activated PDT efficacy (Zheng et al., 2007). This finding validated the main principal of the photodynamic molecular beacons concept demonstrating that selective PDT-induced cell death can be achieved by controlling of the photosensitizer's ability to produce singlet oxygen.

### 3.4 Receptor Tissue Factor (TF)

Tissue factor (TF) is a transmembrane receptor protein that belongs to the class II cytokine receptor family. It is known to bind with high affinity to its endogenous ligand coagulation factor VII (fVII), thus initiating the blood coagulation cascade *via* the extrinsic pathway (Nemerson 1988). In addition to its role in coagulation, accumulating studies suggest that receptor TF regulates intracellular signaling pathway (Spek 2004), play an important role in embryonic development (Pedersen et al., 2005), inflammation (Chu 2005), angiogenesis (Chen et al., 2001) and, tumour growth and metastasis (Versteeg et al., 2004). Many studies revealed that receptor TF is expressed on endothelial cells of pathological blood vessels associated with solid tumours (Chen et al., 2001, Contrino et al., 1996, Hu & Garen 2000, 2001, Hu et al., 1999, Shoji et al., 1998, Tang et al., 2007), wet macular degeneration (wMD) (Bora et al., 2003, Tezel et al., 2007) and endometriosis (Krikun et al., 2010), but not on endothelial cells of normal blood vessels (Contrino et al., 1996, Drake et al., 1989, Hu & Garen 2000, 2001, Hu et al., 1999, Mulder et al., 1995, Osterud 1997, Rao & Pendurthi 1998, Tang et al., 2007). It has also been reported that VEGF protein secreted by tumour cells induces endothelial cells in tumour vasculature to express receptor TF (Clauss et al., 1990, Zucker et al., 1998). All these findings suggest that receptor TF provide accessible and specific therapeutic target for tumour cells and tumour vasculature (Shoji et al., 2008).

According to that, several strategies have been developed to target cancer cells and tumour neovasculature for alternative treatment using fVII as a drug carrier.
Hu *et al.* developed a ligand-targeted photodynamic therapy system by conjugating factor VII protein with verteporfin (Hu et al., 1999). The fVII-targeted verteporfin PDT and non-targeted verteporfin have been tested both *in vitro* and *in vivo* to kill breast cancer cells and VEGF-stimulated vascular endothelial cells, and to inhibit the tumour growth of breast tumours in mouse xenograft model (Hu et al., 2010). Their results showed that: *(i)* fVII protein could be conjugated to verteporfin without affecting its binding activity; fVII-targeted PDT could selectively kill receptor TF-expressing breast cancer cells and VEGF-stimulated angiogenic HUVECs but no side effect on non-receptor TF expressing unstimulated HUVEC, CHO-K1 and 293 cells; *(iii)* fVII targeting enhanced the effect of verteporfin PDT by three to four-fold; *(iv)* fVII-targeted PDT induced significantly stronger levels of apoptosis and necrosis than non-targeted PDT; and *(v)* fVII-targeted PDT had a significantly stronger effect on inhibiting breast tumour growth in mice than non-targeted PDT (Hu et al., 2010). Since receptor TF is expressed in many types of cancer cells including leukemia cells, and selectively on angiogenic vascular endothelial cells, these findings suggest that fVII-targeted PDT could have broad therapeutic applications for cancer treatment.

## 4. Conclusion

Vasculature damage is an important mechanism involved in PDT mediated tumour eradication. Vascular targeted photodynamic therapy (VTP) is developed and designed to further strengthen the vascular photosensitization effect by site-targeted delivery of photosensitizing agents to the vascular target. In addition, selective delivery of therapeutic amounts of photosensitizers in diseased tissues is recognized as an absolute requirement for efficient and safe PDT for the treatment of cancers. It gives a big challenge to extend the application of PDT for the treatment of a broad ranges of tumour types, as such modality present many advantages over the conventional therapies. To achieve this goal, the development in targeted PDT continues to take advantage of the advances in the characterization of molecular mechanisms of tumour development. A large variety of specific molecular targets have been characterized and explored in tumour targeting. Many photosensitizing agents have been elaborated and evaluated through both *in vitro* and *in vivo* studies; nevertheless, only very few have reached clinical evaluation phases. Each photosensitizer has specific characteristics, but none includes all the properties of an ideal photosensitizer. Although third-generation photosensitizers have been widely described for selective targeting, very few have been evaluated for clinical applications as the *in vivo* selectivity was not sufficiently high.

## 5. References

Ahmad M. Z., Akhter S., Jain G. K., Rahman M., Pathan S. A., Ahmad F. J. & Khar R. K. (2010). Metallic nanoparticles: Technology overview and drug delivery applications in oncology. *Expert Opinion on Drug Delivery*, 7, 8, pp. 927-942.

Allen C. M., Sharman W. M., La Madeleine C., Weber J. M., Langlois R., Quellet R. & Van Lier J. E. (1999). Photodynamic therapy: Tumor targeting with adenoviral proteins. *Photochemistry and Photobiology*, 70, 4, pp. 512-523.

Bando H., Weich H. A., Brokelmann M., Horiguchi S., Funata N., Ogawa T. & Toi M. (2005). Association between intratumoral free and total VEGF, soluble VEGFR-1, VEGFR-2 and prognosis in breast cancer. *British Journal of Cancer*, 92, 3, pp. 553-561.

Bechet D., Couleaud P., Frochot C., Viriot M. L., Guillemin F. & Barberi-Heyob M. (2008). Nanoparticles as vehicles for delivery of photodynamic therapy agents. *Trends in Biotechnology*, 26, 11, pp. 612-621.

Bechet D., Tirand L., Faivre B., Plenat F., Bonnet C., Bastogne T., Frochot C., Guillemin F. & Barberi-Heyob M. (2010). Neuropilin-1 targeting photosensitization-induced early stages of thrombosis via tissue factor release. *Pharmaceutical Research*, 27, 3, pp. 468-479.

Bernatchez P. N., S. Rollin, S. Soker & Sirois M. G. (2002). Relative effects of VEGF-A and VEGF-C on endothelial cell proliferation, migration, and PAF synthesis: Role of neuropilin-1. *Journal of Cellular Biochemistry*, 85, 3, pp. 629-639.

Bloemendal H. J., T. Logtenberg & Voest E. E. (1999). New strategies in anti-vascular cancer therapy. *European Journal of Clinical Investigation*, 29, 9, pp. 802-809.

Boisbrun M.,. Vanderesse R, Engrand P., Olie A., Hupont S.,. Regnouf-de-Vains J. B & Frochot C. (2008). Design and photophysical properties of new RGD targeted tetraphenylchlorins and porphyrins. *Tetrahedron*, 64, 16, pp. 3494-3504.

Bora P. S., Hu Z., Tezel T. H., Sohn J. H., Kang S. G., Cruz J. M. C., Bora N. S., Garen A. & Kaplan H. J. (2003). Immunotherapy for choroidal neovascularization in a laser-induced mouse model simulating exudative (wet) macular degeneration. *Proceedings of the National Academy of Sciences of the United States of America*, 100, 5, pp. 2679-2684.

Brooks P. C., Clark R. A. F. & Cheresh D. A. (1994a). Requirement of vascular integrin alpha (v) beta (3) for angiogenesis. *Science*, 264, 5158, pp. 569-571.

Brooks P. C., Montgomery A. M. P., Rosenfeld M., Reisfeld R. A., Hu T., Klier G. & Cheresh D. A. (1994b). Integrin alpha (v) beta (3) antagonists promote tumor regression by inducing apoptosis of angiogenic blood vessels. *Cell*, 79, 7, pp. 1157-1164.

Brown S. B., Brown E. A. & Walker I. (2004). The present and future role of photodynamic therapy in cancer treatment. *Lancet Oncology*, 5, 8, pp. 497-508.

Byrne J. D., Betancourt T. & Brannon-Peppas L. (2008). Active targeting schemes for nanoparticle systems in cancer therapeutics. *Advanced Drug Delivery Reviews*, 60, 15, pp. 1615-1626.

Chaleix V., Sol V., Guilloton M., Granet R. & Krausz P. (2004). Efficient synthesis of RGD-containing cyclic peptide-porphyrin conjugates by ring-closing metathesis on solid support. *Tetrahedron Letters*, 45, 27, pp. 5295-5299.

Chambers A. F. & Matrisian L. M. (1997). Changing views of the role of matrix metalloproteinases in metastasis. *Journal of the National Cancer Institute*, 89, 17, pp. 1260-1270.

Chaudhuri K., Keck R. W. & Selman S. H. (1987). Morphological changes of tumor microvasculature following hematoporphyrin derivative sensitized photodynamic therapy. *Photochemistry and Photobiology*, 46, 5, pp. 823-827.

Chen B., Pogue B. W., Hoopes P. J. & Hasan T. (2006a). Vascular and cellular targeting for photodynamic therapy. *Critical Reviews in Eukaryotic Gene Expression*, 16, 4, pp. 279-306.

Chen B., Pogue B. W., Luna J. M., Hardman R. L., Hoopes P. J. & Hasan T. (2006b). Tumor vascular permeabilization by vascular-targeting photosensitization: Effects, mechanism, and therapeutic implications. *Clinical Cancer Research*, 12, 3 I, pp. 917-923.

Chen B., Crane C., He C., Gondek D., Agharkar P., Savellano M. D., Hoopes P. J. & Pogue B. W. (2008). Disparity between prostate tumor interior versus peripheral vasculature in response to verteporfin-mediated vascular-targeting therapy. *International Journal of Cancer*, 123, 3, pp. 695-701.

Chen H., Chedotal A., He Z., Goodman C. S. & Tessier-Lavigne M. (1997). Neuropilin-2, a novel member of the neuropilin family, is a high affinity receptor for the semaphorins Sema E & Sema IV but not Sema III. *Neuron*, 19, 3, pp. 547-559.

Chen J., Bierhaus A., Schiekofer S., Andrassy M., Chen B., Stern D. M. & Nawroth P. P. (2001). Tissue factor - A receptor involved in the control of cellular properties, including angiogenesis. *Thrombosis and Haemostasis*, 86, 1, pp. 334-345.

Chetty C., Lakka S. S., Bhoopathi P. & Rao J. S. (2010). MMP-2 alters VEGF expression via alpha-v beta-3integrin-mediated PI3K/AKT signaling in A549 lung cancer cells. *International Journal of Cancer*, 127, 5, pp. 1081-1095.

Chu A. J. (2005). Tissue factor mediates inflammation. *Archives of Biochemistry and Biophysics*, 440, 2, pp. 122-131.

Clauss M., Gerlach M., Gerlach H., Brett J., Wang F., Famillettiv, Pan Y. C. E., Olander J. V., Connolly D. T. & Stern D. (1990). Vascular permeability factor: A tumor-derived polypeptide that induces endothelial cell and monocyte procoagulant activity, and promotes monocyte migration. *Journal of Experimental Medicine*, 172, 6, pp. 1535-1545.

Contrino J., Hair G.,. Kreutzer D. L & Rickles F. R. (1996). In situ detection of tissue factor in vascular endothelial cells: Correlation with the malignant phenotype of human breast disease. *Nature Medicine*, 2, 2, pp. 209-215.

Davidson B., I. Goldberg, W. H. Gotlieb, J. Kopolovic, G. Ben-Baruch, J. M. Nesland, A. Berner, M. Bryne & R. (1999). High levels of MMP-2, MMP-9, MT1-MMP and TIMP-2 mRNA correlate with poor survival in ovarian carcinoma. *Clinical and Experimental Metastasis*, 17, 10, pp. 799-808.

Denekamp J. (1999). The tumour microcirculation as a target in cancer therapy: A clearer perspective. *European Journal of Clinical Investigation*, 29, 9, pp. 733-736.

Desgrosellier J. S. & Cheresh D. A. (2010). Integrins in cancer: Biological implications and therapeutic opportunities. *Nature Reviews Cancer*, 10, 1, pp. 9-22.

Dolmans D. E. J. G. J., Fukumura D. & Jain R. K. (2003). Photodynamic therapy for cancer. *Nature Reviews Cancer*, 3, 5, pp. 380-387.

Dougherty T. J., Gomer C. J., Henderson B. W., Jori G., Kessel D., Korbelik M., Moan J. & Peng Q. (1998). Photodynamic therapy. *Journal of the National Cancer Institute*, 90, 12, pp. 889-905.

Drake T. A., Morissey J. H. & Edgington T. S. (1989). Selective cellular expression of tissue factor in human tissues. Implications for disorders of hemostasis and thrombosis. *American Journal of Pathology*, 134, 5, pp. 1087-1097.

Egeblad M. & Werb Z. (2002). New functions for the matrix metalloproteinases in cancer progression. *Nature Reviews Cancer*, 2, 3, pp. 161-174.

Ellis L. M., Liu W., Ahmad S. A., Fan F., Jung Y. D., Shaheen R. M. & Reinmuth N. (2001). Overview of angiogenesis: Biologic implications for antiangiogenic Therapy. *Seminars in Oncology*, 28, 5 SUPPL. 16, pp. 94-104.

Ellis L. M. (2006). The role of neuropilins in cancer. *Molecular Cancer Therapeutics*, 5, 5, pp. 1099-1107.

Favier B., Alam A., Barron P., Bonnin J., Laboudie P., Fons P., Mandron M., Herault J. P., Neufeld G., Savi P., Herbert J. M. & Bono F. (2006). Neuropilin-2 interacts with VEGFR-2 and VEGFR-3 and promotes human endothelial cell survival and migration. *Blood*, 108, 4, pp. 1243-1250.

Ferrara N. & Davis-Smyth T. (1997). The biology of vascular endothelial growth factor. *Endocrine Reviews*, 18, 1, pp. 4-25.

Ferrara N. (2002). VEGF and the quest for tumour angiogenesis factors. *Nature Reviews Cancer*, 2, 10, pp. 795-803.

Ferrara N. (2004). Vascular endothelial growth factor: Basic science and clinical progress. *Endocrine Reviews*, 25, 4, pp. 581-611.

Fingar V. H., Wieman T. J., Wiehle S. A. & Cerrito P. B. (1992). The role of microvascular damage in photodynamic therapy: The effect of treatment on vessel constriction, permeability, and leukocyte adhesion. *Cancer Research*, 52, 18, pp. 4914-4921.

Fingar V. H. (1996). Vascular effects of photodynamic therapy. J*ournal of Clinical Laser Medicine and Surgery* 14, 5, pp. 323-328.

Fingar V. H., Wieman T. J. & Haydon P. S. (1997). The Effects of Thrombocytopenia on Vessel Stasis and Macromolecular Leakage after Photodynamic Therapy Using Photofrin. *Photochemistry and Photobiology*, 66, 4, pp. 513-517.

Fiore E., Fusco C., Romero P. & Stamenkovic I. (2002). Matrix metalloproteinase 9 (MMP-9/gelatinase B) proteolytically cleaves ICAM-1 and participates in tumor cell resistance to natural killer cell-mediated cytotoxicity. *Oncogene*, 21, 34, pp. 5213-5223.

Folkman J. (1971). Tumor angiogenesis: therapeutic implications. *New England Journal of FMedicine*, 285, 21, pp. 1182-1186.

Fritsch C., Goerz G. & Ruzicka T. (1998). Photodynamic therapy in dermatology. *Archives of Dermatology*, 134, 2, pp. 207-214.

Frochot C., Di Stasio B., Vanderesse R., Belgy M. J., Dodeller M., Guillemin F., Viriot M. L. & Barberi-Heyob M. (2007). Interest of RGD-containing linear or cyclic peptide targeted tetraphenylchlorin as novel photosensitizers for selective photodynamic activity. *Bioorganic Chemistry*, 35, 3, pp. 205-220.

Fuh G., Garcia K. C. & De Vos A. M. (2000). The interaction of neuropilin-1 in vascular endothelial growth factor and its receptor Flt-1. *Journal of Biological Chemistry*, 275, 35, pp. 26690-26695.

Fukumura D. & Jain R. K. (2007). Tumor microenvironment abnormalities: Causes, consequences, and strategies to normalize. *Journal of Cellular Biochemistry*, 101, 4, pp. 937-949.

Gilson D., Ash D., Driver I., Feather J. W. & Brown S. (1988). Therapeutic ratio of photodynamic therapy in the treatment of superficial tumours of skin and subcutaneous tissues in man. *British Journal of Cancer*, 58, 5, pp. 665-667.

Grosskreutz C. L., Anand-Apte B., Duplaa C., Quinn T. P., Terman B. I., Zetter B. & D'Amore P. A. (1999). Vascular endothelial growth factor-induced migration of vascular smooth muscle cells in vitro. *Microvascular Research*, 58, 2, pp. 128-136.

Gu C., Limberg B. J., Brian Whitaker G., Perman B., Leahy D. J., Rosenbaum J. S., Ginty D. D. & Kolodkin A. L. (2002). Characterization of neuropilin-1 structural features that confer binding to semaphorin 3A and vascular endothelial growth factor 165. *Journal of Biological Chemistry*, 277, 20, pp. 18069-18076.

Guillemin F., Cosserat-Gerrardin I., Notter D. & Vigneron C. (2001). Diagnosis and treatment of bladder tumors by photodynamic therapy. *Diagnostic et traitement des tumeurs de vessie par thÃ©rapie photodynamique*, 49, 10, pp. 815-823.

Haddada H., Cordier L. & Perricaudet M. (1995). Gene therapy using adenovirus vectors. *Current Topics in Microbiology and Immunology*, 199, III, pp. 297-306.

Haubner R., Wester H. J., Weber W. A., Mang C., Ziegler S. I., Goodman S. L., Senekowitsch-Schmidtke R., Kessler H. & Schwaiger M. (2001). Noninvasive imaging of alpha (v) beta (3) integrin expression using 18F-labeled RGD-containing glycopeptide and positron emission tomography. *Cancer Research*, 61, 5, pp. 1781-1785.

Hu Z. &. Garen A (2000). Intratumoral injection of adenoviral vectors encoding tumor-targeted immunoconjugates for cancer immunotherapy. *Proceedings of the National Academy of Sciences of the United States of America*, 97, 16, pp. 9221-9225.

Hu Z., Sun Y. & Garen A. (1999). Targeting tumor vasculature endothelial cells and tumor cells for immunotherapy of human melanoma in a mouse xenograft model. *Proceedings of the National Academy of Sciences of the United States of America*, 96, 14, pp. 8161-8166.

Hu Z. & Garen A. (2001). Targeting tissue factor on tumor vascular endothelial cells and tumor cells for immunotherapy in mouse models of prostatic cancer. *Proceedings of the National Academy of Sciences of the United States of America*, 98, 21, pp. 12180-12185.

Hu Z., Rao B., Chen S. & Duanmu J. (2010). Targeting tissue factor on tumour cells and angiogenic vascular endothelial cells by factor VII-targeted verteporfin photodynamic therapy for breast cancer in vitro and in vivo in mice. *BMC Cancer*, 10, pp.

Ishida A., Murray J., Saito Y., Kanthou C., Benzakour O., Shibuya M. & Wijelath E. S. (2001). Expression of vascular endothelial growth factor receptors in smooth muscle cells. *Journal of Cellular Physiology*, 188, 3, pp. 359-368.

Ishigami S. I., Arii S., Furutani M., Niwano M., Harada T., Mizumoto M., Mori A., Onodera H. & Imamura M. (1998). Predictive value of vascular endothelial growth factor (VEGF) in metastasis and prognosis of human colorectal cancer. *British Journal of Cancer*, 78, 10, pp. 1379-1384.

Jichlinski P. & Leisinger H. J. (2001). Photodynamic therapy in superficial bladder cancer: Past, present and future. *Urological Research*, 29, 6, pp. 396-405.

Karrer S., Szeimies R. M., Hohenleutner U. & Landthaler M. (2001). Role of lasers and photodynamic therapy in the treatment of cutaneous malignancy. *American Journal of Clinical Dermatology*, 2, 4, pp. 229-237.

Katoh O., Tauchi H., Kawaishi K., Kimura A. & Satow Y. (1995). Expression of the vascular endothelial growth factor (VEGF) receptor gene, KDR, in hematopoietic cells and inhibitory effect of VEGF on apoptotic cell death caused by ionizing radiation. *Cancer Research*, 55, 23, pp. 5687-5692.

Kertes P. J. (2006). Verteporfin therapy of subfoveal minimally classic choroidal neovascularization in age-related macular degeneration: 2-Year results of a randomized, clinical trial - Commentary. *Evidence-Based Ophthalmology*, 7, 1, pp. 42-44.

Keyt B. A.,x Nguyen Y., Berleau L. T., Duarte C. M., Park J., Chen H. & Ferrara N. (1996). Identification of vascular endothelial growth factor determinants for binding KDR and FLT-1 receptors: Generation of receptor-selective VEGF variants by site-directed mutagenesis. *Journal of Biological Chemistry*, 271, 10, pp. 5638-5646.

Kolodkin A. L., Levengood D. V., Rowe E. G., Tai Y. T., Giger R. J. & Ginty D. D. (1997). Neuropilin is a semaphorin III receptor. *Cell*, 90, 4, pp. 753-762.

Konan Y.N., Gurny R., Allémann E. (2002). State of the art in the delivery of photosensitizers for photodynamic therapy. *J Photochem Photobiol B*, 66, 2, pp. 89-106

Konerding M. A., Fait E. & Gaumann A. (2001). 3D microvascular architecture of pre-cancerous lesions and invasive carcinomas of the colon. *British Journal of Cancer*, 84, 10, pp. 1354-1362.

Kremer C., Breier G., Risau W. & Plate K. H. (1997). Up-regulation of flk-1/vascular endothelial growth factor receptor 2 by its ligand in a cerebral slice culture system. *Cancer Research*, 57, 17, pp. 3852-3859.

Krikun G., Hu Z., Osteen K., Bruner-Tran K. L., Schatz F., Taylor H. S., Toti P., Arcuri F.,. Konigsberg W, Garen A., Booth C. J. & Lockwood C. J. (2010). The immunoconjugate "icon" targets aberrantly expressed endothelial tissue factor causing regression of endometriosis. *American Journal of Pathology*, 176, 2, pp. 1050-1056.

Kurohane, K., Tominaga, A., Sato, K., North, J.R., Namba, Y. & Oku, N. (2001). Photodynamic therapy targeted to tumor-induced angiogenic vessels. *Cancer Letters* 167, 1, pp. 49-56

Leinonen T., Pirinen R., Bohm J., Johansson R., Ropponen K. & Kosma V. M. (2006). Expression of matrix metalloproteinases 7 and 9 in non-small cell lung cancer: Relation to clinicopathological factors, beta-catenin and prognosis. *Lung Cancer*, 51, 3, pp. 313-321.

Leung D. W., Cachianes G.,x. Kuang G., Goeddel D. V. & Ferrara N. (1989). Vascular endothelial growth factor is a secreted angiogenic mitogen. *Science*, 246, 4935, pp. 1306-1309.

McDonald D. M. & Choyke P. L. (2003). Imaging of angiogenesis: From microscope to clinic. *Nature Medicine*, 9, 6, pp. 713-725.

Metz J. M. &. Friedberg J. S (2001). Endobronchial photodynamic therapy for the treatment of lung cancer. *Chest Surgery Clinics of North America*, 11, 4, pp. 829-839.

Miao H. Q., Lee P., Lin H., Soker S. & Klagsbrun M. (2000). Neuropilin-1 expression by tumor cells promotes tumor angiogenesis and progression. *FASEB Journal*, 14, 15, pp. 2532-2539.

Moriwaki S. I., Misawa J., Yoshinari Y., Yamada I., Takigawa M. & Tokura Y. (2001). Analysis of photosensitivity in Japanese cancer-bearing patients receiving photodynamic therapy with porfimer sodium (Photofrin). *Photodermatology Photoimmunology and Photomedicine*, 17, 5, pp. 241-243.

Mulder A. B., Blom N. R., Smit J. W., Ruiters M. H. J., Van Der Meer J., Ruud Halie M. & Bom V. J. J. (1995). Basal tissue factor expression in endothelial cell cultures is caused by contaminating smooth muscle cells. Reduction by using chymotrypsin instead of collagenase. *Thrombosis Research,* 80, 5, pp. 399-411.

Nemerson Y. (1988). Tissue factor and hemostasis. *Blood,* 71, 1, pp. 1-8.

Neufeld G., Cohen T., Shraga N., Lange T., Kessler O &. Herzog Y. (2002). The neuropilins: Multifunctional semaphorin and VEGF receptors that modulate axon guidance and angiogenesis. *Trends in Cardiovascular Medicine,* 12, 1, pp. 13-19.

Osterud B. (1997). Tissue factor: A complex biological role. *Thrombosis and Haemostasis,* 78, 1, pp. 755-758.

Pedersen B., Holscher T., Sato Y., Pawlinski R. & Mackman N. (2005). A balance between tissue factor and tissue factor pathway inhibitor is required for embryonic development and hemostasis in adult mice. *Blood,* 105, 7, pp. 2777-2782.

Pepper M. S., Ferrara N., Orci L. & Montesano R. (1992). Potent synergism between vascular endothelial growth factor and basic fibroblast growth factor in the induction of angiogenesis in vitro. *Biochemical and Biophysical Research Communications,* 189, 2, pp. 824-831.

Pepper M. S., Wasi S., Ferrara N., Orci L. & Montesano R. (1994). In vitro angiogenic and proteolytic properties of bovine lymphatic endothelial cells. *Experimental Cell Research,* 210, 2, pp. 298-305.

Pernot M., Vanderesse R., Frochot C., Guillemin F. & Barberi-Heyob M. (2011). Stability of peptides and therapeutic success. *Expert Opinion on Drug Metabolism and Toxicology* in press.

Perret G. Y., Starzec A., Hauet N., Vergote J., Le Pecheur M., Vassy R., Leger G., Verbeke K. A., Bormans G., Nicolas P., Verbruggen A. M. & Moretti J. L. (2004). In vitro evaluation and biodistribution of a 99mTc-labeled anti-VEGF peptide targeting neuropilin-1. *Nuclear Medicine and Biology,* 31, 5, pp. 575-581.

Pham W., Choi Y., Weissleder R. & Tung C. H. (2004). Developing a peptide-based near-infrared molecular probe for protease sensing. *Bioconjugate Chemistry,* 15, 6, pp. 1403-1407.

Plate K. H., Breier G., Weich H. A. & Risau W. (1992). Vascular endothelial growth factor is a potential tumour angiogenssis factor in human gliomas in vivo. *Nature,* 359, 6398, pp. 845-848.

Plouet J., Schilling J. & Gospodarowicz D. (1989). Isolation and characterization of a newly identified endothelial cell mitogen produced by AtT-20 cells. *EMBO Journal,* 8, 12, pp. 3801-3806.

Radu A., Wagnieres G., Van den Bergh H. & Monnier P. (2000). Photodynamic therapy of early squamous cell cancers of the esophagus. *Gastrointestinal Endoscopy Clinics of North America,* 10, 3, pp. 439-460.

Rao L. V. M. & Pendurthi U. R. (1998). Tissue factor on cells. *Blood Coagulation and Fibrinolysis,* 9, SUPPL. 1, pp. S27-S35.

Renno R. Z., Terada Y., Haddadin M. J., Michaud N. A., Gragoudas E. S. & Miller J. W. (2004). Selective photodynamic therapy by targeted verteporfin delivery to experimental choroidal neovascularization mediated by a homing peptide to vascular endothelial growth factor receptor-2. *Archives of Ophthalmology,* 122, 7, pp. 1002-1011.

Rollin S., Lemieux C., Maliba R., Favier J., Villeneuve L. R., Allen B. G., Soker S., Bazan, Y. Merhi N. G. & Sirois M. G. (2004). VEGF-mediated endothelial P-selectin translocation: Role of VEGF receptors and endogenous PAF synthesis. *Blood*, 103, 10, pp. 3789-3797.

Savary J. F.,. Monnier P, Fontolliet C., Mizeret J., Wagnieres G., Braichotte D. & Van Den Bergh H. (1997). Photodynamic therapy for early squamous cell carcinomas of the esophagus, bronchi, and mouth with m-tetra(hydroxyphenyl) chlorin. *Archives of Otolaryngology - Head and Neck Surgery*, 123, 2, pp. 162-168.

Sharman W. M., Allen C. M. & Van Lier J. E. (1999). Photodynamic therapeutics: Basic principles and clinical applications. *Drug Discovery Today*, 4, 11, pp. 507-517.

Sharman W. M., Van Lier J. E. & Allen C. M. (2004). Targeted photodynamic therapy via receptor mediated delivery systems. *Advanced Drug Delivery Reviews*, 56, 1, pp. 53-76.

Sharwani A., Jerjes W., Hopper C., Lewis M. P., El-Maaytah M., Khalil H. S. M., MacRobert A. J., Upile T. & Salih V. (2006). Photodynamic therapy down-regulates the invasion promoting factors in human oral cancer. *Archives of Oral Biology*, 51, 12, pp. 1104-1111.

Shiomi T. & Okada Y. (2003). MT1-MMP and MMP-7 in invasion and metastasis of human cancers. *Cancer and Metastasis Reviews*, 22, 2-3, pp. 145-152.

Shoji M., Hancock W. W., Abe K., Micko C., Casper K. A., Baine R. M., Wilcox J. N., Danave I., Dillehay D. L., Matthews E., Contrino J., Morrissey J. H., Gordon S., Edgington T. S., Kudryk B., Kreutzer D. L. & Rickles F. R. (1998). Activation of coagulation and angiogenesis in cancer: Immunohistochemical localization in situ of clotting proteins and vascular endothelial growth factor in human cancer. *American Journal of Pathology*, 152, 2, pp. 399-411.

Shoji M., Sun A., Kisiel W., Lu Y. J., Shim H., McCarey B. E., Nichols C., Parker E. T., Pohl J., Mosley C. A., Alizadeh A. R., Liotta D. C. & Snyder J. P. (2008). Targeting tissue factor-expressing tumor angiogenesis and tumors with EF24 conjugated to factor VIIa. *Journal of Drug Targeting*, 16, 3, pp. 185-197.

Siemann D. W., Chaplin D. J. & Horsman M. R. (2004). Vascular-targeting therapies for treatment of malignant disease. *Cancer*, 100, 12, pp. 2491-2499.

Siemann D. W., Bibby M. C., Dark G. G., Dicker A. P., Eskens F. A. L. M., Horsman M. R., Marme D. & LoRusso P. M. (2005). Differentiation and definition of vascular-targeted therapies. *Clinical Cancer Research*, 11, 2 I, pp. 416-420.

Soker S., Takashima S., Miao H. Q., Neufeld G. & Klagsbrun M. (1998). Neuropilin-1 is expressed by endothelial and tumor cells as an isoform- specific receptor for vascular endothelial growth factor. *Cell*, 92, 6, pp. 735-745.

Soker S., Miao H. Q., Nomi M., Takashima S. & Klagsbrun M. (2002). VEGF165 mediates formation of complexes containing VEGFR-2 and neuropilin-1 that enhance VEGF165-receptor binding. *Journal of Cellular Biochemistry*, 85, 2, pp. 357-368.

Solban N., Ortel B., Pogue B. & Hasan T. (2005). Targeted optical imaging and photodynamic therapy. *Ernst Schering Research Foundation workshop*, 49, pp. 229-258.

Spek C. A. (2004). Tissue factor: From 'just one of the coagulation factors' to a major player in physiology. *Blood Coagulation and Fibrinolysis*, 15, SUPPL. 1, pp. S3-S10.

Star W. M., Marijnissen H. P. A. & Van den Berg-Blok A. E. (1986). Destruction of rat mammary tumor and normal tissue microcirculation by hematoporphyrin derivative photoradiation observed in vivo in sandwich observation chambers. *Cancer Research*, 46, 5, pp. 2532-2540.

Staton C. A., Kumar I., Reed M. W. R. & Brown N. J. (2007). Neuropilins in physiological and pathological angiogenesis. *Journal of Pathology*, 212, 3, pp. 237-248.

Tang Y., Borgstrom P., Maynard J., Koziol J., Hu Z., Garen A. & Deisseroth A. (2007). Mapping of angiogenic markers for targeting of vectors to tumor vascular endothelial cells. *Cancer Gene Therapy*, 14, 4, pp. 346-353.

Tezel T. H., Bodek E., Sonmez K., Kaliappan S., Kaplan H. J., Hu Z. & Garen A. (2007). Targeting tissue factor for immunotherapy of choroidal neovascularization by intravitreal delivery of factor VII-Fc chimeric antibody. *Ocular Immunology and Inflammation*, 15, 1, pp. 3-10.

Thomas N., Tirand L., Chatelut E., Plenat F., Frochot C., Dodeller M., Guillemin F. & Barberi-Heyob M. (2008). Tissue distribution and pharmacokinetics of an ATWLPPR-conjugated chlorin-type photosensitizer targeting neuropilin-1 in glioma-bearing nude mice. *Photochemical and Photobiological Sciences*, 7, 4, pp. 433-441.

Thomas N., Bechet D. P.Tirand, Vanderesse R., Frochot C., Guillemin F. & Barberi-Heyob M. (2009). Peptide-conjugated chlorin-type photosensitizer binds neuropilin-1 in vitro and in vivo. *Journal of Photochemistry and Photobiology B: Biology*, 96, 2, pp. 101-108.

Thorpe P. E. (2004). Vascular Targeting Agents As Cancer Therapeutics. *Clinical Cancer Research*, 10, 2, pp. 415-427.

Tirand L., Frochot C., Vanderesse R., Thomas N., Trinquet E., Pinel S., Viriot M. L., Guillemin F. & Barberi-Heyob M. (2006). A peptide competing with VEGF165 binding on neuropilin-1 mediates targeting of a chlorin-type photosensitizer and potentiates its photodynamic activity in human endothelial cells. *Journal of Controlled Release*, 111, 1-2, pp. 153-164.

Tirand L., Thomas N., Dodeller M., Dumas D., Frochot C., Maunit B., Guillemin F. & Barberi-Heyob M. (2007). Metabolic profile of a peptide-conjugated chlorin-type photosensitizer targeting neuropilin-1: An in vivo and in vitro study. *Drug Metabolism and Disposition*, 35, 5, pp. 806-813.

Tozer G. M., Kanthou C. & Baguley B. C. (2005). Disrupting tumour blood vessels. *Nature Reviews Cancer*, 5, 6, pp. 423-435.

van Kempen L. C. L., de Visser K. E. & Coussens L. M. (2006). Inflammation, proteases and cancer. *European Journal of Cancer*, 42, 6, pp. 728-734.

Veikkola T., Karkkainen M., Claesson-Welsh L. & Alitalo K. (2000). Regulation of angiogenesis via vascular endothelial growth factor receptors. *Cancer Research*, 60, 2, pp. 203-212.

Verma S.,. Watt G. M, Mai Z. & Hasan T. (2007). Strategies for enhanced photodynamic therapy effects. *Photochemistry and Photobiology*, 83, 5, pp. 996-1005.

Versteeg H. H., Spek C. A., Peppelenbosch M. P. & Richel D. J. (2004). Tissue factor and cancer metastasis: The role of intracellular and extracellular signaling pathways. *Molecular Medicine*, 10, 1-6, pp. 6-11.

Vihinen P., Ala-Aho R. & Kahari V. M. (2005). Matrix metalloproteinases as therapeutic targets in cancer. *Current Cancer Drug Targets*, 5, 3, pp. 203-220.

Woodhams J. H., MacRobert A. J., Novelli M. & Bown S. G. (2006). Photodynamic therapy with WST09 (Tookad): Quantitative studies in normal colon and transplanted tumours. *International Journal of Cancer*, 118, 2, pp. 477-482.

Xu X., Wangv, Chen Z., Sternlicht M. D., Hidalgo M. & Steffensen B. (2005). Matrix metalloproteinase-2 contributes to cancer cell migration on collagen. *Cancer Research*, 65, 1, pp. 130-136.

Yoneda T., Sasaki A., Dunstan C., Williams P. J., Bauss F., De Clerck Y. A. & Mundy G. R. (1997). Inhibition of osteolytic bone metastasis of breast cancer by combined treatment with the bisphosphonate ibandronate and tissue inhibitor of the matrix metalloproteinase-2. *Journal of Clinical Investigation*, 99, 10, pp. 2509-2517.

Zheng G., Chen J., Stefflova K., Jarvi M., Li H. & Wilson B. C. (2007). Photodynamic molecular beacon as an activatable photosensitizer based on protease-controlled singlet oxygen quenching and activation. *Proceedings of the National Academy of Sciences of the United States of America*, 104, 21, pp. 8989-8994.

Zucker S., Mirza H., Conner C. E., Lorenz A. F., Drews M. H., Bahou W. F. & Jesty J. (1998). Vascular endothelial growth factor induces tissue factor and matrix metalloproteinase production in endothelial cells: Conversion of prothrombin to thrombin results in progelatinase A activation and cell proliferation. *International Journal of Cancer*, 75, 5, pp. 780-786.

# 6

# Binary Radiotherapy of Melanoma – Russian Research Results

Victor Kulakov[3], Elena Grigirjeva[2], Elena Koldaeva[2],
Alisa Arnopolskaya[3,1] and Alexey Lipengolts[3,1]
*[1]Federal Medical Biophysical A.I. Burnasyan's Centre of Federal Biomedical Agency of the Russian Federation*
*[2]Russian N.N. Blochin's Cancer Research Centre of Russian Academy of Medical Science*
*[3]Moscow Engineering & Physics Institute (State University)*
*Russian Federation*

## 1. Introduction

Radiotherapy (RT) in its different forms –distance, contact, intraoperative - currently is a powerful means of damaging cancer cells. RT is used both, as a radical monotherapy and in combination with different radiosensitizers or antitumor chemotherapeutic agents. The main problem of radiotherapy is the inevitable effect of ionizing radiation on normal tissues that results in unwanted side effects. Solving this problem was achieved practically by improvement of technical capacities of the ionizing radiation source and planning systems of irradiation procedure. The up-to-date therapeutic devices combine capacities of a medical imaging system (computed tomography) with a radiation therapeutic device. The combination according to the "two-in-one" principle ensures not only an ideal guiding of radiation on the target, but also constantly corrects the guiding, taking into consideration displacement of the target in the process of the patient's breathing, etc. The up-to-date planning systems help to increase reliability of precise guiding of ionizing radiation. Thus, unwanted action of ionizing radiation on normal tissues is reduced to the minimum, but is not excluded completely. In the last 100 years RT has transformed into a separate powerful trend in medicine. RT is equipped with sophisticated therapeutic devices widely used in oncological clinical practice - about 70% of oncological patients need these or those variants of RT. What are the prospects of the further improvement of RT? Obviously, the further technical improvement of therapeutic devices cannot be considered as a single way of RT development.

### 1.1 Binary radio therapy: What is it?

The most real trend of RT development is the development and introduction into clinical practice of Binary radiotherapy (BRT). Currently it is possible to speak about two types of BRT. They are neutron capture therapy (NCT), the idea of which was proposed in 1936 (Locher, 1936) and photon capture therapy (PCT). In English scientific literature is used the term "photon activation therapy". The principles of NCT and PCT (Khokhlov, 2004) are very similar. A malignant tumor is saturated with a preliminarily administered agent containing an element which is highly capable of interacting with the particular external ionizing radiation. Then tumor distant irradiation is carried out and local release of energy directly in the target tumor takes place. The main task is to make the total dose in the tumor to be lethal for its cells, and radiation exposure of normal tissues not to exceed the limits of their radiotolerance. Ideally, this permits to replace sophisticated technical devices for guiding ionizing radiation into the tumor with self targeting system based on biological or pharmacokinetic principles, and to increase considerably specificity and therapeutic effectiveness of radiation treatment technology. It is this circumstance that is the main impetus initiating research in this direction. For implementation of BRT two components are needed - a source of ionizing radiation (flow of neutrons or photons of certain energy) and pharmaceutical which composition includes the elements being highly capable of interaction with ionizing radiation.

### 1.2 Physic principals of binary radio therapy

The basis of BRT are the physical processes occurring as a result of interaction of certain elements, being constituents of composition of special pharmaceuticals, with external ionizing radiation. Let us consider in more details peculiarities of BRT taking as an example boron neutron capture therapy (BNCT), gadolinium neutron capture therapy (GdNCT) and PCT.

$^{10}$B-Neutron Capture Therapy (BNCT) is based on nuclear reaction $^{10}B(n,\alpha,\gamma)^{7}Li$ occurs as the result of interaction between stable isotope $^{10}$B with thermal neutron (En=0.025 eV). That interaction has very high probability ($\sigma$=3890 barn). Also as the result of the following nuclear reaction high energy short range charged particles – nucleus of helium ($\alpha$-particle) and nucleus of lithium are emitted. These particles has high linear energy transfer (LET) to tissue (200 keV for $\alpha$-particle and 350 keV for lithium nucleus) and short path length (about 14 μm) comparable to the diameter of a single cell. Such charged particles are equally lethal for oxygenated cells, hypoxic cells and cells in G0-stage. Sub lethal and potentially lethal damages caused by this kind of particles are nonreparable unlike the damages induced by the photon radiation. That is why BNCT is the most effective in treating tumors with cells are highly capable for DNA reparation. i.e. melanoma and glioblastoma. And if selective accumulation of $^{10}$B in tumor cells is provided then selective radiation exposure could be achieved on the cell level: only tumor cells with $^{10}$B inside would be destroyed leaving healthy tissues undamaged, thus killing all indefinitely small metastasis. In theory BNCT could overcome major limitations of photon radiotherapy: too high radioresistance of some tumor cells and to low radiotolerance of normal tissues.

For successful implementation of BNCT in clinical practice a complex of complicated chemical, medical, biological, physical and engineering problems must be solved. The most important task of them is development of $^{10}$B-containing drug capable to deliver necessary therapeutical amount of $^{10}$B into malignant tumor cells providing $^{10}$B optimum intracellular distribution for a time necessary for neutron irradiation. It was calculated that for a fluence of $10^{13}$ n/cm$^2$ concentration of $^{10}$B should be about 20-35 μg/g or $10^9$ atoms of $^{10}$B per cell. To prevent damage of healthy tissues in the irradiated volume there must be at least 3 times less concentration of $^{10}$B in them than in the tumor tissue. The requirement of the $^{10}$B amount in the tumor cell depends greatly on it's intracellular localization. It's assumed that 2 μg/g of $^{10}$B is enough for successful BNCT in case of it's localization inside the cells nuclei. Therefore the radiobiological efficacy of $^{10}B(n,\alpha,\gamma)^{7}Li$ reaction greatly depends on so called "factor of compound" provided by peculiarities of chemical structure of boron with main substance, it's metabolism and it's distribution among the most important organelles of the tumor cell.

After many years of purposeful searches, two compounds were selected for BNCT - mercaptoundecahydrododecaborate (Sivaev, 2002) - $Na_2B_{12}H_{11}SH$ (BSH) and *p*-(dihydroxybor)-L-phenylalanine (BPA) (Snyder, 1958). As the clinical experience has shown, these compounds are not optimal for BNCT, but nevertheless it is possible to use BSH rather successfully at the combined treatment of brain tumors with BNCT (Japan, USA, countries of EU), and BPA - at the treatment of skin melanoma and its metastases (Japan, USA). Clinical trials are being conducted to study effectiveness of BNCT with BPA in treating brain tumors (Japan, USA). A parallel intensive scientifically grounded search of new, more perfect, boron-containing compounds for BNCT is going on.

An important aspect of the effective conduction of BNCT is also the existence of the methods which are capable to provide the optimal individual planning and control of its conduction. First of all, it is necessary to know the absolute concentration of $^{10}B$, its microdistribution in the process of irradiation, that will allow to choose correctly the time of irradiation, to enhance accuracy of dosimetry and microdosimetry, thereby determining success of BNCT. In this connection of particular value is the development and mastering in clinical setting of the neutron radiation method of determining boron in tumor and normal tissues in real time by (n,γ)-reaction to $^{10}B$, and also a number of other analytical methods allowing to determine intracellular concentration and location of boron, such as quantitative autoradiography of high performance, electron spectroscopy and others. Up to the present the evaluation of boron concentration in tumor at BNCT is conducted as a rule on the basis of preliminarily obtained data, for example, during surgical operation for removal of brain tumor, or indirectly - by the blood level of boron taking into account also preliminarily established ratio of its concentrations tumor/blood.

Interaction of photon radiation with different elements is characterized by dominating in a particular energy range (Fig. 1) of photon absorption by heavy elements (with Z≥53) on absorption by light elements composing biological tissues (H, O, N, C, Na, K, Cl etc.). This difference can be used for local increasing of energy absorption in the target (tumor) by administration or accumulating some heavy element in necessary region of irradiation.

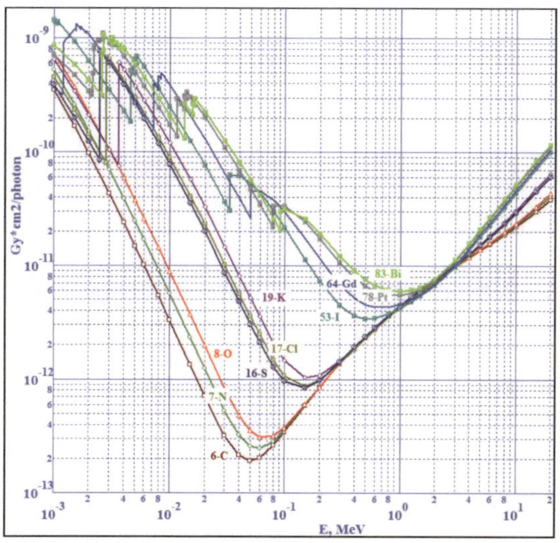


Fig. 1. Energy dependence of specific photon kerma for the basic elements of biological tissue and some heavy elements (Sheino, 2006).

In terms of Radiotherapy such approach can be implemented by administration or accumulation in a tumor volume the necessary amount of a pharmaceutical containing some heavy element with subsequent irradiation of the tumor region with X-rays of certain energy spectrum. As the result of such irradiation local increase of absorbed dose in the tumor occurs. In case of necessary amount of heavy element in the target is provided the increase of absorbed dose can be 2-3 times higher than for the same irradiation but with no drug administered (Karnas, 1999; Sheino, 2006). Emission of short range radiation caused by photoabsorption on heavy elements directly in the irradiated target is effective factor of tumor cell growth suppression. Significant that in PCT absorbed dose in healthy tissues could be lower than it's tolerant dose. Thus radiation influence on healthy tissues is decreasing and selectivity of tumor tissue damage is increasing during irradiation procedure. Such binary technology was called Photon Capture Therapy. Combination of biological self targeting of radiation and it's main localization in target volume makes PCT prospective Radiotherapy technology.

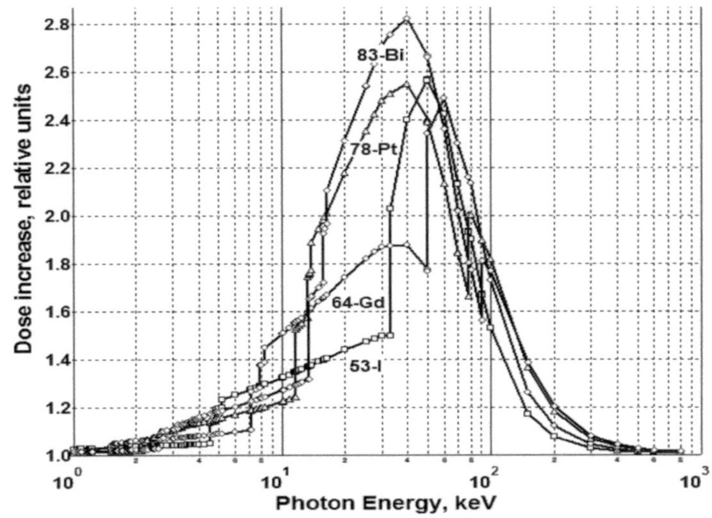


Fig. 2. Relative increase of a dose in a biological tissue for various elements with Z>53 at their concentration of 1% in dependence on energy of photons. (Sheino, 2006).

Calculated estimation show (Sheino, 2006) that proper therapeutic efficacy of PCT could be achieved if the concentration of heavy element is around ~ 10 mg/g. At present there are no drugs with i.v. administration capable to accumulate in tumor tissues in such amount. That is why gadolinium containing MRI-contrast pharmaceutical Dipentast® (Russia) and intratumoral way of administration were used in our primary studies of PCT.

### 1.3 Tasks of research

The chapter presents the results of the preclinical studies on BRT conducted in Russia. Melanoma was chosen as the main object of the research. The studies were carried out in conformity with the effective RF requirements for three main directions: 1. the studies on the B-16 mouse melanoma cell culture; 2. the studies of mice with the transplanted B-16 melanoma; the studies on dogs with spontaneous B-16 melanoma. The similarity of canine and human melanomas permitted to replace the transplanted nude melanomas with the model of canine spontaneous melanoma. The chapter presents the used neutron and photon bundles. It presents the main characteristics of the used pharmaceutical products with $^{10}B$ ([$^{10}B$]-boron phenylalanine in the pharmaceutical form borate ether with D-fructose; [$^{10}B$]-BSH - mercapto-closo-undecaborateas a sodium salt (Sivaev, 2002) and gadopentetat in the pharmaceutical form ensuring delayed elimination of the substance from the injection site). The results of remote consequences of BRT and traditional methods of melanoma treatment - surgical intervention, immune therapy, action of ionizing radiation (neutrons and gamma-radiation) are given. The comparison of therapeutic effectiveness of NCT with $^{10}B$ and Gd used as both monotherapy and in combination with adjuvant immune therapy with interleukin-2 (Roncoleukin®) is presented. Separately there are presented the results of the micropharmacokinetic studies - distribution of BSH and a number of new boron-containing agents across the main organelles of melanoma cell. For the results beyond the scope of the preclinical studies, the references to the published works are given.

## 2. Materials and methods

### 2.1 Irradiation of biological objects

Neutron irradiation was performed on the irradiation facilities of Moscow Engineering and Physics Institute research reactor IRT and research reactor RR-8 of RRC "Kurchatov Institute". The IRT facility includes the irradiation room for positioning cell cultures and laboratory animals including dogs in the neutron beam. The neutron beam delivered to the irradiation room has the following characteristics: thermal neutron flux – $1.1\times10^{9}$ n/cm$^{2}$s, fast neutron flux – $5.8\times10^{7}$ n/cm$^{2}$s, photon dose rate - $1.8\times10^{-4}$ Gy/s. Irradiation room is equipped with video surveillance to observe the state of irradiation object and with the physiological parameters monitoring system (heart and breath frequency, blood pressure, body temperature ) as well as with drug delivery system. IR-8 reactor facility is designed for irradiation small object only - cell cultures and small animals. Thermal neutron flux on IR-8 facility was $1.2\times10^{8}$ n/cm$^{2}$s, fast neutron flux – less than $0.96\times10^{7}$ n/cm$^{2}$s, photon dose rate - $8.3\times10^{-7}$ Gy/s. Small animals were not anesthetized prior the irradiation. At the IR-8 animals were irradiated in Teflon® cages, at IRT animals were situated in lead boxes, which were limiting animal's movements but not interfering feeding and defecations. Local irradiation of transplanted into the rear paw tumor immobilized in advance was performed with dose of 2.5 Gy-Eq. Considering that poor fluence power thermal neutron irradiation was prolonged for time individual group as control for each animal group was used.

X-rays irradiations were performed using radiobiology autoprotective X-rays facility with anode voltage 220 kV and dose rate at the position of cell culture monolayer 2.0 Gy/min for cell culture irradiation and X-rays irradiation of mice bearing B-16 melanoma was performed with an X-ray unit with anode voltage of 150 kV and dose rate of 0.7 Gy/min at treated tumor volume.

### 2.2 Dosimetry

Thermal neutron absorbed dose at NCT was measured with prompt gamma neutron activation analysis (PGNAA). Average dose in tissue without drug was 0.25 Gy/h. Total absorbed dose was determined by 3 nuclear reactions, which provide the major part of absorbed dose (95-97%) during interaction of thermal neutrons with nuclides of biological tissue - $^{1}H(n,\gamma)^{2}H$; $^{14}N(n,p)^{14}C$; $^{10}B(n,\alpha)^{7}Li$.

Dose rate of X-rays in irradiation position was performed using DKS-AT5350/1 dosimeter (Russia) and dosimetric films Gafchromic® EBT. Optical density of dosimetric films was measured on Varian Cary-50 spectrophotometer.

### 2.3 Animals and cell culture

B-16 melanoma cell culture for experiments was received from Blockin's Cancer Research Center (Russia) storage. These cells were grown as monolayer in glass flasks containing mixture of RPM6-1640 and Eagle's nutrient media with 10% calf serum and gentamicyne. Grown cells were suspended in saline. Cell concentration in suspension was 1000 per 1 ml.

Cultural flasks in PCT in vitro studies were divided to experimental and control groups. Both groups were irradiated using X-rays with 10 Gy, 20 Gy, 30 Gy and 40 Gy. Before irradiation Dipentast® was added into experimental flasks for 0.2 mg/ml Gd concentration.

Experiments in vivo were conducted on C57Bl/6 male and female mice bearing subcutaneously transplanted melanoma B-16. All mice were of veterinary certification.

The mice were subcutaneously inoculated into rear paw with $(3.5\text{-}4)\cdot 10^6$ melanoma cells. All NCT and PCT experiments were conducted 10-11 days after transplantation (tumor volume was about 0.9-1.0 $cm^3$).

For NCT studying the mice were injected intraperitoneally with saline solutions of KUG-1 and BSH in amount of 0.2 ml containing 150 mg of boron per kg body weight for BSH and 25 mg of B per kg body weight for KUG-1. After injection of studied compounds ( in 6 hours for BSH and in 24 hours for KUG-1) tumor was locally irradiated.

For PCT the animals were divided into four groups: 1- experimental group irradiated with X-rays and administered with Gd-DTPA before irradiation, 2 – mice only locally irradiated with X-rays but not injected with Gd-DTPA, 3 – nonirradiated mice but only administered with Gd-DTPA with the same amount that the experimental group, 4 – untreated mice. When tumor volume was achieved 1 $cm^3$ 1 and 3 animal groups were intratumorally administrated with 0.175 ml Dipentast®. After administration mice from 1 group were immediately irradiated with X-rays in 20 Gy dose.

For NCT studies Dogs with spontaneous oral cavity melanoma were selected in LLC "Biocontrol" based on the results of clinical examination. The owners of the dogs were agreed on experimental treatment.

60 dogs with oral cavity melanoma were selected for the study . The dogs were examined before and after treatment using clinical and histological methods. The dogs were divided on the following groups: I group - without treatment; II group - surgical treatment; III - distant gamma-therapy, IV group - neutron therapy; V - BNCT; VI - GdNCT ; VII - Complex treatment (NCT with adjuvant immunotherapy with Ronkoleukine®); VIII group - NCT without immunotherapy. BNCT was performed with $[^{10}B]$-BPA in pharmaceutical form of boron ether solution with D-fructose. GdNCT was performed with Dipentast®.

In V group BPA were administered by two routes: in the artery which nourish tumor and intravenously (Fig. 3). Administration of the medicine was controlled by X-ray examination. Irradiation was performed 2.0-2.5 hours after BPA administration

### 2.4 Cell vitality assessment

For cell vitality assessment after irradiation MTT-test (Mosman, T., 1983) and clonogenic test were used. For MTT-test cells were sewed in 96-holes flat-bottomed plates and incubated during 3, 5, 7 days. 2-3 hours before termination 10 µl of (4,5-dimethylthiazoline-2)-2,5 diphenyltetrazoly bromide (final concentration was 1 mg/ml). After incubation cells were centrifuged at 1200 rev/min during 7-10 min. Supernatant was carefully removed. 200 µl of DMSO were added into each hole for formazane solution. Optical density of homogenous solution was determined in "Picon" photometer at 530 nm. Optical density of solution was demonstration of redox-intensivity in cell culture. For clonogenic test cells of both groups were sewed in 6-holes plates with full medium and in 3, 5, 7 days cell colonies were count using LOMO microscope.

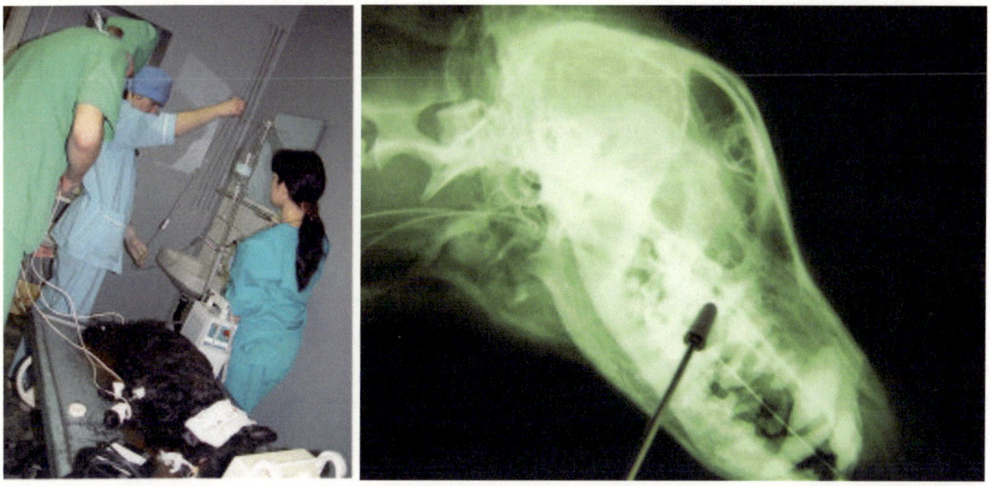

Fig. 3. Preclinical trials of BNCT in dogs with spontaneous malignant melanoma. Infusion of BPA drugs using a feeding pump (left); X-ray control of the compound administration (richt).

### 2.5 Quantification of boron and gadolinium

Boron tumor concentration was measured in vivo with PGNAA (Khokhlov, 2008; Khokhlov, 2009). During irradiation this concentration in tumor varied about 7-8 µg/g for [$^{10}$B]-BSH, 10-20 µg/g for BPA and 10-11 µg/g for KUG-1.

Gd tumor concentration varied about 10-100 mg/cm$^3$, Gd concentration in biological samples was measured with neutron-activation analysis (Zaitsev, 2004 a) or using roentgen fluorescent analysis in X-Art-M concentration analyzer (Comita Ltd, Russia).

### 2.6 Subcellular boron distribution

In 5 min., 1 and 24 h after BSH, KUG-1 administration experimental tumors were excised, rinsed, weighed and homogenized. The cell organelles were prepared using routine techniques of differential centrifugation (De Duve, 1967).

Subcellular fractions (nuclei, mitochondria, lysosomes, cytosol) were received for further boron determination with PGNAA method.

### 2.7 Study of kinetics of B-16 melanoma cell population

Kinetics of B-16 melanoma cell population was studied at determination of melanocytes and DNA-synthesizing cells percentage in total studied tumor cells.

For this purpose tumors of exponential growth phase were used. On 7-th day after subcutaneous inoculation experimental C57BL/6 mice (body weight of 17-20 g; tumor size of 4-5 mm in diameter) were intraperitoneally administrated with 100 mg of BSH per 1 kg of body weight. In 1 hour before euthanasia the mice were administrated with $^{3}H$-thymidin (74 kBq/g of body weigh); as control administration saline was used Excised tumors were used for preparation of cytological preparations. Melanocytes were determined as cells containing more than 5 granules of melanin (Alberts, 1989). Analysis of kinetics of DNA-synthesizing cells was studied in preparations covered with "M" emulsion counting $^{3}H$-labelled melanocytes. These parameters were separately assessed for peripheral and central zones.

### 2.8 Study of cell distribution through the cell cycle

Alterations of the quantitative distribution through the cell cycle were also investigated. The distribution of tumor cells through the cell cycle was studied by flow DNA-cytofluorimetry on ICP-22 cytofluorimeter.

The BSH distribution was investigated in B-16 melanoma bearing male C57Bl/6 mice. The mice had a body weight (BW) of 17-20 g, the tumor was subcutaneously transplanted. BSH was administrated intraperitoneously. 2 dose groups were injected with 50 and 150 mg/kg body weight on 9-11-th day after subcutaneous tumor inoculation. In 3, 12 and 24 hours after administration tumors were excised (3 samples per time point). Tumor samples were used for preparation of cell nuclei suspension. This suspension was dyed with mixture of ethidium bromide and mitramicin (1:1).

### 2.9 Assessment of tumor growth

During experiments with transplanted tumors three reciprocally perpendicular tumor's diameters were daily measured and evaluated tumors volumes taking tumor's shape as ellipse:

$$V=(\pi/6).\,d_1.\,d_2\,.\,d_3 \qquad (1)$$

Where V- tumor volume, d1, d2, d3 – linear dimensions of ellipsoid, cm

For every temporary point tumor volume was normalized to it's volume at the beginning of exposure (V0) and then V1/V0 against time from the beginning of exposure curves were constructed depending on every dose D and for every concrete mouse at adequate control for it (D=0). The parameters of tumor growth delay (Td) and of time of tumor's volume duplication were evaluated from these curves as well as tumor growth index (2).

$$TGI=S_E/S_K \qquad (2)$$

where: $S_{E.}$ – area under tumor growth curve of experimental group, $S_K$ – area under tumor growth curve of experimental group.

Area under tumor growth curve was calculated as following:

$$S=\sum_{i=1}^{n-1}\frac{V_i+V_{i+1}}{2}t_i \qquad (3)$$

where $V_i$ - tumor volume at $i^{th}$ measurement,

n – number of measurements,

$t_i$ – period between nearby measurements.

### 2.10 Drugs

In our studies we have used the following medicines: [$^{10}$B]-BPA (Khoknlov, 2001, Kulakov, 2001, Kulakov, 2002) – 4-(dihidroxyboron)–L-phenilalane (BPA, KatChem, Chehia), Katchem, (Czechia), chemical purity of 98 % , degree of enrichment of $^{10}$B – 99.7 %); borated ethers with D-fructose ([$^{10}$B]-BPA-F) and D-galactose ([$^{10}$B]-BPA-Gal); $Na_2{}^{10}B_{12}H_{11}SH$ - [$^{10}$B]-BSH (Katchem, (Czechia) , chemical purity of 99 % ; degree of enrichment of $^{10}$B – 99.7 %; novel boron-contained compound KUG-1 (this is manufacturing code of compound), chemical purity of 99 % with natural boron and Dipentast® - Gd-DTPA based pharmaceutical with Gd content of 28.11% and semi-elimination period from site of injection - 55±6 min.).

The dogs were intravenously administrated with boron-containing compounds while the mice were administrated with boron-containing compounds intraperitoneally. Dipentast® was administrated intratumorally at uniform distribution (4-6 injection per tumor) both in NCT and PCT studies.

## 3. Results of investigations

### 3.1 Cell pharmacokinetics

In the time interval from 1 to 12 h after the BSH administration relatively high boron content was in subcellular structures of tumor tissue. BSH was preferably accumulated in nuclei and mitochondria. (Table 1). These data suggest the BNCT with BSH might be more effective during time interval from 6 to 12 h after drug administration.

| Subcellular fractions | Time after administration, h | | | | | |
|---|---|---|---|---|---|---|
| | 1 | | 6 | | 12 | |
| | Tumor | Liver | Tumor | Liver | Tumor | Liver |
| Nucleus | 5.7 | 14 | 6.9 | 12.0 | 2.2 | 2.9 |
| Mitochondria | 3.0 | 6.1 | 2.6 | 5.1 | 2.1 | 0.5 |
| Lysosomes | 0.8 | 1.8 | - | 4.9 | 2.0 | 1.2 |
| Cytosol | 1.5 | 1.2 | 0.2 | 1.5 | 0.2 | 1.3 |

Table 1. $^{10}$B concentration in subcellular fractions of B-16 melanoma and liver in C57Bl/6 mice after BSH administration [$^{10}$B μg/g]

In the time interval from 24 to 48 h after the KUG-1 administration maximal boron content was in nuclear fraction. This concentration exceeded necessary and sufficient concentration for successful NCT. Boron content in other subcellular fractions was sufficient for therapeutic efficacy of NCT. (Table 2). Therefore boron subcellular distribution had confirmed clinical perspectives of KUG-1.

| Subcellular fractions | Time after administration, h | | | |
|---|---|---|---|---|
| | 24 | | 48 | |
| | Tumor | Liver | Tumor | Liver |
| Nucleus | 8.13 | 9.1 | 10.9 | 9.3 |
| Mitochondria | 4.59 | 3.17 | 4.29 | 4.56 |
| Lysosomes | 3.48 | 3.83 | 4.58 | 13.5 |
| Cytosol | 3.3 | 5.28 | 1.53 | 5.8 |

Table 2. $^{10}$B concentration in subcellular fractions of B-16 melanoma and liver in C57Bl/6 mice after KUG-1 administration [$^{10}$B μg/g]

### 3.2 Influence on cell cycle and kinetics of cell population of B-16 melanoma

This research was devoted to study the influence of BSH – boron carrier at anticancer neutron capture therapy on cell population of murine melanoma B-16. It was proved that prevalent accumulation of tumor cells in synthetic and premitotic phases (S and G2/M) of cell cycle was caused by BSH effect. Probably this phenomenon of cell proliferation may be linked to compensatory population response on damaging factor of BSH (Ado, 1993).

The detected activity of the latter coupled with its ability to penetrate into the nucleus and mitochondria may be the reason for its efficacy in NCT of melanoma and opens new perspectives of the well known drug. These data are shown in tables 3, 4.

| Days after administration | Peripheria | | Centre | |
|---|---|---|---|---|
| | Control | Experiment | Control | Experiment |
| 1 | 4.0±0.9 | 10.9±1.1 | 9.2±1.3 | 12.0±1.2 |
| 2 | 13.1±1.2 | 15.3±1.3 | 16.7±1.3 | 8.8±1.0 |
| 3 | 22.0±1.5 | 18.9±1.3 | 17.6±1.4 | 12.3±1.2 |

Table 3. Quantity of melanocytes and labeled cells in peripheral and central zones of of B-16 melanoma after BSH administration (100 mg/kg of body weight)

| Time after administration, h | BSH, $^{10}$B μg /kg BW | Phase of cell cycle | | | | |
|---|---|---|---|---|---|---|
| | | $IG_1$ | $IIG_1$ | S | $G_2/M$ | S+ $G_2/M$ |
| 3 | 50 | 19.5±2.0 | 58.4±5.7 | 13.7±1.4 | 8.4±0.9 | 22.1 |
| | 150 | 20.1±2.1 | 57.2±4.5 | 14.3±1.5 | 7.9±0.8 | 22 |
| 12 | 50 | 16.7±1.5 | 56.4±5.4 | 8.9±1.1 | 18.7±2.0 | 27.6 |
| | 150 | 16.2±1.3 | 54.6±5.1 | 16.6±1.3 | 12.7±1.3 | 29.3 |
| 24 | 50 | 17.0±1.8 | 57.9±5.6 | 10.1±1.1 | 15.9±1.6 | 25.1 |
| | 150 | 16.0±1.4 | 57.0±5.5 | 14.3±1.3 | 12.7±1.3 | 27.0 |
| 24 | Control (saline) | 20.1±1.9 | 59.2±5.7 | 14.0±1.5 | 6.7±0.7 | 20.7 |

Table 4. Influence of BSH on cell cycle of B-16 melanoma after BSH administration

So, BSH is the drug of threefold action and this action allows to realize full potential of BSH.

1. BSH is boron carrier to deliver boron into tumor and it's vital structures.
2. BSH stimulates proliferating cells (S+G2/M), increasing sensitivity for all types of irradiation.
3. BSH influences on cell differentiation ( synthesis of melanin is index of cell differentiation for melanoma).

The results of investigations demonstrated most efficacy of NCT during the first 24 h after BSH administration due to both subcellular distribution and influence on cell cycle.

In further searching of new boron compounds for NCT it would be remembered that any chemical agent is probably active agent effecting on cell biology.

### 3.3 In vitro studies of photon capture therapy

On the base of obtained results of MTT-test and clonogenic test curves of dependence " part of survived cells - exposition dose" were constructed. (Fig. 4 and Fig. 5).

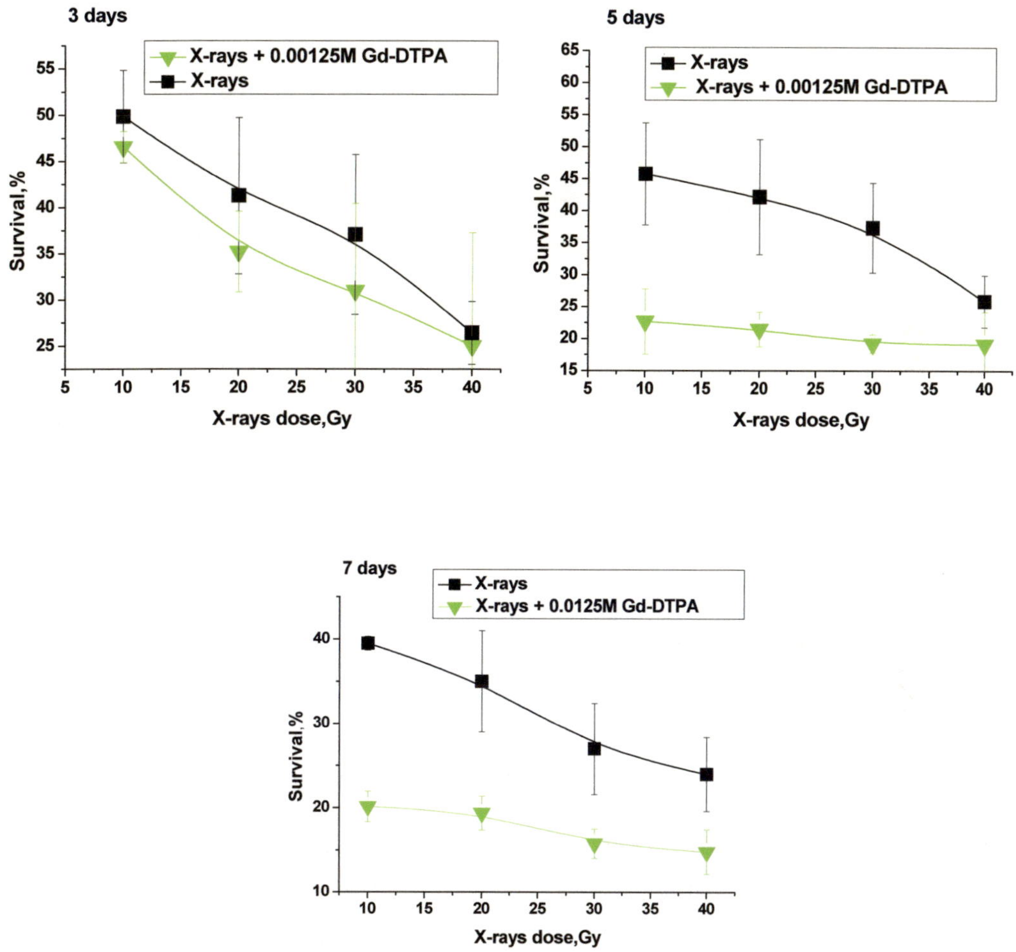


Fig. 4. Cell survival for control and experimental groups (MTT-test data) at 3rd, 5th and 7th days

MTT-test data had shown equal parts of survived cells in both groups on 3-rd day. On 5-th day part survived cells in experimental group was essentially low and was retained at this level to 7-th day. RGG-test data had shown (Fig. 5) practically complete suppression of cell growth in experimental group even at 10 Gy. In control group significant quantity of cell colonies were observed.

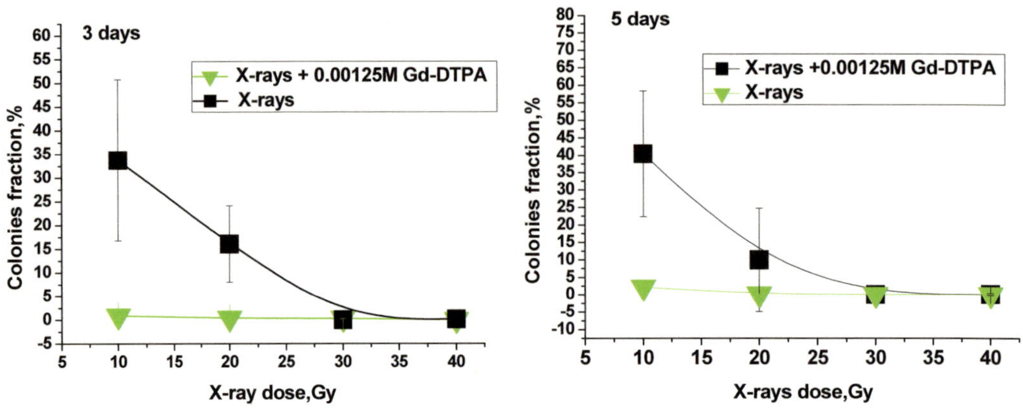


Fig. 5. Cell survival for control and experimental groups (clonogenic test data) , 3-rd and 5-th days.

### 3.4 Radiobiological studies in vivo

Studies of binary radio therapy in animals with potentially suitable for clinical application pharmaceuticals

#### 3.4.1 Boron neutron capture therapy

The therapeutic efficacy of NCT was studied using two compounds: BSH and KUG-1 containing 55% and 20% boron relatively. PGNAA data demonstrated that maximal boron content in tumor (12 µg/g of tissue) was achieved in 1 hour after BSH injection decreasing by 6 hours. Then this level was not varying for 48 hours. On the same time the compound rapidly eliminated from all tissues adjacent to tumor excluding skin. As result in 12-48 hours interval there was sufficient for NCT ratio tumor/adjacent tissue including blood. The boron content suitable for NCT in the case of introduction of KUG-1 was accumulated in 24 hours and was constant not less then 15 hours. It should be noted that the total absorbed dose in tumor was determined from three major nuclear reactions - $(n,\gamma)^{2}H$; $^{14}N(n,p)^{14}C$; $^{10}B(n,\dot{\alpha})^{7}Li$ - contributing essential part in to absorbed dose at interactions between thermal neutrons and nuclides of living tissue and was equal to 95-97%. The time of tumor volume duplication (Td) at NCT with BSH injection was increased to 14-15 days comparatively with 3-4 days for intact animals. In the case of Ph1 injection this time was prolonged to 8-10 days. The injection of Ph2 did not make this parameter differ from control meanings.

The increase of survival of treated mice was equal to 57% in the case of BSH administration and only 14% at KUG-1 administration in spite of KUG-1 accumulation coefficient was more than the same for BSH. It is caused with toxic side effect of KUG-1 (hepatic- and neurotoxicity).

KUG1 is perspective for purposes of NCT but needs a development for eliminations of toxic side effects. Results of irradiation are shown in table 5 and in figure 6.

| B-10-carrier for NCT | KUG-1 | BSH |
|---|---|---|
| Absorbed dose in tumor from reaction on B-10,Gy | 1.76 | 1.23 |
| Absorbed dose in tumor from reaction on N, Gy | 0.42 | 0.79 |
| Absorbed dose in tumor from reaction on H, Gy | 0.45 | 0.36 |
| Total absorbed dose in tumor | 2.63 | 2.38 |
| Concentration of B-10 in tumor, initial, µg/g | 11.3 | 8.3 |
| Concentration of B-10 in tumor, initial, µg/g | 9.9 | 7 |

Table 5. Results of thermal neutron irradiation mice bearing B-16 melanoma

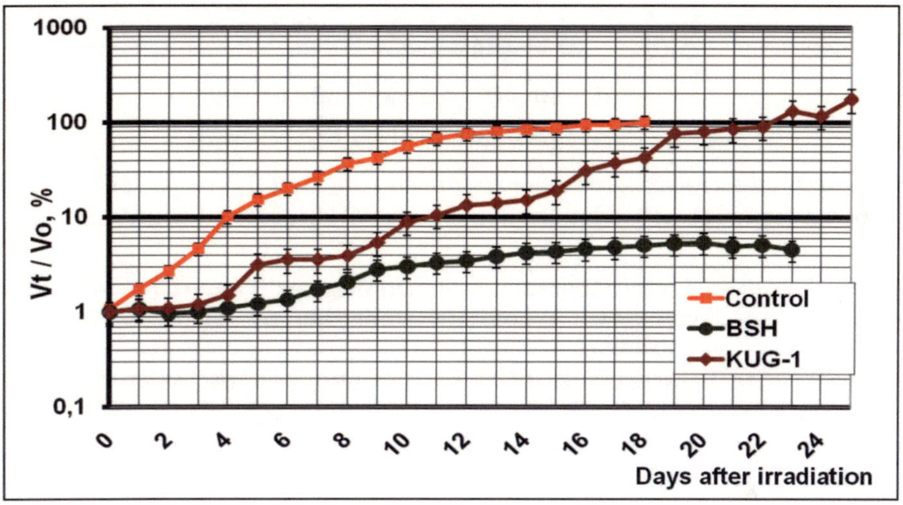


Fig. 6. Growth of transplanted B-16 melanoma in C57bl/6 after thermal neutron irradiation at presence of BSH and KUG-1

### 3.4.2 Photon capture therapy

On the base of obtained results of irradiation curves of tumor growth were constructed. (Fig. 7). Quantitative assessment of efficacy of each force was determined. (Table 6).

| Criterion | Group 1 | Group 2 | Group 3 |
|---|---|---|---|
| Tumor growth delay time, days | 15±1 | 8±1 | - |
| Tumor volume doubling time, days | 16±2 | 11±1 | - |
| Tumor growth index (IG) | 0.1±0.03 | 0.25±0.05 | 0.75±0.05 |

Table 6. Quantitative parameters of effect assessment

Obtained data demonstrate that local irradiation of melanoma containing Dipentast® resulted in significant inhibition of tumor growth in comparison with irradiation only. Administration of Dipentast® without consecutive irradiation didn't result in expressed anticancer effect.

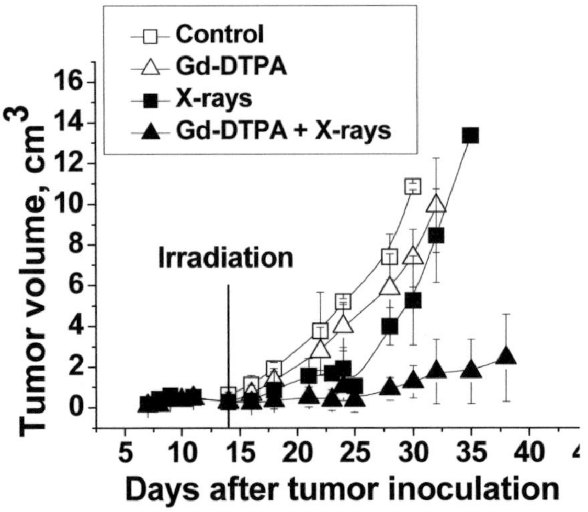


Fig. 7. Tumor volume growth kinetics for irradiated with Gd-DTPA injection group (▲), only irradiated group (■), only administered with Gd-DTPA group (Δ), untreated group (□)

### 3.5 Results of neutron capture therapy studies in dogs with spontaneous melanoma of the oral mucosa. Development of combined radiotherapy scheme on the basis of NCT and adjuvant immunotherapy

The improvement of the technology of neutron capture therapy under the condition of nuclear reactors, conduction of detailed studies with the purpose of comparative evaluation of effectiveness of different variants of neutron capture technology and traditional methods of treatment is an important and topical clinical task. The conduction of preclinical studies will permit to choose the most efficient scheme of treatment of melanoma, since melanoma of the oral mucosa in dogs may be regarded as a correct model of human melanoma.

The studies on effectiveness of BNC technology in treatment of spontaneous melanoma of canine oral mucosa have been conducted for several years. The preclinical study of neutron capture therapy on dogs with the diagnosis of oral mucosa melanoma has yielded the following results.

In group I of the animals which did not receive any treatment, the average animal life expectancy was 38±13.6 days. 100% of the animals were euthanized due to their severe condition. The reason for euthanasia of such animals was local propagation of the tumor and systemic metastasis.

In the group of animals who underwent surgical removal of the oral mucosa tumor, 100% recurrence occurred within the period of 26 ±12.5 days. In group III where the animals received traditional radiotherapy, stabilization of tumor growth was seen in 75% of cases, partial regression in 12.5% of animals and complete regression - also in 12.5% of animals. In 100% of cases resumption of tumor growth within 30±5.5 days was observed.

Thus, both at surgical treatment and at radiotherapy recurrence occurred in 100% of cases. The statistical analysis showed that the duration of the recurrence-free period at the use of these methods of treatment was in fact equal.

This indicates that surgical treatment and radiotherapy are virtually low-effective methods of treating melanoma of oral mucosa in dogs at stage II-III of btumor process. This probably can be explained by the specific location of the tumor when it is impossible to perform radical removal of the tumor. At these stages of tumor process the tumor size appears to be sufficiently large.

To evaluate effectiveness of neutron capture radiotherapy, that is, NCT, the results obtained were compared to the animals subject to the action of neutron bundle alone. In this group (IV, n=5) partial regression was attained in 80% of cases, and complete regression - in 20% of cases. In 100% of cases the continued growth of the tumor within 101±28.8 days was also diagnosed.

In group V, where irradiation with neutron bundle was performed with a preliminary administration of boron agents, that is, BNCT, complete tumor regression was possible to be attained in 78% of cases. (Fig. 8) At BNCT, in cases of complete tumor regression no recurrence was observed. The absence of recurrence in complete tumor regression proves complete destruction of melanoma cells in the primary tumor focus.

In this study the boron product was administered by two routes: intravenously and regionally into the artery feeding the tumor. Having analyzed the results obtained, we got sufficiently significant data on that the route of the product administration exerts no effect on NCT effectiveness. Thus, during further studies of BNCT it is possible to administer 10B BFA intravenously that facilitates conduction of the BNCT procedure.

During conduction of NCT with Dipentast®, that is, GdNCT (group VI), somewhat other results were obtained as compared to BNCT. First, tumor regression took place more slowly in at GdNCT comparing to BNCT, and complete tumor regression was noted only in 46% of cases (Fig.9). In 66.7% of animals recurrence of the tumor was seen 106±7.5 days after the procedure of GdNCT. Nevertheless, the effect of irradiation at GdNCT was sufficiently high that suggested a possibility of development of an effective technology of melanoma treatment on the basis of GdNCT.

Since so far a small number of studies on GdNCT was conducted and there are no data on the optimal concentration of gadolinium inside the tumor which is necessary to achieve the tumoricide dose, we studied the GdNCT effect at different doses of gadolinium in tumor. The studied range of concentrations was from 10 mg/cm$^3$ to 100 mg/cm$^3$. During the clinical trial the regularity was determined at which the best clinical effect of GdNCT was observed at the gadolinium concentration in tumor of up to 12 mg/cm$^3$.

We also conducted the study on investigating distribution of the power of total dose depending on the gadolinium concentration inside tumor. Such study was performed on the basis of the developed model of GdNCT (1).

The study of total dose rate distribution during GdNCT at different concentration showed that at the gadolinium concentration over 12 mg/cm$^3$ the total dose in the tissue sharply decreases by several times. So, at concentrations of 6-12 mg/cm$^3$ the total dose power at the depth of 0.5 cm of tissue is 150-200 cGy/min and does not increase with the growth of the gadolinium concentration in target (Fig. 10). Such effect is due to the fact that isotopes of gadolinium $^{157}$Gd (the content in the natural element 15.68%) have high sections of capture of thermal neutrons. That causes an increase of absorption of thermal neutrons during GdNCT at high concentrations of gadolinium products. The so-called "shielding effect" occurs.

Thus, the analysis of distribution of the total dose, by using the solving of the equation of transfer of neutrons and photons by the method of discrete ordinates according to the RADUGA-5 program, showed that the optimal concentration of $^{157}$Gd is within the range of 6-12 mg of Gd in 1 cm$^3$ of tumor. These conclusions help to optimize subsequently the process of GdNCT for achieving the maximum result.

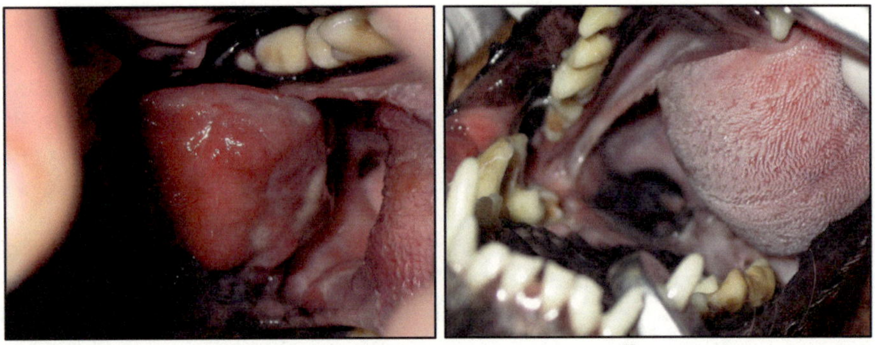

A. B.

Fig. 8. BNCT Results of spontaneous melanoma of the oral mucosa: A - Melanoma before BNCT, B - 2 weeks after procedure BNCT. Full Tumor regression

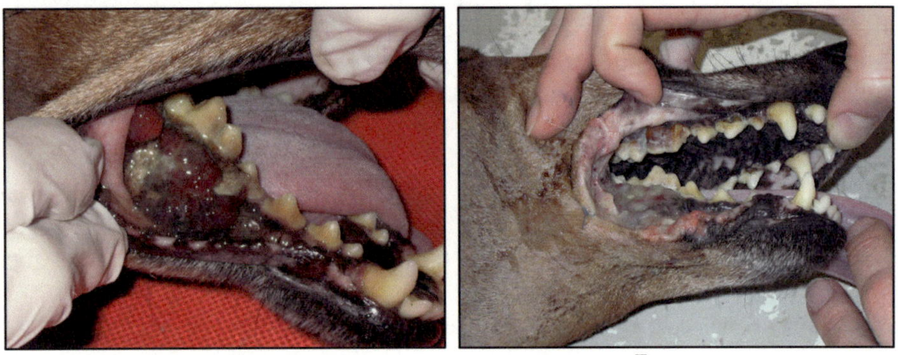

A. B.

Fig. 9. GdNCT Full regression of melanoma. A – Oral Melanoma, B - 1,5 months after GdNCT

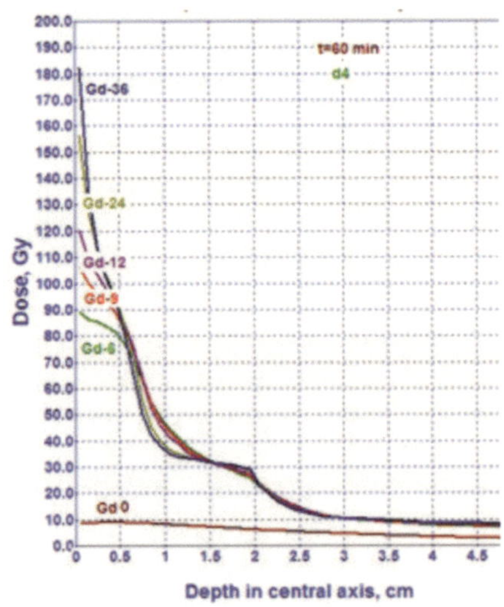


Fig. 10. Tumor dose distribution in different $^{157}$Gd concentration.

Thus, the clinical results agree entirely with the further studies on investigating distribution of the total dose power depending on the gadolinium concentration inside tumor.

Comparing the time of recurrence in control and at GdNCT we found that the time of recurrence at GdNCT (106±7.5 days) significantly exceeds the time of recurrence at surgery (26±12.5 days) and at traditional gamma-therapy (30±5.5 days). Such advantage of the GdNCT method comparing to traditional therapy is explained by a high local dose of irradiation of 80-100 Gy per the irradiated target.

The differences in the results of BNCT and GdNCT, in our opinion, may be explained by two reasons:

the differences in the pharmacokinetic properties of the used products - 10B-boron phenylalanine during BNCT and the complex of gadolinium with DTPA during GNCT;

different products of nuclear and physical reactions of nuclei of $^{10}B$ and Gd with thermal neutrons.

During BNCT there is a selective accumulation of 10B-boron phenylalanine inside the tumor cells. The ratio of $^{10}B$ concentrations in the tumor and in normal tissues is not less than 2.5. The run of alpha-particles which are formed during irradiation is commensurable with the cell diameter, and the nuclei of $^{6}Li$ – less than the cell diameter. Therefore secondary radiation affects predominantly tumor cells, by which a high effect of BNCT effect is achieved. And in the given study during BNCT we observed degree 1-2 of local radiation reactions.

During GdNCT the used product with gadolinium - Dipentast® is mainly in the intercellular space, and accumulation of the product inside tumor is achieved only by intratumoral administration of the product. As a result of absorption of thermal neutrons by the nuclei of 157Gd there are formed high-energy gamma-quanta, low-energy electrons and roentgen radiation. It is secondary radiation that causes death of tumor cells. However, the character of secondary radiation leads to affection of healthy tissues as well. At the use of GdNCT degree 2 of local radiation reactions was diagnosed in all animals, and in one case - stage 4.Such difference in the mechanism clinically should manifest itself in an increase of side effects on healthy tissues during GdNCT. Indeed, during GdNCT the degree of radiation lesions of healthy tissues was somewhat higher (degrees 2 and 4 of local radiation reactions) than at irradiation with neutrons and during BNCT (degree 1-2 of local radiation reactions).

An increase of recurrence rate at GdNCT even in complete regression of tumor shows that at GdNCT it is not always possible to achieve death of all tumor cells. One of the reasons of this result may be the excessive concentration of $^{157}Gd$ inside tumor. As natural gadolinium has the section of neutron capture two orders higher than boron has, at its excessive concentration in tumor the effect of screening on the tumor surface may occur that does not allow to achieve destruction of cells in a deeper layer. During further studies, at improvement of GNCT technology, it is necessary to administer gadolinium product in such way so that the gadolinium concentration in tumor tissue would not exceed 12 mg/cm$^3$.

Despite the conducted treatment, in all animals there was recorded systemic metastasis into the lungs, that is, despite local cure of oral mucosa melanoma, the further generalization of tumor process could not be avoided. Thus, NCT is effective comparing to other methods for local treatment of the primary tumor focus but influences in no way the process of formation of metastases. Therefore the task of this study was not only to evaluate NCT effectiveness during treatment of the primary tumor focus, also development of the multimodality treatment aimed at both the primary tumor focus and prevention of quick metastasis of tumor. We formed two groups of animals - groups VII and VIII in which we determined life expectancy. These groups embraced the animals at one stage of tumor process in which complete regression was achieved as a result of NCT. In this study the adjuvant therapy influence on life expectancy of dogs with oral cavity melanoma (group VII) was investigated by using Ronkoleukin®. For inclusion into the scheme of treatment of melanoma on the basis of BNCT and GdNCT as the means hampering the process of metastasis, the Russian agent Roncoleukin® was chosen which is an immunostimulator, it enhances the antibacterial, antiviral, antifungal and antitumor immune response.

We managed to carry out the study on a small group of animals, but the results obtained show significantly that life expectancy at conduction of immunotherapy increase on the average by three times. So, in the study group of the animals which received successful BNCT at stage II of tumor process and also receive adjuvant immunotherapy, the average life expectancy was about 305 days. In group VIII where BNCT was conducted without immunotherapy, the average life expectancy was 113 days.

Thus, in cases of successful NCT at concomitant conduction of immune therapy we observed the maximum life expectancies, and most such animals were long-living ones.

The studies performed by us have shown that treatment of oral mucosa melanoma should be of multimodality character and be aimed at both combating the primary tumor focus and remote metastases.

During conduction of NCT it is necessary to attain complete regression of tumor, it is in these cases that the maximum life expectancies may be reached.

This approach to the diseases, namely the combination of NCT and adjuvant immune therapy permitted us to gain the maximum results in treating melanoma.

In this chapter the results of complex method of oral canine melanoma are shown, but also we studied the possibility of NCT combination with other methods for canine osteosarcoma treatment. Induction chemotherapy, intraarterious administration of BPhA, bone resection, extracorporal BNCT of bone fragment, radiated bone implantation and adjuvant chemotherapy were included in treatment scheme (Fig. 11). 24 hours after operation dog can lean on the leg. 2.5 months after operation, results of biopsy showed absence of tumor cells in replanted bone. X-ray imaging showed full consolidation of replanted bone with maternal bone, without carcinogenesis signs (Fig. 11, 12), Total life span of the dog was 2.5 years without recurrence.

Results of highly malignant tumors treatment show that, instead of high metastatic activity and low traditional methods efficacy , it is possible to achieve high therapeutic efficacy with application of complex treatment scheme on the basis of NCT.

## 4. Conclusion

There is a large world positive experience of BNCT clinical application in combined treatment of more than 300 patients with brain tumors (Japan, USA, EU countries) and more than 30 patients with melanoma, including metastatic melanoma (Japan, USA), which shows the prospects for future development and optimization of this type of binary therapy. According to Japanese clinical data for 1968-1996, average life span of patients with brain tumors was from 640 till 1811 days, depending on histological type of tumor, without strong mental disorders. 6 patients after BNCT live more than 10 years. Average life span of such

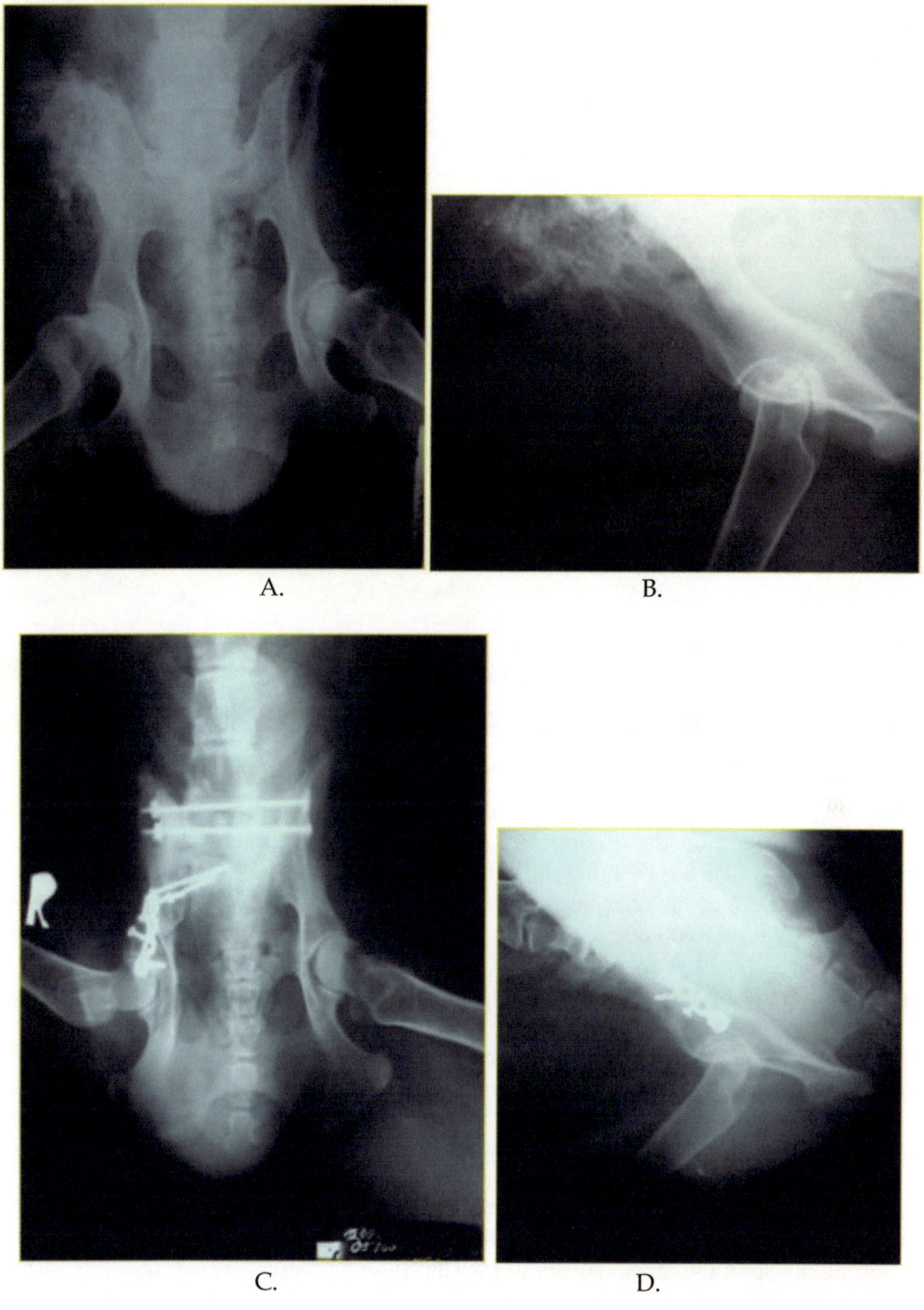


Fig. 11. BNCT of primary osteosarcoma IIb stage. A, B – Roentgenoscopy before operation; C, D - Roentgenoscopy 2.5 months after surgery.

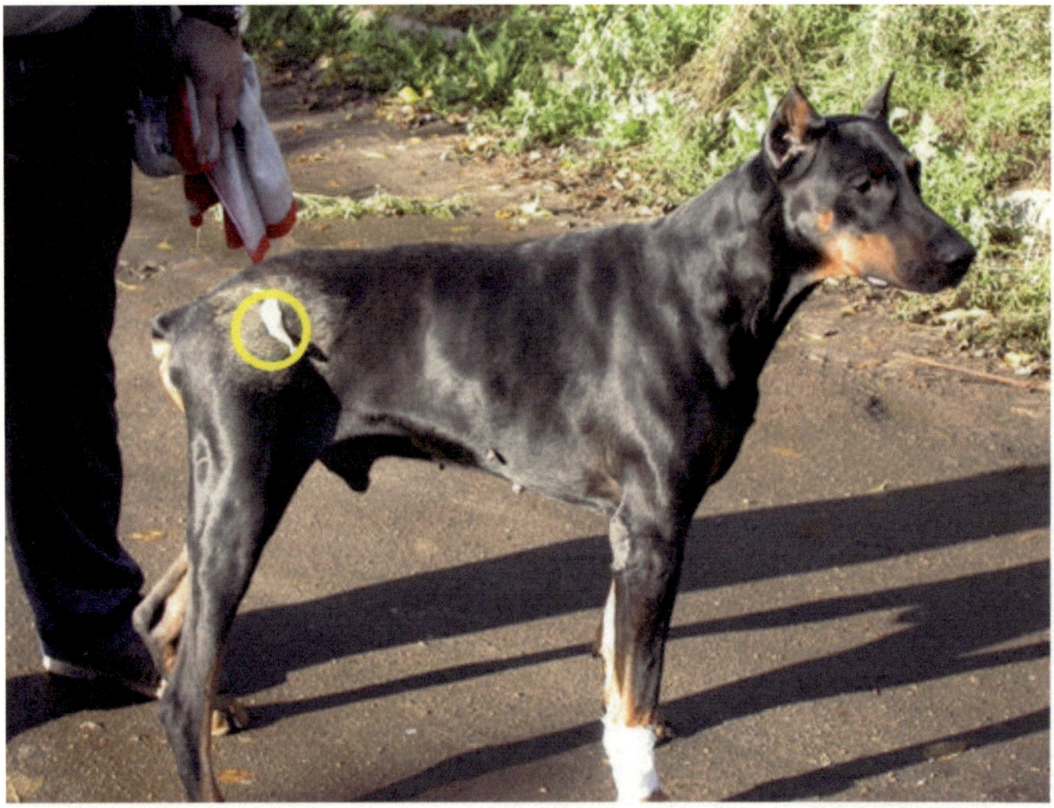

Fig. 12. A dog on walk 2.5 months after BNCT. Surgery region is marked in yellow

patients after traditional methods of treatments was 8-10 months. Doctor Nakagawa Y., taking into consideration BNCT opportunities and analyzing his own clinical experience, supposes, that BNCT is the best method for malignant brain tumors treatment, which needs further development of neutron beams and $^{10}B$-containing drugs (Nakagawa & Hatanaka, 1997; Nakagava et. al., 2003). Preliminary analysis of melanoma treatment clinical results shows, that more than 2 years life span for patients with melanoma was 78%, treatment can be succeed in $T_{3-4}$ $N_0M_0$ melanoma in more than 90% of patients. (Mishima 1996; Busse et al., 1997; Barth et al., 2005).

Achieved by Russian scientists results prove the advantages of BRT in comparison with traditional methods of treatment. BPA is more effective substance for BNCT than BSH and KUG-1. Full tumor regression was reached in 80% of cases with application of BNCT, and in the group of GdNCT full tumor regressions was in 50% of dogs with oral cavity melanoma, while the application of traditional gamma-therapy provides only 12,5 % of full tumor regression. Complex therapy, which combines BNCT with adjuvant immunotherapy with Ronkoleukin® (Interleukin-2) can increase the total life span more than 3 times. To compare with human life span we can speak about possibility of 5-10 years recurrence-free period for humans. As canine melanoma is the correct model of human melanoma, such complex method of treatment significantly more effective than traditional methods of treatment One of the reason of BNCT efficacy with BSH is the capability of BSH to penetrate into the cell nucleus and mitochondrions. This fact opens new prospects for future application of BSH in

BNCT. Complex treatment scheme, which combines traditional methods of treatment with BRT can significantly improve malignancy treatment.
Therapeutic possibilities of BRT are note finally defined, but this method of treatment has low cost and it can be easily installed and transported to other hospital. It makes us to intensify the studies for effective BRT technologies creation, putting more attention for creation of specific pharmaceuticals, which can accumulate in the tumor with tumor/normal concentration gradient more than 3. To minimize resources for new pharmaceuticals selection for further studies we apply developed screening scheme.

## 5. References


Ado, A.D., (1993). *Physiopathology (in rus), Triada-X, Moscow/*

Alberts, B., Bray, D., Lewis, J., Raff, M., Roberts, K., Watson, J.D. (1989). Molecular Biology of the Cell (second edition). Garland Publishing Inc., ISBN 0-8240-3695-6, London

Gabel D., (1989). tumor-seeking compounds for boron neutron capture therapy: synthesis and biodistribution, *Clin Aspects Neutron capture Ther.* pp.233-241. Upton. - New-York-London.

Grigorieva E.Yu., Nikolaeva T.G., Koldaeva E.Yu., Naidenov M.G., Sprishkova RA., (2005). $Na_2{}^{10}B_{12}H_{11}SH$ (BSH) - pharmaceuticall for neutron capture therapy and it's influence on melanoma B-16 cell cycle, *Rossiyskiy Bioterapevtitcheskiy Zhurnal (in rus.).* № 3, pp. 30-33.

De Duve C., 1967. General principles in enzyme Cytology. Ed. by Roodyn, D.B. Academic Press, London.

Karnas, S.J., Yu, E., McGarry, R.C., Battista, J.J. (1999). Optimal photon energies for IUdR K-edge radiosensitization with filtered x-ray and radioisotope sources. Physics in Medicine and Biology, Vol. 44, No. 10, (October 1999), pp. 2537-2549, ISSN 0031-9155.

Khokhlov, V.F., Kulakov V.N., Zaitsev K.N., Riaboukhine Yu.S., Yarmonenko S.P., Deineko O.N., Kornienko V.N. (2001). The Rushian Project on Neutron Capture Therapy for Cancer. Therapy *Frontiers in Neutron Capture, ed. by Hawthorne et al. Kluwer Academic/Plenum Publishers, N-Y,* 2001, p.p. 425-432.

Khokhlov V.F., Kulakov V,N., SheinoI.N., Nasonova T.A. & Mitin V.N. (2004). Patent RF #2270045.

Khoknlov V.F., Zaitsev K.N. , Beliaev V.N., Kulakov V.N., Kvasov V.I., Lipengolts A.A., Portnov A.A. (2008). Prompt Gamma Neutron Activation Analysis of 10B and Gd in Biological Samples at the MEPhI Reactor. Proceedings of 13th International Congress on Neutron Capture Therapy "A new option against cancer". Italy, Florence, November 2-7. ENEA. pp. 415-417.

Khoknlov V.F., Zaitsev K.N., Beliaev V.N., Kulakov V.N., Lipengolts A.A., Portnov A.A. (2009). Prompt gamma neutron activation analysis of 10B and Gd in biological samples at the MEPhI reactor. Applied Radiation and Isotopes. Vol. 67.- Issue 7-8S.- S251–S253.

Koldaeva E.Yu., Grigorieva E.Yu., Kulakov V.N., Sauerwein W. (2010). BSH for BNCT of B-16 Melanoma in a Murine Model. *New Challenges in Neutron Capture Therapy 2010, Proceedings of 14th International Congress on Neutron Capture Therapy,* October 25-29, 2010, Buenos Aires, Argentina, p. 144-146.

Kulakov V.N., Bregadze V.I., Sivaev I.B., Nikitin C.M., Gol'tyapin Yu.V., Khokhlov V.F. (2001). Design of Boron- and Gadolinium- Containig Agents for NCT *Frontiers in Neutron Capture, ed. by Hawthorne et al. Kluwer Academic/Plenum Publishers, N-Y,* 2001, p.p. 843-846.

Kulakov V.N., Khokhlov V.F., Nasonova T.A., Portnov A.A., Zaitsev K.N., Kvasov V.I., Alekseev K.P., Mescherykova V.V., Klimova T.P. (2002) Compounds with $^{10}B$ and Gd in the Russian NCT Project. Research and Development in NCT, *Essen, September 8-13 2002, Ed.: W.Sauerwein, R.Moss, A.Wittig, Monduzzi Editore, Intern. Proceeding Division*, 2002, p. 107-101.

Lipengolts, A.A. Khokhlov V.F., Kulakov V.N., Nasonova T.A., Dobrynina O.A., Sheino I.N. (2010). Photon Capture Therapy - Process Analog of Neutron Capture Therapy. First Experimental Results of Melanoma Treatment in Mice. *New Challenges in Neutron Capture Therapy 2010; Proceedings of 14th International Congress on Neutron Capture Therapy, October 25-29, 2010, Buenos Aires, Argentina, p. 105-106.*

Makarenkov A.S., Terekhov S.M., Kalashnikova E.A., Smirnova T.D. и др., (2003). The Stady of variability of MTT metabolism intensivitity in cell culture at evaluation of death and proliferation of cells with MTT-test. , Cytologija (in rus.), (2003), № 9, pp. 899-903.

Mossman T. (1983). Rapid colorimelric assay for cellular growth and survival: application to proliferation and cytotoxic assays, *J. Immunol. Methods*, Vol. 65, pp. 55-63.

Locher C. (1936). Biological Effects and Therapeutic Possibilities of Neutrons. Am. J. Roentgenol. Radium Ther. Vol. 36, pp. 1.

Mitin V.N., V.N.Kulakov, Khokhlov V.F., Sheino I.N., Kozlovskaya N.G., Zaitsev K.N., Portnov A.A., Arnopolskaya A.M., Bass L.P., Nikolaeva O.V. (2006). GdNCT of Spontaneous Canine Melanoma. Proceedings of ICNCT-12 «Advances in Neutron Capture Therapy 2006». Ed. by Y.Nakagawa, T.Kobayashi, H.Fukuda. Japan, Kagawa. pp 127-130.

Mitin V.N., Kulakov V.N., Khokhlov V.F., Sheino I.N., Arnopolskaya A.M., Kozlovskaya N.G., Zaitsev K.N., Portnov A.A. (2008). Comparison of BNCT and GdNCT Efficacy in Treatment of Canine Cancer. Proceedings of 13th International Congress on Neutron Capture Therapy "A new option against cancer" Italy Florence, November 2-7,.- ENEA.- 2008.- pp.

Sheino I.N., V.N.Kulakov, Mitin V.N. (2005). Dose-supplementary beam therapy of cancer. Proceedings of II Eurasian Congress at Medical Physic and Engineering, Moscow, June 21-24, p.p. 85-86.

Sheino, I.N. (2006). Dose-supplementary therapy of malignant tumors, Proceedings of ICNCT-12 12th International Congress on Neutron Capture Therapy, ISBN 4-9903242-0-X, Kagawa Japan conference location, October 2006.

Sivaev I. B., Bregadze V.I., Kusnetzov N.T. (August 2002). Anion of kloso-dodecaborat in Boron capture therapy. Izvesiya of RAS, chemistry, (in rus.). №8, pp. 1256-1267.

Snyder H.R., Reedy A.J., Lennarz Wm.J. (1958). Synthesis of Aromatic Boronic Acids. aldehydo Boronic Acids and a Boronic Acid Analogue of Tyrosine, J.Am.Chem.Soc. Vol.80, № 4, pp. 835-838.

Strukov A.N., Ivaniva M.A., Nikitin A.K., (2001). *Problems in oncology* (in rus.) vol. 47, № 5, pp. 616-618.

Zaitsev K., Portnov A., Sakharov V., Troshin V., Savkin V., Kvasov V., Mishcherina O., Khokhlov V., Kulakov V.N., Sheino I., Meshcherikova V., Mitin V., Koslovskaya N., Shikunova I. (2004 a). Neutron capture therapy at the MEPhI reactor. *Int. J. Nuclear Energy Science and Technology.* Vol. 1 No. 1, pp. 83-101.

Zaitsev K., Portnov A., Sakharov V., Troshin V., Savkin V., Kvasov V., Mishcherina O., Khokhlov V., Kulakov V.N., Sheino I., Meshcherikova V., Mitin V., Koslovskaya N., Shikunova I. (2004 b). NCT at the MEPhI reactor. Proceedings of Intern. Symposium on Boron Neutron Capture Therapy, *Ed.: S.Taskaev,* Budker Institute of Nuclear Physics, Russia, Novosibirsk, July 7-9, pp. 82-98.

# 7

# Clinical Development Paradigms for Cancer Vaccines: The Case of CIMAvax EGF®

Gisela González, Tania Crombet and Agustín Lage
*Center of Molecular Immunology*
*Cuba*

## 1. Introduction

Scientific progress is inhabited by paradigm shifts. In 1962, Tomas Kuhn popularized the concept of ¨paradigm shift¨ arguing that scientific advancement is not evolutionary, but rather is a "series of peaceful interludes punctuated by intellectually violent revolutions", and in those revolutions "one conceptual world view is replaced by another" (Kuhn, 1962).
Again according to Kuhn, ¨paradigm shifts occur when anomalies in the old paradigm accumulate and cannot be overlooked anymore¨. This is probably the situation today in the treatment of advanced cancer.
However, changes are difficult. Human beings resist changes.
For many years, chemotherapy has been the gold standard of cancer therapy. The era of cancer chemotherapy began in the 1940s with the first use of nitrogen mustards and folic acid antagonist drugs (De Vita et al, 2005) and a major break-through in 1965, when James Holland, Emil Freireich, and Emil Frei hypothesized that cancer chemotherapy should follow the strategy of antibiotic therapy for tuberculosis with combinations of drugs, each with different mechanisms of action (Frei et al, 1965). Cytotoxic chemotherapy in fact succeeded in producing major therapeutic effects, including cures, in hematological malignancies and some solid tumors such as testicular and ovarian cancers. However its contribution to the treatment of most solid tumors has been much less. The success history of chemotherapy in leukemia and lymphoma simply did not repeat in most solid tumors.
Chemotherapy has the disadvantage of its high toxicity, because is an unspecific treatment which effect does not distinguish between normal and tumor cells.
The paradigm of selective killing of cancer cells in a way alike to what antibiotics do for infections, created in turn a standardized procedure for stepwise drug development through conventional Phase I, II and III trials, which was soon adopted and translated into regulations by many drug regulatory authorities. The designs of these clinical trials respond to the need of demonstrating the drug efficacy at its maximal tolerable dose (MTD).
However, although retaining the main concept and adapting to the old paradigm malfunctioning, variants have been introduced for cancer drugs approval: i.e. approvals without randomized trials and approvals based in accelerated approval regulations.
From January 1973 through December 2006, 68 new drugs were approved for cancer therapy from which 31 were approved without 2 arms randomized clinical trials including a control arm with different therapy, supportive care or placebo (Tsimberidou, 2009).

Accelerated approval (AA) regulations were established by the US Food and Drug Administration (FDA) designed to shorten development times of drugs for serious medical diseases, i.e. cancer (Dagher et al, 2004; Richey et al, 2009). According these, drugs received AA based in Phase II trials and sponsors must confirm efficacy in post-approval trials. Since the first AA for an oncology indication was granted between 1995 and 2008, 51 new molecular entities have received FDA approval for cancer therapeutic indications: 32 with regular approval and 19 with AA (Richey et al, 2009).

In some way, regulations have moved towards faster access to patients of even the very toxic chemotherapies.

Biotechnology development has provided new therapeutic weapons for cancer therapy. According Pharma 2009 report, there are currently 633 biotechnology medicines under development, from which 254 are for cancer therapy (109 monoclonal antibodies and 63 cancer vaccines). That means, 40% of worldwide biotechnology is cancer therapy.

These Biotechnological products have the characteristics of being highly specific which in turn causes a low toxicity, long-term usability and usability in combinations.

Biotechnology anticancer drugs are not just more drugs, they are different drugs; and their entrance into cancer therapy high lightened the limitations of the prevalent paradigm for drug development. The enormous differences between the new biotechnological products and chemotherapeutic agents, makes necessary changes in established clinical development paradigms. Specifically, for cancer vaccines, more flexible and focused developmental guidelines are needed to address their unique characteristics (Hoos et al, 2007).

In this report we use the case of CIMAvax-EGF® to illustrate the operation of the emerging paradigms.

## 2. Conventional clinical development paradigm for anti-cancer chemotherapeutics

Cancer drugs development paradigms have been based on criteria adjusted to cytotoxic agents. These criteria were not always transparent in the literature, but they basically are the following:

- Maximizing dose should maximize efficacy.
- Pharmacokinetics is relevant to dose finding.
- Objective response predicts survival (SV) and clinical benefit.
- Tumor shrinkage is expected to occur fast.
- Objective progression indicates treatment failure (drugs are not active if the tumor is growing).
- Drugs to be tested in combination must be active as single agents.
- Patient population for clinical trials must be as homogeneous as possible.
- Drugs must be tested first in advanced disease and moved to "adjuvant setting" (seeking cures).

According these criteria, clinical trials have been designed and classified into different phases, covering the different questions to be answered about drugs under development.

Considering the high toxicity of cytotoxic agents, and considering the concept that maximizing doses should maximize efficacy, Phase I are dose escalation trials, designed for testing pharmacokinetics and MTD. Dose escalation in Phase I trials gives data about the maximal dose which could exert a therapeutic effect without severe damage due to excessive toxicity. The effective time of the drug in circulation has to be studied in pharmacokinetics studies, and this has been an additional goal of Phase I clinical trials.

Once defined the drug dose, a proof of clinical benefit is the next step. Currently, this is measured as objective response (assessing tumor shrinkage), because cytotoxic drugs are expected to decrease the tumor mass. Phase II trials are designed and conducted to find this kind of anti-tumor activity in some specific patient population. These trials are usually not randomized and evaluate the tumor response according to RECIST criteria (Response Evaluation Criteria in Solid Tumors). They include the minimal patient population required to show statistical significance of a given percentage of tumor response which is different from zero.

When the product under study demonstrates to have anti-tumor activity, randomized Phase III trials are then designed to compare the new drug with the currently accepted standard therapy.

If a novel chemotherapeutic agent is more efficient and/or has better safety profile than a previous one, it is considered to substitute the previous therapy or to add on it. Usually, a large number of patients are required to achieve statistical power to detect small differences between randomized groups.

It is this statistical significance of therapeutic effect in Phase III clinical trials which guarantee the Regulatory Approval. Nevertheless, the limitations of this stepwise process have driven regulatory adaptations such as the concept of AA after an obviously successful Phase II Trial. This concept has had diverse expressions and nuances in different regulatory authorities.

## 3. A clinical development paradigm shift is needed for cancer vaccines: Why?

Therapeutic cancer vaccines are active immunotherapy approaches that provoke an immune response against antigens relevant for tumor cell survival or growth (Talucka, 2011). As their action is very specific towards the cancer associated antigen, cancer vaccines has very low toxicity profiles. That makes possible long lasting use as well as combination with other drugs. In general, not tumor shrinkage is expected, but a prolonged patient´s survival as a consequence of disease control with chronic vaccinations compatible with good quality of life (Lage & Crombet, 2010).

In this very different scenario, the development paradigm used for chemotherapeutics is not working well (Table 1):

- In cancer vaccines the MTD is not always the optimal dose.
- Objective response according to RECIST is not always a good predictor of **SV**.
- Therapeutic benefit could be delayed on time.
- Cancer vaccines could be active even beyond progression.
- Combinations can be effective using drugs that are not active as single agents.

The first trials with cancer vaccines are mainly devoted to demonstrate the proof of the therapeutic principle, i.e. immunogenicity of the vaccine preparation, eliciting an immune response to the antigen they are intended to target; and they are also used for testing different formulations, doses, schemes and, by sure, safety. The novel paradigm of clinical development of cancer vaccines makes then Phase I trials better defined as Proof of Principle trials (PPT).

For cytotoxic drugs, tumor reductions are expected and objective responses predict clinical benefit. In cancer vaccines it has been demonstrated that objective response is not always a good SV predictor; and therefore SV remains the appropriate end point. For SV analysis, comparison between randomized vaccine and control groups is required. Then after PPT, cancer vaccines moves directly towards randomized trials to test the efficacy of the product.

| General principles that have ruled oncology drug development. | Why these principles are not well adapted to cancer vaccines |
|---|---|
| The increase in dose should increase efficacy. | Maximal tolerated doses are not optimal doses. Due the low toxicity of cancer vaccines, it is not evident that a maximal tolerable dose will be coincident with the optimal dose to reach the vaccine effect, which could be much lower. |
| Pharmacokinetics is relevant for finding optimal dose. | |
| Objective responses predict clinical benefit. | Objective response is not a good SV predictor. Not necessarily, a patient with objective response has increase SV, which is the most important factor for the cancer patient. |
| A fast tumor reduction is expected. | Therapeutic benefit could be delayed on time. Cancer vaccines require some time to exert their effect, unlike cytotoxic drugs that provokes an immediate cell destruction effect. |
| An objective progression is considered a treatment failure. Drugs are NOT active if the tumor is growing. | Cancer vaccines could be actives even beyond disease progression. Progression doesn´t means less effectiveness of the vaccine, measured by increase in SV, which could be reached by slower progression related with a good quality of life. |
| Drugs assayed in combination must be individually actives. | Therapeutic vaccines can be effectives in combinations with other onco-specific drugs, even when not individually active. They can be used additionally and not instead of other therapies. |

Table 1. Why general principles that direct oncologic drugs development does not apply to cancer vaccines?

As can be realized, these trials do not fulfill the characteristics of classic Phase II trials defined for cytotoxic drugs, firstly because the end point is different, and secondly because are already randomized trials.

In the novel paradigm for cancer vaccines, these trials are called ¨Efficacy trials¨ (ET).

The number of patients in these trials is adjusted to show statistical significance of a therapeutic advantage which is considered medically meaningful. With a wise medical judgment of what is medically relevant these ET could be often smaller to the current Phase III trials of the classic paradigm.

Such an emerging paradigm for the development of cancer vaccines should also translate into the attitude of Regulatory Authorities for granting Registration.

## 4. CIMAvax EGF®: Immune response translates into clinical impact

The need of a new paradigm for cancer vaccine development can be illustrated by the story of CIMAvax EGF®, a therapeutic vaccine recently registered in Cuba for advanced lung cancer (Gonzalez et al, 1998, 2003, 2007, 2011; Lage et al, 2003; Crombet et al, 2006; Gonzalez & Lage, 2007; García et al, 2008; Neninger et al, 2008a, 2008b; Rodriguez et al, 2010).
Endocrine therapy is an old and well validated approach for cancer treatment. Some tumors are considered as hormone-dependent because they require hormone stimulation for the continued growth of the tumor cells. In such cases, cancer bearing patients may benefit from hormone therapy, mainly based in deprivation of hormonal stimulus by different procedures.
But in addition to sex steroid hormones, tumor can be regulated by growth factors, such as EGF, through the binding to their receptors and activation of phosphorilation cascades leading to tumor cell proliferation. Currently, research in new anticancer drugs is increasingly focused in growth factors, their receptors and signal transduction mechanisms. Active and passive immunotherapies can be instrumental in the aim of interfering growth-factor stimulation of cancer cell proliferation. (Gonzalez & Lage, 2007).
The Epidermal Growth Factor(EGF) based cancer vaccine (CIMAvax EGF®) is a conjugate of human recombinant EGF with the P64K protein of *Neisseria meningitides* (acting as a carrier protein) (Rodríguez et al, 2008). It was designed to induce specific anti-EGF antibodies (Abs) which, in turn, recognize and bind circulating EGF, avoiding further binding to the cell membrane receptor (EGF R).
These ligand / Ab unions, forms immune-complexes that are eliminated from the circulation through the liver, as other immune-complexes do (González et al, 1996). As can be realized, it is like an immune-castration effect, more similar to some hormone-therapies approaches aiming to deprive the cells of the hormone, but with the difference that it is the self immune system which deprives the growth factor (EGF).
This vaccine is not meant to destroy the tumor by inducing immune effectors mechanisms, but to inhibit further tumor cell growth. This completely different mechanism of action could not only stop tumor growth, but could shift the balance between uncontrolled proliferation and cell death.
Anti-EGF Abs are then a main marker of response to vaccination. This has been verified in the clinical setting by the observation that patients with higher anti-EGF Ab titers survived significantly more than patients with low anti-EGF Ab titers.

## 5. How CIMAvax EGF® moved through clinical development: Applying the paradigm shift

The clinical development of CIMAvax EGF began in 1995. From then up to date, more than 1000 advanced cancer patients have received this vaccine.
Our very first objective was to demonstrate that the vaccine elicited anti-EGF Abs as it was designed to do. Clinical trials (Table 2) where then designed to demonstrate that the vaccine was immunogenic and provoked a depletion of circulating EGF. All trials have also safety as primary objective.

Different formulations, schemes and doses of the vaccine were tested and related with immunogenicity and safety.
As can be realized, these trials were not designed with the main goals of Phase I trials defined for cytotoxic drugs (pharmacokinetics and definition of maximal tolerable dose). Trials designed for this vaccine can be better called PPT.
Five PPT were performed allowing the selection of the optimal formulation, scheme and doses for moving forward to the ET.
In the first clinical trial, 10 patients with epithelial tumors were enrolled. Patients received two single doses of the vaccine composed by human recombinant EGF coupled to either Tetanus Toxoid (hu-r-EGF-TT) (5 patients) or the recombinant P64K protein from *Neisseria meningitidis* (hu-r-EGF-P6K) (5 patients), both groups used aluminum hydroxide (alum) as adjuvant. Each single dose of the vaccine was given on days 0 and 14.

| Clinical trial | Target population | End point | Reference |
|---|---|---|---|
| PPT<br>Exploratory trial (1) | Solid tumor patients<br>(n=10) | Carrier selection<br>(TT vs. P64) | Ann Oncol<br>1998;9(4):431 |
| PPT<br>Exploratory trial (2) | NSCLC patients<br>(n=20) | Adjuvant selection<br>(Alum vs. Montanide) | Ann Oncol 2003;<br>4(3):461 |
| PPT<br>Exploratory trial (3) | NSCLC patients<br>(n=20) | Cyclphosphamide<br>(CPM) pre-treatment<br>(CPM or not) | Ann Oncol 2003;<br>4(3):461 |
| PPT<br>Exploratory trial (4) | NSCLC patients<br>(n=20) | Dose escalation<br>(2 doses) | Cancer Biol Ther. 2006;<br>5, 15. |
| PPT<br>Exploratory trial (5) | NSCLC patients<br>(n=20) | Schedule evaluation<br>Vaccine-<br>Chemotherapy-<br>Vaccine | J Immunother<br>2009;32:92–99 |
| ET (6) | NSCLC patients<br>(n=80 s) | SV benefit<br>Vaccine vs. BSC<br>(2nd line therapy) | J Clin Oncol. 2008<br>6(9):1452. |
| ET (7) | NSCLC patients<br>(n=579) | SV benefit<br>Vaccine vs. BSC<br>(2nd line therapy) | Ongoing, not<br>published. |

Table 2. Clinical trials of CIMAvax EGF

The main objectives of the trial were to look at safety and immunogenicity of vaccination with self EGF in humans as well as to compare between the 2 carrier proteins: TT and P64K. Following vaccination there were no significant adverse events. Seroconversion (defined in this study as a doubling of Ab titer above baseline) was reported in 6 of the 10 patients included in the trial.

Both Tetanus Toxoid and P64K protein from *Neisseria meningitides* showed carrier effect. In each of both treatment groups 60% of patients developed anti-EGF Ab responses after immunization. However, the Ab response against the TT in the group of patients vaccinated with hu-r-EGF-TT was very high, but not the Ab response against P64K in the group of patients vaccinated with hu-r-EGF-P64K. Trying to avoid any phenomenon related with epitopic suppression, P64K was selected as carrier protein for further trials (Gonzalez et al, 1998).

The second clinical trial was designed to demonstrate the safety and immunogenicity of the EGF based cancer vaccine using two different adjuvants: aluminum hydroxide (alum) or Montanide ISA 51 (Seppic, France). In this case, 20 stages IIIb-IV NSCLC patients were enrolled in the trial one month after concluding their first line chemotherapy, and then randomized for the adjuvant to be used. Ten patients received the conjugated vaccine in alum and 10 patients in Montanide ISA 51 as adjuvant.

A secondary aim of this study was to evaluate the effect of 5 single doses of the vaccine in the induction period (days 0, 7, 14, 21 and 51) so as of re-immunization when antibody titers decreased to, at least, 50% of their peak titer reached at the induction phase. Also the relation between anti-EGF antibody titers and patient's SV was evaluated (Gonzalez et al, 2003).

The third clinical trial had the very same design that the second one, but all patients in both treatment groups, received a low dose CPM as an immune-enhancer, 100 mg/m$^2$ body surface area 3 days before starting vaccination schedule. (Gonzalez et al, 2003).

In both, second and third trials, sera were collected on days 0, 14, 28, 60 and then monthly for anti-EGF Ab titers determination. Tumor response was evaluated on the first month after inclusion and then, every 3 months, by chest X-ray, abdominal ultrasound, and thoracic and abdominal computerized tomography (CT) scan. Objective responses were classified according to the WHO criteria.

Pooled results from both trials were analyzed looking for immunogenicity, safety and effect of EGF vaccination on SV in the different treatment groups. (Gonzalez et al, 2007).

For immunogenicity analysis, two variables were analyzed: % of patients able to develop an Ab response as well as Ab titer levels.

Patients able to develop an Ab response after vaccination were grouped as:

1. Patient that seroconverts.
2. Good Antibody Responders (GAR).
3. Poor Antibody Responders (PAR).

According to this classification, the higher % of either, seroconversion and GAR, were obtained in the groups of patients using Montanide ISA 51 as adjuvant. Cyclophosphamide pre-treatment did not show any improvement regarding % of seroconversion neither % GAR. It was concluded that the use of Montanide ISA 51 as adjuvant with the EGF vaccine improves % of anti-EGF Ab responder's patients.

When analyzing Ab titer levels in responder patients, measured as geometric means of sera dilutions, an improvement was observed when Montanide ISA 51 was used as adjuvant. Pre-treatment with cyclophosphamide also improved the Ab titer levels.

Taken together, the data from both trials indicates that, regarding immunogenicity (% of responders and Ab titer levels), the best results were obtained when using Montanide ISA51 as adjuvant and cyclophosphamide pre-treatment.

The kinetics of anti-EGF Ab response was also studied. Re-immunizations when Ab titers decreased did not provoked a characteristic booster effect (stronger and maintained Ab responses). Ab titers increased after re-immunization but only to the same levels reached as previous maximal values and decreased again in a short period of time. It is likely to confirm that continuous re-immunizations were needed to maintain anti-EGF Ab titer levels.

Results showed a significant increase in SV for GAR as compared with PAR and with an historical control group (Table 3). In pre-clinical studies, we demonstrated a direct relation between anti-EGF Ab titers and SV in tumor challenged mice (González et al, 1996). The results obtained from clinical trials indicate that a similar association occurs in vaccinated cancer patients.

| SV | Mean (months) | Median (months) | p (log rank test) |
|---|---|---|---|
| GAR | 12,41 | 9,41 | P<0,05 |
| PAR | 5,47 | 4,5 | |
| Historical control group | 7,41 | 5,67 | |

Table 3. Relation between Ab titers provoked by vaccination and patient´s survival in 2nd and 3rd clinical trials with the EGF based vaccine.

One of the patients that reached a maintained high anti-EGF Ab response showed a tumor regression on month 12 after receiving the first vaccination. This is a single case and should be looked carefully, but it should be noted that this was one of the patients that developed higher and maintained anti-EGF Ab titers after vaccination.

No evidence of severe clinical toxicity was observed. Secondary reactions were mild or moderated, limited to 14 of 40 patients. Main reactions consisted on chills, fever, vomits, nausea, hypertension, headache, dizziness, flushing, and pain at the site of injection, bone pain, mouth dryness or hot flashes that, in all cases, disappeared after medication. Hematological data and blood chemistry remained within normal ranges during the immunization and follow-up period.

A fourth trial was then designed, in this case an scale up dose Phase I trial, in which patients were randomized to receive a single dose of the conjugate vaccine hu-r-EGF-P64K in alum as adjuvant (10 patients) or a double dose of the same vaccine (in alum also) in 2 injection sites (10 patients). The immunization schedule consisted in 5 immunizations with the vaccine (single or double doses), on days 0, 7, 14, 21 and 28, and then monthly re-immunizations. This trial was further extended to include 0 more patients (10 in each group) (Crombet et al, 2006).

Regarding immunogenicity, improved results were obtained in patients receiving double doses of the vaccine, considering Ab titer levels (sera dilution geometric means).

In this trial, EGF levels in sera were also tested. An inverse correlation was observed between EGF levels in patient sera and anti-EGF Ab titers. This result agrees with the vaccine working hypothesis. Anti-EGF Ab should bind to circulating EGF provoking a decrease in the EGF concentration. Less (or none) EGF is available to bind the EGF receptor, avoiding then the proliferation mechanisms derived from such binding.

Patients in the double dose group reduced more their EGF sera concentration that patients in the single dose group.

Again a significant increase in SV was observed for GAR as compared with PAR (Table 4).

Additionally, in these trials EGF sera levels were measured. A significant increase in SV was directly correlated with decreased EGF blood levels. Vaccinated patients with an EGF sera concentration after vaccination ≤168 pg/mL showed a significant increase in SV as compared with patients with levels >168 pg/mL ( (Table 4). This is also an important result, and could means that EGF levels can be considered as an adequate surrogated marker of anti-tumor response.
There was a trend to increased SV in patients in the double dose group as compared with patients in the single dose group.
According to the results obtained from the previous trials, it was decided to move forward with the vaccine formulation composed by EGF-P64k in Montanide ISA 51 as adjuvant (CIMAVAX EGF) in a scheme including pre-treatment with low dose of cyclophosphamide.
A trial was designed where 80 patients, 1 month after concluding their 1rst line chemotherapy, were randomized in 2 groups, one receiving the vaccine CIMAvax EGF and the other only Best Supportive Care. According to the statistical design, with this small size randomized trial we expected to find a statistical improve in survival of 4 month for vaccinated patients as compared with the non vaccinated controls. An induction step of five single doses were given on days 0, 7, 14, 21 and 51, followed by monthly re-immunizations (Neninger et al, 2008a)

| SV | Mean (months) | Median (months) | p (log rank test) |
|---|---|---|---|
| GAR | 17,1 | 11,87 | <0,05 |
| PAR | 7,84 | 7,07 | |
| EGF sera concentration ≤168 pcg/ml | 15,28 | 11,3 | <0,05 |
| EGF sera concentration >168 pcg/ml | 5,79 | 5 | |

Table 4. Relation between Ab titers, sera EGF concentration and SV in the 4$^{th}$ clinical trial with the EGF based vaccine.

It is evident that this trial design does not correspond with the Phase II trials currently used for testing chemotherapeutics. It was called our first ET.
Results from this trial showed that, the% of patients that seroconverted (2X original anti-EGF antibody levels) or GAR, was significantly greater in vaccinated patients than in controls. The 50% of vaccinated patients were GAR. Serum EGF concentration was significantly lower in vaccinated patients than those in controls. That means, the vaccination generates anti-EGF antibody titers and decreases the EGF sera concentration.
It was also demonstrated that anti-EGF Ab titers correlates with decreasing EGF serum concentration in the vaccine group, but not in the control group.
Again it was corroborated that SV in GAR patients was significantly longer than in PAR patients. Additionally, there was a statistical difference in SV between vaccinated and control patients inside the GAR group but not inside the PAR group
Survival in patients with lower EGF sera concentration was longer than in patients with higher sera EGF concentration. There was a significant increase in SV between patients that

reached EGF sera concentration levels below168 pcg/ml as compared with patients didn´t reached these levels.

There was a trend toward better SV in vaccinated patients as compared with controls, which becomes significant when considered only those patients younger or equal 60 years old. Vaccination efficacy was well demonstrated in this patient cohort.

Differences in SV were much more advantageous for vaccinated patients when considered, for both vaccinated and controls, only those patients' responders to the first line of chemotherapy, but the trial has not a design strong enough to make the difference significant. Also in those patients with performance status (PS) 0 or 1 the effect of vaccination in SV was stronger. Again, the small sample number didn´t allow finding a statistical significance.

Summarizing we were looking an advantage in SV for vaccinated patients over non vaccinated controls that become increased in some patient niches, such as age under 60 years old, response to chemotherapy and PS.

At our experience, once safety of the vaccine is established, PPT needs not to be consecutive. After concluding the patient recruitment in our first ET, we decided to design and perform a new PPT to test the optimal conditions that, up to this date, given the best results regarding immunogenicity (Neninger et al, 2008).

This trial design included:

1. Use of Montanide ISA51 as adjuvant and cyclophosphamide pre-treatment.
2. Four single doses of the vaccine given in 4 different anatomical sites.
3. Time intervals between vaccinations of 14 days.
4. Vaccine-Chemotherapy-Vaccine (V-Ch-V) approach: That means, a previous vaccination induction step on days 0 and 14 (4 single doses in 4 injection sites) is given before the first line of chemotherapy, then, after chemotherapy, vaccinations continue, 4 single doses (in 4 injection sites) each 14 days and then monthly.

With this immunization schedule, a huge improvement in immunogenicity was observed with 95 % of patients reaching the GAR condition and up to 20 fold increase in anti-EGF titers as compared with the levels previously obtained.

Because of the high anti-EGF antibody levels, an additional classification of immune response was considered. Patients were considered super Gar (sGAR) when reached anti-EGF Ab titers of 1:64,000 or more. The 55% of patients in the trial reached this condition while only 2,8% did in the previous Efficacy trial..

The association between Ab response and survival was corroborated in this series, where sGAR patients survived significantly more than GAR patients.

In all patients vaccinated under this V-Ch-V scheme, the EGF sera concentration decreased to 78 pcg/mL (baseline of the detection kit).

All vaccinated patients survived significantly more than the control group of the phase II trial.

From this trial, it was demonstrated the possibility of given 4X the vaccine dose used in the first efficacy trial, and the significant improvement in immunogenicity and EGF depletion that such scheme produced.

It was then designed a new trial, where, taking into account the results from both, the first ET and the fifth PPT, Five hundred and seventy nine patients were selected after being responsive to the first line of chemotherapy and subsequently stratified per age. One hundred ninety eight patients were included in the group of age equal or minor to 60 years old (strata 1) and 381 patients in the group of ages older than 60 years old (strata 2). After

stratification, patients were randomized for receiving vaccination or only Best Supportive Care. All patients received a 4X vaccine dose administered in 4 injection sites.
The sample size was calculated taking into consideration previous results and considering a 3 month of increase in SV for vaccinated patients in the strata 1 and 2 months of increase in survival for vaccinated patients in the strata 2.
As may be noticed, this trial design corresponds to a second ET that aimed to corroborate the results of our first ET results optimized conditions.
This trial is currently ongoing and a partial cut on the results according to the statistical design is very encouraging.
As well as the classical Phase I-II-III paradigm, the new sequence of cancer vaccine clinical trials also approaches the goals of understanding safety and efficacy. In such a way, the commonly called Phase I and Phase II clinical trials matches with PPT, while Phase III trials matches with ET.

## 6. The relationship between clinical trials and "levels of Evidence" CIMAvax EGF® example

In the last decades, as the emergence of new medical technology accelerates, there has been a growing claim to assess and to classify emerging knowledge according to the strengths of the evidence (Elstein, 2004)
A "Level of Evidence" ladder has emerged as follows:
Evidence level Ia: The evidence comes from a meta-analysis of randomized, controlled, well designed trials.
Evidence Level Ib: The evidence comes from, at least, one randomized, controlled trial.
Evidence level IIa: The evidence comes from, at least, one controlled, well designed, not randomized trial.
Evidence Level IIb: The evidence comes from, at least, one study not completely experimental, well designed, as cohort studies. Is referred to the situation when the application of an intervention is out of the investigators control, but whose effect can be assessed.
Evidence Level III: The evidence comes from studies of well-designed non-experimental descriptive, such as comparative studies, correlation studies or case-control studies . Evidence level IV: The evidence comes from documents or opinions of expert committees or clinical experience of prestigious authorities or series of cases.
Levels of evidence then translate into the strength of recommendation that can be assigned to a given new technology.
A: Evidence level I: Highly recommended
B: Evidence level II: Favorable recommendation
C: Evidence level III : Recommendation favorable but not conclusive
D: Evidence level IV: Expert consensus without adequate research evidence.
During the clinical development of CIMAvax EGF®, the vaccine has transited through different stages of clinical trials and through different Evidence levels (Table 5).
We can conclude that CIMAvax EGF has 5 PPT, 2 ET (one ongoing) and has reached a level of evidence Ib that makes it highly recommended for its use in patients.
In summary, the historical development of CIMAvax EGF, illustrates the new development paradigm for cancer vaccines.
Firstly, the vaccine dose and schedule was selected across 5 different PPT, considering the specific immune response and its duration, and not the MTD or pharmacokinetics. The

vaccine was very well tolerated, provoking only grade 1 or 2 of adverse events; the MTD was never achieved.

Secondly, after optimizing dose and schedule, a randomized trial was conducted to assess the preliminary efficacy in terms of survival and not response rate. Tumor shrinkage was rarely observed while all vaccinated patients had a trend toward SV benefit that was significant in those patients with 60 years old or younger. The Kaplan Meier survival curve showed a non-proportional hazard ratio, illustrating the delayed (not immediate) effect of the drug. CIMAVax EGF needed at least 3 months to induce a mature, neutralizing immune response and a consequent survival curve separation.

Finally, vaccination was not stopped at the moment of clinically irrelevant, radiologic progression. Patients received chronic vaccination, which increased their probability of becoming good responders and long survivors (González et al, 2011)

<table>
<tr><th>Stages of clinical trials typically used for clinical development of new chemotherapeutic drugs</th><th>Stages of clinical trials proposed for cancer vaccines development</th><th>Evidence Levels</th><th>CIMAvax EGF trial number</th></tr>
<tr><td rowspan="5">Phase I trials<br>Phase II trials</td><td rowspan="5">PPT</td><td rowspan="5">IIa</td><td>1</td></tr>
<tr><td>2</td></tr>
<tr><td>3</td></tr>
<tr><td>4</td></tr>
<tr><td>5</td></tr>
<tr><td rowspan="2">Phase III trials</td><td rowspan="2">ET</td><td rowspan="2">Ib</td><td>6</td></tr>
<tr><td>7</td></tr>
</table>

Table 5. Relation between clinical trials stages and Evidence Levels

## 7. How to implement the changes in clinical development paradigms for cancer vaccines?

There are clear facts showing that the old paradigms for chemotherapeutics development, no longer apply to cancer vaccines. But paradigms not only differs in contents, but also are the source of methods and normative of solutions accepted by a mature scientific community in a given moment. As a result, receipt of a new paradigm often necessitates a redefinition of the corresponding science.

Moreover, an existing paradigm is shared by members of the scientific community who are engaged with the same. A paradigm shift requires a change not only in tools, but also in the visions of the problem by the related scientific community.

The question is: What is the process by which a new candidate for paradigm replaces its predecessor?

In this case, Axel Hoos et al (Hoos et al, 2007) have firstly described the needs of a paradigm shift for development of cancer vaccines and other related biologics. They have defined new terms or vocabulary according new needs and explained how to apply these new tools in further products development.

Many people working in cancer vaccines development are facing the need of a change in clinical development paradigm as described by Axel Hoos et al and currently been being borne out in practice. As usual in the history of science, crises arise in different places at once, in this case, caused by the emergence of new therapies (cancer vaccines) that do not agree with the mechanism of action of these previously used (cytotoxic antitumor therapies). These people that faced firstly the needs of changes are the pioneers of the new paradigm and have the challenge of ¨converting¨ the rest of the scientific community to the new ideas.
How to induce the conversion and how it resists? Probably the single most common argument put forward by proponents of a new paradigm is that they can solve problems that have led to the old paradigm to crisis. As it has been extensively explained in this chapter, new paradigms proposed for cancer vaccines development solve the problems for which the old paradigms no longer work.
The challenge now is to persuade the whole medical community as well as the Regulatory bodies on the new conceptions, which will result in a more direct development of new drugs and a more rapid availability of the same for patients with cancer.

## 8. Conclusion: A field of science in transition

As Thomas Kuhn said in his book The Structure of Scientific Revolutions: ¨In science occurs as in manufacturing: a change of tools is an extravagance that is reserved for occasions that demand it. The significance of crises is that they provide an indication that it is time to change tools¨ .This is precisely what is going on in the field of cancer vaccines.
Cancer vaccines are, as other biological molecules, product of the development of Biotechnology, a tool of science which opened a new wave of opportunity for cancer immunotherapy. It created the possibility of finding and manufacturing biological molecules with the same purity, reproducibility and scalability of classic chemical pharmaceuticals. These novel therapeutical tools have the attribute of specificity, which means possibility of therapeutic effect with lack of toxicity. That property makes them very different to the cytotoxic tumor drugs approach for cancer treatment.
Because of that, biotechnology drugs claimed for a change in the paradigm through which antitumor drugs has been up to date investigated, developed, and finally approved. This is especially pertinent in the field of therapeutic cancer vaccines.
We are facing times of changes. As soon as new paradigms are implemented for new drugs development, the faster the profits of these new drugs will be available.
This is just the beginning. Cancer therapy is a field of Science in transition. The changes in the paradigm of product development come together with other changes also intrinsic to novel biotechnology drugs attributes.
There are other important differences between cancer vaccines and cytotoxic antitumor drugs: one is that they are intended to restrain tumor growth, not necessarily to reduce tumor mass, and the second is that they can be used long term.
These features connect with another paradigm shift which is going on in medical oncology, which is the transition of advanced cancer from a rapidly fatal disease into a chronic condition, compatible with years of quality life.
Such a transition is not new in the history of medicine. Diabetes Mellitus Type I was also a rapidly fatal disease until the introduction of Insulin in 1923. Now it is a chronic condition, which cannot be cured, but can be controlled long term.

Biotechnology drugs and specially cancer vaccine have the potential to implement an analogous transition in oncology.

A new paradigm for accelerating the development of cancer vaccines should be embraced by the research community. With these therapeutic tools in hand, also a new paradigm for chronic management of advanced cancer should be embraced by the medical community and by Public Health Systems. Two field of Science which are evolving in parallel, and whose evolutions should merge in the near future, for the benefit of cancer patients and Society at large.

## 9. References

Crombet T. Neninger E., Catalá M., García B., Leonard I., Martínez L., González G., Pérez R., Lage A (2006). Treatment of NSCLC Patients with an EGF-Based Cancer Vaccine: Report of a Phase I Trial. *Cancer Biology & Therapy*, Vol. 5, No. 2 (Feb 2006), pp. 145-149.

Dagher R., Johnson J., Williams G., Keegan P., Pazdur,R (2004). Accelerated Approval of Oncology Products: A Decade of experience. *J. Natl. Cancer Inst.* Vol. 96, No. 20, (Oct 2004), pp. 1500-1509.

De Vita V., Lawrence T., Rosemberg S. (2008). Cancer. Principles and Practice of Oncology. By Lippincott William & Wilkins. ISNN-13:978-0-7817-7205-5. Phiadelphia. PA.

Elstein AS (2004). On the origins and development of evidence-based medicine and medical decision making. *Inflamm. Res.* Vol. 53 Suppl 2 (Aug 2004), pp.184–189

Frei E 3rd, Karon M, Levin RH, Freireich EJ, Taylor RJ, Hananian J, Selawry O, Holland J.F., Hoogstraten B., Wolman I.J., Abir E., Sawitsky A., Lee S., Mills S.D., Burgert E.O. Jr, Spurr C.L., Patterson R.B., Ebaugh F.G., James G.W .3rd, Moon J.H. (1965). The effectiveness of combinations of antileukemic agents in inducing and maintaining remission in children with acute leukemia. *Blood.* Vol 26, No. 5, (Nov 1965), pp.642-656.

García B.,Neninger E.,de la Torre A., Leonard I., Martínez R., Viada C., González G., Mazorra Z., Lage A., Crombet T.(2008). Effective Inhibition of the Epidermal Growth Factor / Epidermal Growth Factor Receptor Binding by Anti-Epidermal Growth Factor Antibodies is Related to Better Survival in Advanced Non-Small-Cell Lung Cancer Patients Treated with the Epidermal Growth Factor Cancer Vaccine. *Clinical Cancer Research*, Vol 14, No.3, (Feb 2008), pp. 840-846.

González G., Pardo O.L., Sánchez B., García J.L., Beausoleil I., Marinello P., González Y., Domarco A., Guillén G., Pérez R., Lage A.(1997) Induction of Immune Recognition of Self Epidermal Growth Factor II: Characterization of the Antibody Response and Use of a Fusion Protein *Vaccine Research*, Vol. 5, No.4, pp 91-100.

González G., Crombet T., Catalá M., Mirabal V.,Hernández J.C., González Y., Marinello P., Guillén G., Lage A. A novel cancer vaccine composed of human recombinant epidermal growth factor linked to a carrier protein: Report of a pilot clinical trial(1998). *Annals of Oncology*, Vol 9, No. 4, (Apr 1998), pp. 431-435.

Gonzalez G., Crombet T., Torres F., Catalá M., Alfonso L., Osorio M., Neninger E., García B., Mulet A., Pérez R., Lage A. (2003). Epidermal Growth Factor-based cancer vaccine for non-small cell lung cancer therapy. Ann Onc Vol 14, No 3, (Mar 2003), 461-466.

González G, Crombet T., Neninger E., Viada C., Lage A.(2007). Therapeutic Vaccination with Epidermal Growth Factor /EGF) in advanced Lung Cancer: Analysis of Pooled Data fromThree Clinical Trials. *Human Vaccines*, Vol 3: No.1, (Feb 2007) pp. 8-13.

González G., Lage A., Crombet T., Rodríguez G., García B., Cuevas A., Viña L., Arteaga N., Neninger E.(2009) CIMAvax-EGF: A novel therapeutic vaccine for advanced lung cancer. *Applied Biotechnology*, Vol. 26, No. 4, pp. 345-348.

Gonzalez G., Crombet T., Lage A. (2011) Chronic Vaccination with a therapeutic EGF-based Cancer Vaccine: a Review of Patients Receiving Long Lasting Treatment. *Current Cancer Drug Targets* Vol 11, No. 1, Jan pp 103-110.

González G and Lage A: Cancer Vaccines for Hormone / Growth Factor Immune deprivation: A Feasible Approach for Cancer Treatment (2007). *Current Cancer Drug Targets* Vol 7, No 3, (May 2007), pp 191-201.

Hoos A., Parmiani G., Hege K., Sznol M., Loibner H., Eggermont A., Urba W., Blumenstein B., Sacks N., Keilholz U., Nichol G. (2007). *J Immunotherapy*, Vol 30, No. 1, (Jan 007), pp1-15.

Kuhn T.S. (1962),La Estructura de las revoluciones científicas, (3rd edition), Ed Fondo Cultura Económica, ISBN 978-968-16-7599-8, Mexico.

Lage A., Crombet T., González G. (2003) Targeting epidermal growth factor receptor signaling: early results and future trends in oncology. *Annals of Medicine* Vol35, No.5, 327-336.

Lage A., Crombet T.,(2011). Control of Advanced Cancer: The Road to Chronicity.*Int. J. Environ. Res. Public Health*, Vol 8, pp.683-697.

Neninger E., de la Torre A., Osorio M., Catalá M., Bravo I.,Mendoza M., Abreu D.., Acosta S., Rives R., del Castillo C., González M., Viada C., García B., Crombet T., González G., Lage A.(2008 a): Phase II Randomized Controlled Trial of an Epidermal Growth Factor Vaccine in Advanced Non-Small-Cell-Lung Cancer. *Journal of Clinical Oncology*, Vol. 26, No. 9,( March 2008) pp. 1452-1458.

Neninger E., Verdecia B.G., Crombet T, Viada C., Pereda S.,Leonard I.,Mazorra Z., Fleites G., González M., Wilkinson B., González G, Lage A (2008 b). Combining an EGF-based Cancer Vaccine with Chemotherapy in Advanced Nonsmall Cell Lung Cancer. *J Immunotherapy*, Vol. 32, No. 1, (Jan 2008), 92-99.

Richey E.A., Lyons E.A., Nebeker J.R., Shankaran V., McKoy J.M., Luu T.H., Nonzee N., Trifilio S., Sartor O., Benson A.B., Carson K.R., Edwards B.J., Gilchrist-Scott D., Kuzel T.M., Raish D.W., Tallman M.S., West D.P., Hirchfeld, S. Grillo-López A.J., Bennett C.L. (2009). Accelerated Approval of Cancer Drugs: Improved Access to Therapeutic Breakthroughs or Early Release of Unsafe and Ineffective Drugs? *J. Clin. Oncol.* Vol 7, No.26, (Sept 2009), pp 4398-4405.

Rodríguez G.,Albisa A., Viña L., Cuevas A., García B., García A.T., Portillo A., Calvo L., Crombet T., González G., Chico E. (2008) Manufacturing Process Development for an Epidermal Growth Factor-Based Cancer Vaccine. *Int Biopharm* Vol.21, No. 10, (Oct 2008), pp. 36-42.

Rodríguez P.C., Rodriguez G, González G, Lage A. Clinical Development and perspectives of CIMAvax EGF, Cuban vaccine for Non -Small cell Lung Cancer Therapy (2010). *Meddic Review*, Vol 12, No. 1, (Winter 2010), p.p.17-23.

Talucka K., Hueno H., Banchereau J. (2011). Recent Developments in Cancer Vaccines. J. Immunol. Vol. 186, No. 3, (Feb 2011), 1325-1331

Tsimberidou A.M., Braiteh F, Stewart D.J., Kurzrock R. (2009). Ultimate Fate of Oncology Drugs Aproved by the US Food and Drug Administration Without a Randomized Trial (2009). *J. Clin. Oncol.*Vol 27, No 38, (Dec 2009), pp.6243-6250.

8

# Brain Metastases: Biology and Comprehensive Strategy from Radiotherapy to Metabolic Inhibitors and Hyperthermia

Baronzio Gianfranco[1], Fiorentini Giammaria[2]
Guais Adeline[3] and Schwartz Laurent[4]
*[1]"Metabloc Cancer Center", c/o Centro Medico Kines Castano primo, (Mi)*
*[2]Oncology Unit, Hospital San Salvatore, Pesaro*
*[3]Biorébus, Paris*
*[4]Hôpital Raymond Poincaré, Garches*
*[1.2]Italy*
*[3.4]France*

## 1. Introduction

Metastases to the brain is one of the most feared complication of systemic cancer and its incidence is rising for several reasons. The two most important reasons are the improvement in treatment, with a longer patient life; and the advance in diagnostic and imaging means Magnetic Resonance Image (MRI) and Computed Tomography (CT), Positron Emission Tomography [PET]) that have permitted to detect smaller lesions in asymptomatic patients. These improvement in radiology allows earlier diagnosis and result in better treatment management (Kamar et al., 2010, Rao et al, 2007, Patchell et al. 2003). Single metastases are detected in greater proportion. For example, in the case of ovarian tumors brain metastases are solitary in 43% of the cases (Pectasides et al. 2006). Single metastases appear approximately in one quarter of all patients with brain metastases (Rao et al. 2007). Norden et al. 2005 recently reported that breast, colon and renal cell carcinoma tend to produce single metastases, whereas melanoma and lung cancer have a greater tendency to produce multiple metastases. Single metastases can be treated surgically or by high precise radiotherapy modalities such as Gamma knife and StereoTactic Radiotherapy (SRT) or Conformal Radiotherapy (CRT). SRT was initially used for substituting surgical approach in patients with inaccessible tumor location or with comorbid medical conditions, now is used in many institutions as first approach, peculiarly from breast colon and renal carcinoma. Actually, many patients, refuse surgical approach so the use of SRT or CRT in combination with whole brain irradiation (WBRT) or SRT as a boosting method after WBRT is increasing. Associated to radiotherapy and chemotherapy we suggest and discuss the biological reasons for adding hyperthermia and glycolysis metabolic inhibitors with the aim to obtain a better control of brain metastases.

## 2. Epidemiology, pathology and prognosis of patients with brain metastasis

Brain metastases occur in 20% to 40% of cancer patients. Posner and Chernik, from 1970 to 1976 at the Memorial Sloan-Kettering Cancer Center, autopsied 3219 cancer patients. They found that 24% of these patients had intracranial metastases and the 20% had leptomeningeal metastases (Posner and Chernik 1978). Other studies reported similar percentage even if the methodology is slightly different (Baker et al. 1942, Chason et al 1963, Nussbaum 1996). In decreasing frequency, lung cancer, unknown primary, breast, melanoma, renal, and colon cancers are the most common tumors to metastasize to the brain (Pectasides et al. 2006, Norden et al. 2005, Posner and Chernic 1978, Chason et al 1963, Nussbaum et al. 1996).

### 2.1 Localization of brain metastases

Another important aspect is the precise localization of the metastases in the brain (Globus et al. 1942, Tom et al. 1946, Zimm et al. 1981, Tikhtman et al 1995). Approximately the 80% of metastases are localized in the cerebral hemisphere, 17% in the cerebellum and 3% in the brain stem (Tikhtman et al 1995). Delattre and contributors have also analyzed the localization of metastases in the specific regions of the cerebral hemisphere (Delattre et al. 1988). They found that brain metastases involved the frontal area for 21%, the parietal and the temporoparietal-occipital for 19%. These authors have also outlined that metastasis located preferentially at the junction of gray and white matter. Hwang et al. recently reexamined the importance of the vascular border zone and the gray and white matter junction in the distribution of brain metastases and agreed with Delattre and contributors (Hwang et al. 1988). They found in 302 metastatic brain lesions studied, that gray and white matter junction was the preferred site for 64 % of the brain metastases and the vascular border zones were the site of predilection for the 62%. These results support the notion that metastatic emboli tend to lodge in an area of sudden reduction of vascular caliber (gray/white matter junction) and in the most distal vascular field area (Border zone) (Hwang et al. 1988).

### 2.2 Shape of brain metastases

Most metastases appear round well-demarcated lesions that displace rather than invade the surrounding brain parenchyma. The lesions can vary in size ranging from microscopic to masses of 1-4 centimeters in diameter. The histopathologic features are similar to that of tumor of origin.

Microinvasion is present although the majority of metastatic lesions appear well demarcated and sometimes with reactive astrocytosis surrounding the metastatic area (Shaffrey et al. 2004). A new vasculature can appear at peripheral zones and is part of the edema. In central areas, necrotic areas are present (Nathoo et al. 2005). Meningeal metastases diffuse into the subarachnoid space with accumulation around blood vessels (Shaffrey et al. 2004).

### 2.3 Prognosis of brain metastases

Untreated brain metastases have a dismal prognosis, generally no greater than 1-5 months. Gaspar et al. 2000, studying a RTOG (Radiation Therapy Oncology Group) data base, performed a Recursive - Partitioning Analysis [RPA] on 1200 patients. They identified the factors able to influence the prognosis of these patients (Gaspar et al. 2000, D'Ambrosio et al. 2007). Among the several prognostic factors, Karnofsky Performance Status (KPS) has been identified as the most important. The other important factors were: status of primary tumor, age and the presence or absence of systemic metastases. Stratifying the patients according these criteria they have been able to obtain the following prognostic factors. Patients with KPS = 70%, with age = 65 with controlled primary tumor and absence of systemic metastases had a median survival of 7.1 months, whereas the survival was reduced to 2.3 months for patients with KPS < 70. The presence of uncontrolled tumor and systemic metastases even if with a KPS = 70% reduced the median survival to 4.2 months (Gaspar et al. 1997, 2000). The survival was not different between patients with undiagnosed primary lesion and thosewith diagnosed primary tumor (6 and 4.5 months, respectively; p = 0.097) as reported in a recent study by D'Ambrosio (D'Ambrosio et al. 2007).

### 2.4 Brain metastases biology

Researchers have gained insight into the mechanisms by which metastatic cells arise from certain primary tumors (i.e. breast, melanoma) and metastasize to brain. These findings have been obtained in a mouse model (Kang et al. 2004, Nicolson 1993, Beasley et al. 2011). These authors have outlined that metastases formation are not due to patterns of initial cell arrest, motility, or invasiveness, but rather to the ability of metastatic tumor cells to grow in that environment, this in agreement with the Paget hypothesis of seed and soil. In other words, the formation of metastasis requires the right cells with the compatible environment (Fidler 2002, 2010, Deichman 1998).

Metastatic process is a high selective non-random process consisting in a series of linked sequential steps. In a heterogeneous population of primitive tumor cells only some are able to survive and to lodge at distant sites (Shaffrey et al. 2004). The outcome of cancer metastases depends on multiple interactions between metastatic cells and homeostatic mechanisms. Each metastatic step is selective and if the various steps are not completed, the metastatic process may fail. This is probably why only 0.01% of the cells that reach the circulation form a metastatic colony (Shaffrey et al. 2004, Kang et al 2004).

For tutorial purpose we can divide the metastatic process to the brain in the following steps (Fidler 2010, Deichman 1998):

A) process of selection among the heterogeneous tumor cells of origin into an aggressive and able to mobilize subpopulation; B) penetration of this selected subpopulation into the host circulation; C) localization into the microvasculature of the brain; D) crossing of Blood Brain Barrier (BBB); D) migration and growth in the brain structure.

The process of selection (A) is the result of different pressures exerted by the tumor microenvironment and the genetic instability intrinsic to the tumor cells living in that environment. For different pressures we intend: tumor hypoxia, different metabolic advantageous tumor micro-area, immunologic pressure, presence or absence of an angiogenesis process. These different pressures can select among cells genetically unstable, cells able to survive in a different environment, to mobilize and to reach the blood stream (Deichman 1998). To gain access to the general circulation and to colonize to distant organs metastatic cells must invade tumor associated vasculature. The molecular mechanisms controlling the penetration of blood vessels are not completely understood (Beasley et al 2011, Fidler 2002, 2010, Deichman 1998). Once these cells have reached the blood vessels, various mechanisms are needed to survive both the immune system and the shear stress. To avoid the identification the immune cells, metastatic cells shielded under an agglomerate of platelets and red blood cells (Deichman 1998)]. Other important mechanisms are the resistances by metastatic cells to the apoptotic effects of reactive oxygen radicals produced by macrophages and neutrophils and the production of prostaglandins of E type (Fidler 2002). Furthermore the adhesion of the platelets on the metastatic cells induces a hypercoagulable state that increases the metastatic potential. In fact this adhesion increases the resistance to both the immune system and the shear stress (Kehrli 1999).

The most common metastatization to brain occurs by hematogenous route. One route is via the general circulation. In fact in the resting state, the brain receives 15% to 20% of the body's blood flow, thus making it likely that circulating tumor cells will reach the brain. The second, via the vertebral venous system (Batson's plexus) which explains the absence of lung metastases found in certain patients with lung cancer. This spreading way is disputed and not confirmed by all authors (Deeken et al. 2007).

Once metastatic cells have survived the circulatory stream, they may adhere to the endothelium, extravasate into the organ and then begin to proliferate in the new parenchyma. The arrest in the microcirculatory system is regulated by several factors, among them the multiple vascular adhesion molecules and the size of circulating emboli. Among adhesion molecules two families seem to be implicated: the selectins and the products of Immunoglobulin (Ig) genes and the integrins (Deeken et al. 2007). Integrins are major adhesion and signaling receptors that mediate cell migration and invasion (Shaffrey et al. 2004). In the case of human non small lung cancer (NSLC) the block of adhesion molecules integrin $\alpha 3\beta 1$ has been demonstrated to significantly decrease the brain metastasis (Nathoo et al 2005).

After reaching the brain capillaries, the metastatic cells must cross the BBB, degrade the brain Extracellular Matrix (ECM) and invade the brain parenchyma. This interaction is tight regulated by the paracrine and autocrine growth mechanisms present in the brain (Nicolson 1993). BBB is constituted by brain endothelial cells associated with pericytes and astrocyte foot processes. Brain endothelial cells have continuous tight junction, no fenestrations and is highly selective in its permeability (Perides et al. 2006). In experimental melanoma the fibrinolytic system facilitates tumor cell migration across the BBB as demonstrated by Perides and his group (Perides et al. 2006). For metastasis to the brain from breast tumor, the cooperation between metastatic cells and astrocyte is of importance (Weil et al. 2005).

To determine why certain tumors produce site-specific metastases to the brain, Fidler and collaborators studied cellsfrom K-175 melanoma syngeneic to C3H/HeN mice and the B16 melanoma syngeneic to C57 Bl/6 mice (Fidler 1999, 2002, 2007). Regardless of the route of injection (internal carotid arteries-or directly into the cerebrum) K-175 produced melanocytic metastases in the brain parenchyma, whereas B16 cells produced lesions in the meninges and ventricles. These researches tried to understand which factors were responsible for the growth the melanoma cells in the specific areas (brain parenchyma, meninges). Some important aspects have been elucidated. For example B16 cells did not produce measurable gelatinase A activity whereas K- 175 cells did. The presence of gelatinase theoretically can facilitate cells extravasation and the growth into the parenchyma. However studies with hybrids of B16 and K-1735 able to produce gelatinase A, failed to grow into brain parenchyma. Fidler switched his research on the different growth factors present in the brain. He studied growth factors such as Epidermal Growth Factor (EGF), basic Fibroblast Growth Factor (bFGF), Platelet Derived Growth Factor (PDGF), however only Transforming Growth Factor-beta 2 (TGF-$\beta_2$ )showed a greater concentration in the brain and was able to inhibit the growth of B16 and B16/K-1735 hybrid cells explaining the incapacity of these hybrids in producing intraparenchymal brain metastases (Fidler 1999).

Whether the progressive growth of brain metastases depends on neovascularisation is also unclear. As outlined by Bucana: "immunohistochemical and morphometric analyses show that the density of blood vessels within experimental metastases in the brains of nude mice, or within brain metastases derived from human lung cancer, is lower than in the adjacent, tumor-free brain parenchyma. However, blood vessels associated with brain metastases are dilated and contain many dividing endothelial cells. Immunohistochemical analysis also reveals that tumor cells located less than 100 micrometer from a blood vessel are viable, whereas more distant tumor cells undergo apoptosis. The blood-brain barrier is intact in and around experimental brain metastases smaller than 0.25 mm in diameter, but is leaky in larger metastases "(Bucana et al. 1999). Regarding melanoma other authors have found that neurotrophins (NTs) can promote brain metastases. NTs enhance the production of ECM degradation enzymes such as heparanases. Heparanases do not only degrade ECM but also the basement membrane of BBB Nathoo et al 2005, Menter et al 1994, Marchetti et al 2003, Denkins et al. 2004).

The potential of angiogenesis in breast metastases has been further been studied. VEGF has been reported to increase the penetration of metastatic MDA-MB-231 breast carcinoma and to play a role in brain metastases dormancy in the absence of inhibitory antiangiogenic factors (Kim et al. 2004, Santarelli et al 2007, Palmieri et al. 2007, Yano et al,. 2000, Kaplan et al. 2005, Chen et al. 2007). Yano and collaborators however do not agree regarding the importance of VEGF on brain metastases and in an experimental mouse model using six different human cancer cell lines has reported that VEGF expression was necessary but not sufficient for the production of brain metastasis (Yano et al. 2000).

Recently, the idea of premetastatic niche is leading the way (Kaplan et al 2006). Some authors support that the arrival of bone marrow-derived hematopoietic progenitors cells in distant sites represent early changes in the local environment (premetastatic niche) that dictates the pattern of metastatic spread and explains tumor dormancy (Kaplan et al. 2005,2006). Santarelli et al. 2007, outline that the reactive monocytosis and activated microglia present in the premetastatic niche increase the local inflammatory response and can induce the growth of tumor cells transplanted to the brain. Furthermore these authors outline that it is plausible that the brain is able to generate the adequate environment in anticipation and preparation of the ensuing metastatic colonization (Santarelli et al. 2007). Other studies have evidenced new mechanistic insights regarding some kind of tumors such as breast cancer and melanoma.

**Her-2 receptor**. Overexpression of Her-2 receptor in breast carcinoma seems not only correlated to a poor prognosis but also to an increased colonization to the brain as demonstrated by Palmieri et al. (2007).

**Metabolic factors.** Regarding only breast carcinoma, Chen et al (2007) have evidenced by proteomic analysis, that brain- metastasizing cancer cells over expressed enzymes involved in aerobic glycolysis and tricarboxylic acid cycle (TCA) cycle. From this study the authors outline that breast cancer that colonize the brain are able to adapt to the energy metabolism of the brain or develop metabolism able to survive in that specific environment.

**Stat3.** In melanoma, the activation and over expression of Stat3 (Signal Transducer and Activator of Transcription 3), as reported by Tong-Xin is associated to brain metastases and might be considered a new potential target in this clinical situation (Tong et al 2006).

**Metastasis suppressor genes.** Recently seven Metastasis Suppressor Genes (MSGs) have been identified. These genes have no effect on the growth of primary tumors but have the

ability to suppress metastases *in vivo*. Proteins that regulate different functions such as adhesion, migration, growth and differentiation are coded by these MSGs. These genes have been described for breast carcinoma (Seraj et al. 2000), melanoma (Leone et al. 1991) and prostate cancer (Dong et al. 1995).
Notwithstanding all these progresses the entire process of brain colonization remains actually poorly understood and better human and animal models are to be tried. It is our hypothesis that the peculiar metabolism of the normal brain with its high glucose uptake may explain the large incidence of metastases.

## 3. Current methods of treatment of brain metastases

The treatment of brain metastasis is multidisciplinary and different medical (surgeons, radiotherapists, chemotherapists) and non-medical figures (specialized nurses, health physicists, and radiotherapy technics) are interested. The clinical treatment consists in a combination of surgery, radiotherapy and chemotherapy.
For describing the current therapies of brain metastases we have followed the suggestions of the "American College of Surgical oncology CNS Working Group" (2005) and some recent reviews on the argument (Shaffrey et al. 2004, Eichler A. F. and Loeffler J. S 2007, Ngguyen and De Angelis 2004). The criteria used by the American college of Surgical Oncology are the following: age, Karnofsky Index, presence or absence of non-Central Nervous System (CNS) metastasis. Using these criteria and the predictive study [RPA] of Gaspar et al. (1997, 2000) it is possible to calculate the median survival. For patients falling in the RPA 1 with median survival = 7.1 months, an aggressive approach is suggested. It is out of doubt that the improvement in imaging techniques has changed the treatment options, and that the survival of patients with brain metastasis is dependent on the status of their systemic disease (Kamar et al. 2010, Rao et al. 2007, Patchell 2003, Eichler A. F. and Loeffler J. S 2007).

### 3.1 Surgery

Surgical approach has changed the survival and the quality of life of many patients. The most convincing evidence of this benefit is reported for Non-Small Lung Cancer (NSLC) patients with a single brain metastasis. Different authors have reported a 5-years survival ranging from 0% to 45% (Hankins et al. 1988, Wronski et al. 1995). As outlined by Nguyen and De Angelis (2004) this variation on survival is accounted by two factors: a) variation on treatment aggressiveness of primary lung tumor, b) variation on the incidence of systemic disease burden among those series.
Surgical resection is generally followed by Whole - Brain Radiation Therapy (WBRT). WBRT has demonstrated palliation of neurologic symptoms and extension on survival (see studies of Patchell et al. 1990 and Vecht et al. 1993). Surgery for single metastases has shown benefit for melanoma (Buchsbaum et al. 2002), prostate cancer (McCutcheon et al. 1999), colorectal cancer (Hammoud et al. 1996), ovarian ( Cormio et al. 2003) and cervical cancer (Tajran et al. 2003).
Surgery for multiple brain metastases is a relatively new approach supported by the important retrospective study of University of Texas M.D. Anderson Cancer Center. In this study were treated 56 patients with no more than 3 metastases. No more than 3 craniotomies were performed and the group was divided in two subgroups according to the extension of the surgical resection. For one group [A] of 30 patients the complete resection was not possible, for a second group [B] of 26 patients the multiple metastases were completely

resected. In a third Group [C], 26 patients were resected for single metastasis and this group was used as control. From the comparison of the various subgroups the following results emerged: Group C and Group B obtained the same survival time and a multivariate analysis demonstrated that the only variables significantly affecting the survival were the groups of patients and the extent of the primary tumor (Bindal et al. 1993). The recurrence was similar in group B and C suggesting that an aggressive surgical approach may be useful. This approach has been confirmed by another study on 138 patients (Iwadate et al 2000). This study included other two variables: age and Karnofsky index. Age >60 years and Karnofsky < 70 and incomplete removal were significant factors.

### 3.2 Radiation therapy

Radiotherapy is the mainstay therapy of brain metastases. Currently there are three major categories of radio therapeutic treatments of brain metastasis: WBRT, radiosurgery, stereotactic radiotherapy. There are two options for radiosurgery: Gamma knife, Linac - based radiosurgery.

*WBRT* has been demonstrated by Patchell 1990 and Vecht 1993 to increase life survival in association with surgery. The WBRT is a palliative procedure which aim is to achieve life prolongation, local control and improvement in quality of life. WBRT has been also used prophylactically, aimed to treat malignancies having high brain metastasizing affinity, such as small cell lung carcinoma (SCLC), leukemia and lymphoma (Meert et al. 2001, Brown et al. 2005). The most frequently applied doses range from 20 Gy to 30 Gy in 5-10 sessions. Doses from 30 to 36 Gy are used as prophylaxis in the case of SLC and from 12-18 for hematologic diseases (Alexander et al. 1995, Brown et al. 2005). The combination of WBRT with radiosurgery will be discussed later.

**Radiosurgery** is now possible because of the availability of CT and MRI and computer planning makes possible the delivery of high dose of radiation to a precise target tumor area. This delivering of precise high dose of radiation energy to a tumor is called radiosurgery. It can be achieved combining 3 elements: 1) stereotactic localization of metastatic lesion; 2) precise collimation of the radiation energy and 3) administration of the total dose coming from different points in space and intersected in a single target volume. The peculiarity of radiosurgery is the fall of dose at the target edges, this permit to concentrate the dose to the target tumor area sparing everything possible the healthy tissue surrounding the tumor (Lunsford et al. 1990). Two radiosurgical treatment facilities exist: **Gamma Knife, Linac radiosurgery**.

Historically, LeKsell in Sweden was the first to apply radiosurgery. Initially low energy x-rays (280 kV) were used and concentrated stereotactically to the intracranial target. The technique was first accepted with skepticism; however after the initial studies by Lunsford et al. (1990) (University of Pittsburgh), radiosurgery has gained a considerable acceptance. Lately in 1967, Leksell, in collaboration with Larsson, developed according to the same principle of radiosurgery the first cobalt - 60 gamma unit (Gamma Knife).

The **Gamma Knife** contains 201 cobalt sources of gamma rays arrayed in a hemisphere within a shielded structure. A primary collimator, forces all the emitted sources to a common focal area, then a secondary collimator adapts this primary focal beam to sizes from 4 to 18 mm, through computer software, to target to the corresponding size of brain metastasis. In this case the limiting size of this device are brain metastases with a major diameter = 18 mm or tumor volume ranged from 0.5 to 33 $cm^3$ (Alexander et al. 1995, Lunsford et al. 1990).

Following the same principle several authors (Betti et al. 1991, Colombo et al. 1985, Hartman et al. 1985, Giller and Berger 2005, Shoshan et al. 2005, Sperduto 2003, Valk and Dillon 1991) in the late 1980 developed **LINAC** based radiosurgical method. Linac radiosurgical treatment relies upon the following aspects: a) a collimated X-ray is directed stereotactically to the target area; b) the gentry of the linear accelerator rotates over the patient producing an arc of radiation oriented on the target. In this manner different arc or multiple non-coplanar intersecting arcs of radiation are used. Some important aspects of Linac therapeutic methodology are to be evidenced, they are: size, dose, toxicity.

### 3.2.1 Size of target tumor volume

Brain metastases have been considered ideal targets for radiosurgery and stereotactic radiotherapy due to their small spherical size, non-infiltrative borders, and location in non-eloquent areas of the brain. In terms of stereotactic radiosurgery, the superiority of one energy source over another depends primarily on the dose distribution capabilities, which in turn depend on the target's volume, location, and shape. For small lesions (= 5 $cm^3$), the dose distributions produced by the gamma knife are essentially identical to those achievable with LINAC units. When the target lesion is non -spherical or of intermediate size ( =5 or = 25 $cm^3$), LINAC units may have an advantage over Gamma Knife units, due to their ability to treat larger lesions without requiring multiple isocenters (which makes treatment planning difficult), and the ability to shape the dose using collimated fields (Giller and Berger 2005).

### 3.2.2 Dose fractionation

Standard radiobiological principles suggest that fractionating radiation therapy (i.e., delivery in multiple sessions) will reduce both early and late toxicities to surrounding normal tissues. Radiotherapy can be delivered in a single session and is called radiosurgery, or in different sessions and is called: Stereotactic radiotherapy (SRT) or Conformal RadioTherapy (CRT) (Giller and Berger 2005, Shoshan et al. 2005, Sperduto 2003, Valk and Dillon 1991).

### 3.2.3 Toxicity (radioprotection)

Radiosurgery, notwithstanding its precision is not devoid of severe side effects on brain parenchyma, the worse being radionecrosis.CNS damage occurs in three different stages. The acute post radiation stage is usually well tolerated and consists in headache, nausea and somnolence. These symptoms are related to the cerebral edema and can be controlled with corticosteroids. A sub-acute stage caused by transient demyelization mediated damage to oligodendrocytes. This demyelization is clinically manifested by numbness, irritability, anorexia, somnolence and sometimes dysfunction of electric conduction. These symptoms occur approximately 10 weeks after cranial irradiation. Late effects (radionecrosis) become manifest from 6 to 9 months later and can evolve for a number of years following cranial irradiation. The process is associated with glia proliferation, mononuclear cell / astrocyte activation, and astrocyte secreted protein loss and cytokines production (Baker and Krochak 1989, Michalowsky 1986). The endothelium damage is the principal target of irradiation, is irreversible and progressive and determines an increase in the blood brain permeability

(Valk and Dillon 1991). The leakier endothelium determines an increment in the quantity of fluid in the interstitium, an excessive production of free radicals due to the iron loss by red blood cells and an increased production of proinflammatory prostaglandins and cytokines (see Fig.1) (Michalowsky 1986, St Clair and Given 2003, Wong and Van der Kogel 2004). An interesting study by Kureshi et al. (1994) on frozen specimen obtained by patients with radionecrosis has shown that all specimen were infiltrated with both CD4+ and CD8+ cells and activated macrophages (CD11c+, HLA-DR+). Furthermore they analyzed a panel of cytokines and found that Tumor Necrosis Factor- α (TNF-α) and Interleukin-6 immunoreactivity was prominent in majority of the specimen (75%) and were predominately produced by macrophages. TGF-[beta] astrocytic and macrophage immunoreactivity was present at moderate levels in all cases. Other authors have outlined that radiation injury is not only maintained by the inflammatory reaction elicited by radiation but is self maintained by the induction of apoptosis of endothelial cells (Wong and Van der Kogel 2004). These authors have also outlined the importance of hypoxia and VEGF production and of increased release of nitric oxide (NO) (Wong and Van der Kogel 2004). Belka et al. 2001, in agreement with us have outlined that radiation injury is the result of a complex alterations and that no single mechanism is responsible of the event. At least four factors contribute to central nervous system toxicity: (1) damage to vessel structures, (2) deletion of oligodendrocytes, (3) deletion of neural stem cells, (4) generalized alterations of cytokine expression (Kureshi et al. 1994). Actually no definitive therapies exist for radionecrosis (Valk and Dillon 1991, Belka et al 2001, Nieder et al 2007), however high dosage of corticosteroids, stem cell transplantation or erythropoietin (EPO) have been suggested. Pleiotropic functions of EPO on CNS have been recognized such as: inhibition of apoptosis, anti-inflammatory anti oxidative effects, prevention of glutamate-induced toxicity and stimulation of angiogenesis (Wong and Van der Kogel 2004). Other authors have proposed melatonin as radioprotective agent (Vijayalaxmi et al. 2004). Hyperbaric oxygen has been also proposed, however as outlined by Wong and Van der Kogel (2004), has not demonstrated a benefit. Since 1999, for brain metastases, a radioprotector formed by an association between bioflavonoids (silymarin) and omega three fatty acids has been suggested by an Italian group to decrease the risk ratio of developing brain necrosis and to improve significantly survival time (Gramaglia et al 1999). Omega 3 fatty acids have demonstrated to decrease the synthesis of proinflammatory prostaglandins (Fig.1) and cytokines, to have antitumoral activity and to change many tumor environmental parameters (Baronzio et al. 1994) whereas bioflavonoids have elicited protection of neuronal cells from oxidative stress and glutamate (Ishige et al 2001). A recent review on silymarin by Agarwaal et al. (2006) has outlined that this bioflavonoid has important anti-inflammatory and antiangiogenic activity. A vision of the various point of activity of these two natural drugs is illustrated in Fig.1.

As previous described, **Linac radiosurgery** technology delivers high doses of ionizing radiation to small intracranial targets. SRT or CFRT requires: adequate a) **patient immobilization**, b) accurate **three - dimension dose calculation TP** (treatment planning); c) **X-rays collimation**.

a. **The patient immobilization.** SRT is done using a frame fixed to patient's skull using four pins. These pins are anchored into the periosteum and afford an excellent immobilization. The method is not devoid of side effects such infections and pain. Anesthetic is used during the procedure to control this last side effect. For treatment that last several weeks the immobilization device should be reproducible and in this case an individual customized thermoplastic mould is built.

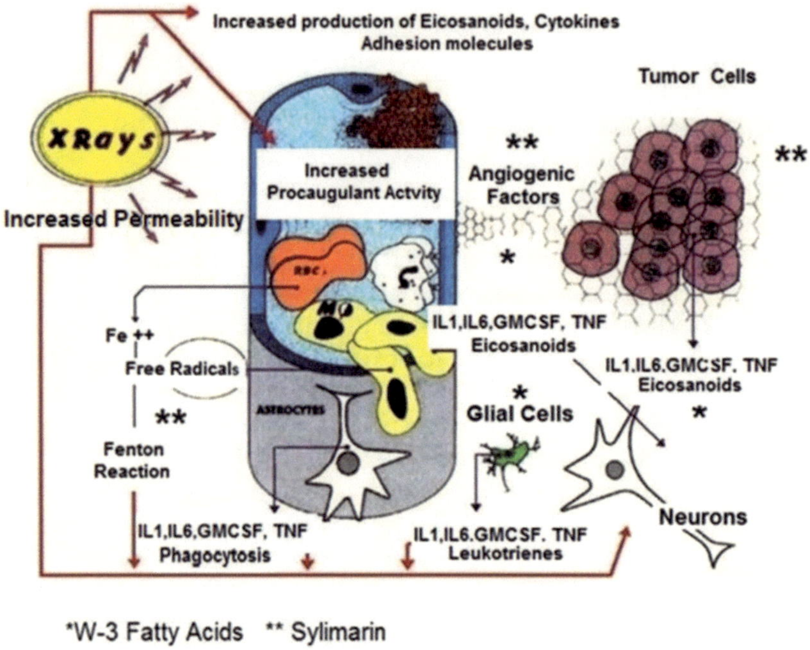


Fig. 1. In this figure, the effects of Radiotherapy on Brain structure, the reactions produced and the targets of radioprotectors such as Sylimarin ** and omega 3 fatty acids (W-3) * are illustrated.

b. **Treatment Planning.** After careful positioning the patient, is immobilized with thermoplastic moulds or with stereotactic frame undergoes to a contrast enhanced brain Computed Tomography (CT) or to a Brain Magnetic Resonance (MRI) scans with 2-5 mm slice thickness and 2-5 mm separation. Once obtained the CT/MR data, these are processed using a computerized treatment planning. CT/MRI images are fused using image fusion software and the Gross Tumor Volume (GTV) is defined and contoured manually. In some departments an integration of images with metabolic information such as Single Photon Emission Computed Tomography (SPECT) is also used (Mongioj et al 1999).This permits sometimes to obtain more accurate tumor visualization. The fusion of images is obtained by commercial software (i.e. package SRS PLATO®) consisting of three principal algorithms: (1) a module dedicated to the localization of each tomographic section on stereotactic space; (2) a CT/MR dedicated module for the creation of regions of interest (ROIs) for each slice and (3) a 3D- visualization module. Once the GTV is obtained, a margin over these countered borders must be defined to take into account the possible microscopic extension of the tumor not evidenced on the CT/MR scans. These margins are generally 10-20 mm around the GTV obtaining the Planned Target Volume (PTV). After PTV determination, a new contour is done ensuring PTV coverage by 95% isodose line with the aim for obtaining uniform dose homogeneity.

c. **Collimator.** The major problem in radiosurgery is treating irregularly shaped lesions. The use of overlapping spherical treatments results in some shaping advantages but the increased time used to reproduce this technique determines a non-homogeneous dose deposition and an increase on side effects. Improved tumor dose homogeneity can be obtained using a field shaping device able to form an optimal field shape for each beam direction (Kurup et al 2007). To obtain the best dose distribution different devices have been set up (i.e. 3D line®, Radionics ®) (Gauer et al. 2008, urie et al. 2001). Generally, these collimator devices consist of two opposing banks tungsten leaves and allows shaping of a radiation field up to a size of 11 x 10 $cm^2$ at the isocenter. Mechanical and dosimetric evaluations are performed to test the stability of the mechanical isocenter and to determine leaf leakage, penumbra width, and accuracy of leaf positions and uniformity of leaf speed. Several multileaf collimators are commercially available and differ from each other by many aspects such as: Leaf pairs, field size, leaf width, leaf transmission, maximum speed and total weight. As example, in table 1 we report some of the characteristics of 3D line® and that of Radionics ®.

| | Radionics | 3Dline |
|---|---|---|
| Leaf pairs | 31 | 24 |
| Field size( $cm^2$) | 10x12 | 11x10 |
| Leaf Width (mm) | 4 | 4.5 |
| Focused design | Single | Double |
| Total weight (Kg) | 35 | 35 |
| Maximum speed (cm/s) | 2.5 | 1 |

Table 1. Comparison of Some Characteristics of Radionics ® and 3Dline ® multileaf Collimator

## 4. Current debates on the best treatment options

An important question arises: is SRT efficacious as surgery in achieving local control (Rao et al. 2007)? As reviewed by Sperduto (2003), SRT is as good as or even better than surgical resection in term of local control. Another prospective study has addressed this question (Mucacevic et al. 2006). Mucacevic et al. 2006 found that local control was superior in SRT treated patients compared to surgery, and that SRT group had a greater improvement in quality of life even if a higher rate of distant brain failure was present.

Another question is: can SRT be used only for multiple brain metastases? Previous studies suggested that use of radiosurgery for brain metastases should be limited to patients with three or fewer lesions (Gupta 2005, Andrews et al. 2004). A recent randomized trial, compared whole-brain radiation therapy (WBRT) plus radiosurgery boost to metastatic foci. This trial has demonstrated a significant advantage of radiosurgery boost over WBRT alone in terms of freedom from local failure, and that the result also present among patients with 2, 3, or 4 metastases (Andrews et al. 2004). Survival also did not depend on number of metastases. The drawback of this technique is the risk of radiation necrosis. Chang et al. (2000) found that radionecrosis occurred in the 5.4% of patient treated and only 7 tumors required subsequent surgical resection. Regarding toxicity by adding SRT + WBRT however, Aoyama et al. (2006) found no difference between the group treated with SRT alone or the group treated with SRT + WBRT. Furthermore they found that the patients in whom WBRT was omitted had a higher rate of failure in the brain (76%vs. 48%) and required salvage therapy more often for recurrent brain metastases.

Study by Hidefumi et al. 2006, has clearly evidenced that WBRT associated to SRT improve the survival of patients with 1 to 4 brain metastases. Furthermore these authors outlined that intracranial relapse occurred more frequently in patients who did not receive WBRT. A recent study however indicate that SRT boost after WBRT for single brain metastases improves survival in select patients, whereas for patients up to four metastases the association improves local control not overall survival (Eichler and Loeffler 2007). Patchell et al. (1998) and Sneed et al. (2002) however disagree and from their retrospective and prospective data suggest that omitting WBRT does not result in shorter survival. They outline that the status of systemic disease is the predominant determinant of patient's prognosis. To our opinion WBRT can omitted on selected patients with high risk of radionecrosis (increased accumulation of gadolinium in tumor area, neuro cognitive deterioration, persistence of headache and peritumoral edema) or if a close follow-up can be ensured to the patients treated with SRT. If patients do not show increased risk of radionecrosis, have a Karnofsky index > 70% and the systemic
disease is minimal WBRT is however mandatory.

### 4.1 Chemotherapy

As outlined by Nguyen and De Angelis 2004, chemotherapy has a limited role in treating brain metastases and is used after failure of surgery and or radiation therapy. Many chemotherapy drugs do not cross the blood-brain barrier but can reach malignant tumors in the brain, presumably through a local breakdown in the blood-brain barrier. In some chemotherapy-sensitive tumors like, lymphoma, small cell lung cancer (SCLC) and breast cancer (Eichler and Loeffler 2007), chemotherapy can induce remissions, but its routine use is still under evaluation. But for most tumors, chemotherapy for brain metastases is ineffective, may be because of the existence of the BBB. In fact, many drugs do not cross easily BBB, and do not remain in the brain long enough or at high concentration to ensure adequate cancer killing effect (Tosoni et al. 2004). Drugs active on primary tumors may not be as active on metastases (Chang et al. 2007, Cavaliere and Shiff 2007). On the contrary other authors outline that brain metastases are as responsive as primary systemic cancer. This has been demonstrated by numerous phase II studies (Tosoni et al. 2004).

Different chemotherapeutic regimens have been used for treating brain metastases from SCLC [52, 101]. Drugs have been used as single agent or combined to other drugs or associated with WBRT or SRT. The most active single drugs are cisplatinum (CCP), and temozolomide (TMZ) (Nguyen and De Angelis 2004). Cisplatinum alone has shown a response rate (RR) of 30% (Tosoni et al. 2004). A better response of 50% rate has been obtained combining to cisplatinum, etoposide, cyclophosphamide, methotrexate, and 5 fluouracil (Tosoni et al. 2004). The association with WBRT was better in term of overall survival and in treatment response (57% vs 22%) compared to patients who had received only WBRT (Postmus et al. 2000).

Breast cancer is sensitive to chemotherapy (Cavaliere and Shiff 2007). Rosner et al (1986) have shown a 50% response rate among 100 women treated with different regimens. The most common agents are: cyclophosphamide, doxorubicin, 5-fluorouracil, methotrexate, and vincristine. All these agents do not cross BBB notwithstanding a response by metastatic foci have been obtained. This outlines that BBB is not so important and that the appropriate regimen and the chemosensitivity of the metastases are more important. Boogerd et al. 1992, reported a 59% RR, and according to Rosner et al. (1986), suggest that chemotherapeutics may cross BBB at a sufficient concentration to achieve a clinical effect. Another interesting and a standard drug on breast cancer is doxorubicin. Doxorubicin does not cross easily BBB however when encapsulated in liposomes its penetration can increase (Siegal et al. 1995). Caraglia et al. (2006) used liposomal doxorubicin and temozolomide (TMZ) in 19 patients with brain metastases. This association resulted in a RR of 37%; furthermore 8 patients had complete response and 2 a partial response. Temozolamide has limited activity against breast cancer so the majority of the response may be attributed to doxorubicin (Cavaliere and Shiff 2007).

The incidence of metastases in breast cancer increases with the increase in HER2 overexpression. HER2 is an 185KDa transmembrane tyrosine kinase with extensive homology to the epidermal growth factor receptor. Trastuzumab is a monoclonal antibody (MOaBs) now approved as a first line chemotherapy in patients with positivity for HER2 receptors. After its introduction however an increased incidence in brain metastases has been noted. Retrospective studies documented an incidence between the 25% and the 40%, suggesting that HER-2 positive tumors have a biological predisposition to metastasize to brain (Lin and Winer 2007). The reasons for this increased incidence, as reported by Lin and Winer (2007), are multifactorial and include biological and treatment related factors. This last factor seems linked to the low penetration across BBB of Trastuzumab. Recently, to overcome this problem, Lapatinib has been suggested. Lapatinib has a dual inhibitor activity on epidermal growth factor and on HER2 and in preliminary has shown an objective response in two patients among 39 treated (Lin et al. 2006). Other studies with lapatinib and other HER2 inhibitors are currently been tested (Lin and Winer 2007).

The incidence of brain metastases in melanoma is high and can reach the 43%. Melanoma is relatively chemoresistant. The various biological treatments such as interferon or interleukin-2 and chemotherapeutics (dacarbazine) have shown a limited activity. Temozolomide (TMZ) has demonstrated a relatively important response against brain metastases from melanoma. TMZ is a third generation alkylating agent that can be taken orally. Its small size and lipophilic properties, allows TMZ to cross easily BBB. CNS concentrations can reach 30% of the plasma concentrations. When it has reached the CNS, TMZ is converted to the active metabolite (MTIC). TMZ has been used as a single agent or combined with WBRT (Cavaliere and Shiff 2007). For example, in a phase II study on 151 patients ( Agarwala et al. 2004), , 39 patients (26%) showed a stable disease. Other authors have reported similar results, futhermore the association of TMZ with WBRT resulted in a better overall survival compared to TMZ alone (9 months versus 5 months) (Hoffman et al. 2006).

### 4.2 Hyperthermia and metabolic inhibitors, the future?

Multiple attempts have been made to improve the results of WBRT alone or combined with SRT/CFRT, by adding radiosensitizing agents. All the trials failed to demonstrate any benefit either in local control or in survival (Eichler and Loeffler 2007). When brain metastases reach a critical mass > 1-2 $mm^3$ ($10^6$ cells) and a distance from host nutritive vessel > of 100-200 μm develop area of hypoxia and angiogenesis. Hypoxia results in radioresistance (Wouters et al. 2007). Actually, no definitive clinical therapies exist for overcoming tumour hypoxia out of hyperthermia (HT) (Pontiggia et al. 1990, Baronzio et al. 2006). HT is a treatment raising the temperature of tumor - loaded tissue to 40-43 degrees C. It is deprived of important side effects and has shown to enhance the effects of radiotherapy and to potentiate the efficacy of certain drugs, such as nitrosurea, cisplatinum, metothrexate (Baronzio et al. 2006, Dewey et al 1977). HT combined with radiation has been reported to yield higher complete and durable responses than radiation alone in superficial tumors. Despite difficulties in increasing human tumor temperatures, recent clinical trials have shown that a combination of hyperthermia with radiation is superior to radiation alone in controlling many human tumors (Dewey et al. 1977, Gabriele and Roca 2006). The increased effect seen by combining cytotoxic agents with hyperthermia is complex, but may be due to altered drug pharmacokinetics such as increased solubility (e.g. nitrosureas and alkylating agents), altered plasma protein binding (e.g. cisplatinum) and activation of enzymatic processes (e.g. anthracyclines) (Luk and Hulse 1980, Gerweek 1985). Hyperthermia does not usually cause marked increase in radiation side effects. Regarding brain, Seegenschmiedt et al. (1995), in their review affirmed that treatment toxicity to brain, is relatively low and long-term side effects are similar to that observed to RT alone. Ikeda et al. (1994), studied the toxicity of radiofrequency interstitial HT in dog and found alteration of Blood Brain Barrier (BBB). Other authors outlined that the maximum tolerated heat dose to CNS lies in the range of 40-60 min at 42-42.5°C or 10-30 min at 43°C (Gerweek 1985). A recent review by Sharma and Hoopes (2003) has reported that HT specifically alters the mammalian CNS. The morphological alterations for temperature in the range 40°C to 42 °C for 4 hours has been demonstrated for the axons, the glial cells and the vascular endothelium. Sneed and Stea 1995, demonstrated in a randomized study that HT has an acceptable toxicity, in fact no grade 5 toxicity was found outside 4 patients on 112 ( 3.5% ) with grade 2 and 7 (Sneed et al. 1995).

There are only a small number of studies on brain metastases with HT. In an interesting study reported by Pontiggia on 17 patients with lung cancer,the patients were treated with nitrosurea and capacitive HT for 60′. Sixteen patients out of 17 responded with clinical improvement and radiological regression of the disease. The survival time was in median 12.7 months (Pontiggia et al. 1995).

Hyperthermia is a useful adjunct to chemotherapy and radiotherapy; however, new therapeutic strategies easily applicable in many institutions are to be developed.

The search for functional characteristics that allow cancer cells to spread to brain and development of new animal models will open new opportunities in target and drug discovery (Gril et al. 2010). Metabolic profiles of cells with metastatic propensity to brain may be one of these targets. In fact, studies by proteomics have demonstrated that breast cancer cells that metastasize to brain , have a unique protein profile consistent with increased expression of enzymes involved in glycolysis, tricarboxylic acid cycle, and oxidative phosphorylation pathways, permitting to these cells to have an enhanced proliferation and adaptation (Chen et al. 2007). Studies by Blasberg et al. (1985), using 14C-deoxyglucose and quantitative autoradiography in metastatic walker 256 brain tumors confirm that glucose utilization is of primary importance in metastatic cells and that brain metastases consume glucose in presence of a low oxygen tension, the so called aerobic glycolysis or "Warburg effect" (Warburg 1956).

Palmieri et al. 2009 have confirmed the "Warburg effect" analyzing resected human brain metastases of breast cancer through real time PCR. They demonstrated an upregulation of hexokinase-2, an enzyme that mediates the first step of glucose metabolism, its upregulation is associated with a poor prognosis (Palmieri et al.2009). Hennipman et al. (1988) suggested an association of an increasing rate of enzymes implicated in glycolysis in breast cancer metastases and that their activities were higher in metastases compared to the primary tumors (Richardson et al. 2008). Another study on MCF10 model of mammary carcinoma by Richardson, confirms the major shift toward aerobic glycolysis (Gambhir et al. 2001). Increased glycolysis at metastatic site has been confirmed by [18F] 2-fluoro-2-deoxy-D-glucose positron emission tomography (PET) (Richardson et al. 2008, Gambhir et al. 2001, Gillies et al. 2008, and Lee et al. 2008).

Our group (Guais et al. 2010) has developed a drugs combination able to alter two different steps of tumor metabolism (pyruvate dehydrogenase and ATP citrate lyase). The first drug is α-lipoic acid (ALA), which, as is the case for dichloroacetate, inhibits the enzyme Pyruvate Dehydrogenase Kinase-1 (PDHK1). Inhibition of PDHK1 can restore the activity of pyruvate dehydrogenase, thus possibly redirecting aerobic glycolysis to respiration and thus decreasing the amount of lactate produced. The second drug is hydroxycitrate (HCA), which inhibits ATP citrate lyase. The efficacy of this combination appears in animals to be similar to conventional chemotherapy (cisplatin or 5-FU), as it results in both significant tumor growth inhibition and enhanced survival (Schwartz et al. 2010). Similar results have been obtained in one case of pancreatic patient metastatic to liver (Guais et al. 2010). An unpublished result, of a patient with head and neck cancer with brain metastases treated with ALA and HCA and chemotherapy has shown a complete disappearance of brain metastases (personal communication).

Immunohistochemistry studies on several specimens of primitive and metastatic human cancers, such as colon, breast, lung, ovarian and pancreas, have, also revealed an overexpression of hypoxia- inducible factor 1 (HIF) (Zhong et al. 1999). This overexpression supports two basic biological behavior of cancer and its metastases, an altered glucose transport and a limited diffusion of $O_2$, glucose and nutrients (Liu et al. 2002). Hypoxic tumor cells become hypersensitized to glycolytic inhibitors (Liu et al. 2002) and to hyperthermia (Baronzio et al. 2006), reinforcing our hypotheses on metabolic treatment of metastatic cancer.

## 5. Discussion and conclusions

Patients with brain metastases have usually a short survival. Historical studies have demonstrated that with no treatments the survival is of the order of one - two months, due to systemic progression in sites other than brain. Although brain metastases incidence is increasing, there is no consensus for their treatment. Currently, treatment options include WBRT, surgery, chemotherapy and SRT/CRT. WBRT has the advantage of being easily and widely available and is able to extend survival to three to six months. In the case of solitary metastases, the addition of surgical resection to WBRT has doubled the survival, in the range of 10 - 12 months (Patchell et al. 1990, Heilbrun and Adler 2010). However, many patients have metastases in locations not amenable to surgical resection. STRT, for these patients has demonstrated in terms of survival and palliation to be a reliable clinical tool

(Brown and Pollock 2005). For larger lesions surgery could be considered when feasible in alternative to STRT even though in our opinion the SRT as first attempt could avoid the risk of seeding and partial resection. Surgery, in our institution, showed its major role in two different settings, i.e. for solitary brain disease with a controlled disease outside the brain and for resection of large necrotic masses, as result of previous STRT (mainly for lesions of more than 45 mm of diameter). A recent work has confirmed that previous surgical treatments have a negative impact on survival, suggesting that intervention must follows SRT (Vijayalaxmi et al 2004). As outlined by De Angelis (1994), another biological aspect, favoring the use SRT compared to WBRT, relies on that, approximately half of patients have single metastases and 20% of patients have only two metastatic lesions at the moment of their diagnosis. This aspect suggests that metastases to brain must be considered and treated as a local disease process. We suggest that the correct approach to patients bearing brain metastases should have to consider palliation as first intent. SRT, which reach this need faster than WBRT, is to be considered the treatment of choice mainly for patients bearing up to 3 lesions at first diagnosis, reserving WBRT as adjuvant to SRT and for palliation attempt to those with more than 3 lesions. Surgery must be used for patients without evident primary tumor and for necrotic lesions following aggressive radiotherapy. Furthermore, the altered glucose metabolism of metastases, suggests that the metabolic treatment is a promising line of research that could have significant therapeutic applications in a near future.

## 6. References

Agarwal R, Agarwal C, Ichikawa H et al: Anticancer potential of silymarin: from bench to bed side. Anticancer Res. 2006; 26:4457-98.

Agarwala SS, Kirkwood JM, Gore M, et al: Temozolomide for the treatment of brain metastases associated with metastatic melanoma: a phase II study. J Clin Oncol. 2004; 22 :2101-2107.

American College of Surgical oncology CNS Working Group: The management of brain Metastases. In Principles of Neuroncology. David Schiff and Brian Patrick O'Neill Editors. pp553-579, 2005 McGraw- Hill, New York, London, Toronto.

Alexander EIII, Moriarty T.M., Davis R.B., et al: Stereotactic Radiosurgery for the definitive, non invasive treatment of brain metastasis. J Natl Cancer Inst 1955; 37: 34-40.

Andrews D.W., Scott C.B., Sperduto P.W., et al: Whole brain radiation therapy with or without stereotactic radiosurgery boost for patients with one to three brain metastases: phase III results of the RTOG 9508 randomized trial: The Lancet 2004, 363:1665-1672.

Aoyama H, Shirato H, Tago M, et al: Stereotactic radiosurgery plus whole brain radiotherapy vs. stereotactic radiosurgery alone for treatment of brain metastases: a randomized controlled trial. JAMA 2006;295: 2483-2491.

Baker AB: Metastatic tumors to the nervous system. Arch Pathol 1942;24: 495-537.

Baker D.G. and Krochak R.J.: The response of microvascular system to radiation. A review. Cancer Investigation 1989;7: 287-294.

Baronzio G:F.,Freitas i, Griffini P; et al: Omega-3 fatty acids can improve radioresponse modifying tumor interstitial pressure, blood rheology and membrane peroxidability. Anticancer res 1994,14.1145-1154.

Baronzio G.F., Cerreta V, Baronzio A;, et al: Thermo chemo-radiotherapy association: Biological rationale, Preliminary observations on its use on Malignant brain tumors. "Hyperthermia in Cancer treatment: A primer" Baronzio G.F. and Hager D editors, Landes / Springer 2006, pp:123-151.

Belka C, Budach W, Kortmann R.D. et al: Radiation induced CNS toxicity-molecular and cellular mechanisms. British J Cancer 2001,85:1233-1239.

Beasley KD, Toms SA. The molecular pathobiology of metastasis to the brain: a review. Neurosurg Clin N Am. 2011 Jan;22(1):7-14.

Betti O.O., Galmarini D, Derechinsky V. radiosurgery with a linear accelerator. Methodologic Aspects. Stereotac Func Neurosurg 1991;57.87-98.

Bindal R.K., Sawaya R, Leavens M.E., et al: Surgical treatment of multiple brain metastases. J Neurosurg 1993;79:210-216.

Blasberg RG, Shinohara M, Shapiro WR, Patlak CS, Pettigrew KD, Fenstermacher JD.Apparent glucose utilization in Walker 256 metastatic brain tumors. J Neurooncol. 1985;3(2):153-64.

Boogerd W, Dalesio O, Bais E.M. et al: response of brain metastases from breast cancer to systemic chemotherapy. Cancer 1992; 69: 972-980.

Brown P.D. and Pollock B.E. Principles of Radiotherapy and Radiosurgery In Principles of Neuroncology. David Schiff and Brian Patrick O'Neill Editors . pp553-579, 2005 McGraw- Hill, New York, London, Toronto.

Bucana CD, Yano S, Reynolds D, Fidler IJ.: 22 morphometric investigation of immunostained blood vessels in brain metastasis in nude mice.J Histochem Cytochem. 1999 ; 47:1647C-1648.

Buchsbaum J.C., Suh J.H., Lee S.Y., et al: Survival by radiation therapy oncology group recursive partitioning analysis class and treatment modality in patients with brain metastases from malignant melanoma: a retrospective study. Cancer 2002;94: 2265-2272.

Caraglia M, Addeo R, Costanzo R et al: Phase II study of temozolamide plus pegylated liposomal doxorubicin in the treatment of brain metastases from solid tumors. Cancer Chemother Pharmacol. 2006; 57: 34-39

Cavaliere R and Schiff D: Chemotherapy and cerebral metastases: Misperception or reality? Neurosurg Focus 2007, 22 : 1.9.

Chang S.D., Lee E, Gordon R.N.;et al: Stereotactic radiosurgery in patients with multiple brain metastases. Neurosurg Focus 2000; 9: 1-5.

Chang J.E., Robins H.I., Mehta M.P.: Therapeutic advances in the treatment of brain metastases. Clinical advances in Hematology & Oncology. 2007; 5: 54-64.

Chason JL, Walker FB, Landers JW: Metastatic carcinoma in the central nervous system and dorsal root ganglia. A prospective autopsy studied. Cancer 1963;16:781-787.

Chen E, Hewell J, Krueger J, et al: Adaptation of energy metabolism in breast cancer brain metastases. Cancer Res. 67: 1472-1486.

Chenyu Zhang and Dihua Yu : Microenvironment Determinants of Brain Metastasis. Cell & Bioscience 2011, 1:8 .

Colombo F, Benedetti A, Pozza F., et al: Stereotactic radiosurgery utilizing a linear accelerator. Appl Neurophysiol 1985;48:133-145

Cormio G, Maneo A, Colamaria A, et al. : Surgical resection of solitary brain metastasis from ovarian carcinoma: an analysis of 22 cases. Gynecol Oncol. 2003;89: 116-119.

D'Ambrosio A, Agazzi S: Prognosis in patients presenting with brain metastases from an undiagnosed primary tumor. Neurosurg Focus. 2007;22:1-7.

Delattre JY, Krol G, Thaler HT, et al.: Distribution of brain metastases. Arch Neurol. 1988;45:741-744.

DeAngelis LM. Management of brain metastases. Cancer Invest. 1994;12(2):156-65.

Deeken J-F- and Löscher W: The blood brain barrier and cancer: transporters, treatment, and Trojan horses. Clin Cancer Res. 2007,13.1663-1674.

Deichman GI: Natural host resistance and in vivo selection of malignant tumour cells. Cancer Surveys 1998. 7:675-690.

Denkins Y, Reiland J, Roy M et al. Brain metastases in melanoma: roles of neurotrophins. Neuro-Oncology 2004;6:154-165

Dewey WC, Hopwood LE Sapareto SA et al. :Cellular responses to combinations of hyperthermia and radiation. Radiology 1977;123: 463-474.

Dong J.T., Lamb P.W., Rinker-Schaeffer C.W., et al: KA11, a metastasis suppressor gene for prostate cancer on human chromosome 11p11.2. Science 1995, 268.884-886.

Eichler A. F., Loeffler J. S.: Multidisciplinary management of brain metastases. The Oncologist 2007;12: 884-898.

Fidler IJ, Schackert G, Zhang RD, Radinsky R, Fujimaki T. The biology of melanoma brain metastasis. Cancer Metastasis Rev. 1999;18(3):387-400.

Fidler IJ, Yano S, Zhang RD,ety al: The seed and soil hypothesis: vascularisation and brain metastases. Lancet Oncol. 2002;3:53-7.

Fidler IJ. Critical determinants of metastasis. Semin Cancer Biol. 2002; 12:89-96. Gupta G.P.and Massagué J: Cancer metastasis: Building a framework. Cell.2006;17: 679-695.

Fidler IJ, Kim S-J and Langley R.R.: The role of the organ environment in the biology and therapy of cancer metastasis. J. Cell. Biochem. 2007;101:927-936.

Fidler IJ, Balasubramanian K, Lin Q, Kim SW, Kim SJ. The brain microenvironment and cancer metastasis. Mol Cells. 2010 Aug;30(2):93-8.

Gabriele P and Roca C:Results of hyperthermia alone with radiation therapy and or / chemotherapy. In "Hyperthermia in Cancer treatment: A primer" BAronzio G.F. and Hager D editors, Landes/Springer 2006, pp:114-119.

Gambhir SS, Czernin J, Schwimmer J, Silverman DH, Coleman RE, Phelps ME.: A tabulated summary of the FDG PET literature. J Nucl Med. 2001 May;42(5 Suppl):1S-93S.

Gaspar L, Scott C, Rotman M, Asbell S, Phillips T, et al. Recursive partitioning analysis (RPA) of prognostic factors in three Radiation Therapy Oncology Group (RTOG) brain metastases trials.Int J Radiat Onc ol Biol Phys. 1997 ;37(4):745-51.

Gaspar LE, Scott C, Murray K, Curran W. Validation of the RTOG recursive partitioning analysis (RPA) classification for brain metastases. Int J Radiat Oncol Biol Phys. 2000;47:1001-6.

Gauer T, Sokoll J, Cremers F, Harmansa R, Luzzara M, Schmidt R.Characterization of an add-on multileaf collimator for electron beam therapy.Phys Med Biol. 2008 Feb 21;53(4):1071-85.

Gerweck L. E.: Hyperthermia in Cancer Therapy: The Biological Basis and Unresolved Questions[1] *Cancer Research* 1985, 45, 3408-3414.

Gillies RJ, Robey I, Gatenby RA. : Causes and consequences of increased glucose metabolism of cancers. J Nucl Med. 2008 Jun;49 Suppl 2:24S-42S.

Giller C.A., and Berger B.D.: New frontiers in radiosurgery for the brain and body. BUMC Proceedings. 2005; 18:311-319.

Globus JH, Meltzer T. Metastatic tumors of the brain. Arch Neurol Psychiatr. 1942;482:163-226.

Gramaglia A, Loi G.F., Mongioj V, and Baronzio G.F.: Increased survival in brain metastatic patients treated with stereotactic radiotherapy, omega three fatty acids and bioflavonoids. Anticancer res 1999; 19. 5583-5586.

Gril B, Evans L, Palmieri D, Steeg PS.: Translational research in brain metastasis is identifying molecular pathways that may lead to the development of new therapeutic strategies. Eur J Cancer. 2010 May;46(7):1204-10.

Guais A, Baronzio G, Sanders E, Campion F, Mainini C, Fiorentini G, Montagnani F, Behzadi M, Schwartz L, Abolhassani M.: Adding a combination of hydroxycitrate and lipoic acid (METABLOC™) to chemotherapy improves effectiveness against tumor development: experimental results and case report. Invest New Drugs. 2010 Oct 8.

Gupta T: Stereotactic radiosurgery for brain oligometastases: good for some, better for all. Annals of oncology 2005; 16:1749-54.

Hammoud M.A., McCutcheon I.E:, Elsouki R, et al: Colorectal carcinoma and brain metastasis: distribution, treatment, survival. Ann Surg Oncol 1996; 3: 453-463.

Hankins J.R., Miller J.E., Salcman M, et al: Surgical management of lung cancer with solitary cerebral metastasis. Ann. Thorac. Surg. 1988;46:24-28.

Hartmann G.H., Schlegel W, Strum V,et al: Cerebral radiation surgery using moving field irradiation at a linear accelerator facility. Int J Radiat Oncol Biol Phys.1985,11.1185-1192.

Heilbrun MP, Adler JR. The 2009 devaluation of radiosurgery and its impact on the neurosurgery-radiation oncology partnership. J Neurosurg.2010,Jul;113(1):10-5.

Hennipman A, van Oirschot BA, Smits J, Rijksen G, Staal GE. : Glycolytic enzyme activities in breast cancer metastases. Tumour Biol. 1988;9(5):241-8.

Hidefumi A, Hiroki, Masao T, et al: Stereotactic Radiosurgery Plus Whole-Brain Radiation Therapy vs Stereotactic Radiosurgery Alone for Treatment of Brain Metastases *JAMA*. 2006;296:2089-2090.

Hofmann M, Kiecker F, Wurm R et al: Temozolomide with or without radiotherapy in melanoma with unresectable brain metastases. IJ Neurooncol 2006; 76: 59-64.

Hwang TL, Close TP, Grego JM et al: Predilection of brain metastases in gray and white matter junction and vascular border zones. Cancer 1996;77:1551-11555.

Ikeda N, Hayashida O, Kameda H et al: Experimental study on thermal damage to dog normal brain. Int. J. Hyperthermia. 1994;10:553-561.

Ishige K, Shubert D, Sagara Y: Flavonoids protect neuronal cells from oxidative stress by three distinct mechanisms. Free radical Biology & Medecine 2001;30: 433-446.

Iwadate Y, Namba H, Yamaura A: Significance of surgical resection for the treatment of multiple brain metastases. Anticancer Res 2000;20: 573-577.

Kamar FG, Posner JB. Brain metastases. Semin Neurol. 2010 Jul;30(3):217-35.

Kang M, Fujimaki T, Yano S and Fidler I: Biollogy of brain metastasis from: Contemporary cancer Research: Brain Tumors, 2004: pp 91-106, Edited by Ali-Osman F Humana Press Inc., Totowa ,NJ.

Kaplan R.N., Rafti S, Lyden D: preparing the soil: the premetastatic niche. Cancer Res. 2006; 66:11089-11093.

Kaplan R.N., Riba R.D., Zachaurolis S, et al: VEGFR1-positive haemopoietic progenitor cells initiate the premetastatic niche. Nature 2005; 438:820-827.

Kehrli P.: Biologie des métastases cérébrales. Neurochirurgie. 1999,45:364-368.

Kim LS, Huang S, Lu W et al: Vascular endothelial growth factor expression promotes the growth of breast cancer brain metastasis in nude mice. Clin Exp Metastasis. 2004,21:107-118.

Kleisbauer J.P:, Guerin J.C., Arnaud A et al: Chemotherapy with high dose cisplatin in brain metastases of lung cancer.Bull Cancer 1990;77:661-665.

Kureshi S. A.; Hofma, F; Schneider J. H.; et al: Cytokines and delayed radiation necrosis. Neurosurgery. 1994; 35:822-830.

Kurup P.G.G., Murali V, Sankar A.: Advantages of minimultileaf in stereotactic radiotherapy. Journal of Medical Physics 2007;32: 12-17.

Leone A, Flatow U, King C.R., et al: Reduced tumor incidence , metastatic potential, and cytokine responsiveness on nm23-transfected melanoma cells. Cell 1991;65:25-35.

Lin N.U., Carey L.A., Liu M.C. et al: Phase II trial of lapatinib for brain metastases in patients with HER2+ breast cancxer. J Clin Oncol 2006;3s.

Lin N.U:,and Winer E.P:: Brain metastases: The HER2 paradigm. Clin Cancer Res 2007; 13: 1648-1655.

Liu H, Savaraj N, Priebe W, Lampidis TJ. Hypoxia increases tumor cellsensitivity to glycolytic inhibitors: a strategy for solid tumor therapy (ModelC). Biochem Pharmacol. 2002 Dec 15;64(12):1745-51.

Luk K.H. and Hulse R. M. : Hyperthermia in Cancer Therapy. West J Med. 1980; 132: 179–185.

Lunsford L.D., Flickinger J, Coffey R.J.: Stereotactic gamma knife radiosurgery. Initial North American experience in 207 patients. Arch Neurol 1990;47:797-803.

Marchetti D, Denkins Y, Reiland J et al: Brain-metastatic melanoma. A neurotrophic perspective. Pathology oncology Research 2003:3: 147-158.

Menter d.G., Hermann J.L., Marchetti D et al: Involvement of neurotrophins and growth factors in brain metastasis formation. Invasion Metastasis 1994-1995;14:372-384.

Meert A.P., Paesmans M, Berghmans T, et al: Prophylactic cranial irradiation in small cell lung: a systematic review of the literature with meta-analysis. BMC Cancer 2001;1:5

McCutcheon I.E., Eng D.Y., Logothetis C.J. : Brain metastasis from prostate carcinoma: ante mortem recognition and outcome after treatment. Cancer 1999; 86:2301-2311.

Michalowsky A: the pathogenesis of late side-effects of radiotherapy. Clinical radiology 1986;37:203-207.

Mongioj V, Brusa A, Loi G.F. et al: Accuracy evaluation of fusion of CT, MR, and SPECT images using commercially available software packages (SRS Plato and IFS). Int, J. Radiation Oncology, Biol. Phys. 1999;43: 227-234.

Muacevic A, Wowra B, Kreth F, et al.: a randomized trial of surgery and radiotherapy versus radiosurgery alone in the treatment of single metastasis to the brain. Doc OP256, Deutscher Krebscongress. Berlin, Deutscher Krebscongress, 2006.

Nash G.F:, Turner L.F., Scully M.F. et al: Platelets and cancer. Lancet Oncol. 2002, 3:425-430.

Nathoo N, Chahlavi A, Barnett GH, et al: Pathobiology of brain metastases. J Clin Pathol. 2005; 56:237-242.

Nicolson G: paracrine and autocrine growth mechanisms in tumor metastasis to specific sites with particular emphasis on brain and lung metastasis. Cancer Metastasis Rev 1993.12: 325-343.

Nieder C, Andratschke N and Asner S.T:: Experimental concepts for toxicity prevention and tissue restoration after cental nervous system irradiation. Radiation Oncology. 2007,2:23-33.

Norden AD, Wen PY, Kesan S: Brain metastases. Current Opinion In Neurology.2005; 18:654-661.

Ngguyen T and DeAngelis L.M.: Treatment of brain metastases. The Journal of Supportive Oncology. 2004; 2: 405-416.

Nussbaum ES, Djalilian HR, Cho KH et al: Brain metastases. Histology, multiplicity, surgery and survival. Cancer 1996;78:1781-1788.

Palmieri D, chambers BF, Huang S et al: The biology of the metastasis to a sanctuary site. Clin Cancer Res. 2007;13: 16561662.

Palmieri D, Fitzgerald D, Shreeve SM, Hua E, Bronder JL, Weil RJ, Davis S, Stark AM, Merino MJ, Kurek R, Mehdorn HM, Davis G, Steinberg SM, Meltzer PS, Aldape K, Steeg PS.: Analyses of resected human brain metastases of breast cancer reveal the association between up-regulation of hexokinase 2 and poor prognosis. Mol Cancer Res. 2009 Sep;7(9):1438-45.

Patchell R.A., Tibbs P.A., walsh J.W:, et al. : A randomized trial of surgery in the treatment of single metastases to the brain. N. Engl J Med. 1990;322:494-500.

Patchell R.A., Tibbs P.A., Regine W.F.; et al: postoperative radiotherapy in the treatment of single metastases to the brain. A randomized trial. JAMA 1998,280.1485-1489

Patchell R A: The management of brain metastases. Cancer Treat Rev. 2003 ;29: 533-40.

Pectasides D, Pectasides M, Economopoulos T : Brain metastases from epithelial ovarian cancer:A review of the literature. The Oncologist2006;11:252-260

Perides G, Zhuge Y, Lin T et al: the fibrinolytic system facilitates tumor cell migration across the blood-brain barrier in experimental melanoma brain metastasis. BMC Cancer 2006, 6: 56-65.

Pontiggia P, McLaren JR, Baronzio GF, Freitas I: The biological responses to heat. Adv Exp Med Biol. 1990;267:271-91.

Pontiggia P, Cuppone Curto F, Rotella G, et al : Hyperthermia in the treatment of brain metastases from lung cancer. Experience on 17 cases. Anticancer Res. 1995; 15: 597-601.

Postmus P.E., Haaxama –Reiche H, Smit E.F. et al: Treatment of brain metastases of small cell lung cancer: comparing teniposide and teniposide with whole brain radiotherapy-a phase III study of European Organization for the research and treatment of Cancer Lung Cancer cooperative group. J. Clin. Oncol. 2000,18: 3400-3408.

Posner JB, Chernic NL: intracranial metastases from systemic cancer. Adv Neurol 1978; 19: 589-592

Rao R, Brown P, Buckner JC: Innovation in management of brain metastases. Oncology 2007; 21:473-481.

Richardson AD, Yang C, Osterman A, Smith JW. Central carbon metabolism in the progression of mammary carcinoma. Breast Cancer Res Treat. 2008

Rosner D, Nemoto T, Warren W.L.: Chemotherapy induces regression of brain metastases in breast carcinomas. Cancer 1986;58: 832-839.

Santarelli J.G., Sarkissaian V, Hou L et al: Molecular events of brain metastasis. Neurosurg Focus 2007; 22: E1-E5.

Seegenschmiedt MH, Feldmann HJ, Wust P et al: Hyperthermia- Its actual role in Radiation Oncology, part IV Thermoradiotherapy for malignant brain tumors. Strhlentherapie und Onkologie 1995;171:560-572.

Seraj M.J., Samant R.S., Verderame M.F., et al: Functional evidence for a novel human breast carcinoma metastasis suppressor,BRMS1, encoded at chromosome 11q13. Cancer Res 2000;60:2764-2769.

Shaffrey M.E., Mut M., Asher A.L., et al: Brain metastases Curr Probl Surg 2004;41:665-741

Sharma HS and Hoopes PJ: Hyperthermia induced pathophysiology of the central nervous system. Int. J Hyperthermia. 2003;19:325-354.

Shoshan Y.,Wygoda M and Umansky F.: Stereotactic radiosurgery and fractionated stereotactic radiotherapy: background, definition, applications. IMAJ 2005;7: 597-599.

Siegal T, Horowitz A, Gabizon A: Doxorubicin encapsulated in sterically stabilized liposomes for the treatment of a brain tumor model: biodistribution and Therapeutic efficacy. J Neurosurg. 1995; 83: 1029-1037.

Sminia P, Van Der Zee J, Wondergem J et al: Effect of hyperthermia on central nervous system: a review. Int. J. Hyperthermia 1994;10: 1-30.

Sneed PK and Stea B: Thermoradiotherapy for brain tumors. Appeared in "Thermoradiotherapy and Thermochemotherapy" MH Seegenschmiedt , P. Fessenden and C.C. Vernon editors. Springer Verlag, Berlin, Heidelberg,New York 1995; pp 159-175.

Sneed P.K., Suh J.H., Goetch S.J, et al: a multi-institutional review of radiosurgery alone vs. Radiosurgery with whole brain radiotherapy as the initial management of brain metastases. Int J Radiat. Oncol. Biol. Phys. 2002,53.519-526.

Sperduto P.W.: A review of stereotactic radiosurgery in the management of brain metastases. Technology in Cancer Research treatment 2003;2: 105-109Weil R.J, Palmieri D.C., Bronder J.L.et al: Breast cancer metastasis to the central nervous system. Am J Pathol 2005,16: 913-920.

St. Clair W.H:, Given C.A.: Stereotactic Radiosurgery associated neurotoxicity. Technology in Cancer Research treatment 2003;2: 147-151.

Schwartz L, Abolhassani M, Guais A, Sanders E, Steyaert JM, Campion F, Israël M.: A combination of alpha lipoic acid and calcium hydroxycitrate is efficient against mouse cancer models: preliminary results. Oncol Rep. 2010 May;23(5):1407-16.

Shaffrey ME, Mut M, Asher AL, Burri SH, Chahlavi A, et al: Brain metastases. Curr. Probl. Surgery.2004;4:665-741.

Tajran D, Berek J.S.: Surgical resection of solitary brain metastasis from cervical cancer Int J Gynecol cancer. 2003;13:368-370.

Tikhtman AJ, Patchell RA: Brain metastases. In: Morantz RA, Walsh JW, editors. Brain tumors: Marcel Dekker, Inc 1995;553-556.

Tom MI: Metastatic tumors of the brain. Can Med Assoc J. 1946;54.265-268.

Tong-xin Xie, feng-ju H., Aldape K.D:, et al: Activation of Stat3 in human melanoma promotes brain metastases. Cancer Res 2006; 66: 3188- 3196

Tosoni A, Ermani M, Brandes A.A:. The pathogenesis and treatment of brain metastases: a comphrensive review. Critical reviews in Oncology /Hematology. 2004; 52:199-215.

Urie MM, Lo YC, Litofsky S, FitzGerald TJ. Miniature multileaf collimator as an alternative to traditional circular collimators for stereotactic radiosurgery and stereotactic radiotherapy. Stereotact Funct Neurosurg. 2001;76(1):47-62.

Valk P..E. and Dillon W.P.: Radiation injury of the brain. AJR 1991,156: 689-706.

Vecht C.J., Haaxma-Reich H, Noordjik E. et al: Treatment of single brain metastases: radiotherapy alone or combined with neurosurgery. Ann Neurol 1993; 33: 583-590.

Vijayalaxmi, Reiter R.J., Dun-Xian T.; et al: Melatonin as a radioprotective agent: a review. Int. J. Radiation oncology Biol. Phys. 2004, 59: 639-653.

Warburg O.: On the origin of cancer cells. Science. 1956 Feb 24;123(3191):309-14.

Wong CS, Van der Kogel AJ.: Mechanisms of radiation injury to the central nervous system: implications for neuroprotection. Mol Interv. 2004 Oct;4(5):273-284.

Wouters A, Pauwels B, Lardon F, et al: Review: Implications of In Vitro Research on the Effect of Radiotherapy and Chemotherapy Under Hypoxic Conditions The Oncologist 2007; 12: 690-7129

Wronski M,Arbit E, Burt M, et al: Survival after surgical treatment of brain metastases from lung cancer: a follow-up study of 231 patients treated between 1976 and 1991. J Neurosurg 1995;83: 605-616.

Yano S, Shinoara H, Herbst RS et al: Expression of vascular endothelial growth factor is necessary but not sufficient for production and growth of brain metastasis. Cancer Res 2000; 60.4959-4967.

Zimm S, Wampler GL, Stablein D, et al: Intracerebral metastases in solid tumor patients, natural history and result of treatment. Cancer. 1981; 48:384-394.

Zhong H, De Marzo AM, Laughner E, Lim M, Hilton DA, Zagzag D, Buechler P,Isaacs WB, Semenza GL, Simons JW. Overexpression of hypoxia-inducible factor 1alpha in common human cancers and their metastases. Cancer Res. 1999 Nov 15;59(22):5830-5.

# Part 2

# Cancer Signaling, Mechanisms and Targeted Therapy

9

# Survivin: Identification of Selective Functional Signaling Pathways in Transformed Cells and Identification of a New Splice Variant with Growth Survival Activity

Louis M. Pelus[1] and Seiji Fukuda[2]
[1]*Department of Microbiology and Immunology*
*Indiana University School of Medicine, Indianapolis, IN*
[2]*Department of Pediatrics, Shimane University School of Medicine, Shimane*
[1]*USA*
[2]*Japan*

## 1. Introduction

Survivin is a member of the inhibitors of apoptosis (IAP) family of highly conserved proteins implicated in regulation of mitosis, cytokinesis, cell cycle and apoptosis (Altieri, 2003a; Altieri, 2003b; Fukuda & Pelus, 2006). It is expressed during development but down regulated in most adult tissues. However, Survivin is over-expressed in the majority of solid tumors and leukemias, and is usually associated with higher proliferative index, reduced apoptosis, resistance to chemotherapy and increased rate of tumor recurrence, making it an attractive therapeutic target. We have previously shown that Survivin is expressed and growth factor regulated in normal hematopoietic cells and regulates apoptosis and cell cycle entry (Fukuda et al., 2002; Fukuda et al., 2004; Fukuda & Pelus, 2001; Fukuda & Pelus, 2002). Antagonizing Survivin impairs mouse progenitor cell production in vitro (Fukuda et al., 2002; Fukuda et al., 2004) and loss of function upon conditional deletion in vivo leads to bone marrow ablation as a consequence of loss of stem cell function (Leung et al., 2007). While Survivin is tightly regulated in normal hematopoietic cells, deregulated expression is frequently observed in hematologic diseases particularly those characterized by stem cell expansion. Survivin is aberrantly over expressed in acute myeloid leukemia (Adida et al., 2000; Carter et al., 2001) but down regulated in aplastic anemia where hematopoietic stem and progenitor cells are reduced (Badran et al., 2003). It is now clear that Survivin can regulate cell growth under both physiological and pathological conditions. Therefore, identification of differential signaling cascades between normal and abnormal cells downstream of Survivin is required in order to identify cancer cell specific targets without toxicity to normal cells.

## 2. Survivin mediates aberrant proliferation of hematopoietic progenitor cells transformed by ITD-Flt3

Internal tandem duplication (ITD) mutations of the Flt3 tyrosine kinase receptor are found in many patients with acute leukemia, and are an unfavorable prognostic factor (Fukuda et al.,

2009; Gilliland & Griffin, 2002; Levis et al., 2005). We reported that the combination of Flt3 ligand (FL), stem cell factor (SCF) and thrombopoietin (TPO) induces Survivin expression in human CD34+ cells (Fukuda & Pelus, 2001), suggesting that Survivin lies downstream of Flt3 signaling. We therefore evaluated the effects of constitutive ITD-Flt3 signaling on Survivin expression. Survivin is up regulated by ITD-Flt3 in whole cells, as well as cells in $G_0/G_1$ phase of the cell cycle (Figure 1) as determined by intracellular flow cytometric analyses. This suggests that up regulation of Survivin is not a consequence of cell cycle progression. Similarly, Survivin mRNA was up regulated in Ba/F3 cells by ITD-Flt3 compared to wild-type Flt3 following IL3 withdrawal. Up regulation of Survivin by ITD-Flt3 was associated with growth factor independent proliferation of Ba/F3 cells (Fukuda et al., 2009). We next evaluated whether Survivin plays a role in aberrant growth factor-independent primary HPC proliferation upon transformation by ITD-Flt3. Over expression of human wild-type Flt3 in CFU-GM from control Survivin $^{fx/fx}$ or Survivin $^{fx/fx}$ mice harboring a tamoxifen-inducible Cre recombinase (Cre-ER$^{TM}$) failed to proliferate in vitro, whereas ectopic expression of ITD-Flt3 resulted in significant growth of CFU-GM in the absence of added growth factors. Treatment with 4OH-Tamoxifen to delete Survivin resulted in a significant reduction in the growth factor-independent proliferation of CFU-GM induced by ITD-Flt3 (Figure 2). Identical results were observed in the immunophenotypically defined c-kit$^+$, Sca-1$^+$, Lineage $^{negative}$ (KSL) population of cells enriched for mouse stem and progenitor cells. These findings suggest that Survivin is involved in the growth factor-independent proliferation of HPC induced by ITD-Flt3 and that antagonizing Survivin may be therapeutically beneficial for acute myeloid leukemia (AML) expressing ITD-Flt3.

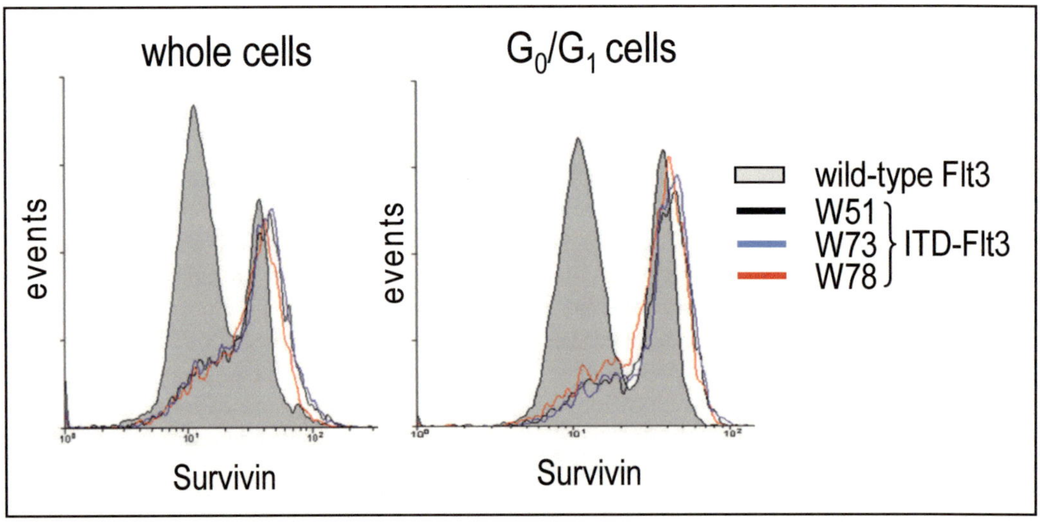


Fig. 1. BaF3 cells expressing wild-type Flt3 or ITD-Flt3 were fixed and stained for Survivin and DNA in whole cells (left) and cells with 2N DNA representing $G_0/G_1$ cells (right).

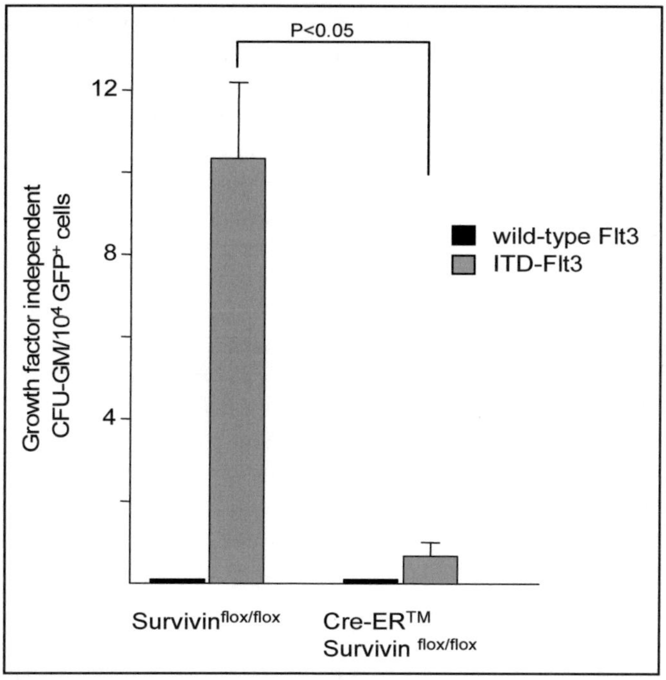


Fig. 2. Wild type Flt3 or ITD-Flt3 were retrovirally transduced into marrow cells from Cre ER Survivin $^{fx/fx}$ or control Survivin $^{fx/fx}$ mice. Following transduction, cells were plated in a CFU assay in agar with 30% FBS and 1uM 4OH tamoxifen in the absence of hematopoietic growth factors for 2 weeks. Treatment with 4OH-TM significantly reduced growth factor independent CFU-GM induced by ITD-Flt3 in Cre-ERTM Survivin $^{fx/fx}$ marrow cells.

## 3. Survivin regulated genes

While it is clear that antagonizing Survivin may reduce the aberrant proliferation of hematopoietic progenitor cells transformed by ITD-Flt3 and that ITD-Flt3 mutations are present in human leukemic stem cells (LSC) (Levis et al., 2005) , studies from our group and others indicate that Survivin is a normal regulator of hematopoietic stem and progenitor cells (HSPC) (Fukuda et al., 2002; Fukuda et al., 2004; Leung et al., 2007). This suggests that Survivin targeted therapies will likely result in hematopoietic toxicity. Therefore, identification of differential signaling cascades downstream of Survivin between normal HSPC and cancer stem cells (CSC) or LSC are required to pinpoint targets that can effectively eradicate CSC/LSC with acceptable toxicity to normal HSPC. In order to identify Survivin regulated genes associated with ITD-Flt3 signaling but not normal Flt3 signaling, we evaluated human ITD-Flt3 transformed KSL cells from conditional Survivin knockout mice as a model of normal and leukemic stem cells. We identified 1096 transcripts differentially regulated by Survivin in ITD-Flt3 transformed stem cells [Tables of Survivin regulated genes can be found in (Fukuda et al., 2011)]. Classification of these genes based upon biological process and molecular function defined by Gene Ontology Term using David 2008 showed significant regulation of biological processes, notably phosphate metabolic processes, cell cycle, cell division response to DNA stimulus, RNA biosynthetic processes and transcription. When evaluated based upon molecular function, iron binding, nucleotide binding, DNA binding and protein kinase activity were the functions most significantly affected by Survivin deletion. Although Survivin is known to inhibit caspases 3, 7 and 10 that mediate apoptosis (Altieri, 2003a; Altieri, 2003b; Fukuda & Pelus, 2006), we did not observe significant changes in genes that mediate apoptosis, suggesting that Survivin can regulate ITD-Flt3 transformed KSL cell fate independent of its ability to inhibit caspase activity. However, microarray analysis was performed on lineage marker negative viable cells that express GFP and stem cell markers and survived in culture, perhaps explaining lack of effects on genes involved in apoptotic pathways. The finding that Survivin deletion affected transcription was surprising since there is no direct evidence that Survivin regulates gene transcription. However, this is consistent with the fact that the *Caenorhabditis elegans* Bir1 Survivin homologue regulates transcription, most likely through effects on histone phosphorylation by Aurora kinase (Kostrouchova et al., 2003). Survivin is essential for activation of Aurora kinase that phosphorylates histone H3 (Bolton et al., 2002; Chen et al., 2003), an event required for transcriptional regulation (Cheung et al., 2000; Li et al., 2002; Nowak & Corces, 2000) and cytokinesis (Wei et al., 1999). Furthermore, modulation of Survivin affects transcription in cancer cells (Asanuma et al., 2004; Balkhi et al., 2008; Takizawa et al., 2007) and transgenic Survivin expression alters gene expression in bladder cells (Salz et al., 2005). Overexpression of Survivin also leads to phosphorylation of the Sp1 transcription factor (Asanuma et al., 2004).

## 4. Survivin modulates expression of genes deregulated in human AML LSC

The facts that Survivin is required for the self-renewal of ITD-Flt3 transformed KSL cells and ITD-Flt3 is present in leukemic stem cells (LSC) suggests that Survivin is important for LSC fate decisions. When the 1,096 differentially expressed genes in Survivin deleted ITD-Flt3$^+$ KSL cells was compared with the deregulated gene expression database for human AML stem cells (Majeti et al., 2009), 137 genes were identified in common. Survivin deletion resulted in down-regulation of 79 genes, while 58 genes were up-regulated, implying that these genes are conversely increased and decreased by the presence of Survivin. In contrast, 92 genes were upregulated and 45 genes were downregulated in LSC. Among the 79 genes downregulated by Survivin deletion, 55 were upregulated while 24 genes were downregulated in LSC. Among the 58 transcripts upregulated by Survivin deletion, 21 were downregulated and 37 upregulated in LSC.

Classification of these genes into functional annotation groups using DAVID program identified significantly ($p<0.05$) enriched functional groups annotated as phosphoprotein, nucleus, acetylation, cell cycle, ATP binding, regulation of EGF signaling pathway, and cell adhesion, with a number of genes showing shared function, suggesting enrichment of gene groups with redundant function. Among the molecules most frequently shared within the functional groups included BGLAP [bone gamma carboxyglutamate protein 1($\Delta$ -10.7)], Chrac1 [chromatin accessibility complex 1 ($\Delta$ -4.3), Hmgb1 [high mobility group box 1 ($\Delta$ -3.4)] and Smarce1 [SWI $\Delta$ -2.9)]. Phosphoprotein, acetylation, DNA binding, ATP binding and DNA replication were significantly enriched when the 76 genes upregulated or downregulated both by Survivin deletion and LSC were classified (Figure 3).

Comparison of the 1,096 differentially Survivin-regulated genes against the mouse HSC database (Ivanova et al., 2002) identified 94 differentially expressed genes. This included 45 genes regulated by Survivin in ITD-Flt3+ HSC whose expression was selectively enriched in HSC compared to other populations. Notably, Crem, Emp1, Hmga2, Lrrn1, Maff, Myef2,

Rps4x and Sos1 are known to be deregulated in LSC. Comparison of the human LSC associated 137 genes regulated by Survivin in ITD-Flt3+KSL cells with differentially regulated genes in normal CD34neg KSL cells from control and Survivin deleted mice indicated that coincident with reduction of Survivin expression (10-fold in CD34neg KSL cells from CreER™-Survivin fx/fx mice compared to control Survivin fx/fx in two independent experiments) out of 137 genes, Arg2, Med25, Pmaip1, Pola2, Ube3b, Ephb2 and Rab18 were differentially regulated in both ITD-Flt3+ KSL cells and normal CD34neg KLS cells. In contrast, Cenpa, Cpd, Myef2, Nmt2, Taf1b and Tmpo were down regulated in ITD-Flt3+ KSL cells while they were upregulated in normal CD34neg KSL cells. These findings suggest that 124 genes are regulated by Survivin exclusively in ITD-Flt3+ KSL cells but not in normal CD34neg KSL cells (The complete list of the genes regulated by Survivin in CD34neg KSL cells will be reported elsewhere). However, these data clearly indicate that Survivin contributes to deregulation of gene expression in AML stem cells via effects on selective signaling pathways that are distinct from normal HSC that can be potentially targeted for more selective anti-Survivin anti-cancer therapies.

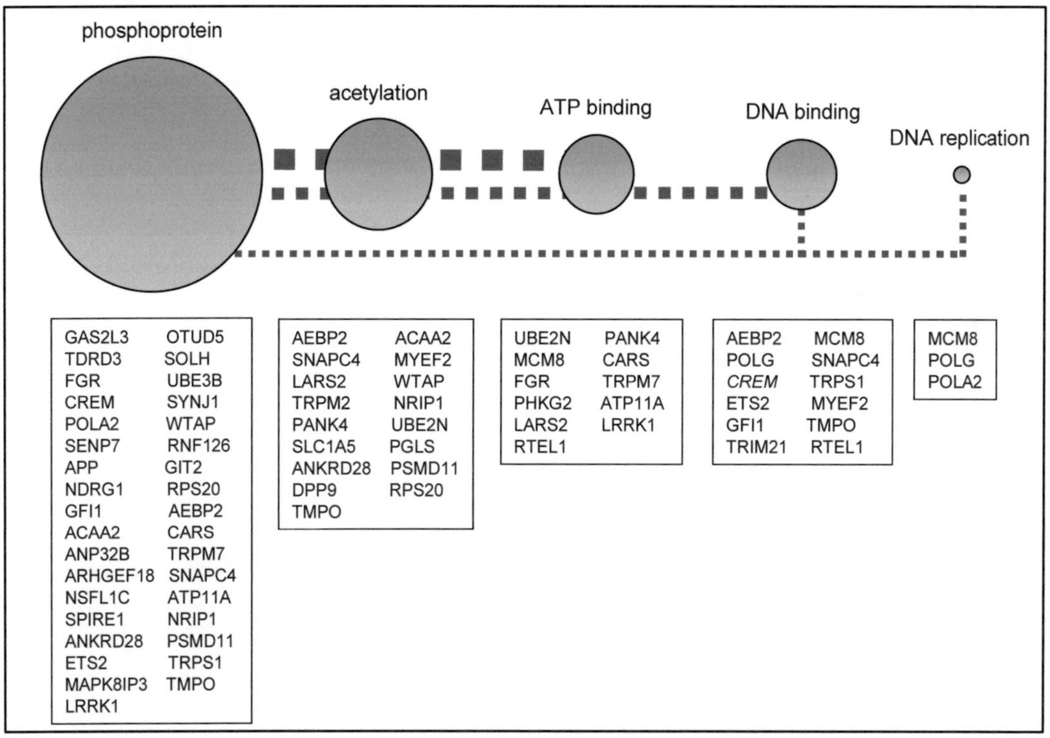


Fig. 3. Genes regulated in common by Survivin and LSC. The 76 genes up-regulated or down regulated by Survivin and LSC were functionally classified by DAVID software. The size of each circle represents the number of genes involved in each functional categories and the thickness of the line indicates the number of genes shared with any function. Functional classification was performed based on Swissprot Keywords. Genes annotated in each functional category are shown in the text box.

## 5. Survivin modulates gene expression in LSC that connects through an EGFR signaling pathway

Functional annotation analysis indicates that genes related with dorso-ventral axis formation or epidermal growth factor receptor signaling pathway (EGFR) are significantly enriched in the shared genes associated with LSC and Survivin signaling in the KEGG database (http://www.genome.jp/kegg/) (P<0.03). Similarly, genes associated with regulation of EGFR signaling pathway are enriched in the Gene Ontology database (P<0.02). Our analysis shows that molecules shared by LSC and Survivin signaling are mapped on a functional signaling network that connects through the EGFR pathway (Figure 4). EGFR signaling

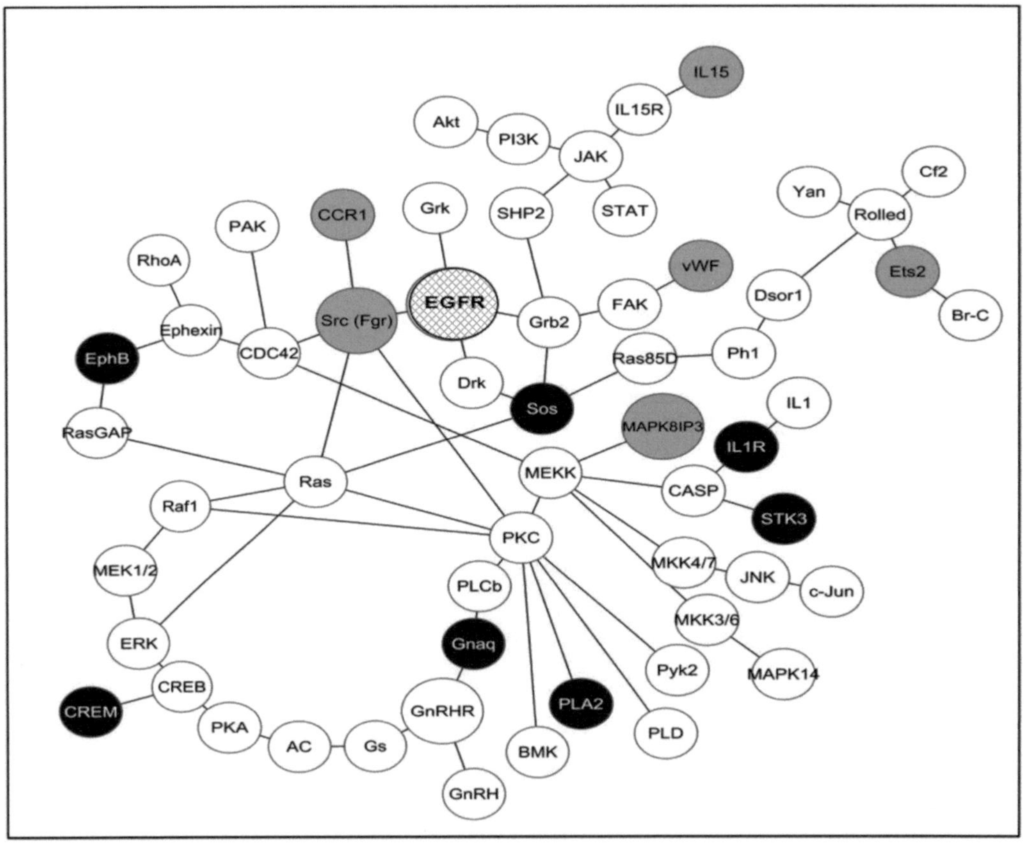


Fig. 4. Genes regulated by Survivin in ITD-Flt3+ KSL cells and deregulated in LSC are mapped on a functional signaling network associated with the epidermal growth factor receptor signaling pathway. Epidermal growth factor receptor signaling pathway (EGFR) is significantly enriched in the shared genes associated with LSC and Survivin signaling by pathway enrichment analysis in KEGG and Gene Ontology databases. Our analysis shows that 13 molecules shared by LSC and Survivin signaling are mapped on a functional signaling network associated with EGFR. The network was created based on the KEGG database using Cytoscape software. Gray and black circle represents down regulation and up regulation by Survivin gene deletion, respectively. The hatched circle shows EGFR.

activates signaling cascades involved in cell proliferation, such as Src, Sos and MAP-kinases and is known to be dysregulated in a number of solid tumors (Alvarez et al., 2010; Harris & McCormick, 2010). These findings suggest a potential role of EGFR signaling downstream of Survivin in AML stem cells, despite the fact that EGFR is not usually up regulated in AML cells (Hahn et al., 2009). However, recent studies indicate an anti-neoplastic effect of an EGFR inhibitor in AML via off-target effects (Boehrer et al., 2008; Hahn et al., 2009). Thus, our data would support EGFR signaling as a candidate pathway for treatment of patients with AML, even though the number of molecules detected that associates with EGFR signaling is small.

## 6. Survivin splice variants

Survivin, like many genes, is alternatively spliced and variants having both similar or opposite activities have been identified, some of which are of prognostic significance (Fukuda & Pelus, 2006; Sampath & Pelus, 2007) . Spliced variants identified to date include Survivin 2α (Caldas et al., 2005; Mahotka et al., 2002) , 2B, ΔEx3 (Ling et al., 2005; Mahotka et al., 1999; Mahotka et al., 2002; Song & Wu, 2005) and 3B (Badran et al., 2004), and some of these variants have been evaluated for their anti- or pro-apoptotic function and ability to interact with wild-type Survivin and other chromosomal passenger proteins (CPC) in some model systems. More recently, several new Survivin splice variants were found in the expressed sequence tag (est) database or described based on RT-PCR using RNA from Molt-4 cells (Li & Ling, 2006; Mola et al., 2007), however the biological functions of these new variants are not known. Overall, with most all the variants reported to date, there is still a considerable lack of understanding of their biology and their function and prognostic value is only now being realized (Sampath & Pelus, 2007). In order to better understand the biology of human Survivin splice variants, we cloned each variant and evaluated their antiapoptotic functions. In the process, we identified a new splice variant we termed Survivin 3γ that is similar to Survivin 3B (Figure 5). To determine if this was truly a novel variant, a forward primer specific for all splice variants and a splice variant specific reverse primer were designed and used to amplify cDNA using a polydT reverse transcribed cDNA library from HL60, K562 and Mo7e-Bcr-abl cells, the products resolved on an agarose gel and ~400bp bands excised, cloned and sequenced. Sequence analysis confirmed the presence of the novel splice variant. Survivin 3γ contains 12 new amino acids at the C-terminus compared to wild-type Survivin and differs from all of the previously reported Survivin splice variants. Secondary structure prediction using Jpred suggests that Survivin 3γ is structurally similar to wild-type Survivin, with the new amino acids predicted to be capable of forming a C-terminal helix that could potentially form the coiled coil domain, even though the length of this helix would be smaller than wild-type Survivin.

## 7. Expression of Survivin 3γ

Survivin 3γ expression in primary cancer tissues was determined by quantitative RT-PCR on primary breast and prostate tumor samples obtained in an array format. In contrast to most cancers where wild-type Survivin is the predominant transcript, Survivin 3γ was expressed at higher levels in benign prostate tissue and at equivalent levels in breast cancer cells. In primary breast cancer samples a statistically significant increase in wild-type Survivin expression at stages 1, 2 and 3 compared to control normal breast tissue was observed, with no significant difference observed between wild-type Survivin expression at stage 1 compared to later stages. In 7 normal breast tissue samples wild-type Survivin and Survivin 3γ were expressed at the same level. However, in contrast to expression of wild-type Survivin, Survivin 3γ expression remained relatively constant at all stages of disease, resulting in statistically significant ($p<0.005$) lower relative expression to wild-type Survivin.

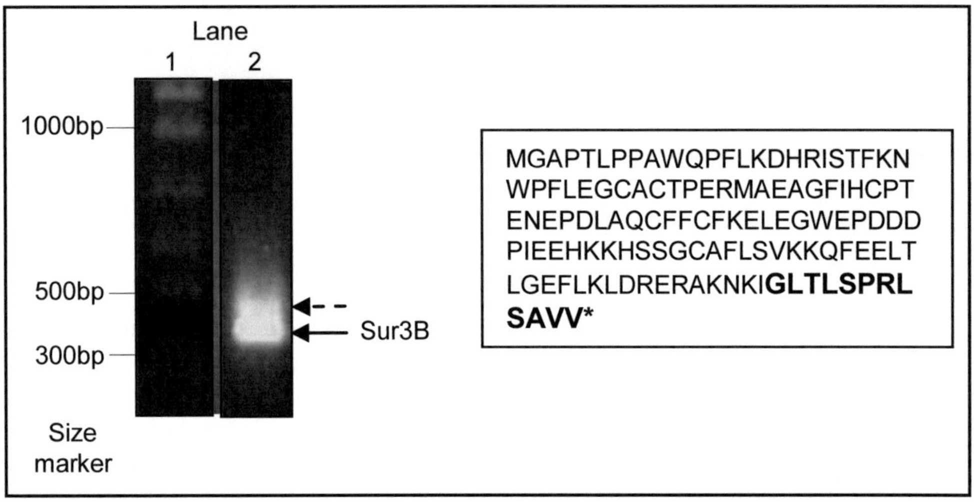


Fig. 5. Agarose gel electrophoresis of cDNA amplified from HL60 cells (lane 2). The Survivin-3B variant is indicated by a solid arrow, the dotted arrow points to the slower migrating band. Amino acid sequence of Survivin-3γ is shown on the right. Bold letters indicate novel sequence distinct from wild-type Survivin. The stop codon is indicated by the *.

In 48 prostate cancers at different stages of the disease, wild-type Survivin expression was higher in stage 1 prostate cancer compared to benign hyperplasia; however sample size was too small to evaluate statistical significance. No clear over-expression of wild-type Survivin was seen at higher stages, except for a single stage 4 sample. The expression of Survivin 3γ was higher than wild-type Survivin in benign hyperplasia tissue and comparison of the relative expression of wild-type Survivin and Survivin 3γ at each stage of prostate cancer indicated that Survivin 3γ transcripts remained higher than wild-type Survivin at all stages except stage 1. To our knowledge, the higher expression of Survivin 3γ in benign prostate hyperplasia is the first demonstration of a Survivin splice variant expressed at higher levels than wild-type Survivin and suggest that it may play a role in normal cell function.

The finding that Survivin 3γ expression was higher than wild-type Survivin in benign prostate hyperplasia (BPH) samples and did not change with stage of disease is consistent with one study (Kaur et al., 2004) where Survivin expression was detected by immunohistochemistry. However, other reports show increased Survivin with stage of disease either at the RNA level by standard RT-PCR and gel electrophoresis (Kishi et al., 2004; Krajewska et al., 2003) or by immunohistochemistry (Krajewska et al., 2003). The difference between our study and those reported using standard RT-PCR could be due to differences in sensitivity of the method used. SYBR green quantitative RT-PCR is more sensitive and efficient in amplifying smaller amplicons than conventional RT-PCR. We also show that expression of wild-type Survivin and Survivin 3γ were comparable in normal breast tissues and that the expression of Survivin increased at stage 1 and remained high at all stages, whereas a recent report (Sohn et al., 2006) showed Survivin expression increased gradually at all disease stages. This difference could again be due to different methodologies and sensitivity between RNA analyses versus immunohistochemistry. Since the Survivin 3γ splice variant was identified in the human HL-60 promyelocytic cell line, we evaluated its expression in other hematopoietic cells by quantitative RT-PCR using SYBR Green. While wild-type Survivin was the predominant transcript identified in all cell lines tested, Survivin 3γ transcripts represented ~0.7-6% of the total Survivin transcripts detected. The absolute expression of Survivin 3γ was lowest in growth factor dependant cells and highest in growth factor independent cells. Analysis of Survivin 3γ in primary umbilical cord blood (UCB) $CD34^+$ cells that are enriched for hematopoietic stem and progenitor cells showed that Survivin 3γ was expressed at significantly higher levels than wild-type Survivin. This is in contrast to most splice variants that are expressed at lower levels than wild-type Survivin in these cells. However, growth factor stimulation induced a dramatic increase in expression of wild-type Survivin after 48 hours consistent with our previous findings (Fukuda et al., 2002; Fukuda & Pelus, 2001; Fukuda & Pelus, 2002), whereas the expression of Survivin 3γ increased only slightly, therefore relative levels compared to wild-type Survivin decreased by ~2-fold. This suggests perhaps that Survivin 3γ may play a role in hematopoietic stem cell maintenance.

## 8. Survivin 3γ demonstrates antiapoptotic activity

To evaluate the function of the novel Survivin 3γ splice variants, we stably expressed human (Hu) wild-type Survivin with or without an N-terminal Flag-tag or Survivin 3γ with an N-terminal HA-tag in murine YAC-1 lymphoma cells. Wild-type HuSurvivin, wild-type Flag-HuSurvivin and HA-Survivin 3γ were all expressed, although their levels of expression varied, with wild-type HuSurvivin expressing at 31-fold, whereas wild-type Flag-HuSurvivin and HA-Survivin 3γ were expressed at 76- and 63-fold higher levels, respectively than the empty vector control cells at the RNA level. Western blot analysis using a rabbit anti-Survivin polyclonal antibody that recognizes both the human and the murine Survivin showed background levels of murine Survivin as well as the presence of each of the transduced Survivins, indicating that each of the splice variants was translated. Analysis of band intensity indicated that wild-type HuSurvivin was expressed at the highest level followed by wild-type Flag-HuSurvivin with HA-Survivin 3γ expressed at a lower level. The same pattern of expression was observed with a mouse anti-Survivin monoclonal antibody that recognizes predominantly human Survivin.

As a measure of anti-apoptotic function we evaluated resistance of YAC-1 cells transduced with wild-type Survivin, wild-type Flag-Survivin and HA-Survivin 3γ to the chemotherapeutic drugs Etoposide and Taxol at their optimal therapeutic dose. Treatment of cells with Taxol showed that, as expected, over expression of either wild-type Survivin or wild-type Flag-Survivin provided 2.7- and 2.8-fold resistance to Taxol-induced cell death, respectively, compared to YAC-1 cells transduced with vector control (Figure 6). Ectopic expression of HA-Survivin 3γ provided 2.6-fold resistance. In multiple experiments, the $IC_{50's}$ for wild-type HuSurvivin, wild-type Flag-HuSurvivin and HA-Survivin 3γ were significantly higher than control (2.85 ± 0.32; $P<0.05$). YAC-1 cells expressing wild-type

Survivin also showed significant resistance to Etoposide. Wild-type Flag-Survivin and HA-Survivin 3γ conferred resistance to Etoposide in YAC-1 cells to a similar degree as wild-type Survivin. These studies suggest that expression of Survivin 3γ could potentially contribute to drug resistance. Expression levels of murine wild-type Survivin and the only known murine Survivin splice variant, Survivin-121 (Conway et al., 2000) were unchanged (not shown), indicating that changes in endogenous murine Survivin levels were not involved in the increase in resistance to chemotherapeutic compounds. These findings suggest that wild-type and Survivin 3γ proteins possess equivalent anti-apoptotic function. Since crystal structure of wild-type Survivin indicates that the C-terminal helix could be involved in protein-protein interaction (Chantalat et al., 2000) and required for interaction with the chromosomal passenger protein, INCEP (Wheatley et al., 2004), whereas the N-terminus of wild-type Survivin was unordered (Chantalat et al., 2000), we hypothesized that addition of a C-terminal tag would hinder protein-protein interactions, therefore we engineered N-terminal tags into all the Survivin cDNAs. The presence of HA-tag at the N-terminus of the Survivin coding region did not affect activity since they were equivalent to N-terminal Flag-tagged wild-type Survivin, which itself behaved similar to wild-type Survivin at least for drug sensitivity. The facts that Survivin 3γ confers drug resistance/anti-apoptotic function to two different classes of chemotherapeutic drugs Taxol, a microtubule destabilizing agent, and Etoposide, a topoisomerase II inhibitor, as well as growth factor independence similar to wild-type Survivin, and that it may be preferentially associated with maintenance of stem cell quiescence, makes it an interesting potential therapeutic target .

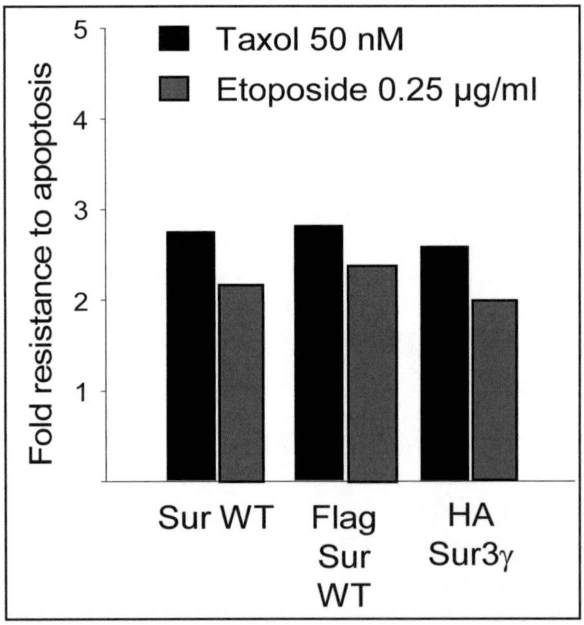


Fig. 6. Response of YAC1 cells over expressing wild-type human Survivin (SurWT), wild-type human Flag-Survivin (Flag-Sur WT) and HA Survivin 3γ (HA-Sur3γ) to chemotherapeutic drugs. Fold resistance of stable transduced YAC-1 cells treated with 50 nM Taxol or 0.25 µg/ml Etoposide.

## 9. Summary

We have shown that ITD-Flt3 mutations increase expression of Survivin, which regulates development of ITD-Flt3+ acute leukemia, clearly indicating a potential therapeutic benefit for antagonizing Survivin in patients with ITD-Flt3+ AML (Fukuda et al., 2009; Fukuda et al., 2011; Sampath & Pelus, 2007). However, we have shown that Survivin also regulates normal HSPC function (Fukuda et al., 2004; Fukuda & Pelus, 2002; Leung et al., 2007; Sampath & Pelus, 2007); raising caution that targeting Survivin can have hematopoietic toxicity. Therefore, identification of differential signaling cascades downstream of Survivin between normal hematopoietic cells versus cancer and leukemia stem cells is required to pinpoint targets that can lead to effective anti-malignant therapies with acceptable normal stem cell toxicity. Our genetic profiling using normal and ITD-Flt3 transformed cells from conditional Survivin knockout mice has identified a panel of genes that are specifically regulated by Survivin in ITD-Flt3 transformed cells and known to be deregulated in human LSC that can be potentially targeted for selective anti-leukemia therapy.

Inherited and acquired changes in pre-mRNA splicing have been documented to play a significant role in human disease development and loss of fidelity or variation of the splicing process may play a major role in carcinogenesis (Fackenthal & Godley, 2008; Matlin et al., 2005; Skotheim & Nees, 2007) . Splice variants that are found predominantly in tumors have clear diagnostic value (Brinkman, 2004; Caballero et al., 2001) and may provide potential drug targets. Splice variants of Survivin have been reported but their prognostic value is not clear, partially based upon detection methods that are not sufficiently specific (Sampath & Pelus, 2007), or due to lack of information on biological function. We have identified a novel Survivin splice variant with anti-apoptotic activity similar to wild-type Survivin, at least with respect to sensitivity to chemotherapeutic drugs. We characterized its expression in several transformed cell lines, and similar to other Survivin splice variants, wild-type Survivin is the predominant transcript. However, in contrast to wild-type Survivin, Survivin 3γ expression does not change with increasing stage/severity of primary prostate and breast cancers. In addition, unlike other Survivin splice variants, Survivin 3γ is expressed at higher levels than wild-type Survivin in primary HSPC, and their lack of increase with cell proliferation suggests that they may play a role in stem cell maintenance. Since Survivin 3γ was cloned from and found to be highly expressed in hematopoietic cells, it will be particularly interesting to evaluate its expression in hematopoietic malignancies and their correlation with disease/stage/survival. Furthermore, since ITD-Flt3 mutations increase Survivin expression, it will be interesting to determine if they also modulate Survivin 3γ expression and how this relates to disease progression and prognostic value. Given the specific genes regulated by Survivin in leukemic stem cells, it will also be of interest whether Survivin 3γ elicits overlapping or divergent gene products that can be utilized for development of anti-leukemia therapies.

## 10. References

Adida, C. et.al (2000). Expression and prognostic significance of survivin in de novo acute myeloid leukaemia. *Br J Haematol*, Vol.111:196-203.

Altieri, D.C. (2003a). Survivin, versatile modulation of cell division and apoptosis in cancer. *Oncogene*, Vol.22:8581-8589.

Altieri, D.C. (2003b). Validating survivin as a cancer therapeutic target. *Nat Rev Cancer*, Vol.3:46-54.

Alvarez, R.H.; Valero, V. & Hortobagyi, G.N. (2010). Emerging targeted therapies for breast cancer. *J Clin Oncol*, Vol.28:3366-3379.

Asanuma, K. et.al (2004). Survivin enhances Fas ligand expression via up-regulation of specificity protein 1-mediated gene transcription in colon cancer cells. *J Immunol*, Vol.172:3922-3929.

Badran, A. et.al (2004). Identification of a novel splice variant of the human anti-apoptopsis gene survivin. *Biochem Biophys Res Commun*, Vol.314:902-907.

Badran, A. et.al (2003). Expression of the anti-apoptotic gene survivin in myelodysplastic syndrome. *Int J Oncol*, Vol.22:59-64.

Balkhi, M.Y. et.al (2008). AML1/ETO-induced survivin expression inhibits transcriptional regulation of myeloid differentiation. *Exp Hematol*, Vol.36:1449-1460.

Boehrer, S. et.al (2008). Erlotinib exhibits antineoplastic off-target effects in AML and MDS: a preclinical study. *Blood*, Vol.111:2170-2180.

Bolton, M.A. et.al (2002). Aurora B kinase exists in a complex with survivin and INCENP and its kinase activity is stimulated by survivin binding and phosphorylation. *Mol Biol Cell*, Vol.13:3064-3077.

Brinkman, B.M. (2004). Splice variants as cancer biomarkers. *Clin Biochem*, Vol.37:584-594.

Caballero, O.L. et.al (2001). Alternative spliced transcripts as cancer markers. *Dis Markers*, Vol.17:67-75.

Caldas, H.; Honsey, L.E. & Altura, R.A. (2005). Survivin 2alpha: a novel Survivin splice variant expressed in human malignancies. *Mol Cancer*, Vol.4:11-

Carter, B.Z. et.al (2001). Cytokine-regulated expression of survivin in myeloid leukemia. *Blood*, Vol.97:2784-2790.

Chantalat, L. et.al (2000). Crystal structure of human survivin reveals a bow tie-shaped dimer with two unusual alpha-helical extensions. *Mol Cell*, Vol.6:183-189.

Chen, J. et.al (2003). Survivin enhances Aurora-B kinase activity and localizes Aurora-B in human cells. *J Biol Chem*, Vol.278:486-490.

Cheung, P. et.al (2000). Synergistic coupling of histone H3 phosphorylation and acetylation in response to epidermal growth factor stimulation. *Mol Cell*, Vol.5:905-915.

Conway, E.M. et.al (2000). Three differentially expressed survivin cDNA variants encode proteins with distinct antiapoptotic functions. *Blood*, Vol.95:1435-1442.

Fackenthal, J.D. Godley, L.A. (2008). Aberrant RNA splicing and its functional consequences in cancer cells. *Dis Model Mech*, Vol.1:37-42.

Fukuda, S. et.al (2011). Survivin selectively modulates genes deregulated in human leukemia stem cells. *J Oncol*, Vol.2011:doi:10.1155/2011/94936-

Fukuda, S. et.al (2002). The antiapoptosis protein survivin is associated with cell cycle entry of normal cord blood CD34(+) cells and modulates cell cycle and proliferation of mouse hematopoietic progenitor cells. *Blood*, Vol.100:2463-2471.

Fukuda, S.; Mantel, C.R. & Pelus, L.M. (2004). Survivin regulates hematopoietic progenitor cell proliferation through p21WAF1/Cip1-dependent and -independent pathways. *Blood*, Vol.103:120-127.

Fukuda, S. Pelus, L.M. (2001). Regulation of the inhibitor-of-apoptosis family member survivin in normal cord blood and bone marrow CD34(+) cells by hematopoietic growth factors: implication of survivin expression in normal hematopoiesis. *Blood*, Vol.98:2091-2100.

Fukuda, S. Pelus, L.M. (2002). Elevation of Survivin levels by hematopoietic growth factors occurs in quiescent CD34+ hematopoietic stem and progenitor cells before cell cycle entry. *Cell Cycle*, Vol.1:322-326.

Fukuda, S. Pelus, L.M. (2006). Survivin, a cancer target with an emerging role in normal adult tissues. *Mol Cancer Ther*, Vol.5:1087-1098.

Fukuda, S. et.al (2009). Survivin mediates aberrant hematopoietic progenitor cell proliferation and acute leukemia in mice induced by internal tandem duplication of Flt3. *Blood*, Vol.114:394-403.

Gilliland, D.G. Griffin, J.D. (2002). The roles of FLT3 in hematopoiesis and leukemia. *Blood*, Vol.100:1532-1542.

Hahn, C.K. et.al (2009). Proteomic and genetic approaches identify Syk as an AML target. *Cancer Cell*, Vol.16:281-294.

Harris, T.J. McCormick, F. (2010). The molecular pathology of cancer. *Nat Rev Clin Oncol*, Vol.7:251-265.

Ivanova, N.B. et.al (2002). A stem cell molecular signature. *Science*, Vol.298:601-604.

Kaur, P. et.al (2004). Survivin and Bcl-2 expression in prostatic adenocarcinomas. *Arch Pathol Lab Med*, Vol.128:39-43.

Kishi, H. et.al (2004). Expression of the survivin gene in prostate cancer: correlation with clinicopathological characteristics, proliferative activity and apoptosis. *J Urol*, Vol.171:1855-1860.

Kostrouchova, M. et.al (2003). BIR-1, a Caenorhabditis elegans homologue of Survivin, regulates transcription and development. *Proc Natl Acad Sci U S A*, Vol.100:5240-5245.

Krajewska, M. et.al (2003). Elevated expression of inhibitor of apoptosis proteins in prostate cancer. *Clin Cancer Res*, Vol.9:4914-4925.

Leung, C.G. et.al (2007). Requirements for survivin in terminal differentiation of erythroid cells and maintenance of hematopoietic stem and progenitor cells. *J Exp Med*, Vol.204:1603-1611.

Levis, M. et.al (2005). Internal tandem duplications of the FLT3 gene are present in leukemia stem cells. *Blood*, Vol.106:673-680.

Li, F. Ling, X. (2006). Survivin study: an update of "what is the next wave"? *J Cell Physiol*, Vol.208:476-486.

Li, J. et.al (2002). Involvement of histone methylation and phosphorylation in regulation of transcription by thyroid hormone receptor. *Mol Cell Biol*, Vol.22:5688-5697.

Ling, X. et.al (2005). Differential expression of survivin-2B and survivin-DeltaEx3 is inversely associated with disease relapse and patient survival in non-small-cell lung cancer (NSCLC). *Lung Cancer*, Vol.49:353-361.

Mahotka, C. et.al (2002). Differential subcellular localization of functionally divergent survivin splice variants. *Cell Death Differ*, Vol.9:1334-1342.

Mahotka, C. et.al (1999). Survivin-deltaEx3 and survivin-2B: two novel splice variants of the apoptosis inhibitor survivin with different antiapoptotic properties. *Cancer Res*, Vol.59:6097-6102.

Majeti, R. et.al (2009). Dysregulated gene expression networks in human acute myelogenous leukemia stem cells. *Proc Natl Acad Sci U S A*, Vol.106:3396-3401.

Matlin, A.J.; Clark, F. & Smith, C.W. (2005). Understanding alternative splicing: towards a cellular code. *Nat Rev Mol Cell Biol*, Vol.6:386-398.

Mola, G. et.al (2007). Exonization of Alu-generated splice variants in the survivin gene of human and non-human primates. *J Mol Biol*, Vol.366:1055-1063.

Nowak, S.J. Corces, V.G. (2000). Phosphorylation of histone H3 correlates with transcriptionally active loci. *Genes Dev*, Vol.14:3003-3013.

Salz, W. et.al (2005). A survivin gene signature predicts aggressive tumor behavior. *Cancer Res*, Vol.65:3531-3534.

Sampath, J. Pelus, L.M. (2007). Alternative splice variants of survivin as potential targets in cancer. *Curr Drug Discov Technol*, Vol.4:174-191.

Skotheim, R.I. Nees, M. (2007). Alternative splicing in cancer: noise, functional, or systematic? *Int J Biochem Cell Biol*, Vol.39:1432-1449.

Sohn, D.M. et.al (2006). Expression of survivin and clinical correlation in patients with breast cancer. *Biomed Pharmacother*, Vol.60:289-292.

Song, Z. Wu, M. (2005). Identification of a novel nucleolar localization signal and a degradation signal in Survivin-deltaEx3: a potential link between nucleolus and protein degradation. *Oncogene*, Vol.24:2723-2734.

Takizawa, B.T. et.al (2007). Downregulation of survivin is associated with reductions in TNF receptors' mRNA and protein and alterations in nuclear factor kappa B signaling in urothelial cancer cells. *Cancer Invest*, Vol.25:678-684.

Wei, Y. et.al (1999). Phosphorylation of histone H3 is required for proper chromosome condensation and segregation. *Cell*, Vol.97:99-109.

Wheatley, S.P. et.al (2004). Aurora-B phosphorylation in vitro identifies a residue of survivin that is essential for its localization and binding to inner centromere protein (INCENP) in vivo. *J Biol Chem*, Vol.279:5655-5660.

# 10

# Signalling Pathways Leading to TRAIL Resistance

Roberta Di Pietro
*G. d'Annunzio University*
*Department of Medicine and Aging Sciences, Chieti*
*Italy*

## 1. Introduction

One fundamental problem of most malignancies, including those of haematological origin, is the development of multiple mechanisms of resistance, which progressively reduce or suppress the therapeutic efficacy of conventional radio-chemotherapy. In recent years novel compounds have been identified to overcome this major hurdle. Among these, TNF-related apoptosis-inducing ligand (TRAIL) generated considerable enthusiasm for its anticancer therapeutic effectiveness, selectively targeted to a wide range of cancer cells without affecting cells derived from normal tissues and organs. A number of preliminary studies sustain the use of TRAIL-Receptors agonistic antibodies (TRAs) instead of rTRAIL (recombinant TRAIL) in the treatment of tumour cells protected from rTRAIL-induced apoptosis by the expression of cell surface decoy receptors. Although the early clinical trials are promising and well tolerated, the efficacy of these novel approaches is restricted to patients with TRAIL-sensitive tumours. In addition, TRAIL-Rs loss or mutations that can often occur in neoplastic diseases can compromise expected therapeutic results. To overcome TRAIL resistance, novel strategies based on the combination of TRAIL with radio-chemotherapy, or with proteasome or histone deacetylase or NF-κB inhibitors have been developed. In light of this complex background, this chapter will discuss the current knowledge of the signalling pathways leading to TRAIL resistance and promising targeted therapies in the treatment of haematological malignancies.

## 2. The TRAIL/TRAIL-Rs system as a novel avenue in anticancer treatment

In recent years novel compounds have been identified to overcome emergence of cancer cells resistance to conventional radio-chemotherapy. Among these, TRAIL generated considerable enthusiasm for its anticancer therapeutic effectiveness, selectively targeted to a wide range of cancer cells without affecting cells derived from normal tissues and organs. TRAIL, also known as Apo-2 Ligand (Apo-2L) (Pitti et al., 1996), is a member of the TNF super-family of cytokines including structurally related proteins that play important roles in regulating cell death, immune response and inflammation. The story of TRAIL begins when a new member of the TNF super-family capable of inducing apoptosis was identified and characterized by virtue of its sequence homology to CD95/Fas/Apo1L (FasL) and TNF (Wiley et al., 1995).

TRAIL/Apo-2L consists of 281-291 amino acids in the human and murine forms, respectively, which share 65% amino acid identity. Like other members of the TNF family, TRAIL is a type II membrane protein having an intracellular amino-terminal portion, an internal trans-membrane domain, and an external carboxyl-terminus that forms a soluble molecule upon proteolytic cleavage (Mariani & Krammer, 1998). To facilitate biological studies, an epitope-tagged soluble form of TRAIL was constructed and identified with SDS-PAGE with an apparent molecular weight of 28 kDa (Wiley et al., 1995). Gel filtration analysis of the purified soluble TRAIL disclosed that the native molecule was multimeric in solution with a size of ~80 kDa. Since then, a lot of rTRAIL preparations have been obtained and commercialized so that the variety of techniques of construction/purification employed may justify some data inconsistencies (LeBlanc & Ashkenazi, 2003). Both TRAIL and FasL exist as full-length membrane-bound molecules and as shorter soluble forms (Almasan & Ashkenazi, 2003) and induce apoptosis in a wide variety of transformed cell lines of diverse origin (Walczak & Krammer, 2000), although the membrane-bound form with a greater efficiency (Schneider et al., 1997). What immediately distinguished TRAIL both from FasL and TNFα was its ability to induce apoptosis in various continuous cell lines and primary tumour cells, displaying minimal or no toxicity on most normal cells and tissues (Ashkenazi & Dixit, 1999). Significant levels of TRAIL transcripts have been detected in many human tissues and expressed constitutively in some cell lines (Wiley et al., 1995; Pitti et al., 1996), suggesting that TRAIL, unlike FasL, must not be cytotoxic to most tissues *in vivo*. Actually, accumulating evidences indicate that TRAIL plays important roles in the immune response to viruses, self-antigens and allergens and in the immune surveillance of tumours and metastases (Falschlehner et al., 2009).

### 2.1 The TRAIL receptor family and regulation

The biological effects induced by TRAIL are mediated by interactions with cell surface TRAIL-Receptors (TRAIL-Rs). Several studies have demonstrated an extreme complexity of TRAIL-Rs expression and function (Mellier et al., 2010; Mahmood & Shukla, 2010)). In fact, at least five TRAIL receptors belonging to the apoptosis-inducing TNF-receptor family have been described so far. TRAIL-R1 (death receptor DR4; TNFRSF10a) (Pan et al., 1997a) and TRAIL-R2 (DR5; TNFRSF10b) (Pan et al. 1997b) transduce apoptotic (Ozören & El-Deiry, 2003; Huang & Sheikh, 2007) as well as non-apoptotic signals (Di Pietro & Zauli, 2004; Park et al., 2005) upon TRAIL binding, while TRAIL-R3 (DcR1; TNFRSF10c) (Pan et al., 1997b) and TRAIL-R4 (DcR2; TNFRSF10d) (Marsters et al., 1997) as well as osteoprotegerin (OPG; TRAIL-R5; TNFRSF11b) (Emery et al., 1998) are homologous to TRAIL-R1 and TRAIL-R2 in their cysteine-rich extracellular domain but they lack the intracellular death domain (DD) and apoptosis inducing capability (Almasan & Ashkenazi, 2003).

#### 2.1.1 TRAIL death receptors

TRAIL-R1 (Pan et al., 1997a) and TRAIL-R2 (Pan et al. 1997b) are type I trans-membrane proteins exposing the N-terminal TRAIL-binding domain and exerting pro-apoptotic signals through the cytoplasmic death domain. The cytoplasmic domain of TRAIL-R1/R2 shares a significant homology to the DD of different death receptors (DRs), such as CD95 and TNF-R1. Upon TRAIL binding to appropriate cognate receptors (TRAIL-R1 and TRAIL-R2), there is aggregation of TRAIL-Rs on the cell surface followed by the activation of both extrinsic and intrinsic intracellular death signalling pathways (Cretney et al., 2007). Shortly after addition of the ligand, the death-inducing signalling complex (DISC) is assembled (Kischkel et al., 1995). TRAIL DISC resembles that of Fas since the adaptor protein Fas associated death domain (FADD) and the apoptosis initiator caspase-8 are recruited to TRAIL-R1 and/or TRAIL-R2 (Sprick et al., 2000). Although initial studies have attributed a central role to caspase-8 in mediating the apoptotic signal of TRAIL, subsequent studies have demonstrated that apoptosis can be triggered independently through TRAIL-R1 or TRAIL-R2 and proteolytic activation of effector caspases either directly by apical caspase-8 or -10 (Kischkel et al., 2001) and/or indirectly through Apaf-1-mediated activation of caspase-9 (Green, 2000). Similarly to CD95L, the response to TRAIL is cell-type specific and might be characterized by two distinct cell death pathways (LeBlanc & Ashkenazi, 2003). In the type I extrinsic pathway, extrinsic signals lead to the activation of large amounts of caspase-8 and to the rapid cleavage of executioner caspase-3 prior to loss of mitochondria trans-membrane potential. As a consequence, in type I cells (including leukaemia cells) Bcl-2 over-expression blocks the mitochondrial changes associated with cell death but does not prevent apoptosis that occurs upon death receptors activation. Recent studies have suggested that death receptor induction of apoptosis may depend on the degree of receptor aggregation/multimerization, which may, in turn, depend on the concentration of the death ligand, its form (i.e. soluble versus membrane-bound), the relative DR expression on the cell surface and the array of growth factors and cytokines to which the cells are exposed (Abdulghani & El-Deiry, 2010; Mellier et al., 2010). In the type II intrinsic pathway of apoptosis, intrinsic signals, like DNA damage, growth factor withdrawal or cytokine deprivation, affect the function of Bcl-2 family members (Roos & Kaina, 2006). In fact, in type II cells the extrinsic pathway activated by death receptors is ineffective to recruit, at the DISC level, enough caspase-8 to activate effector caspases. However, through homotypic aggregation at the DISC, caspase-8 is stabilized in an active form and released into the cytosol, where it cleaves its target proteins, most notably the pro-apoptotic Bcl-2 homology domain (BH3)-only protein Bid (BH3-interacting-domain death agonist) (Kelley & Ashkenazi, 2004), thus connecting the "intrinsic" mitochondrial pathway to the "extrinsic" DR pathway (Sprick & Walczak, 2004). In turn, truncated Bid (tBid) is able to bind anti-apoptotic Bcl-2 family members like Bcl-2, Bcl-XL, Bcl-W and A1 allowing the pro-apoptotic Bcl-2 family members Bax and Bak to engage the mitochondria and induce the release of mitochondrial cytochrome c and Smac (second mitochondria-derived activator of caspases)/DIABLO into the cytosol, where these latter factors promote caspase activation. Actually, cytochrome c forms the "apoptosome" complex with the adaptor protein Apaf-1 resulting in the activation of the apoptosis-initiating protease caspase-9, which then stimulates effector caspases (Green, 2000). Instead, Smac/DIABLO binds to inhibitors of apoptosis proteins (IAPs), preventing their negative-regulatory binding to caspase-9 and -3 and then augmenting apoptosis induction (Salvesen & Abrams, 2004). In this scenario, oncogenic mutations affecting molecules involved in the intrinsic mitochondrial pathway might cause resistance emergence in type II cells, while mutations in the DR pathway could confer resistance to DR-dependent apoptosis especially in type I cells (Fig. 1).

It has been demonstrated that the expression pattern of the two killer receptors is broad and partly overlapping, suggesting that they may serve as an alternate or "backup" system, allowing the immune system to control aberrant cells even if one of the two receptors had failed (Greil et al., 2003). Although further investigations are needed to assess differences between DR signalling and regulation, some interesting observations have been reported so far. For example, it has been shown that TRAIL-R1 is activated both by the soluble and the membrane-bound form of the ligand (MacFarlane et al., 2005) whereas TRAIL-R2 is activated by cross-linked soluble and membrane-bound TRAIL ligand but not by the soluble non-cross-linked ligand (Wajant et al., 2001). We previously found a selective radiation-induced up-regulation of TRAIL-R1 in different cell lines of haematological origin that sensitized cells to TRAIL cytotoxic activity (Di Pietro et al., 2001), whereas other investigators have suggested a key role for TRAIL-R2 in p53-dependent apoptosis in response to DNA damage both *in vitro* and *in vivo* (Burns et al., 2001). Similarly, TRAIL-R2 was up-regulated in B-CLL (chronic lymphocytic leukaemia) cells in response to the small molecule Nutlin-3 in a p53-dependent manner (Coll-Mulet et al., 2006). By means of receptor-selective TRAIL mutant ligands, MacFarlane et al. (2005) demonstrated that CLL cells signal to apoptosis primarily through TRAIL-R1, whereas cross-linked agonistic TRAIL-R2 antibodies facilitate signalling via TRAIL-R2 (Natoni et al., 2007). Other authors have shown different responses of DRs in their cytoplasmic domains that may account for the differences in the activation of these receptors (Thomas et al., 2004). These authors postulated that the binding of ligand and agonistic antibody to the extracellular domain exposes the FADD-binding region differently in the cytoplasmic domain of TRAIL-R1 and TRAIL–R2 to enhance caspase-8 binding and cleavage while promoting recruitment of ancillary proteins. In addition, one more recent paper indicates TRAIL-R2 as a mediator of anoikis of colorectal carcinoma cell lines through the preferential recruitment of the "extrinsic" pathway of apoptosis (Laguinge et al., 2008).

### 2.1.2 TRAIL decoy receptors

Unlike TRAIL death receptors, TRAIL-R3 and TRAIL-R4 have been originally proposed as "decoy" receptors able to inhibit apoptosis by sequestering TRAIL from the death-inducing TRAIL-Rs or by aggregating with TRAIL death receptors upon binding to the trimeric ligand (Ashkenazi & Dixit, 1999). Nevertheless, it has been demonstrated in primary human CD8+ T cells that the inhibition of TRAIL-induced apoptosis by TRAIL-R4 critically depends on its ligand-independent association with TRAIL-R2 via the NH2-terminal preligand assembly domain overlapping the first partial cysteine-rich domain of both receptors (Clancy et al., 2005). In addition, it has been shown that expression of TRAIL-R1 and/or TRAIL-R2 was necessary but not always sufficient to mediate apoptosis, while expression of TRAIL-R3 and/or TRAIL-R4 often did not correlate with normal and tumour cells resistance to TRAIL effects (Di Pietro & Zauli, 2004). In fact, a number of evidences, based on the use of TRAIL-R agonists rather than over-expression models, have pointed at the primary role of intracellular mechanisms in controlling TRAIL resistance in a number of cell types (Griffith & Linch, 1998; Leverkus et al., 2000), thus cutting down the importance of control at decoy receptors level, whose ability to modulate TRAIL-mediated apoptosis is still controversial. In this regard, particularly intriguing is the role of soluble OPG (Corallini et al., 2008; Secchiero & Zauli, 2008). OPG was initially characterized for its ability to inhibit RANKL-stimulated osteoclastogenesis (Emery et al., 1998), but more recent studies highlighted the capability of OPG to counteract the pro-apoptotic activity of TRAIL in a variety of neoplastic cell types, at least *in vitro* (Schaefer et al., 2007). Of note, the interplay between OPG, RANKL and TRAIL is an important issue in bone and bone marrow biology as well as in the physiopathology of haematological malignancies and in particular of multiple myeloma (MM) (Secchiero & Zauli, 2008).

## 3. Molecular mechanisms of TRAIL resistance

The response of individual leukaemia cell lines to TRAIL may depend on which of pro-apoptotic or pro-survival pathways is dominant. In fact, the sensitivity of leukaemia cell lines to TRAIL is highly variable, with some cell lines demonstrating a marked resistance. In this respect, the large majority of primary haematological tumours are TRAIL-resistant, basically due to the activation of anti-apoptotic signalling pathways (such as Akt and NF-κB), over-expression of anti-apoptotic proteins (such as FLIP, Bcl-2, X-IAP), reduced expression of TRAIL death receptors or increased expression of decoy receptors (Testa, 2010; Mellier et al., 2010) (Fig. 1).

### 3.1 TRAIL-receptors

Defects in either of the different molecules involved in TRAIL signalling can lead to TRAIL resistance. With regard to the relationship between TRAIL-receptors expression and TRAIL-resistance, the data reported in the literature are often contradictory (Russo et al., 2010). An interesting characteristic in the family of DRs is that normal cells are TRAIL resistant, but the molecular basis for TRAIL tumour selectivity is still unclear. In fact, as many chemotherapeutic drugs, TRAIL is not universally active against tumour cell lines, especially primary tumour cells, even expressing DRs on their surface. Dysfunctions of TRAIL-R1/R2 due to oncogenic mutations have been found in different tumours and in different cancer patients (breast, lung, head and neck cancer and non-Hodgkin lymphoma) (Lee et al., 1999; 2001). In particular, most tumours mutations map the intracellular domain of TRAIL-R2 that binds the adaptor protein FADD (Shin et al., 2001), known for being essential together with caspase-8 for the DISC assembly. It has been reported that post-translational modifications, such as O-glycosylation, at the receptor level are essential for TRAIL-R1/R2 full functionality (Wagner et al., 2007), since protein glycosylation could enhance ligand-mediated receptor clustering. Thus, the glycosylation status of TRAIL-R1/R2 has been proposed as a marker of TRAIL sensitivity (Russo et al., 2010).

TRAIL resistance has also been linked to the presence of decoy receptors, although their physiological role as well as their impact on normal and cancer cells signalling is still poorly understood. It has been demonstrated that under experimental conditions decoy receptors over-expression could sequester TRAIL, decreasing the functional binding to TRAIL-R1/R2 and attenuating the apoptotic signalling, but experiments under physiological conditions are still missing (Russo et al., 2010). Initially, the preferential expression of TRAIL-R3/-R4 mRNA in normal cells, including peripheral blood lymphocytes, spleen and thymus, was related to the absence of TRAIL cytotoxicity in normal cells, but subsequent studies, using specific monoclonal antibodies (MoAbs), demonstrated that TRAIL sensitivity was not correlated with the relative expression of TRAIL death or decoy receptors (Griffith et al., 1999). It is now accepted that the simple expression of a death or decoy receptor is not an essential feature for apoptosis sensitivity.

### 3.2 PI3K/Akt, MAPK, c-FLIP

Another molecular mechanism responsible for TRAIL resistance emergence is considered the constitutive activation of pro-survival pathways, including Akt pathway. Akt, also known as protein kinase B (PKB), is a serine/threonine kinase that acts as a transducer of many functions initiated by the growth factor receptors that activate phosphatidylinositol 3-kinase (PI3K). In this respect, Akt and PTEN (phosphatase and tensin homologue deleted on chromosome 10) constitutive phosphorylation has been linked to TRAIL resistance of acute lymphoblastic leukaemia (ALL) cell lines (Didaa et al., 2008) and acute myeloid leukaemia (AML) patient blasts (Martelli et al., 2006). Interestingly, TRAIL itself can paradoxically

activate Akt and downstream targets, like CREB/ATF transcription factors, in leukaemia cells sensitive to its cytotoxic action, loosing to some extent its pro-apoptotic effect (Zauli et al., 2005; Caravatta et al., 2008). Constitutively active Akt is an important regulator of TRAIL sensitivity in prostate cancer (Chen et al., 2001) and protects HL60 leukaemia cells from TRAIL-induced apoptosis by activating the transcriptional factor NF-κB and up-regulating c-FLIP (cellular FADD-like interleukin-1beta-converting enzyme-inhibitory protein) (Bortul et al., 2003). c-FLIP acts as an important intracellular inhibitor of TRAIL sensitivity and delivers growth signals by activating NF-κB and ERK signalling pathways (Almasan & Ashkenazi, 2003). It is structurally related to caspase-8 (but is devoid of enzymatic activity) since it possesses two death domains that facilitate the binding to the death domain of FADD, thereby preventing association of caspase-8 with the DISC. Over-expression of c-FLIP correlates with TRAIL resistance in several types of cancer, especially in type I cells (MacFarlane et al., 2002). Although it is considered as one of the non-apoptotic NF-κB target genes, downwards the anti-apoptotic PKB/Akt and MAPK pathways, it has not been confirmed as a molecular switch between life and death in the same cell (Park et al., 2005).
More controversial is the TRAIL-R1/R2-induced activation of PKB/Akt and MAP kinases (Falschlehner et al., 2007). The three key enzymes of MAPK pathway, i.e. ERK, p38-MAPK and JNK, have been often associated with the anti-apoptotic function of TRAIL receptors. Paradoxically, pro-apoptotic effects connect TRAIL and MAPK pathways in different cell models (Frese et al., 2003; Jurewicz et al., 2006). The existence of a death domain alternative DISC complex has also been suggested to explain the TRAIL-dependent activation of MAPK pathways. FADD, caspase-8, RIP (receptor-interacting protein) and TRAF2 (TNF receptor-associated factor 2) might form a cytoplasmic complex upon TRAIL stimulation leading to p38 and JNK activation (Lin et al. 2000). In HUVECs (human umbilical vein endothelial cells) (Zauli et al., 2003) and synovial fibroblasts (Morel et al., 2005), TRAIL has a direct effect on cell survival and proliferation stimulating the PI3K-dependent phosphorylation and activation of PKB/Akt kinase without activation of NF-κB. Of note, the activation of an ERK-dependent pathway has been linked to TRAIL-induced maturation of erythroid cells (Secchiero et al., 2004a).

### 3.3 NF-κB/ IκB

A number of studies of different groups of investigators, including ourselves, have outlined the importance of NF-κB activation in determining the resistance/susceptibility of target cells to TRAIL cytotoxicity (Ehrhardt et al., 2003; Zauli et al., 2005), possibly by modulating c-FLIP levels (Bortul et al., 2003). Mounting experimental evidences highlight in TRAIL-resistant cells the activation of NF-κB following engagement of TRAIL-R1, -R2, or -R4 (Zauli et al. 2005; Henson et al., 2008). TRAIL activation of NF-κB is mediated via TRADD (TNF-R1-associated death domain protein), TRAF2 and RIP and occurs independently of caspase-8/-10 activation (Mühlenbeck et al., 1998; MacFarlane, 2003) (Fig. 1). Importantly, the level of NF-κB activation has been related to resistance of leukaemia (Ehrhardt et al., 2003) and neuroblastoma cell lines (Yang & Thiele, 2003) to TRAIL cytotoxicity and its aberrant activation has been involved in promoting tumour migration and dissemination. These findings are consistent with the pleiotropic activity of NF-κB transcription factors, which are implicated in the control of cell survival and tumorigenesis (Rayet & Gelinas, 1999). Activation and regulation of Rel/NF-κB proteins are tightly controlled by IκB proteins, which mask the nuclear localization signal (NLS) of NF-κB family members, thereby preventing their nuclear translocation (Baeuerle &

Baltimore, 1996). In response to many stimuli, such as TNFα, lipopolysaccharide (LPS) or interleukin-1 (IL-1), IκB kinase (IKK) is activated and can phosphorylate IκBs, which, in turn, can be poly-ubiquitinated and rapidly degraded by the proteasome, allowing the release of sequestered NF-κB. After its translocation into the nucleus, NF-κB is able to activate its target genes, which, depending on the physiological circumstances (Barkett & Gilmore, 1999), can mediate cell survival or apoptosis. It has been reported, for example, that the TRAIL-mediated recruitment of apical caspase-8/-10 was able to induce the simultaneous activation of both effector caspases (-3, -6, -7) and of NF-κB pathway in TRAIL-sensitive myeloid leukaemia cells (Secchiero et al., 2002). As a consequence, the TRAIL cytotoxic/cytostatic activity mediated by effector caspases was reduced by the concomitant pro-survival effect exerted by NF-κB. Interestingly, NF-κB activation was causally linked to the induction of maturation of the surviving leukaemia cells along the monocytic pathway (Secchiero et al., 2002). Moreover, NF-κB activation was paralleled by the absence of degradation and by the nuclear translocation of IκBα in Jurkat T leukaemia cell lines sensitive to the cytotoxic action of TRAIL (Zauli et al., 2005), whereas in TRAIL-resistant primary human erythroblasts NF-κB activation was concomitant with IκBα cytoplasmic localization (unpublished observations). The dual function of NF-κB, as an inhibitor or activator of apoptosis, would depend on the relative levels of RelA and c-Rel subunits (Chen et al., 2003). In fact, over-expression of RelA or a transcriptional-deficient mutant of c-Rel inhibits TRAIL-induced apoptosis in mouse embryonic fibroblasts, whereas depletion of RelA increases cytokine-induced apoptosis (Chen et al., 2003).

### 3.4 IAP, Bcl-2, caspases

Among the anti-apoptotic genes up-regulated by NF-κB are included cellular inhibitors of apoptosis proteins 1 and 2 (c-IAP1 and c-IAP2), TRAF1 and TRAF2, c-FLIP and Bcl-XL (Wang et al., 1998). Some of these (e.g. survivin, X-IAP, Bcl-2, Bcl-XL) have been shown to be associated with poor prognosis in AML (Tamm et al., 2000; Paydas et al. 2003). Over-expression of Bcl-2, Bcl-XL, or Mcl-1, loss of Bax or Bak function, increased expression of IAPs and reduced release of Smac/DIABLO from the mitochondria to the cytosol are all events resulting in TRAIL resistance in type II cancer cells (Vogler et al., 2008)(Fig. 1) . Another important mechanism through which haematological malignancies can escape TRAIL cytotoxicity is inactivation of the intracellular pro-apoptotic pathways (Ashkenazi et al., 2008). This allows malignant cells not only to escape from TRAIL-induced apoptosis, but also to take advantage of the pro-survival signals induced by TRAIL, which paradoxically may act as a survival cytokine (Fig. 1). In this respect, a possible interplay between the Akt and caspase pathways has been already described in several cell systems (Cardone et al., 1998; Jones et al., 2002; Milani et al., 2003). The picture emerging from these studies is that, when survival signals dominate, Akt impairs the activation of the apical caspases, by directly phosphorylating caspase-9 (Cardone et al., 1998) or by inhibiting the recruitment of procaspase-8/-10 to the DISC (Jones et al., 2002). On the other hand, when pro-apoptotic signals prevail, apical caspase-8/-10 activates downstream caspases, which cleave and inactivate Akt as well as other anti-apoptotic molecules (Milani et al., 2003).

All these findings underline the complexity of the TRAIL-mediated intracellular signals, which simultaneously activate pro-apoptotic and anti-apoptotic pathways. The fate of individual malignant cells would depend on which of these pathways prevail within the cell. These effects should be carefully evaluated in the individual assessment of eligibility of cancer patients to TRAIL-based therapy.

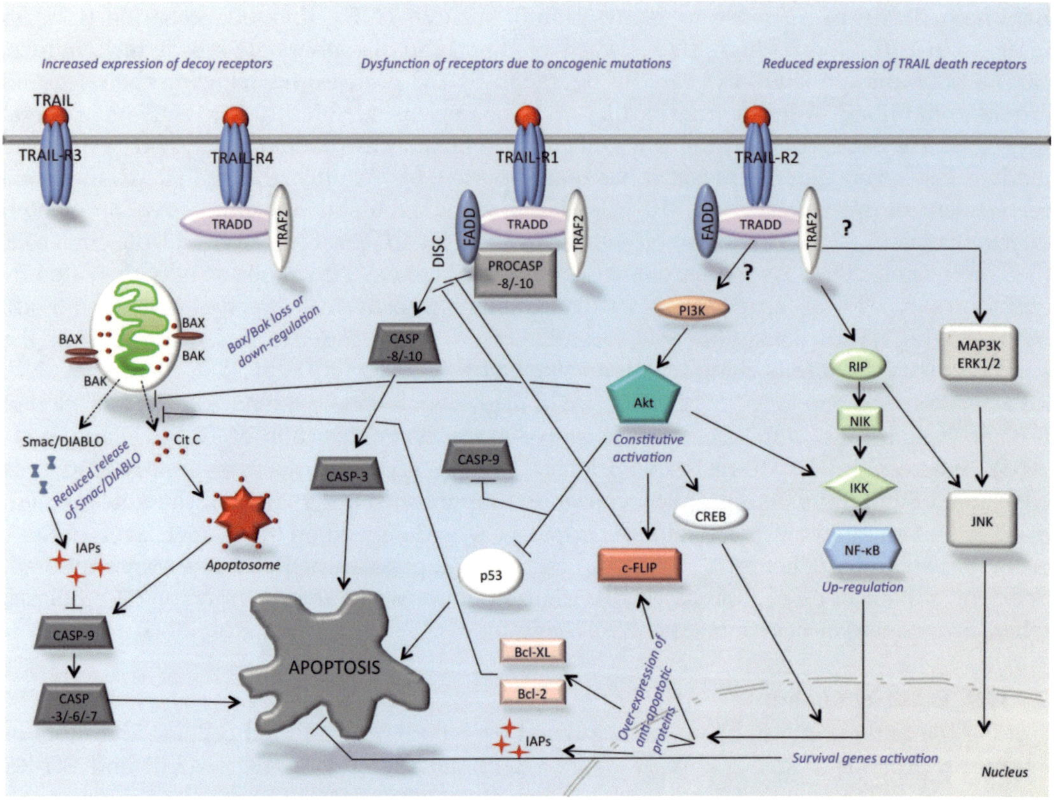


Fig. 1. Schematic representation of key mechanisms involved in TRAIL resistance of haematological malignancies. Activation of TRAIL-Rs can trigger both death and survival pathways, depending on the cell system and environmental conditions. TRAIL-R1 and TRAIL-R2 can lead to apoptotic cell death through the recruitment of FADD and the following cleavage of caspase-8 and -10. Both DRs together with the "decoy" TRAIL-R4 are also involved in the priming of survival genes through the activation of a) NF-κB and JNK pathways triggered by the engagement of TRAF2 and RIP; b) PI3K/Akt and MAPK/ERK1/2 pathways, by means of still unclear mechanisms (highlighted with a question mark). Other mechanisms leading to TRAIL resistance include different caspase or PI3K physiological inhibitors.

## 4. TRAIL treatment of haematological malignancies

It has been shown that TRAIL induces growth arrest and apoptosis in cancer cells independently of $^{wt}$p53 function, Bcl-2 and Bcl-XL (Walczak & Krammer, 2000) and MDR gene expression (Snell et al., 1997). Thus, TRAIL may offer an alternative or complementary approach to conventional anticancer therapy. Unlike other members of the TNF super-family, such as CD95L and TNFα, that are precluded from use in systemic anticancer therapy due to their severe toxic side effects (Tartaglia and Goeddel, 1992), TRAIL is effective in selectively killing both *in vitro* and *in vivo* a vast array of tumour cells from lung, breast, kidney, colon, prostate, thyroid and skin cancers (Walczak & Krammer, 2000; Papenfuss et al., 2008), without causing significant organ toxicity and inflammation *in vivo*.

Moreover, TRAIL exerts a variable cytotoxic activity on haematological malignancies (Snell et al., 1997) and synergistically cooperates with: i) chemotherapeutic drugs, such as etoposide, campthotecin-11, doxorubicin, 5-fluorouracil, taxol (Sabatini et al., 2004; Henson et al., 2008); and ii) ionizing radiation (Chinnaiyan et al., 2000; Di Pietro et al., 2001), causing substantial regression or complete ablation of solid (colon and mammary) cancers in animal models. Besides acting as a tumour suppressor *in vivo* in primary tumours, TRAIL could play a substantial role in suppressing tumour metastasis. In fact, it has been observed that this cytokine may partially limit the formation of hepatic metastases of a variety of mouse tumours (Seki et al., 2003). A study performed in TRAIL -/- null mice demonstrated that the incidence of spontaneous lymphoid malignancies was increased by 25% in comparison with control animals (Zerafa et al., 2005), suggesting a crucial role of TRAIL in the immune-surveillance against lymphoid malignancies. Although it is not established whether TRAIL causes liver toxicity in humans (Jo et al., 2000; Lawrence et al., 2001), pre-clinical studies performed in mice and non-human primates indicated that rTRAIL protein promotes potent apoptosis-inducing activity against tumour cells without a relevant systemic toxicity (Walczak et al., 1999). Phase I and phase II clinical trials in patients with advanced solid tumours or non-Hodgkin lymphoma (NHL) appeared to go in the same direction, indicating that both rTRAIL and TRAs are safe and well tolerated (Koschny et al., 2007; Tolcher et al., 2007). Therefore, TRAIL ligand and TRAs are strong candidates for an effective but tolerable treatment of solid cancers, either used alone or in combination with radio-chemotherapy.

### 4.1 Acute myeloid leukaemia (AML)

The cytotoxic activity of TRAIL has been evaluated in haematological diseases by different groups of investigators, including our research group (Secchiero & Zauli, 2008; Sancilio et al., 2008; Impicciatore et al., 2010). Overall the activity of TRAIL as a single treatment in acute and chronic leukaemia is poor. Unlike the poor outcome of TRAIL treatment in primary AML blasts, continuous cell lines derived from AML display a pronounced sensitivity to the apoptotic action of TRAIL (Snell et al., 1997; Secchiero et al., 2004b). Moreover, when TRAIL is used in combination with chemotherapeutic agents (fludarabine, cytosine arabinoside or daunorubicin) additive or super-additive apoptotic effects are obtained, due to the ability of these agents to activate apical caspase-8/-10 (Jones et al., 2003). In line with these findings, other authors demonstrated that triterpenoids, natural and synthetic compounds with demonstrated anti-tumour activity, induced a substantial increase in cell death in both B-CLL and AML blasts, by inducing a concentration-dependent decrease in the levels of FLIP protein (Suh et al., 2003; Pedersen et al., 2002). A recent report has related the poor response of AML to the simultaneous expression of death and decoy receptors (Inukai et al., 2006), whereas co-expression of death receptors with the decoy receptor TRAIL-R3 resulted in significant shortened overall survival of AML patients (Chamuleau et al., 2011). Another weak point in leukaemia treatment is represented by p53 gene deletions or mutations, that usually occur in less than 15% of AML cases. To augment the poor response of AML to TRAIL cytotoxicity, Secchiero et al. (2007) have recently adopted the strategy to combine rTRAIL with Nutlin-3, a potent non-genotoxic activator of the p53 pathway (Impicciatore et al., 2010). In this investigation Nutlin-3 synergized with TRAIL in inducing apoptosis both in AML cell lines and primary M4-type and M5-type AML blasts, but not in $^{mut}$p53 AML cells, suggesting that the combined treatment of Nutlin-3 plus TRAIL might offer a novel therapeutic strategy for $^{wt}$p53 AML cells.

### 4.2 Acute lymphoblastic leukaemia (ALL)

Clodi et al. (2000) demonstrated that TRAIL has a modest activity in primary ALL since it killed a maximum of 29% of precursor-B-cell blasts within 18 hours treatment against the 75% of the sensitive Jurkat cell line. Childhood T-ALL is frequently accompanied by hyperleukocytosis at disease presentation, suggesting that T-ALL tends to acquire mechanisms for escaping immune surveillance of the hosts that promote its rapid clonal expansion. Clinically, dramatic advances have been made in the treatment of childhood T-ALL. However, despite the use of intensive risk-adapted chemotherapy, treatment failure occurs in approximately 25% of patients (Goldberg et al., 2003). Since the prognosis of relapsed T-ALL remains dismal, the development of a new therapeutic modality is urgently required. In a recent report on T-ALL cell lines and primary samples of childhood T-ALL the failure of anti-leukaemic activity of soluble rTRAIL was linked to the low cell surface expression levels of TRAIL-R1 and TRAIL-R2, which could not be modified by the demethylating agent 5-aza2'deoxycytidine (Akahanea et al., 2010).

### 4.3 Chronic myeloid leukaemia (CML)

Only few studies have investigated the effects of rTRAIL on CML blasts. An interesting study of Tanaka et al. (2007) demonstrated increased levels of serum TRAIL and TRAIL mRNA in neutrophils of CML patients during IFNα therapy, suggesting a novel antineoplastic role of neutrophils mediated by the expression/release of TRAIL. Since neutrophils, unlike activated lymphocytes, display a low susceptibility to TRAIL cytotoxicity (Meurette et al., 2006), these findings are of particular value. Other studies have shown that TRAIL, used as a single agent, significantly reduces the number of myeloid colonies and clusters from patients affected with CML and myelodysplastic syndromes (MDS) (Zang et al., 2001; Uno et al., 2003), while normal human stem cells treated with high doses of TRAIL maintain a repopulating potential when transplanted into NOD/SCID mice (Zang et al., 2001). Moreover, it was recently demonstrated that the loss of Bcr-Abl in imatinib-resistant CML cells leads to the down-regulation of c-FLIP and the subsequent increase in TRAIL sensitivity, suggesting that TRAIL could be an effective strategy for the treatment of imatinib-resistant CML with loss of Bcr-Abl (Park et al., 2009).

### 4.4 B-type chronic lymphocytic leukaemia (B-CLL)

A pressing need for the identification of novel therapeutic approaches regards B-CLL disease. It is known in fact that B-CLL patients may have initial clinical responses to alkylating agents, such as chlorambucil, or adenosine analogs, such as fludarabine, but they ultimately become refractory to therapy. Preliminary studies, carried out on cell lines and a modest number of primary samples, have shown a low cytotoxic activity of TRAIL on low-grade B-CLL (MacFarlane et al., 2002). Collectively, low-grade B-cell malignancies constitute one of the most common form of potentially lethal cancer in Europe and North America, with B-CLL representing the most prevalent of these disorders (Reed et al., 2002). B-CLL is characterized by the accumulation of mature non-proliferating B cells defective in apoptotic mechanisms and resistant to anticancer therapy. A number of molecular defects and biologic features have been identified in this pathology. Olsson et al. (2001) revealed a higher constitutive expression of the long form of FLIP (FLIP-L) in B-CLL as compared to normal tonsillar B cells. MacFarlane et al. (2002) demonstrated that resistance to TRAIL was upstream of caspase-8 activation, since little or no caspase-8 was processed in TRAIL-treated

B-CLL cells. As a consequence, the possibility of sensitizing B-CLL cells to TRAIL-mediated cytotoxicity could reside in the modulation of c-FLIP levels or in the up-regulation of DR surface expression. In consistence with this hypothesis, the combination of TRAIL with anti-CD95 ligand has proved effective in inducing apoptosis of CD40-activated B-CLL cells (Dicker et al., 2005). A more recent study, aimed at evaluating molecular mechanisms of TRAIL resistance of B-CLL, identified a different TRAIL sensitivity of Zap-70low and Zap-70high B-CLL subsets, proposing this negative prognostic marker as responsible to redirect TRAIL signallling from pro-apoptotic to pro-inflammatory pathway (Richardson et al., 2006).

### 4.5 Lymphoma

The potential therapeutic use of TRAIL has been also explored in the therapy of refractory diffuse large B-cell lymphoma (DLBCL) (Cillessen et al., 2006), cutaneous T-cell lymphoma (CTCL) (Braun et al., 2007), mantle B cell lymphoma (MCL) (Roue et al., 2007) and plasmacytoid dendritic cell (PDC) leukaemia (Blum et al., 2006), which shows a particularly aggressive clinical course. In particular, Cillessen et al. (2006) have shown that 12 out of a total of 22 DLBCL samples, including 7 clinically chemotherapy-refractory lymphomas, were sensitive to TRAIL-mediated apoptosis. TRAIL cytotoxic effects were also detected in CD4+CD56+ PDC leukaemia (Blum et al., 2006), as well as in the majority of MCL cell lines and primary cultures investigated by Roue et al. (2007), whose research group used TRAIL in combination with the IκB kinase inhibitor BMS-345541 to overcome resistance of MCL samples. In a recent review (Sancilio et al., 2008), we suggested the possibility to combine two biologically active and well-tolerated agents with different mechanisms of action, such as rituximab and agonist MoAbs against DRs, as an attractive treatment strategy for patients affected with B-cell lymphoma. The *in vivo* mechanisms through which rituximab mediates its effects have not been fully elucidated, though ADCC (antibody-dependent cellular cytotocxicity), CMC (complement-mediated cytotoxicity) and apoptosis have been suggested and supported by several studies (Bonavida, 2007). By contrast, a number of *in vitro* experimental evidences have been obtained in B-NHL cell lines as a model system (Bonavida, 2007). The findings here described demonstrate that rituximab treatment is able to modulate different signalling pathways, like p38-MAPK, Raf-1/MEK/ERK1/2 and NF-κB, leading to the down-regulation of Bcl-2/Bcl-XL gene products, known players of the intrinsic apoptotic pathway. Through this mechanism, chemo-sensitization of drug-resistant B-NHL cell lines to various drug-induced apoptosis could be achieved.

### 4.6 Multiple myeloma (MM)

A number of studies from several groups of investigators have allowed clearly establishing that myeloma is the most susceptible haematological malignancy to rTRAIL used as a single agent (Secchiero et al., 2004b). In particular, Gazitt (1999) demonstrated for the first time that TRAIL induces substantial apoptosis in freshly isolated, flow-sorted myeloma cells obtained from different MM patients. Subsequently, the same group of investigators (Liu et al., 2003) demonstrated that TRAIL is a potent inducer of apoptosis, independent of Bcl-2. Moreover, consistently with the potential role of NF-κB and Akt pathways in counteracting apoptosis induction by either chemotherapy or TRAIL, the cell permeable nuclear factor NF-κB inhibitor SN50 sensitized TRAIL-resistant MM cells to TRAIL cytotoxicity (Mitsiades et al., 2002) and the Akt inhibitor IL-6-Hydroxymethyl-chiro-inositol 2-(R)-2-O-methyl-3-O-octadecylcarbonate-induced cell death of both Dex- and Doxo-sensitive and -resistant cell clones. Interestingly, also thalidomide, which holds great promise as a new anti-neoplastic agent for the treatment of refractory MM, triggers activation of caspase-8 and down-regulates NF-κB activity and c-FLIP (Mitsiades et al, 2002). These studies form the basis for clinical trials of these agents, alone and coupled with conventional and novel therapies, to improve outcome in MM. It is worth underlining that while the potential therapeutic use of rTRAIL or TRAs in most myeloid and lymphoid malignancies is still to be evaluated, rTRAIL appears to be a very promising candidate for the therapy of MM, either alone or in combination with valproic acid, a histone deacetylase inhibitor, arsenic trioxide, IFNγ, or with the low-molecular-weight Smac mimetic LBW242 (Secchiero & Zauli, 2008). Moreover, the use of specific anti-TRAIL-R1 or anti-TRAIL-R2 agonistic antibodies, more than the treatment with TRAIL itself (Locklin et al., 2007), has proved an effective strategy to counteract OPG-mediated effects and increase TRAIL-induced apoptosis of MM cells (Secchiero & Zauli, 2008). Of note, other preclinical studies aimed at targeting the RANK/RANKL/OPG pathway have paved the way to clinical experimentation likely to lead to new therapeutic approaches (Buckle et al., 2010).

## 5. Novel strategies to overcome TRAIL resistance

During the last decades, a better understanding of cancer biology has led to the development of new promising therapeutic approaches, based on "molecular targeted" drugs, directed against specific "target" molecules playing a key role in tumour maintenance (Urruticoechea et al., 2010). Based on the principle that inhibiting as many targets as possible reduces the emergence of drug resistance, the use of combined therapies or multi-target inhibitors is gaining field in the design of new treatments. A number of chemical and physical anticancer strategies have been developed to bypass TRAIL resistance, based on the combination of rTRAIL or agonistic antibodies with chemotherapeutic agents, irradiation, or targeted small molecules, like proteasome, histone deacetylase or NF-κB inhibitors (Testa, 2010; Russo et al., 2010). The agents used in combination with TRAIL either enhance TRAIL-R1/-R2 expression or decrease expression of anti-apoptotic proteins (c-FLIP, X-IAP, Bcl-2) (Mellier et al., 2010) (Fig. 2). Many of these combinatorial therapies hold promise for future developments in the treatment of haematological malignancies since they may reduce excessive systemic toxicity toward normal cells and resistance of tumour cells after recurrent treatments. We and other authors have demonstrated that TRAIL-mediated cytotoxicity is increased by ionizing radiation and chemotherapy in both myeloid and erythroid leukaemia cell lines as well as in T lymphoma cell lines (Gong & Almasan, 2000; Di Pietro et al., 2001; Sabatini et al., 2004; Zauli et al., 2005; Caravatta et al., 2008; Impicciatore et al., 2010; Signore et al., 2011). Although an increasing number of drugs warrant further investigation as potential new strategies for the treatment of solid tumours or AML in combination with soluble rTRAIL (Suh et al., 2003), only in few cases the efficacy of the combined treatments has been proved *in vivo* and a general consensus on how chemotherapy and radiotherapy may synergize with TRAIL therapy is far to be reached (Russo et al., 2010).

### 5.1 TRAIL-death receptor-targeted treatment

A number of receptor-specific TRAIL-variants and agonistic antibodies have been recently developed. Some of these soluble rTRAIL and MoAbs targeting TRAIL-R1 and/or TRAIL-R2 (TRAIL receptor agonists, TRAs) are progressing to phase I/II clinical trials (Mahmood &

Shukla, 2010). The clinical use of TRAs is a very promising and innovative approach to increase selectivity and reduce undesired toxicity of cancer treatments in comparison with modern anticancer drugs (protein kinase inhibitors or MoAb agonists for growth receptors) (Russo et al., 2010). These compounds were generated to selectively bind and activate their respective DRs without affecting decoy receptors or OPG. DRs engagement, using recombinant death ligands or agonistic antibodies, leads to the activation of both extrinsic and intrinsic apoptosis pathways, while, generally, chemotherapy or radiotherapy triggers the mitochondrial/intrinsic pathway (Fig. 2). Therefore, the conventional therapeutic approach could be implemented by DR-induced apoptosis when DRs are expressed and functional on tumour cells. As already mentioned, although soluble rTRAIL as well as TRAs are not completely free from toxicity, both reagents elicit a significant lower hepatotoxicity when administered systemically compared to CD95 receptor agonists (Lawrence et al., 2001). Besides the advantage of an improved specificity and a lower toxicity of TRAs over TRAIL ligand, pharmacokinetic studies performed in primates and humans have shown that these agents have a longer half-life (around 15 days) than soluble TRAIL (30 min) that makes them easier to dose and administer (Duiker et al., 2006). Preclinical studies performed *in vitro* in cultured human cell lines and *in vivo* in murine xenograft cancer models (Cretney et al., 2007) showed favourable results when TRAs were used as single agents and enhanced cytotoxicity when they were combined with chemotherapy or radiotherapy (Marini et al., 2006). In particular, HGS-ETR1 (anti-TRAIL-R1, mapatumumab) as well as HGS-ETR2 (anti-TRAIL-R2, lexatumumab) was able to induce apoptosis in primary and cultured lymphoma cells increasing cell death when associated either with conventional chemotherapy (doxorubicin) or novel drugs like proteasome inhibitors (bortezomib) (Georgakis et al., 2005). As well, multiple solid tumours including lung, colon and renal carcinoma were found responsive to TRAs treatment used alone or in combination with chemotherapy (Pukac et al., 2005). To date, the fully humanized MoAbs HGS-ETR1, HGS-ETR2 and HGS-TR2J (anti-TRAIL-R2) (all three from Human Genome Sciences, Rockville, MD) are used in ongoing trials for the treatment of advanced solid tumours, lymphoma or MM (Mahmood & Shukla, 2010). A number of excellent reviews on different therapeutic approaches to specifically target TRAIL and DR pathways have been recently published (Ashkenazi et al., 2008; Papenfuss et al., 2008; Mahmood & Shukla, 2010; Russo et al., 2010).

Of particular interest is the current use of rTRAIL and TRAs for the treatment of B cell malignancies (Mahmood & Shuka, 2010). As shown by other authors, the DR pathway is intact and functional in various types of cancers, including B-cell lymphomas (Snell et al., 1997; Georgakis et al., 2005). B-cell sensitivity to TRAs is a fundamental requirement for therapeutic efficacy, since TRAIL-R1 and TRAIL–R2 mutations, observed in NHL as well as in other human tumours (Lee et al., 2001), make neoplastic B cells insensitive to TRAIL and, presumably, to agonistic antibodies mimicking its action. TRAIL-R1 and TRAIL-R2 map to human chromosome 8p21-22, a site of frequent allelic loss in tumours. This led to the hypothesis that, as potential tumour suppressors, TRAIL-Rs may also harbour somatic mutations in human tumours. The most frequent mutations identified so far concern TRAIL-R2 and affect the intracellular domain of the receptor, i.e. the FADD-binding domain, and, as a consequence, its capability of inducing apoptosis (Bin et al., 2007). Although still poor is the knowledge of how TRAIL-Rs mutations affect signalling events, it is predictable that a patient displaying a TRAIL-R2 mutation would not benefit from treatment with either rTRAIL or an anti-TRAIL-R2 antibody but from treatment with mapatumumab or a modified version of rTRAIL able to target only one death receptor (MacFarlane et al., 2005). Similarly to TRAIL, TRAs (mapatumumab and lexatumumab) are capable of inducing anti-lymphoma effects both *in vitro* and *in vivo* (Motoki et al., 2005). In particular, it has been recently demonstrated that mapatumumab can trigger apoptosis through caspase-8 activation via the extrinsic apoptotic pathway (Maddiplata et al., 2007). Various groups of investigators have shown that the activation of the TRAIL-Rs by either ligands or MoAbs sensitizes cancer cells to the effects of various chemotherapeutic and/or biological agents (Secchiero et al., 2007), although in a recent report no correlation between the degree of anti-tumour *in vitro* activity of mapatumumab and TRAIL-R1 antigen density has been shown (Maddiplata et al., 2007). To explain their results these investigators hypothesized differences in the receptor hetero-dimerization between various B-cell lymphoma cells upon TRAIL-R1 binding to mapatumumab. In fact, it has been published that following *in vitro* exposure to TRAIL ligand or TRAIL-R1 agonists, other DRs are recruited via trimerization, leading to signal transduction and apoptosis (Cretney et al., 2007). Depending on the type of DR undergoing trimerization upon TRAIL-R1 binding the intensity and type of response could change. In theory, the same principle could justify the absence of anti-tumour activity of lexatumumab despite ample surface expression of TRAIL-R2 in the cell lines tested *in vitro* (Maddiplata et al., 2007). Further studies are needed to address this issue.

### 5.2 Proteasome and histone deacetylase inhibitors

Inhibition of NF-κB (e.g. with mutant forms of IκBα or proteasome inhibitors) has also been shown to increase TRAIL responsiveness (Sayers & Murphy, 2006). In this respect, besides the clinical use of bortezomib (Velcade, PS-341) for the treatment of multiple myeloma (Sayers & Murphy, 2006), it has been recently reported that treatment with the proteasome inhibitors MG-132 and PS-341 is associated with the up-regulation of TRAIL and its death receptors, TRAIL-R1/TRAIL-R2, in primary B-CLL cells and in the Burkitt lymphoma cell line, BJAB (Kabore et al., 2006). Interestingly, the combined treatment with TRAIL or TRAs and proteasome inhibitors leads to a significant apoptosis induction in B-CLL but not in normal B cells (Kabore et al., 2006). DRs up-regulation by PS-341 was attributed to TRAIL-R2 mRNA stabilization and the consequent increased receptor half-life (Kamdasamy & Kraft, 2008). In addition to the proteasome inhibitors, inhibition of histone deacetylase (HDAC) class I sensitizes B-CLL to TRAIL-induced apoptosis (Hamilton et al., 2010). An aberrant regulation of gene expression due to alterations in histone acetyltransferase (HAT) or HDAC recruitment and activity has been constantly found in both solid and haematological tumours (Mai & Altucci, 2009). Therefore HDAC can be considered as potential therapeutic targets of human malignancies. Interestingly, the reduction of TRAIL protein degradation has been recently observed in thyroid cancer cells and proposed as a novel action of HDAC inhibitors (Borbone et al., 2010). It is worth outlining that HDAC inhibitors exert anti-tumour effects at doses that are well tolerated by the patients. Hydroxamic acids, such as SAHA (Vorinostat, Zolinza), were recently approved by the US FDA for the treatment of cutaneous manifestations in patients affected with advanced refractory CTCL. In fact, similarly to what has been seen in B-CLL, CTCL cell lines show pronounced resistance to TRAIL cytotoxicity (Braun et al., 2007). Lastly, a phase I study, currently recruiting participants, will use vorinostat in combination with cytarabine and etoposide for the treatment of patients with relapsed and/or refractory acute leukaemia, MDS or myeloproliferative disorders (see for details http://clinicaltrials.gov).

### 5.3 Small molecules and natural compounds

Besides oncogenes over-expression and cell cycle control mechanisms disruption, mutations in apoptotic regulators (namely p53) are very frequent in cancer cells and represent for them a way to escape toxic effects inducible with radio-chemotherapy. As an alternative strategy to restoring transcriptional activation to mutant p53 proteins in solid tumours, small molecule selective inhibitors of p53/MDM2 interaction (Nutlins) are emerging as an innovative tool in the treatment of malignancies expressing $^{wt}$p53 including haematological disorders (Secchiero et al., 2008; Impicciatore et al., 2010). Nutlins were the first potent and selective small molecules, antagonists of the p53/MDM2 interaction, to be identified 7 years ago (Vassilev et al., 2004). Since then several classes of small-molecule inhibitors with distinct chemical structure have been reported (Shangary & Wang, 2009), although only Nutlin-3 has been extensively evaluated for its therapeutic potential and mechanism of action in human cancer and represents a promising therapeutic candidate for drug development (Shangary & Wang, 2009). Several authors have investigated the effects of Nutlins, used alone or in combination with other therapeutic agents, on primary cells, different cell lines and tumour xenografts (Kojima et al., 2005; Lehmann et al., 2007). In particular, it has been reported that the active enantiomer Nutlin-3a induces i) increased levels of p53, ii) p53- and p21-dependent cell cycle arrest and iii) p53-dependent apoptosis in a number of solid tumours and haematological malignancies including primary AML (Kojima et al., 2005), MM (Stuhmer et al., 2005), B-CLL (Coll-Mulet et al., 2006) and Hodgkin lymphomas (HL) (Drakos et al., 2007). Unlike radiation and conventional chemotherapy, MDM2 inhibitors induce accumulation and activation of p53 in cancer and normal cells without inducing DNA damage or post-translational modifications of p53. Nutlins in fact restore p53 function in $^{wt}$p53 tumour cells without inducing p53 phosphorylation and with limited effects on primary cells (Vassilev et al., 2004). Interestingly, when used at concentrations higher than 10 mM, Nutlin-3, MI-63 and MI-219 are able to inhibit cell proliferation even in cancer cells lacking $^{wt}$p53 (Shangary & Wang, 2009). In response to Nutlin-3 treatment TRAIL-R2 is up-regulated in B-CLL cells in a p53-dependent manner (Coll-Mulet et al., 2006). Moreover, Nutlins reduce the MDM2 ability to stimulate p53 degradation and represent a promising approach for improving radiotherapy effects especially for tumours over-expressing MDM2 such as sarcomas, solid tumours (Momand et al., 1998) and NHL (Finnegan et al., 1994).

Besides the use of a broad range of protein inhibitors, chemotherapeutic agents or irradiation to exert synergistic effects with TRAIL action (Mahalingam et al., 2009), more recently the use of natural compounds, including polyphenols, has gained increasing interest due to their relative safety and anti-tumour efficacy in preclinical models (Jacquemin et al., 2010). Actually, it has been demonstrated that a number of natural compounds are able to enhance TRAIL-induced apoptosis in leukaemia cells (Fas et al., 2006; Russo et al., 2007; Hussain et al., 2008; Sung et al. 2010). In particular, it has been shown that wogonin, derived from a popular Chinese herb, attenuates NF-κB activity (Fas et al., 2006), whereas curcumin, responsible for the yellow colour of the spice turmeric, up-regulates TRAIL-R2 expression and inactivates NF-κB in a ROS-dependent manner in a number of solid tumours including Burkitt's lymphoma (Hussain et al., 2008). Moreover, Russo et al. (2007) reported that leukaemia cell lines were efficiently sensitized by quercetin and TRAIL co-treatment through the inhibition of the Akt pathway, while Sung et al., 2010 observed other survival proteins down-regulation after TRAIL and triterpenoids co-treatment. Taken together, these findings demonstrate that nongenotoxic natural molecules or small compounds enhance TRAIL-mediated killing of tumour cells with reduced side effects compared to conventional radio-chemotherapy.

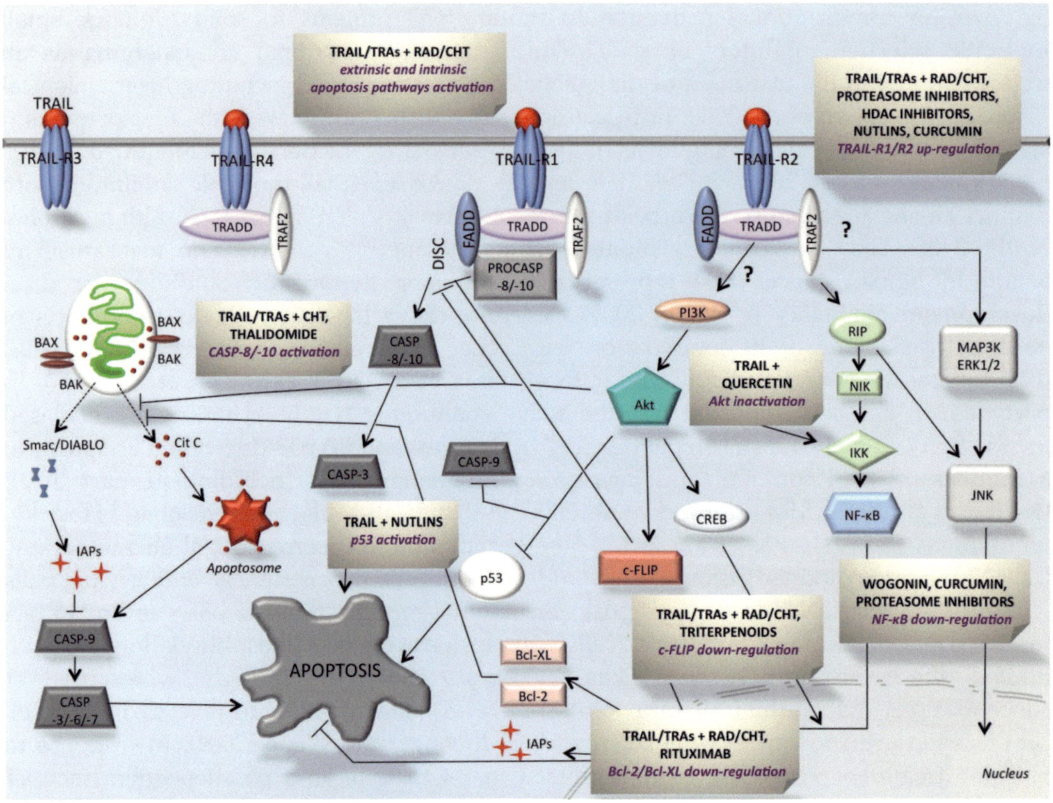


Fig. 2. Schematic representation of molecular mechanisms of novel strategies aimed at restoring TRAIL sensitivity of haematological malignancies. RAD: radiotherapy; CHT: chemotherapy. See text for other abbreviations.

## 6. Conclusion

A number of preliminary studies sustain the use of TRAs instead of rTRAIL in the treatment of tumour cells protected from TRAIL-induced apoptosis by the expression of cell surface decoy receptors. Although the early clinical trials are promising and well tolerated, it is worth outlining that the utility of both rTRAIL and agonistic anti-TRAIL-Rs antibodies therapies is restricted to patients with TRAIL-sensitive tumours. To restore TRAIL sensitivity in cancer cells novel compounds have been identified and are currently used in combined protocols with TRAIL ligand/TRAs or conventional radio-chemotherapy. Once mechanisms of action/resistance to TRAIL signalling are better understood, approaches to predict patient response and optimize combination regimens may be developed to overcome primary and acquired resistance on the trail to a personalized treatment of cancer.

## 7. Acknowledgment

The author wishes to thank Dr. Francesca Gambacorta for helpful assistance in the artwork.

## 8. References

Abdulghani, J. & El-Deiry, W.S. (2010). TRAIL receptor signaling and therapeutics, *Expert Opin Ther Targets* 14(10):1091-1108.

Akahanea, K., Inukaia, T., Zhanga, X., Hirosea, K., Kurodaa, I., et al. (2010). Resistance of T-cell acute lymphoblastic leukemia to tumor necrosis factor-related apoptosis-inducing ligand-mediated apoptosis, *Exp Hematol* 38:885–895.

Almasan, A. & Ashkenazi, A. (2003). Apo2L/TRAIL: apoptosis signaling, biology, and potential for cancer therapy, *Cytokine Growth Factor Rev* 14(3-4):337-348.

Ashkenazi, A. & Dixit, V.M. (1999). Apoptosis control by death and decoy receptors, *Curr Opin Cell Biol* 11:255-260.

Ashkenazi, A, Holland, P. & Eckhardt, S.G. (2008). Ligand-based targeting of apoptosis in cancer: the potential of recombinant human apoptosis ligand 2/tumor necrosis factor–related apoptosis-inducing ligand (rhApo2L/TRAIL), *J Clin Oncol* 26:3621–3630.

Baeuerle, P.A. & Baltimore, D. (1996). NF-kappa B: ten years after, *Cell* 87(1):13-20.

Barkett, M. & Gilmore, T.D. (1999). Control of apoptosis by Rel/NF-kappaB transcription factors, *Oncogene* 18:6910-6924.

Bin, L., Thorburn, J., Thomas, L.R., Clark, P.E., Humphreysm R. & Thorburn, A. (2007). Tumor-derived mutations in the TRAIL receptor DR5 inhibit TRAIL signalling through the DR4 receptor by competing for ligand binding, *J Biol Chem*, 38: 28189-28194.

Blum, A., Chaperot, L., Molens, J.P., Foissaud, V., Plantaz, D. & Plumas, J. (2006). Mechanisms of TRAIL-induced apoptosis in leukemic plasmacytoid dendritic cells, *Exp Hematol* 34:1655–1662.

Bonavida, B. (2007). Rituximab-induced inhibition of antiapoptotic cell survival pathways: implications in chemo/immunoresistance, rituximab unresponsiveness, prognostic and novel therapeutic interventions, *Oncogene* 26(25): 3629-3636.

Borbone, E., Berlingieri, M.T., De Bellis, F., Nebbioso, A., Chiappetta, G. et al., (2010). Histone deacetylase inhibitors induce thyroid cancer-specific apoptosis through proteasome-dependent inhibition of TRAIL degradation, *Oncogene* 29:105-116.

Bortul, R., Tazzari, P.L., Cappellini, A., Tabellini, G., Billi, A.M., et al. (2003). Constitutively active Akt1 protects HL60 leukemia cells from TRAIL-induced apoptosis through a mechanism involving NF-kappaB activation and cFLIP(L) up-regulation, *Leukemia* 17:379–389.

Braun, F.K., Fecker, L.F., Schwarz, C., Walden, P., Assaf, C., et al. (2007). Blockade of death receptor-mediated pathways early in the signaling cascade coincides with distinct apoptosis resistance in cutaneous T-cell lymphoma cells, *J Invest Dermatol* 127(10):2425-2437.

Buckle, C.H., Neville-Webbe, H.L., Croucher, P.I. & Lawson, M.A. (2010). Targeting RANK/RANKL in the treatment of solid tumours and myeloma, *Curr Pharm Des* 16(11):1272-1283.

Burns, T.F., Bernhard, E.J. & El-Deiry, W.S. (2001). Tissue specific expression of p53 target genes suggests a key role for KILLER/DR5 in p53-dependent apoptosis in vivo, *Oncogene* 20(34):4601-4612.

Caravatta, L., Sancilio, S., di Giacomo, V., Rana, R., Cataldi, A. & Di Pietro, R. (2008). PI3-K/Akt-dependent activation of cAMP-response element-binding (CREB) protein in Jurkat T leukemia cells treated with TRAIL, *J Cell Physiol* 214(1):192-200.

Cardone, M.H., Roy, N., Stennicke, H.R., Salvesen, G.S., Franke, T.F., et al. (1998). Regulation of cell death protease caspase-9 by phosphorylation, *Science* 282(5392):1318-1321.

Chamuleau, M.E., Ossenkoppele, G.J., van Rhenen, A., van Dreunen, L., Jirka, S.M., et al. (2011). High TRAIL-R3 expression on leukemic blasts is associated with poor outcome and induces apoptosis-resistance which can be overcome by targeting TRAIL-R2, *Leuk Res* 35(6):741-749.

Chen, X., Thakkar, H., Tyan, F., Gim, S., Robinson, H., et al. (2001). Constitutively active Akt is an important regulator of TRAIL sensitivity in prostate cancer, *Oncogene* 20:6073–6083.

Chen, X., Kandasamy, K. & Srivastava, R.K. (2003). Differential roles of RelA (p65) and c-Rel subunits of nuclear factor kappa B in tumor necrosis factor-related apoptosis-inducing ligand signalling, *Cancer Res* 63:1059-1066.

Chinnaiyan, A.M., Prasad, U., Shankar, S., Hamstra, D.A., Shanaiah, M., et al. (2000). Combined effect of tumor necrosis factor-related apoptosis-inducing ligand and ionizing radiation in breast cancer therapy, *Proc Natl Acad Sci U S A* 97:1754–1759.

Cillessen, S.A., Meijer, C.J., Ossenkoppele, G.J., Castricum, K.C., Westra, A.H., et al. (2006). Human soluble TRAIL/Apo2L induces apoptosis in a subpopulation of chemotherapy refractory nodal diffuse large B-cell lymphomas, determined by a highly sensitive in vitro apoptosis assay, *Br J Haematol* 134:283–293.

Clancy, L., Mruk, K., Archer, K., Woelfel, M., Mongkolsapaya, J., et al. (2005). Preligand assembly domain-mediated ligand independent association between TRAIL receptor 4 TR4 and TR2 regulates TRAIL-induced apoptosis, *PNAS* 102(50):18099–18104.

Clodi, K., Wimmer, D., Li, Y., Goodwin, R., Jaeger, U., et al. (2000). Expression of tumor necrosis factor (TNF)-related apoptosis-inducing ligand (TRAIL) receptors and sensitivity to TRAIL-induced apoptosis in primary B-cell acute lymphoblastic leukaemia cells, *Br J Haematol* 111:580-586.

Coll-Mulet, L., Iglesias-Serret, D., Santidrián, A.F., Cosialls, A.M., de Frias, M., et al. (2006). MDM2 antagonists activate p53 and synergize with genotoxic drugs in B-cell chronic lymphocytic leukemia cells, *Blood* 107(10):4109-4114.

Corallini, F., Rimondi, E. & Secchiero, P. (2008). TRAIL and osteoprotegerin: a role in endothelial physiopathology?, *Front Biosci* 1;13:135-147.

Cretney, E., Takeda, K. & Smyth, M.J. (2007). Cancer: novel therapeutic strategies that exploit the TNF-related apoptosis-inducing ligand (TRAIL)/TRAIL receptor pathway, *Int J Biochem Cell Biol* 39(2):280-286.

Di Pietro, R., Secchiero, P., Rana, R., Gibellini, D., Visani, G., et al. (2001). Ionizing radiation sensitizes erythroleukemic cells but not normal erythroblasts to tumor necrosis factor-related apoptosis-inducing ligand (TRAIL)-mediated cytotoxicity by selective up-regulation of TRAIL-R1, *Blood* 97(9): 2596-2603.

Di Pietro, R. & Zauli, G. (2004). Emerging non-apoptotic functions of tumour necrosis factor-related apoptosis-inducing ligand (TRAIL)/Apo2L, *J Cell Physiol* 201: 331-340.

Dicker, F., Kater, A.P., Fukuda, T. & Kipps, T.J. (2005). Fas-ligand (CD178) and TRAIL synergistically induce apoptosis of CD40-activated chronic lymphocytic leukemia B cells, *Blood* 105(8):3193-3198.

Didaa, F., Lia, Y., Iwaoa, A., Deguchia, T., Azumaa, E. & Komada, Y. (2008). Resistance to TRAIL-induced apoptosis caused by constitutional phosphorylation of Akt and PTEN in acute lymphoblastic leukemia cells, *Exp Hematol* 36:1343–1353.

Drakos, E., Thomaides, A., Medeiros, L.J., Li, J., Leventaki, V., et al. (2007). Inhibition of p53-murine double minute 2 interactions by nutlin 3-A stabilizes p53 and induces cell cycle arrest and apoptosis in Hodgkin Lymphoma, *Clin Cancer Res* 13: 3380-3387.

Duiker, E.W., Mom, C.H., de Jong, S., Willemse, P.H., Gietema, J.A., et al. (2006). The clinical trail of TRAIL, *Eur J Cancer* 42(14):2233-2240.

Ehrhardt, H., Fulda, S., Schmid, I., Hiscott, J., Debatin, K-M. & Jeremias, I. (2003). TRAIL induced survival and proliferation in cancer cells resistant towards TRAIL-induced apoptosis mediated by NF-kappaB, *Oncogene* 22:3842-3852.

Emery, J.G., McDonnell, P., Burke, M.B., Deen, K.C., Lyn, S., et al. (1998). Osteoprotegerin is a receptor for the cytotoxic ligand TRAIL, *J Biol Chem* 273:14363-14367.

Falschlehner, C., Emmerich, C.H., Gerlach, B. & Walczak, H. (2007). TRAIL signalling: decisions between life and death, *Int J Biochem Cell Biol* 39:1462–1475.

Falschlehner, C., Schaefer, U. & Walczak, H. (2009). Following TRAIL's path in the immune system, *Immunology* 127(2):145-154.

Fas, S.C., Baumann, S., Zhu, J.Y., Giaisi, M., Treiber, M.K. et al. (2006). Wogonin sensitizes resistant malignant cells to TNFalpha- and TRAIL-induced apoptosis, *Blood* 108:3700-3706.

Finnegan, M.C., Goepel, J.R., Royds, J., Hancock, B.W. & Goyns, M.H. (1994). Elevated levels of MDM-2 and p53 expression are associated with high grade non-Hodgkin's lymphomas, *Cancer Lett* 11: 215-221.

Frese, S., Pirnia, F., Miescher, D., Krajewski, S., Borner, M.M., et al. (2003). PG490-mediated sensitization of lung cancer cells to Apo2L/TRAIL-induced apoptosis requires activation of ERK2, *Oncogene* 22:5427–5435.

Gazitt, Y. (1999). TRAIL is a potent inducer of apoptosis in myeloma cells derived from multiple myeloma patients and is not cytotoxic to hematopoietic stem cells, *Leukemia* 13(11):1817-1824.

Georgakis, G.V., Li, Y., Humphreys, R., Andreeff, M., O'Brien, S., et al. (2005). Activity of selective fully human agonistic antibodies to the TRAIL death receptors TRAIL-R1 and TRAIL-R2 in primary and cultured lymphoma cells: induction of apoptosis and enhancement of doxorubicin- and bortezomib-induced cell death, *Br J Haematol* 130: 501–510.

Goldberg, J.M., Silverman, L.B., Levy, D.E., Dalton VK, Gelber RD, et al. (2003). Childhood T-cell acute lymphoblastic leukemia: the Dana-Farber cancer institute acute lymphoblastic leukemia consortium experience, *J Clin Oncol* 21:3616–3622.

Gong, B. & Almasan, A. (2000). Genomic organization and transcriptional regulation of the human Apo2L/TRAIL gene, *Biochem Biophys Res Commun* 278:747-752.

Green, D. (2000). Apoptotic pathways: paper wraps stone blunts scissors. *Cell* 102:1-4.

Greil, R., Anether, G., Johrer, K. & Tinhofer, I. (2003). Tracking death dealing by Fas and TRAIL in lymphatic neoplastic disorders: pathways, targets, and therapeutic tools, *J Leukoc Biol* 74(3):311-330.

Griffith, T.S. & Lynch, D.H. (1998). TRAIL: a molecule with multiple receptors and control mechanisms, *Curr Opin Immunol* 10(5):559-563.

Griffith, T.S., Rauch, C.T., Smolak, P.J., Waugh, J.Y., Boiani, N., et al. (1999). Functional analysis of TRAIL receptors using monoclonal antibodies, *J Immunol* 162:2605.

Hamilton, A., Gallipoli, P., Nicholson, E. & Holyoake, T.L. (2010). Targeted therapy in haematological malignancies, *J Pathol* 220:404-418.

Henson, E.S., Johnston, J.B. & Gibson, S.B. (2008). The role of TRAIL death receptors in the treatment of hematological malignancies, *Leukemia & Lymphoma* 49(1): 27–35.

Huang, Y. & Sheikh, M.S. (2007). TRAIL death receptors and cancer therapeutics, *Toxicol Appl Pharmacol*; 224(3):284-289.

Hussain, A.R., Ahmed, M., Al-Jomah, N.A., Khan, A.S., Manogaran, P., et al. (2008). Curcumin suppresses constitutive activation of nuclear factor-kappa B and requires functional Bax to induce apoptosis in Burkitt's lymphoma cell lines, *Mol Cancer Ther* 7:3318–3329.

Impicciatore, G., Sancilio, S., Miscia S. & Di Pietro, R. (2010). Nutlins and ionizing radiation in cancer therapy, *Curr Pharm Des* 16(12):1427-1442.

Inukai, T., Zhang, X., Goto, M., Hirose, K., Uno, K., et al.(2006). Resistance of infant leukemia with MLL rearrangement to tumor necrosis factor-related apoptosis-inducing ligand: a possible mechanism for poor sensitivity to antitumor immunity, *Leukemia* 20(12):2119-2129.

Jacquemin, G., Shirley, S. & Micheau, O. (2010). Combining naturally occurring polyphenols with TNF-related apoptosis-inducing ligand: a promising approach to kill resistant cancer cells? *Cell Mol Life Sci* 67:3115–3130.

Jo, M., Kim, T.H., Seol, D.W., Esplen, J.E., Dorko, K., et al. (2000). Apoptosis induced in normal human hepatocytes by tumor necrosis factor-related apoptosis-inducing ligand, *Nat Med* 6:567.

Jones, R.G., Elford, A.R., Parsons, M.J., Wu, L., Krawczyk, C.M., et al. (2002). CD28-dependent activation of protein kinase B/Akt blocks Fas-mediated apoptosis by preventing death-inducing signaling complex assembly, *J Exp Med* 196(3):335-348.

Jones, D.T., Ganeshaguru, K., Mitchell, W.A., Foroni, L., Baker, R.J., et al. (2003). Cytotoxic drugs enhance the ex vivo sensitivity of malignant cells from a subset of acute myeloid leukaemia patients to apoptosis induction by tumour necrosis factor receptor-related apoptosis-inducing ligand, *Br J Haematol* 121(5):713-720.

Jurewicz, A., Matysiak, M., Andrzejak, S. & Selmaj, K. (2006). TRAIL-induced death of human adult oligodendrocytes is mediated by JNK pathway, *Glia* 53:158–166.

Kabore, A.F., Sun, J., Hu, X., McCrea, K., Johnston, J.B. & Gibson, S.B. (2006). The TRAIL apoptotic pathway mediates proteasome inhibitor induced apoptosis in primary chronic lymphocytic leukemia cells, *Apoptosis* 11:1175–1193.

Kamdasamy, K. & Kraft, A.S. (2008). Proteasome inhibitor PS-341 (VELCADE) induces stabilization of the TRAIL receptor DR5 mRNA through the 3′-untranslated region, *Mol Cancer Ther* 7(5):1091-1100.

Kelley, S.K. & Ashkenazi, A. (2004). Targeting death receptors in cancer with Apo2L/TRAIL, *Curr Opin Pharmacol* 4(4):333-339.

Kischkel, F.C., Hellbardt, S., Behrmann, I., Germer, M., Pawlita, M., et al. (1995). Cytotoxicity-dependent APO-1 (Fas/CD95)-associated proteins form a death-inducing signaling complex (DISC) with the receptor, *EMBO J* 14:5579-5588.

Kischkel, F.C., Lawrence, D.A., Tinel, A., Virmani, A., Schow, P., et al. (2001). Death receptor recruitment of endogenous caspase-10 and apoptosis initiation in the absence of caspase-8, *J Biol Chem* 276:46639-46646.

Kojima, K., Konopleva, M., Samudio, I.J., Shikami, M., Cabreira-Hansen, M., et al. (2005). MDM2 antagonists induce p53-dependent apoptosis in AML: implication for leukemia therapy, *Blood* 106: 3150-3159.

Koschny, R., Walczak, H. & Ganten, T.M. (2007). The promise of TRAIL-potential and risks of a novel anticancer therapy, *J Mol Med* 85(9):923-935.

Laguinge, L.M., Samara, R.N., Wang, W., El-Deiry, W.S., Corner, G., et al. (2008). DR5 receptor mediates anoikis in human colorectal carcinoma cell lines, *Cancer Res* 68(3):909-917.

Lawrence, D., Sdhahroth, Z., Marsters, S., Achilles, K., Shih, D., et al. (2001). Differential hepatocyte toxicity of recombinant Apo2L/TRAIL versions, *Nat Med* 7:383-385.

LeBlanc, H.N. & Ashkenazi, A. (2003). Apo2L/TRAIL and its death and decoy receptors, *Cell Death Differ* 10:66-75.

Lee, S.H., Shin, M.S., Kim, H.S., Lee, H.K., Park, W.S., et al. (1999). Alterations of the DR5/TRAIL receptor 2 gene in non-small cell lung cancers, *Cancer Res* 59:5686.

Lee, S.H., Shin, M.S., Kim, H.S., Lee, H.K., Park, W.S., et al. (2001). Somatic mutations of TRAIL-receptor 1 and TRAIL-receptor 2 genes in non-Hodgkin's lymphoma, *Oncogene* 20:399–403.

Lehmann, B.D., McCubrey, J.A., Jefferson, H.S., Paine, M.S., Chappel, W.H. & Terrian, D.M. (2007). A dominant role for p53 dependent cellular senescence in radiosensitization of human prostate cancer cells, *Cell Cycle* 6: 595-596.

Leverkus, M., Neumann, M., Mengling, T., Rauch, C.T., Bröcker, E.B., et al. (2000). Regulation of tumor necrosis factor-related apoptosis-inducing ligand sensitivity in primary and transformed human keratinocytes, *Cancer Res* 60(3):553-559.

Lin, Y., Devin, A., Cook, A., Keane, M.M., Kelliher, M., et al. (2000). The death domain kinase RIP is essential for TRAIL (Apo2L)-induced activation of IkappaB kinase and c-Jun N-terminal kinase, *Mol Cell Biol* 20:6638–6645.

Liu, Q., Hilsenbeck, S. & Gazitt, Y. (2003). Arsenic trioxide-induced apoptosis in myeloma cells: p53-dependent G1 or G2/M cell cycle arrest, activation of caspase-8 or caspase-9, and synergy with APO2/TRAIL, *Blood* 101(10):4078-4087.

Locklin, R.M., Croucher, P.I., Russell, R.G. & Edwards, C.M. (2007). Agonists of TRAIL death receptors induce myeloma cell apoptosis that is not prevented by cells of the bone marrow microenvironment, *Leukemia* 21(4):805-812.

MacFarlane, M., Harper, N., Snowden, R.T., Dyer, M.J., Barnett, G.A., et al. (2002). Mechanisms of resistance to TRAIL-induced apoptosis in primary B cell chronic lymphocytic leukaemia, *Oncogene* 21(44):6809-6818.

MacFarlane, M. (2003). TRAIL-induced signaling and apoptosis, *Toxicol Lett* 139:89-97.

MacFarlane, M., Kohlhaas, S.L., Sutcliffe, M.J., Dyer, M.J. & Cohen, G.M. (2005). TRAIL receptor-selective mutants signal to apoptosis via TRAIL-R1 in primary lymphoid malignancies, *Cancer Res* 65(24):11265-11270.

Maddipatla, S., Hernandez-Ilizaliturri, F.J., Knight, J. & Czuczman MS. (2007). Antibodies Targeting TRAIL-R1and CD20, *Clin Cancer Res* 13(15): 4556-4564.

Mahalingam, D., Szegezdi, E., Keane, M., Jong, S. & Samali, A. (2009). TRAIL receptor signalling and modulation: are we on the right TRAIL? *Cancer Treat Rev* 35:280–288.

Mahmood, Z. & Shukla, Y. (2010). Death receptors: targets for cancer therapy, *Exp Cell Res* 316:887-899.

Mai, A. & Altucci, L. (2009). Epi-drugs to fight cancer: from chemistry to cancer treatment, the road ahead, *Int J Biochem Cell Biol* 41: 199-213.

Mariani, S.M. & Krammer, P.H. (1998). Differential regulation of TRAIL and CD95 ligand in transformed cells of the T and B lymphocyte lineage, *Eur J Immunol* 28(3):973-982.

Marini, P., Denzinger, D., Schiller, S., Kauder, S., Welz, R., et al. (2006). Combined treatment of colorectal tumours with agonistic TRAIL receptor antibodies HGS-ETR1 and HGS-ETR2 and radiotherapy: enhanced effects in vitro and dose-dependent growth delay in vivo, *Oncogene* 25: 5145-5154.

Marsters, S.A., Sheridan, J.P., Pitti, R.M., Huang, A., Skubatch, M., et al. (1997). A novel receptor for Apo2L/TRAIL contains a truncated death domain, *Curr Biol* 7:1003-1006.

Martelli, A.M., Nyakern, M., Tabellini, G., Bortul, R., Tazzari P.L. et al. (2006). Phosphoinositide 3-kinase/Akt signaling pathway and its therapeutical implications for human acute myeloid leukemia, *Leukemia* 20, 911–928.

Mellier, G., Huang, S., Shenoy, K. & Pervaiz, S. (2010). TRAILing death in cancer, *Mol Aspects Med* 31(1):93-112.

Meurette, O., Fontaine, A., Rebillard, A., Le Moigne, G., Lamy, T., et al. (2006). Cytotoxicity of TRAIL/anticancer drug combinations in human normal cells, *Ann N Y Acad Sci* 1090:209-216.

Milani, D., Zauli, G., Rimondi, E., Celeghini, C., Marmiroli, S., et al. (2003). Tumour necrosis factor-related apoptosis-inducing ligand sequentially activates pro-survival and pro-apoptotic pathways in SK-N-MC neuronal cells, *J Neurochem* 86(1):126-135.

Mitsiades, N., Mitsiades, C.S., Poulaki, V., Chauhan, D., Richardson, P.G., et al. (2002). Biologic sequelae of nuclear factor-kappaB blockade in multiple myeloma: therapeutic applications, *Blood* 99(11):4086.

Momand, J., Jung, D., Wilczynski, S. & Niland, J. (1998). The MDM2 gene amplification database, *Nucleic Acid Res* 26: 3453-3459.

Morel, J., Audo, R., Hahne, M. & Combe, B. (2005). Tumor necrosis factor-related apoptosis inducing ligand (TRAIL) induces rheumatoid arthritis synovial fibroblast proliferation through mitogen-activated protein kinases and phosphatidylinositol 3-kinase/Akt, *J Biol Chem* 280:15709–15718.

Motoki, K., Mori, E., Matsumoto, A., Thomas, M., Tomura, T., et al. (2005). Enhanced apoptosis and tumor regression induced by a direct agonist antibody to tumor necrosis factor-related apoptosis-inducing ligand receptor 2, *Clin Cancer Res* 11:3126-3135.

Mühlenbeck, F., Haas, E., Schwenzer, R., Schubert, G., Grell, M., Smith, C., et al. (1998). TRAIL/Apo2L activates c-Jun NH2-terminal kinase (JNK) via caspase-dependent and caspase-independent pathways, *J Biol Chem* 273:33091-33098.

Natoni, A., MacFarlane, M., Inoue, S., Walewska, R., Majid, A., et al. (2007). TRAIL signals to apoptosis in chronic lymphocytic leukaemia cells primarily through TRAIL-R1 whereas cross-linked agonistic TRAIL-R2 antibodies facilitate signalling via TRAIL-R2, *Br J Haematol* 39(4):568-577.

Olsson, A., Diaz, T., Aguilar-Santelises, M., Osterborg, A., Celsing, F., et al. (2001). Sensitization to TRAIL-induced apoptosis and modulation of FLICE-inhibitory protein in B chronic lymphocytic leukemia by actinomycin D, *Leukemia* 15(12):1868-1877.

Ozören, N. & El-Deiry, W.S. (2003). Cell surface death receptor signaling in normal and cancer cells, *Semin Cancer Biol* 13(2):135-147.

Pan, G., O'Rourke, K., Chinnaiyan, A.M., Gentz, R., Ebner, R., et al. (1997a). The receptor for the cytotoxic ligand TRAIL, *Science* 276:111-113.

Pan, G., Ni, J., Wei, Y.F., Yu, G., Gentz, R. & Dixit, V.M. (1997b). An antagonist decoy receptor and a new death domain-containing receptor for TRAIL, *Science* 277:815-818.

Papenfuss, K., Cordier, S.M. & Walczak, H. (2008). Death receptors as targets for anti-cancer therapy, *J Cell Mol Med* 12:2585.

Park, S.M., Schickel, R. & Peter, M.E.(2005). Nonapoptotic functions of FADD-binding death receptors and their signaling molecules, *Curr Opin Cell Biol* 17(6):610-616.

Park, S.J., Kim, M.J., Kim, H.B., Kang, C.D. & Kim, S.H. (2009). Sensitization of imatinib-resistant CML cells to TRAIL-induced apoptosis is mediated through down-regulation of Bcr-Abl as well as c-FLIP, *Biochem J* 28;420(1):73-81.

Paydas, S., Tanriverdi, K., Yavuz, S., Disel, U., Sahin, B. & Burgut, R. (2003). Survivin and aven: two distinct antiapoptotic signals in acute leukemias. *Ann Oncol* 14(7):1045.

Pedersen, I.M., Kitada, S., Schimmer, A., Kim, Y., Zapata, J.M., et al. (2002). The triterpenoid CDDO induces apoptosis in refractory CLL B cells, *Blood* 100(8):2965-2972.

Pitti, R.M., Marsters, S.A., Ruppert, S., Donahue, C.J., Moore, A. & Ashkenazi, A. (1996). Induction of apoptosis by Apo-2 ligand, a new member of the tumor necrosis factor cytokine family, *J Biol Chem* 271(22):12687-12690.

Pukac, L., Kanakaraj, P., Humphreys, R., Alderson, R., Bloom, M., et al. (2005). HGS-ETR1, a fully human TRAIL receptor 1 monoclonal antibody, induces cell death in multiple tumour types in vitro and in vivo, *Br J Cancer* 92: 1430–1441.

Rayet, B. & Gelinas, C. (1999). Aberrant *rel/nfkb* genes and activity in human cancer, *Oncogene* 18:6938-6947.

Reed, J.C., Kitada, S., Kim, Y. & Byrd, J. (2002). Modulating apoptosis pathways in low-grade B-cell malignancies using biological response modifiers, *Semin Oncol* 29(1 Suppl 2):10-24.

Richardson, S.J., Matthews, C., Catherwood, M.A., Alexander, H.D., Carey, B.S., et al. (2006). ZAP-70 expression is associated with enhanced ability to respond to migratory and survival signals in B-cell chronic lymphocytic leukemia (B-CLL), *Blood* 107:3584–3592.

Roos, W.P. & Kaina, B. (2006). DNA damage-induced cell death by apoptosis, *Trends Mol Med* 12:440–450.

Roue, G., Perez-Galan, P., Lopez-Guerra, M., Villamor, N., Campo, E. & Colomer, D. (2007). Selective inhibition of IkappaB kinase sensitizes mantle cell lymphoma B cells to TRAIL by decreasing cellular FLIP level, *J Immunol* 178:1923–1930.

Russo, M., Mupo, A., Spagnuolo, C. & Russo G.L. (2010). Exploring death receptor pathways as selective targets in cancer therapy, *Biochem Pharmacol* 80:674–682.

Russo, M., Nigro, P., Rosiello, R., D'Arienzo, R. & Russo, G.L. (2007). Quercetin enhances CD95- and TRAIL-induced apoptosis in leukemia cell lines, *Leukemia* 21:1130–1133.

Sabatini, N., Di Pietro, R., Rapino, M., Sancilio, S., Comani, S. & Cataldi, A. (2004). PI-3-kinase/NF-κB mediated response of Jurkat T leukemic cells to two different chemotherapeutic drugs, Etoposide and TRAIL, *J Cell Biochem* 93(2):301-311.

Salvesen, G.S. & Abrams, J.M. (2004). Caspase activation - stepping on the gas or releasing the brakes? Lessons from humans and flies, *Oncogene* 23(16):2774-2784.

Sancilio, S., Grill, V. & Di Pietro, R. (2008). A combined approach with rituximab plus anti-TRAIL-R agonistic antibodies for the treatment of haematological malignancies, *Curr Pharm Des* 14(21):2085-2099.

Sayers, T. J. & Murphy, W. J. (2006). Combining proteasome inhibition with TNF-related apoptosis-inducing ligand (Apo2L/TRAIL) for cancer therapy. *Immunol Immunother* 55:76–84.

Schaefer, U., Voloshanenko, O., Willen, D. & Walczak, H. (2007). TRAIL: a multifunctional cytokine, *Front Biosci* 12:3813-3824.

Schneider, P., Bodmer, J.L., Thome, M., Hofmann, K., Holler, N. & Tschopp, J. (1997). Characterization of two receptors for TRAIL, *FEBS Lett* 416:329-334.

Secchiero, P., Gonelli, A., Mirandola, P., Melloni, E., Zamai, L., et al. (2002). Tumor necrosis factor-related apoptosis-inducing ligand induces monocytic maturation of leukemic and normal myeloid precursors through a caspase-dependent pathway, *Blood* 100:2421-2429.

Secchiero, P., Melloni, E., Heikinheimo, M., Mannisto, S., Di Pietro, R., et al. (2004a). TRAIL regulates normal erythroid maturation through an ERK-dependent pathway, *Blood* 103(2):517-522.

Secchiero, P., Vaccarezza, M., Gonelli, A. & Zauli, G. (2004b). TNF-related apoptosis-inducing ligand (TRAIL): a potential candidate for combined treatment of hematological malignancies, *Curr Pharm Des* 10(29):3673-3681.

Secchiero, P., Zerbinati, C., Melloni, E., Milani, D., Campioni, D., et al. (2007). The MDM-2 antagonist nutlin-3 promotes the maturation of acute myeloid leukemic blasts, *Neoplasia* 9(10):853-861.

Secchiero, P. & Zauli, G. (2008). Tumor-necrosis-factor-related apoptosis-inducing ligand and the regulation of hematopoiesis, *Curr Opin Hematol* 15(1):42-48.

Seki, N., Hayakawa, Y., Brooks, A.D., Wine, J., Wiltrout, R.H., et al. (2003). Tumor necrosis factor-related apoptosis-inducing ligand-mediated apoptosis is an important endogenous mechanism for resistance to liver metastases in murine renal cancer, *Cancer Res* 63(1):207-213.

Shangary, S. & Wang, S. (2009). Small-molecule inhibitors of the MDM2-p53 protein-protein interaction to reactive p53 function: a novel approach for cancer therapy, *Annu Rev Pharmacol Toxicol* 49: 223-241.

Shin, M.S., Kim, H.S., Lee, S.H., Park, W.S., Kim, S.Y., et al. (2001). Mutations of tumor necrosis factor-related apoptosis-inducing ligand receptor 1 (TRAIL-R1) and receptor 2 (TRAIL-R2) genes in metastatic breast cancers, *Cancer Res* 61:4942–4946.

Signore, M., Ricci-Vitiani, L & De Maria, R. (2011). Targeting apoptosis pathways in cancer stem cells, *Cancer Lett* [Epub ahead of print], doi:10.1016/j.canlet.2011.01.013

Snell, V., Clodi, K., Zhao, S., Goodwin, R., Thomas, E.K., et al. (1997). Activity of TNF-related apoptosis-inducing ligand (TRAIL) in haematological malignancies, *Br J Haematol* 99:618-624.

Sprick, M.R., Weigand, M.A., Rieser, E., Rausch, C.T., Juo, P., et al. (2000). FADD/MORT1 and caspase-8 are recruited to TRAIL receptors 1 and 2 and are essential for apoptosis mediated by TRAIL receptor 2, *Immunity* 12:599-609.

Sprick, M.R. & Walczak, H. (2004). The interplay between the Bcl-2 family and death receptor-mediated apoptosis, *Biochim Biophys Acta* 1644:125–132.

Stuhmer, T., Chatterjee, M., Hildebrandt, M., Herrmann, P., Gollasch, H., et al. (2005). Nongenotoxic activation of the p53 pathway as a therapeutic strategy for multiple myeloma, *Blood* 106: 3609-3617.

Suh, W.S., Kim, Y.S., Schimmer, A.D., Kitada, S., Minden, M., et al. (2003). Synthetic triterpenoids activate a pathway for apoptosis in AML cells involving downregulation of FLIP and sensitization to TRAIL, *Leukemia* 17(11):2122-2129.

Sung, B., Park, B., Yadav, V.R. & Aggarwal, B.B. (2010). Celastrol, a triterpene, enhances TRAIL-induced apoptosis through the down-regulation of cell survival proteins and up-regulation of death receptors, *J Biol Chem* 285:11498–11507.

Tamm, I., Kornblau, S.M., Segall, H., Krajewski, S., Welsh, K., et al. (2000). Expression and prognostic significance of IAP-family genes in human cancers and myeloid leukemias, *Clin Cancer Res* 6(5):1796-1803.

Tanaka, H., Ito, T., Kyo, T. & Kimura, A. (2007). Treatment with IFNalpha in vivo up-regulates serum-soluble TNF-related apoptosis inducing ligand (sTRAIL) levels and TRAIL mRNA expressions in neutrophils in chronic myelogenous leukemia patients, *Eur J Haematol* 78(5):389-398.

Tartaglia, L.A. & Goeddel, D.V. (1992). Two TNF receptors. *Immunol Today* 13:151-153.

Testa, U. (2010). TRAIL/TRAIL-R in hematologic malignancies, *J Cell Biochem* 110(1):21-34.

Thomas, L.R., Henson, A., Reed, J.C., Salsbury, F.R. & Thorburn, A. (2004). Direct binding of Fas-associated death domain (FADD) to the tumor necrosis factor-related apoptosis-inducing ligand receptor DR5 is regulated by the death effector domain of FADD, *J Biol Chem* 279(31):32780-32785.

Tolcher, A.W., Mita, M., Meropol, N.J., von Mehren, M. & Patnaik, A. et al. (2007). Phase I pharmacokinetic and biologic correlative study of mapatumumab, a fully human monoclonal antibody with agonist activity to tumor necrosis factor-related apoptosis inducing ligand receptor-1, *J Clin Oncol* 25:1390–1395.

Uno, K., Inukai, T., Kayagaki, N., Goi, K., Sato, H., et al. (2003). TNF-related apoptosis-inducing ligand (TRAIL) frequently induces apoptosis in Philadelphia chromosome-positive leukemia cells, *Blood* 101(9):3658-3667.

Urruticoechea, A., Alemany, R., Balart, J., Villanueva, A., Viñals, F. & Capellá G. (2010). Recent advances in cancer therapy: an overview, *Curr Pharm Des* 16(1):3-10.

Vassilev, L.T., Vu, B.T., Graves, B., Carvajal, D., Podlaski, F., et al. (2004). In vivo activation of the p53 pathway by small-molecule antagonists of MDM2, *Science* 303: 844-848.

Vogler, M., Walczak, H., Stadel, D., Haas, T.L., Genze, F., et al. (2008). Targeting XIAP bypasses Bcl-2-mediated resistance to TRAIL and cooperates with TRAIL to suppress pancreatic cancer growth in vitro and in vivo, *Cancer Res* 68:7956–7965.

Wagner, K.W., Punnoose, E.A., Januario, T., Lawrence, D.A., Pitti, R.M., et al. (2007). Death-receptor O-glycosylation controls tumor-cell sensitivity to the proapoptotic ligand Apo2L/TRAIL, *Nat Med* 13:1070–1077.

Wajant, H., Moosmayer, D., Wüest, T., Bartke, T., Gerlach, E., et al. (2001). Differential activation of TRAIL-R1 and -2 by soluble and membrane TRAIL allows selective surface antigen-directed activation of TRAIL-R2 by a soluble TRAIL derivative, *Oncogene* 20(30):4101-4106.

Walczak, H., Miller, R.E., Ariail, K., Gliniak, B., Griffith, T.S., et al. (1999). Tumoricidal activity of tumor-necrosis factor-related apoptosis-inducing ligand in vivo, *Nat Med* 5:157-163.

Walczak, H. & Krammer, P.H. (2000). The CD95 (APO-1/Fas) and the TRAIL (APO-2L) Apoptosis Systems, *Exp Cell Res* 256:58-66.

Wang, C.Y., Mayo, M.W., Korneluk, R.G., Goeddel, D.V. & Baldwin Jr, A.S. (1998). NF-kappaB antiapoptosis: induction of TRAF1 and TRAF2 and c-IAP1 and c-IAP2 to suppress caspase-8 activation, *Science* 274:782-784.

Wiley, S.R., Schooley, K., Smolak, P.J., Din, W.S., Huang, C.P., et al. (1995). Identification and characterization of a new member of the TNF family that induces apoptosis, *Immunity* 3(6):673-82.

Yang, X. & Thiele, C.J. (2003). Targeting the tumor necrosis factor-related apoptosis-inducing ligand path in neuroblastoma, *Cancer Lett* 197(1-2):137-143.

Zang, D.Y., Goodwin, R.G., Loken, M.R., Bryant, E. & Deeg, H.J. (2001). Expression of tumor necrosis factor-related apoptosis-inducing ligand, Apo2L, and its receptors in myelodysplastic syndrome: effects on in vitro hemopoiesis, *Blood* 98(10):3058-3065.

Zauli, G., Pandolfi, A., Gonelli, A., Di Pietro, R., Guarnieri, S., et al. (2003). Tumor necrosis factor-Related Apoptosis-Inducing Ligand (TRAIL) sequentially upregulates nitric oxide and prostanoid production in primary human endothelial cells, *Circ Res* 92(7):732-740.

Zauli, G., Sancilio, S., Cataldi, A., Sabatini, N., Bosco, D. & Di Pietro, R. (2005). PI-3K/Akt and NF-kappaB/IkappaBalpha pathways are activated in Jurkat T cells in response to TRAIL treatment, *J Cell Physiol* 202: 900-911.

Zerafa, N., Westwood, J.A., Cretney, E., Mitchell, S., Waring, P., et al. (2005). TRAIL deficiency accelerates hematological malignancies, *J Immunol* 175: 5586–5590.

# 11

# Therapeutical Cues from the Tumor Microenvironment

Stefano Marastoni, Eva Andreuzzi,
Roberta Colladel, Alice Paulitti, Alessandra Silvestri,
Federico Todaro, Alfonso Colombatti and Maurizio Mongiat
*Experimental Oncology Division 2, CRO-IRCCS, Aviano*
*Italy*

## 1. Introduction

The tumor can be considered a complex organ where transformed cells characterized by high genomic instability and altered gene expression are interconnected and communicate with the surrounding microenvironment. The microenvironment (Fig. 1) is composed of a large variety of stromal cells including inflammatory, stem and progenitor cells, fibroblasts, myofibroblasts, perycites, endothelial and mural cells of the blood vessels which are interconnected with the components of the extracellular matrix (ECM). The crosstalk between these components and cancer cells deeply affects their survival and proliferation. Due to the critical role of these interactions in cancer progression, each cellular or molecular component represents a potential target for the development of useful drugs in cancer treatment. The cells of the microenvironment are more genetically stable compared to the

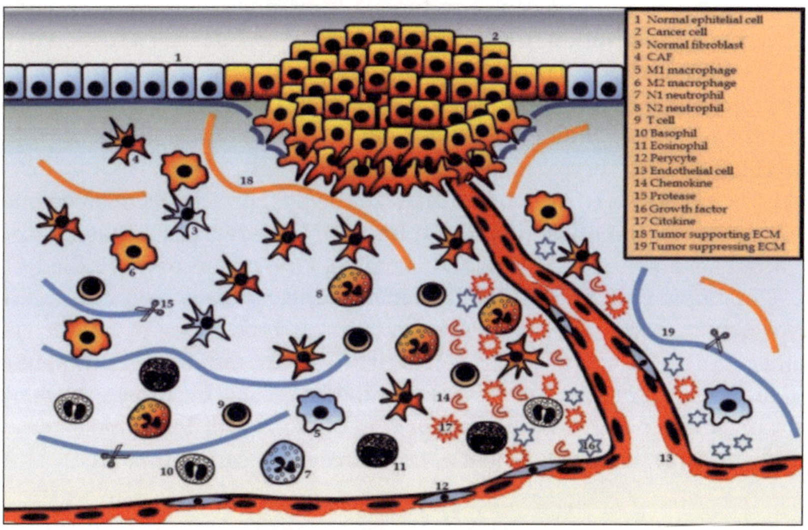


Fig. 1. Schematic representation of the tumor microenvironment; CAF: Cancer Associated Fibroblasts; ECM: extracellular matrix.

tumor cells, and a combinatorial treatment targeting both cancer cells and components of the microenvironment holds the potential for a more successful outcome. In this chapter will list some examples of molecular cues from tumor cells and the surrounding microenvironment that are important for tumor growth and progression and due to their key role in this process are targets for therapeutic drugs under investigation or in clinical use. We will focus on tumor cells and the regulation of proliferation and survival by receptor tyrosine kinases and apoptosis. A number of cellular components of the tumor microenvironment involved in the process of angiogenesis and how ECM affects this process will be taken into account and the effects of some ECM molecules directly affecting tumor cell survival and growth will be also discussed.

### 1.1 Cell signaling: Receptor tyrosine kinases

Networks of protein-protein and protein-metabolite interactions are commonly found in biological systems where signals must be passed from one location or component within the microenvironment to another. Receptor tyrosine kinases (RTKs) have the critical function of transducing signals derived from extracellular ligands to several intracellular pathways. Regulation of such networks is often achieved by transient, reversible modifications of the components involved. To date, more than 200 different types of post translational modifications (PTMs) have been identified, but by far the best appreciated and among the most important involve phosphorylation of serine, threonine and tyrosine residues. Phosphorylation is one of the most studied PTM because it is vital for a large number of protein functions and characterizes many cellular processes spanning from signal transduction, cell differentiation and development to cell cycle control and metabolism. A primary role of phosphorylation is to act as a switch to turn "on" or "off" a protein activity or a cellular pathway in an acute and reversible manner (Hunter, 1995).

Each RTK is composed of an extracellular N-terminal segment able to bind a specific extracellular ligand, a transmembrane domain and an intracellular C-terminal segment containing the enzymatic domain and a series of tyrosin phosphorylation sites. After ligand binding, the dimerization of the receptor induces a trans-phosphorylation of the intracellular domain followed by the activation of the catalytic subunit and the transduction of the signal at intracellular level. The intracellular domain phosphotyrosines are recognized by downstream signal proteins, generally through Src homology-2 (SH2) or phosphotyrosine-binding (PTB) domains and their binding induces the activation of the intracellular signaling cascade (Hubbard & Miller, 2007). The two main pathways through which RTKs act are the MAPK pathway and the PI3K-AKT, although other pathways can be activated under specific situations. After receptor dimerization an adaptor protein allows its coupling with a G protein that in turn activates a series of intracellular kinases. One of the most studied G proteins is called Ras. Mutations that constitutively activate this protein and induce an aberrant stimulation of the pathway are often observed in several types of cancer. Besides Ras, numerous other proteins involved in the RTKs pathway are mutated in different cancer cells, indicating that these proteins retain a fundamental role in tumor development and progression. Considering the central function it is obvious that these molecules represent a fundamental channel for the development of novel drugs for cancer therapy.

### 1.2 Apoptosis

A key process profoundly influencing tumor progression is apoptosis. Apoptosis is the process of programmed cell death occurring in multicellular organisms and is characterized by morphological changes including cell shrinkage, membrane blebbing, cromatine condensation and nuclear fragmentation. Factors such as cellular stress, oncogene activation and dysregulation of cell growth all lead to the activation of p53, which either arrest the cell cycle or activates apoptosis. Apoptosis regulates the proper tissue cell number eliminating damaged or excessive cells and it is also triggered by radiation and chemoterapeutic drugs used for cancer treatment (Sato et al., 1999). Two distinct intercommunicating apoptotic pathways have been described; the intrinsic and the extrinsic. The intrinsic pathway is activated following DNA damage and other severe cellular stresses. The intracellular signals hinge on the mitochondria with the release of cytochrome c which in turn binds to the cytosolic protein Apaf-1 to form the so called apoptosoma decisive for caspase activation. Caspases are a network of proteases that ultimately destroy the cellular structures and induce DNA fragmentation leading to cell death. The extrinsic apoptotic pathway is a receptor-mediated pathway and is activated by extracellular cues upon engagement of the so called death receptors by specific secreted ligands such as Apo2L/TRAIL. Upon activation the receptors for TRAIL activate the caspases specific of the extrinsic apoptotic pathway which ultimately leads to cell death (Jin & El-Deiry, 2005).

### 1.3 Cells of the tumor microenvironment

None of the cells of the tumor microenvironment except tumor cells are per se malignant; however the interactions with each other and directly or indirectly with the cancer cells may lead to the acquisition of an abnormal phenotype and expression pattern. Numerous studies have reported that the cells of the tumor microenvironment not only respond to and support carcinogenesis, but also can actively contribute to tumor initiation, progression, and metastasis. It has been demonstrated that stromal cells can cause transformation of the adjacent cells through transient signaling that, in some cases, leads to the disruption of homeostatic regulation, including control of tissue architecture, adhesion, cell death, and proliferation (Hu & Polyak, 2008).

Fibroblasts in particular are important members of the stromal microenvironment, as they maintain the adjacent epithelia homeostasis through the secretion of growth factors and direct mesenchymal–epithelial cell interactions. It is becoming increasingly clear that fibroblasts are also prominent modifiers of cancer progression. Knowledge of the role of resting and activated fibroblasts in cancer is still evolving. A subpopulation of fibroblasts, the so-called cancer-associated fibroblasts (CAFs), is increasingly recognized as an important promoter of tumor growth and development. CAFs directly stimulate tumor cell proliferation and angiogenesis through paracrine secretion of growth factors, hormones and cytokines in a context-dependent manner (Rasanen & Vaheri, 2010). Many of the CAF-secreted factors acting in isolation are sufficient to induce transformation of epithelial cells, indicative of a tumor-initiating capability of CAFs (Pietras & Ostman, 2010). Moreover CAFs can affect cancer progression by secreting and organizing altered ECM within the tumor stroma (Kalluri & Zeisberg, 2006).

Inflammatory cells can also deeply affect cancer cells behavior. Tumor associated macrophages (TAMs), which represent the major inflammatory component of the stroma of many tumors, are strongly associated with tumor progression and metastasis. In contrast to the reactive macrophages which are characterized by a so-called M1 phenotype, TAMs are alternatively activated and acquire an M2 phenotype, thus promoting tumor growth, angiogenesis, metastasis, as well as suppressing potential anti-tumor immune activities. TAMs affect vascular density and ECM by secreting a vast array of pro-angiogenetic factors and proteolytic enzymes including VEGF, FGF, PDGF, TNF-α, MMPs, plasmin, urokinase-type plasminogen activator (uPA) and the uPA receptor (uPAR) (Guruvayoorappan, 2008; Allavena et al., 2008). One key role for the microenvironment that has gained prominent recognition is neoangiogenesis. Tumors simply cannot progress without concomitant growth and organization of the stromal endothelial cells (EC) and pericyes. Malformed "leaky" tumor vessels contribute to tumor hypoxia, acidosis, and increased interstitial fluid pressure. The tumor in turn responds with a unique repertoire of gene expression, which in turn acts to alter cell growth, invasion, and ultimately metastasis (Li et al., 2007).

### 1.4 Tumor angiogenesis and ECM

Investigations into the roles of the tumor stroma have established that the ECM plays an important role in tumor vascularization (Wernert, 1997). Due to the accumulation of several gene mutations, cancer cells have the ability to be self-sufficient in growth signaling, insensitive to antigrowth signals, unresponsive to apoptotic events and capable of limitless replication. Although all of these neoplastic properties are necessary for tumor development, they are not sufficient to become clinically relevant malignancies, unless the tumor is able to recruit its own blood supply. In most tumors new blood vessels are formed through a process called angiogenesis, in which new blood vessels sprout from the preexisting vasculature (Folkman & Klagsbrun, 1987). Following EC proliferation newly formed vessels differentiate into arterioles and venules, necessary to provide blood supply to the growing tumors. In fact, solid tumors will not grow beyond the size of 1-2 mm, unless they induce the formation of new blood vessels to provide the oxygen and the nutrients necessary for their relentless growth and expansion (Campbell et al., 2010). During the different stages of angiogenesis, temporal and spatial regulation of ECM remodeling leads to local changes in net matrix deposition or degradation, which in turn contribute to control of EC growth, migration and differentiation. ECM remodeling is regulated by pro- and anti-angiogenic factors, matrix-degrading proteases and cell-ECM interactions (Sottile, 2004). In this context discovering the roles played by novel ECM proteins in vascularization is a crucial step in the process of creating new treatments for pathological angiogenesis.

### 1.5 ECM and tumor development

The ECM composition and the stroma's mechanical properties are other important characteristics that profoundly affect tumor cell behavior. The ECM tensile strength or stiffness can regulate cell growth, differentiation and migration, as well as the recruitment of other types of tumor-associated cells. Moreover, the stiffness and the increased interstitial pressure of the tumor stroma influences drug diffusion through the tumor and also the intrinsic drug sensitivity of malignant cells (Augsten et al., 2010).

On the other end, tumor invasion and metastasis are accomplished through ECM breakdown mainly due to matrix metalloproteinases (MMPs) activation. The ECM disruption promotes abnormal inter- and intra- cellular signaling leading to dysregulation of cell proliferation, growth and cytoskeleton reorganization. In turn, the ECM degradation gives rise to an increase of growth factors and ECM-derived molecules that modulate the properties of the different tumor-resident cell types.

An important event in tumor progression is the acquisition by cancer cells of the capability to dissociate from their original site and invade adjacent and distant tissues. Invasion involves the breaching of several barriers, including the basement membrane and the stromal matrix. Tumor cell invasion and metastasis is a compelling issue of cancer treatment accounting for ~ 90% of cancer related deaths, hence the targeting of tumor invasion is increasingly recognized as a fundamental therapeutic approach. Other key elements of the tumor microenvironment are the single ECM components. The ECM is mainly composed by an intricate interlocking mesh of fibrillar and non-fibrillar collagens, elastic fibers, non-collagenous glycoproteins such as proteoglycans (PGs) and glycosaminoglycans as hyaluronan (HA). Within these structural elements, the stroma is made also of matricellular proteins, a group of extracellular proteins that do not contribute directly to the formation of structural elements but serve to modulate cell-matrix interactions and cell function (Steeg, 2006; Brooks et al., 2010). Tumors often display an altered ECM composition due to the factors produced by tumor and stromal cells. Most solid tumors exhibit a profoundly different ECM-protein profile compared to their normal counterparts. Many of these proteins, though the integrins or other cell surface molecules, affect tumor cells behavior in terms of proliferation, apoptotic rate and migration.

## 2. Potential therapeutic targets

### 2.1 Receptor tyrosine kinases

RTKs are specifically activated by several extracellular molecules including growth factors, cytokines, and hormones. Most of the targeted inhibitors under development or already in clinical use are molecules with high affinity for growth factors RTKs, such as the Fibroblast Growth Factor Receptor (FGFR), the Vascular Endothelial Growth Factor Receptor (VEGFR), the Platelet-Derived Growth Factor Receptor (PDGFR), the tyrosine-protein kinase Kit receptor (c-Kit) and the Epidermal Growth Factor Receptor (EGFR). The FGF family contains 22 related peptides able to bind four different FGF receptors (FGFR 1-4). FGFs have been implicated in both physiological and pathological angiogenesis, vasculogenesis and blood vessel remodeling, influencing proliferation and differentiation of different cell types. FGF2 (aka bFGF) is a potent mitogen and chemotactic factor for endothelial and smooth muscle cells and stimulate pericyte formation. It also stimulates the production of the urokinase-type plasminogen activator (uPA) and MMP expression inducing vessel destabilization and ECM breakdown. Receptor dimerization and the presence of heparin or heparan sulfate proteoglycans are necessary for its activation as well as internalization of the ligand to achieve full activation. FGFR1 is the best characterized FGF receptor and it was found to be amplified in 8-10% of breast cancers (Elbauomy et al., 2007). FGFR1 is over-expressed and occasionally amplified also in oral and esophageal squamous carcinomas (Ishizuka et al., 2002)), prostate cancer (Sahadevan et al., 2007), and in a number of bladder carcinomas (Simon et al., 2001). Amplifications have also been observed in ovarian tumors (Gorringe et al., 2007). The EGFR/ERBB family was one of the first to be linked to cancer development and progression. EGFRs regulate cell proliferation, migration and differentiation. Moreover, their signaling is a key driver of the Epithelial-Mesenchimal Transition (EMT) which is a major event involved in the metastatic dissemination of tumor cells (Wilkins-Port & Higgins, 2007). The EGFR family comprises four different receptors, EGFR/HER1 (ERBB1), HER2 (ERBB2), HER3 (ERBB3) and HER4 (ERBB4) and all of them have been implicated in the development of several tumor types. The EGFR downstream signaling cascade includes the Ras-MAP kinase pathway (Herbst, 2004). Over-expression of EGFRs or mutations in their downstream pathways has been linked to poor response to

chemotherapy whereas its correlation with prognosis has not been demonstrated due to contrasting results.
VEGF is an essential growth and survival factor for ECs promoting their survival, proliferation, migration and morphogenesis into functional tubular structures. Moreover, its activity influences vascular permeability (Roskoski, Jr., 2007). The critical role of VEGF in the formation of a new vasculature in growing tumors with the recruitment of circulating ECs and progenitor cells to the sites of neovascularization is well known and plays an important role in tumor progression (Folkman, 1971). In several tumor types including colorectal cancer, VEGF expression has been linked with tumor aggressiveness, poor disease-free and overall survival, distant metastatic spread and decreased response to preoperative radiotherapy (Giatromanolaki et al., 2006; Giralt et al., 2006; Nozue et al., 2001; Zlobec et al., 2005). There are five human VEGF family members and three VEGF receptors. Each VEGF molecule displays a characteristic receptor binding pattern; VEGF-A binds to both VEGFR1 and VEGFR2; VEGF-B and PlGF (Placental Growth Factor) bind to VEGF1, instead VEGF-C and VEGF-D bind to VEGFR3. The activation of VEGFR2 though the binding VEGF-A plays a pivotal role in the regulation of EC function and angiogenesis and for this reason VEGFR2 is one of the most studied receptors of this family. Another important cytokine is the PDGF which is involved in the control of the proliferation, survival and motility of several mesenchymal cell types.
In addition, it is important for the maintenance of the perivascular structures that surround and support tumor blood vessels. For this reason PDGF receptors are under investigation as targets for anti-angiogenic cancer therapy. Two isoforms of the PDGF receptors are known, PDGFRα and PDGFRβ. Both can form homo- or heterodimers and stimulate cell proliferation, but only PDGFRββ and PDGFRαβ dimers can mediate smooth muscle cell and fibroblast chemotaxis. After their activation PDGF receptors activate the Ras/MAPK pathway modulating cell proliferation, migration and differentiation and the PI3K/AKT pathway promoting cell survival. Another member of the PDGFR family is KIT, which was shown to be over-expressed in many tumors, including gastrointestinal stromal tumors (GISTs), mast cell tumors, melanomas, endometrial and ovarian carcinomas and small cell carcinomas of the lung. The binding of stem cell factor to KIT induces receptor dimerization and activation of the intracellular signaling mediated by the PI3K, Ras/MAPK, JAK/STAT pathways to stimulate cell survival (Sattler & Salgia, 2004).

### 2.2 Apoptotic molecules

The life and death decision at the cellular level is controlled by environmental cues including the presence or absence of growth factors and physical stimuli such as mechanical stress or radiation. Moreover, cells sense their three dimensional location through specific interactions with the ECM as well as with neighboring cells and these contacts are essential for cell survival. In particular, the lack of appropriate cells/ECM interactions leads to a peculiar form of cell death named anoikis (Gilmore, 2005). The life and death decision is also profoundly influenced by the components of the ECM, which can change dynamically during differentiation, development and other tissue-remodeling events. As mentioned above, cells' anchorage is essential for survival (Meredith, Jr. et al., 1993) which is maintained through the activation PI3K Kinase-AKT pathway granted by integrin engagement; should this interaction be disrupted cells undergo apoptosis (Frisch & Screaton, 2001). For example the use of competitors for integrin binding such as Arginin,

Glicine, Aspartate-based (RGD-based) peptides can induce apoptosis by directly activating caspases (Adderley & Fitzgerald, 2000). ECs are highly susceptible to survival anchorage dependent stimuli (Scatena et al., 1998). As mentioned, also the loss of cell-cell contacts leads to the activation of a default death programmed in a variety of cell types. For instance, deficiency or truncation of VE-cadherin which mediates adhesion between ECs (Hermiston & Gordon, 1995) induces ECs' apoptosis and abolishes transmission of the survival signal by VEGF-A to AKT Kinase and Bcl2 (Carmeliet et al., 1999) and this profoundly affects the angiogeneic potential. Given the importance of adhesion in maintaining cell survival, altered expression of glycoproteins in the tumor microenvironment leads to an impairment of cell survival. For example, PGs expression is markedly altered during malignant transformation and tumor progression and is influenced by cancer cells-derived secreted factors and this may either facilitate or counteract the growth of solid tumors. PGs, such as versican, perlecan and small leucine-rich PGs affect cancer cell signaling, growth and survival, as well as cell adhesion, migration and angiogenesis. Furthermore, expression of cell-surface-associated PGs, such as syndecans and glypicans, is also modulated in both tumor and stromal cells. Cell-surface-associated PGs bind various factors that are involved in cell signaling, thereby affecting cell proliferation, adhesion and motility. An important mechanism of action is offered by a proteolytic processing of cell-surface PGs known as ectodomain shedding of syndecans; this facilitates cancer and EC motility, protects matrix proteases and provides a chemotactic gradient of mitogens. However, syndecans on stromal cells may be important for stromal cell/cancer cell interplay and may promote stromal cell proliferation, migration and angiogenesis. The abnormal PG expression by cancer and stromal cells may be exploited to evaluate tumor progression and patient survival (Theocharis et al., 2010). It is known that heparan sulphate proteoglycans (HSPGs), represent an important reservoir of chemochines, cytochines and enzymes (Bishop et al., 2007; Sasisekharan et al., 2002). Heparanase, can cleave HS side chains from HSPGs and release a multitude of bioactive molecules including bFGF and Hepatocyte Growth Factor (HGF) (Ogasawara et al., 1996). bFGF enhances EC and tumor cell proliferation and this was demonstrated to contribute to hepatocellular carcinoma progression (Pang & Poon, 2006). Heparanase expression is closely related with apoptosis of several tumors cells, including HCC (Ikeguchi et al., 2003b; Ginath et al., 2001) and there is a significant positive correlation between the mRNA expression levels of heparanase and the percentages of apoptotic hepatocytes in liver tissues (Ikeguchi et al., 2003a). Besides affecting EC proliferation bFGF is also responsible for a direct effect on tumor cells protecting them from apoptosis. Cell surface HSPGs act as co-receptors for formation of high-affinity bFGF-receptor complexes, and in this context the HS chains play a leading role (Chua et al., 2004). In this context, the heparanase-induced alteration of cell surface HSPGs, might down-regulate bFGF pro-survival effects resulting in tumor cell apoptosis. In addition, there is also a group of ECM molecules that have been shown to directly impair cell viability. Among these proteins CCN1, a secreted ECM-associated heparin binding protein, can either induce or suppress apoptosis: it can promote EC survival but also induce fibroblast apoptosis mediated by integrin $\alpha_6\beta_1$ and the heparan sulfate proteoglycan sydecan 4. The mechanism involves the activation of Bax which leads to cytochrome-c release and activation of caspase-9 and -3 activation (Todorovicc et al., 2005).

Another ECM protein playing, among other functions in tumor development, an active role in the control of apoptosis is the Secreted Protein Acidic and Rich in Cystein (SPARC).

SPARC is an important regulator of cell growth and malignancy and enhances apoptosis in various tumors including ovarian cancer, where its absence significantly diminished cell death. The mechanism is still elusive but involves the activation of caspase-8, the initiator caspase of the extrinsic apoptotic pathway independently of death receptor activation and leads to downstream involvement of Bid. Interestingly, this effect results from the interaction between SPARC and the N-terminus of the procaspase-8 DED-containing domain (Tang & Tai, 2007). The secreted small leucine-rich proteoglycan decorin has also been shown to inhibit cancer growth by impairing EGFR function and triggering apoptosis through caspase-3 activation (Seidler et al., 2006).

EMILIN2, another ECM glycoprotein, adopts a peculiar mechanism in affecting tumor development and apoptosis. Elastin Microfibril Interface-Located proteINs (EMILINs) constitute a family of ECM glycoproteins characterized by the presence of an EMI domain at the N-terminus and a gC1q domain at the C-terminus (Doliana et al., 2000; Mongiat et al., 2000). Recent studies show that this molecule affects tumor cell survival leaving normal cells unharmed; the mechanism involves the direct activation of the death receptors and in particular DR4. The activation of the extrinsic apoptotic pathway leads to a dramatic decrease of tumor cell viability associated with DNA fragmentation and caspase-8 and caspase-3 activation. More recently a discrete sequence of this molecule was found to be involved in these anti-tumorigenic effects (Mongiat et al., 2007; Mongiat et al., 2010).

### 2.3 Cells of the microenvironment

*Cancer associated fibroblasts (CAFs)* Several studies have demonstrated that normal fibroblasts contribute to maintaining epithelial homeostasis by suppressing proliferation and oncogenic potential of adjacent epithelia. Once they are recruited to the tumor, most of them switch to a permanently activated phenotype, and become CAFs. The phenotype of CAFs resembles that of normal fibroblasts during wound healing where they are activated and generate ECM components and pro-inflammatory cytokines. After the wound is healed, the normal phenotype is restored; on the contrary, in the tumor microenvironment their status remains permanently activated and for this reason tumors are frequently termed as "wounds that do not heal". By creating an altered microenvironment through the overexpression of cytokines such as TGFβ, PDGF, FGF and connective tissue growth factors, a growing tumor can co-opt fibroblasts and turn them into CAFs (Erez et al., 2010).

CAFs are not only target cells whose activity is modulated by environmental factors, but also active cells that significantly contribute to tumorigenesis and metastasis. Abundant growth-promoting factors have been found in the conditioned media of CAFs isolated from metastatic colon cancer patients, compared to the conditioned media taken from normal skin fibroblasts (Xing et al., 2010). In addition, CAFs are able to induce epithelial cells transformation following injection of normal human breast epithelial cells mixed with irradiated or not-irradiated fibroblasts in immunocompromised mice (Kuperwasser et al., 2004). The tumorigenic potential of CAFs depends also on the production of the mutagenic reactive oxygen species (ROS) under conditions of pH and hypoxia that characterize the tumor microenvironment. CAFs are known to produce Insulin-like Growth Factor-1 and -2 (IGF-1 and -2), thus promoting tumor growth providing survival signals allowing tumor cells to evade programmed cell death. CAFs are also supporters of tumor angiogenesis being an important source of VEGF (Li et al., 2007). Finally, CAFs produce high levels of the Stomal cell-Derived Factor 1α (SDF-1α), the ligand of C-X-C chemokine Receptor type 4

(CXCR4), which is highly expressed by cancer cells. Once activated, CXCR4 can promote mammary epithelial proliferation, migration and invasion and angiogenesis (Orimo et al., 2005).

Another important role of CAFs is their active participation in ECM remodeling during tumor development. The increase production of fibronectin, collagens, proteoglicans and glicosaminoglicans promote survival stimuli from integrin engagement and impair apoptosis induced by chemotherapeutic drugs. Another event affecting the drugs uptake is the increased interstitial fluid pressure. The deposition of a dense ECM network leads to fibroblasts' proliferation which may acquire a contractile phenotype to become myofibrobrast. This results in a constant increase in tension within the tumor connective network and increase of interstitial fluid pressure leading to an impaired uptake of therapeutic agents (Bouzin & Feron, 2007).

It has been demonstrated that in some cases increased fibronectin expression correlates with tumorigenicity amplifing integrin survival signaling (Han et al., 2004; Marastoni et al., 2008). Collagen I also contributes to the decrease of the uptake and regulates the sensitivity of tumor cells to these drugs.

The ECM remodeling by MMPs is one of the most crucial steps for cancer progression where the equilibrium between MMPs and their inhibitors is completely disrupted. It has been shown that CAFs secrete various matrix-degrading proteases as well as their activators such as uPA, thus promoting tumor invasion. The breakage of the basement membrane allows the epithelial cancer cells to intravasate into the circulation system and also in this context the cross-talk between the cancer cells and CAFs seems to be crucial.

*Tumor associated macrophages (TAMs) and inflammatory cells.* It is known that tumors are generally infiltrated by immune cells with which the host tries to contrast tumor progression, a process known as immune surveillance. Several studies report a correlation between the inflammatory infiltrates and an improved prognosis or a better lifespan for patients. However, some evidences contradict this paradigm identifying the presence of immune cells as a negative prognostic factor particularly for breast, prostate, ovarian and cervical cancers (Whiteside, 2007). The association between a chronic inflammation and cancer was first formulated by Dr. Virchow in 1863. This concept has been recently reconsidered when specific inflammatory cell types and in particular TAMs, the major inflammatory component of the stroma of many tumors, have been associated to neoplastic transformation (Houghton, 2010). In less than 10% of the cases, the presence of TAMs is associated with good prognosis. A possible explanation to this apparent paradox is that tumor cells are able to recruit immune cells and, similarly to what happens with CAFs, to activate their status. The cytokine profile in the tumor microenvironment is considered extremely important in determining the phenotype of the local inflammatory cells (Pollard, 2004).

Compared to reactive macrophages, TAMs are alternatively activated, acquiring an M2 phenotype, thus promoting tumor growth, angiogenesis, metastasis and suppressing potential anti-tumor immune activities, a phenomenon known as immunoediting.

A central event determining TAMs activity is NF-kB activation. In response to different pro-inflammatory signals TAMs display defective NF-kB activation that causes impaired expression of cytotoxic mediators, such as Nitric Oxide (NO), Tumor Necrosis Factor α (TNFα), and Interleukin 1 and 12 (IL1 and IL12), (Mantovani et al., 2006). In a normal tissue, pathogenic infection or a wound healing triggers the local expression of an array of inflammatory cytokines and growth factors, such as Colony Stimulating Factor 1 (CSF-1),

Granulocyte–Macrophage CSF (GM-CSF), Macrophage-Stimulating Protein (MSP) and Transforming Growth Factor β1 (TGF-β1). These factors, together with the products of tissue breakdown, recruit circulating monocytes which are stimulated to differentiate into macrophages. Macrophages, in turn, mediate immune responses, kill pathogens, stimulate angiogenesis and participate in tissue repair (Pollard, 2004). This physiological phenomenon is uncontrolled in tumors given the persistent stimuli from both tumor cells and CAFs. CSF-1, the main growth factor responsible for survival, proliferation, differentiation and chemotaxis of macrophages, is over-expressed in different types of cancers. In addition tumor-derived anti-inflammatory molecules such as IL4, IL10, TGFβ-1, and prostaglandin E2 are essential for TAMs' function and this finding suggested that exposure to IL4 and IL10 may induce monocytes to develop into polarized M2 macrophages (Mantovani et al., 2002).

TAM infiltration positively correlates with tumor cell proliferation in breast, endometrial and renal cell carcinoma. In fact, various studies have shown that these cells express a number of factors that stimulate tumor cell proliferation and survival, including EGF, PDGF, TGF-β1, HGF, and bFGF. TAMs are also important supporters of tumor angiogenesis being a source of VEGF; TAMs cluster in avascular areas, recruited by chemokines that are secreted in response to hypoxia. This condition up-regulates hypoxia-inducible factor-2α (HIF-2α) which, in turn, induces VEGF expression. VEGF expression by TAMs is induced by CSF-1 and the cytokine in a positive feedback loop recruits other macrophages thus increasing the rate of vascularization (Lewis & Pollard, 2006). TAMs also produce other pro-angiogenetic factors and proteolitic enzymes including IL8, FGF, PDGF, TNF-α, MMP-2, MMP-7, MMP-9, MMP-12, and cyclooxygenase 2 (COX-2) (Lewis & Pollard, 2006). TAMs enhance the invasive capacity of cancer cells (Lewis & Pollard, 2006). This effect may depend on the expression of MMPs and uPA and its receptor uPAR which enhances the motility and invasion of cancer cells (Guruvayoorappan, 2008).

*Neutrophils.* Once recruited to the tumor microenvironment, neutrophils have also been demonstrated to change their phenotype and promote tumor progression. Various transgenic mice models and clinical data show that the presence of tumor-associated neutrophils often correlates with poor prognosis, given their ability to stimulate tumor growth, angiogenesis and metastasis. IL8, which is frequently over-expressed by tumor and stromal cells, is a strong chemokine for neutrophils, which express the IL8 receptors CXCR-1 and -2. Once inside the tumors, neutrophils can secrete factors such as HGF and oncostatin M which induces tumors cells to enhance the VEGF expression and increases their invasiveness. IL8 also stimulates neutrophil degranulation with the release of MMP9 (Gregory & Houghton, 2011; Murdoch et al., 2008).

Neutrophil elastase (NE) is an important protease released by neutrophils. Recent data show that it promotes tumor growth via an alteration of tumor cell signaling that ultimately leads to PI3K hyperactivity (Gregory & Houghton, 2011; Houghton, 2010). Reactive Oxygen Species (ROS) produced by neutrophils as a host defense against microorganisms could act as pro-tumorigenic agents. As CAFs and TAMs, neutrophils can also facilitate tumor cells metastasis. It is likely that the neutrophils phenotypic switch, which is defined N1-N2 polarization similarly to the M1-M2 polarization of macrophages, is mediated by the key cytokine TGFβ (Fridlender et al., 2009).

*Tumor ECs and pericytes.* Vessels are a requisite for tumor growth and also are necessary for tumors to metastasize. Thus, the ability to recruit vessels is an important and growth limiting step for tumors. The release of pro-angiogenetic factors in the tumor microenvironment results in the recruitment and enhanced proliferation of ECs. Members of

VEGF family and their receptors are considered the major key mediators of angiogenesis. The binding of VEGF to VEGFR triggers an intracellular signaling that is mainly mediated by MAPK and PI3K/Akt/mTOR pathways. This results in the expression of HIF-1α and induction of PDGF, FGF, G-CSF, TGFβ and angiopoietins, thus enhancing angiogenesis (Boehm et al., 2010).

Another important cellular component of the blood vessels are pericytes whose recruitment is highly dependent on PDGFβ-R expression as well as on the production of PDGFβ ligand by ECs (Pietras & Ostman, 2010). Tumor pericytes are rarely dispersed and loosely along the vessels compared to their normal counterparts and their role in tumor development is not yet well defined. Some studies have demonstrated that increased coverage of pericytes enhances tumor growth, by promoting neo-vascularization. In contrast, other cancer models show a pericyte-mediated angiostatic effect, thus the outcome of pericyte-derived signals appears to be highly context dependent (Pietras & Ostman, 2010).

### 2.4 ECM proteins and tumor angiogenesis

The network of fibrous proteins and glycosaminoglycans (GAGs) of the ECM affects tumor vessel formation both in direct and indirect way. The GAGs carbohydrate polymers of the proteoglycans are involved in both keeping the ECM and surrounding cells hydrated and trapping and storing growth factors. Therefore, GAG molecules may exert a variety of regulatory effects on the accessibility of angiogenic factors (Rouet et al., 2005). Heparan Sulfate (HS) GAGs include the syndecans, glypicans, perlecans and agrins. HSGAGs that are present on the EC surface have the ability to either inhibit or promote neovascularization by mediating signalling through VEGF receptors (Iozzo & San Antonio, 2001) or bFGF (Walker et al., 1994).

Most of the ECM proteins, such as fibronectin, collagen and laminin, mediate angiogenesis through integrin-binding RGD motifs. In a resting quiescent state ECs exhibit the lowest cell mitotic index of all the cells of the body (Folkman, 2006). Induction of angiogenesis and ECM remodeling is characterized by an increased proliferation and permeability as well as cytoskeletal and cell-to-cell contact changes which results in newly formed focal contacts primarily mediated by integrins. Fibronectin is produced by both activated ECs and smooth muscle cells (SMC), and its levels are augmented during angiogenesis as fibronectin leaks from the blood due to the increased vascular permeability. The RGD domain of fibronectin binds to the integrin $\alpha_5\beta_1$, which is markedly up-regulated during angiogenesis and is over-expressed in ECs within the tumors. The collagen integrin receptors $\alpha_1\beta_1$ and $\alpha_2\beta_1$ also play a positive role during angiogenesis. Moreover, $\alpha_1$ chain laminin peptides mediate angiogenesis *in vitro* (Malinda et al., 1999). As previously mentioned, the proteolytic activity triggered during angiogenesis facilitates degradation of the basement membrane, matrix remodeling and cell migration and invasion which are essential for the development of novel blood vessels, hence this process is tightly regulated. There are two major classes of enzymes: the PA/plasmin system and MMPs. There are at least 20 members of the MMP family most of them being implicated in tumorigenesis and a large number of these proteases degrade the vascular basement membrane and matrix in order to allow vascular sprouting (Pepper, 2001). The activity of these proteases is regulated by endogenous tissue inhibitors of metalloproteinases (TIMPs) which generally display anti-angiogenic properties. By degrading the matrix, MMPs not only provide physical space within the matrix for cell migration, but also provide ECs with proliferation and differentiation signals due to the release of cryptic sites present on ECM molecules and the release of soluble growth factors.

Various MMPs cleave heparin bound growth factors such as VEGF and bFGF, thus stimulating the formation of new blood vessels (Lee et al., 2005; Hawinkels et al., 2008). Stromal recruitment of fibroblasts and immune cells such as macrophages can also affect angiogenesis as analyzed above. Recently it was found that loss of PTEN signaling in stromal fibroblasts results in the induction of ECM remodeling through the increase of the transcriptional factor Ets2 which is an upstream target of MMP-9 (Trimboli et al., 2009). Protease-mediated cleavage of the ECM also results in the release of cryptic domains that regulate angiogenesis. Cleavage of collagen XVIII and the α1, α2 and α3 chains of collagen IV release the angiogenic inhibitors endostatin, arrestin, canstatin and tumstatin, respectively (Kalluri, 2003). For this reason MMP inhibitors have an impact on tumor angiogenesis. For instance, TIMP-1 over-expression suppresses tumorigenesis, in part due to its effects on the tumor vasculature. Treatment of ECs with TIMP-1 alters the formation of tubules on Matrigel while proliferation is not affected. TIMP-2 decreases EC' proliferation and inhibits angiogenesis *in vivo* (Seo et al., 2003). TIMP-3 has also been shown to decrease angiogenesis, particularly through EC disaggregation and impairment of Matrigel tubulogenesis (Chetty et al., 2008).

Another group of ECM proteins which have been recently linked to tumor angiogenesis are the membrane-associated disintegrin and metalloproteinases (ADAMs), including those carrying Thrombospondin Motifs (ADAMTs) which are instead secreted in the microenvironment (Dunn et al., 2006). These proteins regulate angiogenesis directly or through expression of MMPs. For instance, ADAM-17 alters EC' morphology of decreases cell proliferation. ADAMTS1 and ADAMTS8 contain the thrombospondin antiangiogenic domain (TSR1) and inhibit EC proliferation and suppress growth factor induced vascularization (Vazquez et al., 1999).

The Bone Morphogenic Proteins (BMPs) have also gained recognition for their potential role in tumor angiogenesis. BMPs belong to the TGFβ superfamily of proteins and were found to influence angiogenesis by stimulating the secretion of proangiogenic growth factors such as VEGF (Deckers et al., 2002). BMP expression correlates with increased EC migration and tubulogenesis on Matrigel (Rothhammer et al., 2007). The role of BMPs in angiogenesis is controversial and some reports demonstrate an anti-angiogenic effect. Further understanding of the role played by BMPs in the ECM and tumor angiogenesis will benefit therapeutic studies which target angiogenesis, tumour growth, and metastatic spread of disease.

### 2.5 ECM proteins involved in invasion and metastasis

The main cause of cancer related deaths is the metastatic disease, which is due to the widespread dissemination is often impossible to successfully eradicate. Metastasis results from a complex molecular cascade comprising many steps, all of which are interconnected through a series of adhesive interactions and invasive processes as well as responses to chemotactic stimuli, through which cancer cells leave the site of the primary tumor mass and disseminate to distant anatomic sites where they proliferate and form secondary tumor foci. To complete this process tumor cells must invade the tissue surrounding the primary tumor, enter either the lymphatics or the bloodstream, survive and eventually arrest in the circulation, extravasate into a tissue and grow in the new site. A crucial element in the metastatic process is the ECM whose composition, structure and biophysical forces exerted may influence cell invasion and migration.

*ECM and invasion.* Most solid tumors exhibit a distinctive ECM-protein profile, compared to the normal counterparts and many of these proteins interact directly with tumor cells influencing their migration and invasion ability. A number of proteins, such as tenascin-C (TNC), fibronectin, and SPARC are consistently up-regulated in tumors (Allen & Louise, 2011). TNC is a multifunctional protein expressed at low levels in normal adult tissues but over-expressed in conjunction with cell migration occurring for instance during embryogenesis, wound healing or cancer development. TNC is highly expressed in a variety of invasive and metastasizing cancers, including breast, colon, lung and brain (Guttery et al., 2010). Multiple alternatively-spliced isoforms of TNC are known and seem to be tumor-specific. For example, the full length protein is expressed in pancreatic and prostate cancers, while in breast and ovarian carcinomas the domain A and D containing isoforms are the most abundant. Besides its composition, also the tensile strength of ECM can regulate epithelial cell growth, transformation and migration; the tumor-associated stroma is usually more stiff than the normal tissue, and this peculiar characteristic of the tumor microenvironment may influence tumor progression (Tilghman et al., 2010). For example, the reduction of ECM stiffness can inhibit the malignancy of transformed mammary epithelial cells (Allen & Louise, 2011). One way in which tensile strength can be modulated is the cross-linking of collagens and elastin due to lysil oxidase activity (LOX). Studies conducted using mouse models of breast cancer allowed to correlate the high LOX expression, increased collagen cross-linking and elevated ECM stiffness with the invasive progression of the disease. The role of LOX has been well established in colorectal (Baker et al., 2011) and breast (Erler & Giaccia, 2006) cancer progression, in this last case it was demonstrated that hypoxic primary tumor cells increase LOX expression and secretion, enabling cell movement to more oxygenated and thus nutrient-rich areas. LOX increases cell invasion and migration through regulation of cell-matrix adhesion and focal adhesion kinase (FAK) activity. LOX may be involved in the cell-matrix adhesion interactions required for intravasation and extravasation and, finally, is required for the formation of a mature ECM at the secondary site, allowing survival signaling and possibly bone marrow derived cells recruitment.

The fibrillar collagens surrounding tumors are often remodeled and this is associated with the metastatic progression. The linearization and reorientation of collagen fibers at the invasive front of cancer cells is a classic example of malignant transformation and metastatic dissemination (Cox & Erler, 2011).

In most human tumors there is abundant accumulation of HA. A large number of studies performed during the last three decades have demonstrated a close correlation between malignancy and hyaluronan-rich ECM, as well as with the expression of some specific variants of its CD44 receptor (Misra et al., 2011). The CD44 present at the surface of cancer cells interacts with HA-rich microenvironments, thus affecting cell signaling pathways and enabling malignant cells to migrate, invade basal membranes and ECM and to lodge at distant sites from the primary tumor. The HA content in the tumor stroma impacts on the overall outcome of the disease and correlates with tumor grade and poor prognosis. HA, HA synthetases, hyaluronidases and HA receptors are involved in a wild range of carcinomas, as breast, lung, skin, and gastrointestinal (Sironen et al., 2011).

*Cell-cell and cell-ECM interactions.* Invasion, which characterizes the metastatic process, consists of changes in tumor cell adherence to the other cells and to the ECM and is accompanied by the proteolytic degradation of the surrounding tissue and by the motility that propels tumor cells through the tissue.

Loss of cell-cell adhesion within the primary tumor mass permits disaggregation of tumor cells and hence aids the initial dissemination. Compared with normal epithelial cells, cancer cells show diminished cell-cell adhesiveness, due to the alteration of cadherin/catenin expression. The process leading from a polarized epithelial non-motile phenotype to a more motile and non-polarized phenotype is called epithelial to mesenchymal transition (EMT). This event is associated with the cadherin switch consisting in the loss of E-cadherin expression, normally present on the epithelial cell surface, and the gain of N-cadherin expression which associates with a metastatic phenotype. The loss of E-cadherin expression has been shown in several types of epithelial cancers including breast, gastrointestinal, lung, stomach, prostate, and kidney (Hazan et al., 2004).

The interaction between tumor cells and the stroma is mostly mediated by integrins, which not only mediate cell-ECM adhesion, but also play a role in intracellular signaling stimulating events as proteolysis and angiogenesis (Brooks et al., 2010). Integrins are emerging as important factors in metastatic progression and their expression levels correlate with pathological outcomes, for example colon, breast and prostate cancers often display altered integrin expression which can vary considerably between normal and tumor tissues (Desgrosellier & Cheresh, 2010). Most notably, integrins $\alpha_V\beta_3$, $\alpha_5\beta_1$ and $\alpha_V\beta_6$, are expressed at low levels in most adult epithelia but can be highly up-regulated in tumors. On the other end, $\alpha_2\beta_1$, is down-regulated in cancer leading to an increase of tumor cell dissemination; when this integrin is re-expressed in breast cancer cells, the phenotype is reverted, suggesting that it behaves as a tumor-suppressor integrin.

*Proteases.* The engagement of integrins and other adhesion molecules is accompanied by the recruitment of proteases which degrade the ECM and help providing a pathway for invasion. During the metastatic dissemination of tumor cells, the degradation of components of the ECM is achieved through the action of several hydrolytic enzymes which are released either by the tumor cells themselves or by cells surrounding the tumor. The enzymes play a role during metastasis include MMPs, cathepsines, uPA and heparanases. All these molecules once exogenously over-expressed increase cell invasion (Brooks et al., 2010). The proteolityc activity of these enzymes facilitates the migration of tumor cells in different ways; physical barriers of dense matrix are removed, latent proteases, growth factors and chemotactic agents are often activated, integrin-binding sites within the ECM molecules are exposed and transmit migratory and survival signals, finally bioactive ECM fragments are generated as, for example, from collagen IV and laminin-5 (Geho et al., 2005).

The expression and role of the different MMPs is quite diverse during cancer progression. They can promote or inhibit cancer development depending on the tumor stage, tumor site, enzyme localization and substrate profile. For example, MMP-9 functions as a tumor promoter during carcinogenesis but at later stages of the disease and under specific conditions it can also function as an anticancer enzyme (Gialeli et al., 2011).

Another important regulator of tumor invasion is the uPA system consisting of the specific protease uPA and its cellular receptor uPAR. The enzyme is released by tumor or tumor-associated cells, it binds to the receptor leading to plasmin activation. This mechanism results in the amplification of ECM proteolysis by both the degradative ability of plasmin and the initiation of an activation cascade involving MMPs. Elevated levels of uPA have been reported in many types of cancer, and anti-uPAR targeting therapy is currently being attempted (Brooks et al., 2010).

*The pre-metastatic niche.* Once tumor cells reach the secondary site, they undergo apoptosis, lie dormant or proliferate to form the secondary tumor. Recent evidences suggest that distant sites, called pre-metastatic niches, may be pre-conditioned to become a fertile ground for the establishment of metastasis (Coghlin & Murray, 2010). Hematopoietic cells migrate through the tissues and cause the remodeling of the ECM and growth factors milieu. Such altered microenvironment can attract tumor cells and support their proliferation (Brooks et al., 2010). Elevated fibronectin expression by resident fibroblasts at the pre-metastatic site represents a critical factor in the development of the pre-metastatic niche. The key tumor-secreted factors that determine the formation of this niche have yet to be identified, although TNF, TGF-β and VEGF are likely to be involved (Erler et al., 2009). ECM remodeling enzymes like MMPs and LOX seem to play a role also in the pre-metastatic niche formation. For example, the primary tumor-driven VEGFR-1 activation is required for the secretion of MMP-9 by the ECs and macrophages, thus deeply affecting the metastatic environment of the lungs. This is thought to make the lung microenvironment more hospitable for the subsequent invasion and survival of metastatic cells. The activity of tumor-secreted LOX is essential for the recruitment of bone marrow derived cells, because of ECM remodeling and MMPs' activation induced by collagen cross-linking. Exactly what determines the site of the pre-metastatic niche remains elusive, although some recent studies have proposed that they might occur in sites exposed to frequent mechanical strain (Cox & Erler, 2011).

## 3. Therapeutic strategies

### 3.1 Receptor tyrosine kinase inhibition

Given the critical role that RTKs play in signal transduction profoundly affecting tumor progression, several molecules to block the aberrant activation of these pathways have been developed (Zwick et al., 2002). Due to the high level of complexity of these pathways, investigators have attempted to interfere at different levels of the signaling cascade, from the extracellular ligands, to the membrane receptors, to the intracellular non-receptor tyrosine kinases (Fig.2). Several modalities are currently employed to inhibit kinase activity such as small inhibitors, molecular antibodies, but also peptide mimetics and antisense oligonucleotides (Dancey & Sausville, 2003; Imai & Takaoka, 2006).

*Small molecule tyrosine kinase inhibitors* - Tyrosin kinases are present in an active or inactive form. Active kinases are characterized by high structural homology whereas the structures of the inactive forms are dissimilar. This characteristic suggests that molecules able to recognize and bind to the inactive form of the enzyme, could present higher efficacy because of lower cross-reactivity and increased specificity. Despite the fact that more specific inhibitors allow to precisely control cellular activity, several studies have demonstrated the importance of inhibiting multiple critical nodes in order to increase treatment response. Most cancers in fact are characterized by multiple aberrant signaling pathways and thus may require inhibition of a number of signaling endpoints for an optimal response. In addition, the ability of multi-targeted drugs to inhibit different kinases can represent an advantage in case of the development of drug resistance. In some occasions cells treated with a selective kinase inhibitor activate alternative pathways to maintain their activity. Hence, a chemical compound able to simultaneously inhibit several kinases bares the potential to be less prone to drug resistance. On the other hand, the use of multitargeted inhibitors is usually accompanied by worse side effects and limits on the maximum dose that can be used for treatment, thus limiting the real benefits. Most of the small molecule kinase inhibitors currently in preclinical development and in clinical use are ATP-competitive inhibitors. These molecules are characterized by a high affinity for the kinase ATP-binding sites and their interaction with these sites prevents ATP binding and therefore kinase activation. One of the limitations of this kind of inhibitors is represented by the susceptibility to mutations that enhance target kinase activity, which is common in several types of cancer. In addition to ATP-competitive inhibitors, several non-competitive inhibitors have also been developed. These molecules bind to an allosteric site distant from the ATP-binding site and induce a conformational change of the receptor thus preventing the ATP binding. These kinds of inhibitors are active independently on the ATP binding site sequence, thus maintaining their efficacy also in the presence of mutant proteins.

*Monoclonal antibodies* - An alternative approach to impair the RTKs' activation is represented by the use of blocking monoclonal antibodies (mAbs) (Hinoda et al., 2004). These antibodies act directly preventing the ligand-receptor interaction and therefore inhibiting ligand-mediated intracellular signaling and increasing RTK down-regulation and internalization. In addition, mAbs act also indirectly by stimulating the immune response. Following their binding to the cell surface receptors the subsequent activation of the immune system causes antibody-dependent cellular cytotoxicity through the activation of macrophages or natural killer cells. Finally, recent studies demonstrated that some monoclonal antibodies are able to influence tumor growth by modulating the receptor signaling activity and therefore altering the intracellular signaling inducing apoptosis and/or growth inhibition.

Compared to the small molecule inhibitors, mAbs are more expensive to produce and, due their large molecular weight, the tissue penetration, tumor retention and blood clearance is less efficient especially in some tissues such as the brain. Moreover, because of their inability to penetrate through the cellular membrane, they can only be used to target cell surface molecules and not intracellular proteins. Despite these limitations, in clinical trials the mAbs have encountered higher approval success rates compared to new drugs, including small-molecule agents (Reichert et al., 2005). It must be pointed out that the activation of the immune system is likely crucial to efficiently eliminate tumor cells and for this reason, the use of small molecule inhibitors in combination with mAbs should maximize the therapeutic effects.

*RTKs as Antiangiogenic targets* - The prevention of angiogenesis is a potentially successful mean to impair tumor growth and progression. In contrast to standard chemotherapy, inhibition of angiogenesis generally does not lead to tumor regression but induces long-term stable disease creating a favorable window of opportunity for radiotherapy or chemotherapy to exert stronger tumor-killing effects. Growth factors such as VEGF-A, FGF2, IL8 and PDGF play an important role in promoting blood vessels formation and several antiangiogenic molecules have been developed to target either growth factors or their receptors.

The use of Bevacizumab (Avastin®), a humanized mAb able to specifically bind to VEGF-A and blocking its interaction with VEGFR2, in combination with 5-fluorouracil-based chemotherapy was approved for the first-line treatment of metastatic colorectal cancer (CRC) by FDA in February 2004 (Ferrara et al., 2005). Sunitinib (Sutent®) is an orally active small molecule inhibitor of VEGFR2, PDGFRβ, KIT and FLT3 (Mendel et al., 2003; Abrams et al., 2003) and is used in clinical trials for patients with advanced solid malignancies (Motzer et al., 2006; Motzer & Bukowski, 2006).

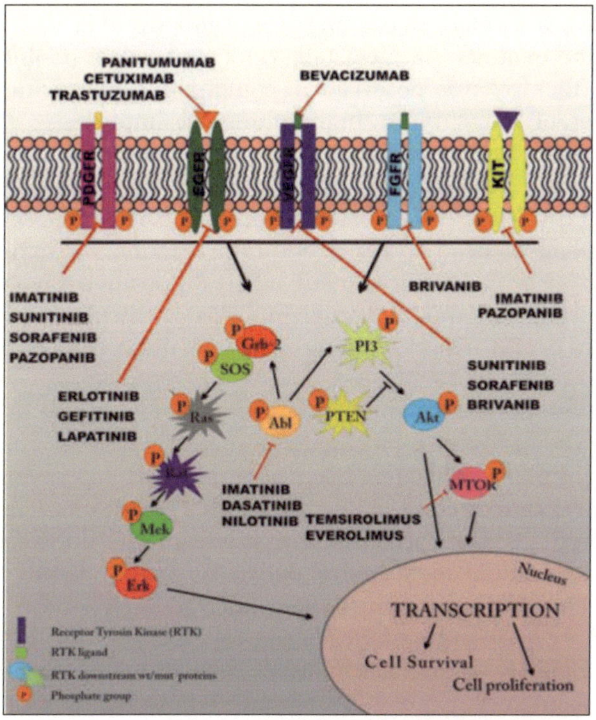


Fig. 2. Schematic representation of the therapeutic strategies targeting receptor tyrosine kinases; PDGFR: Platelet-derived growth factor Receptor; EGFR: Epidermal Growth Factor Receptor; VEGFR: Vascular Endothelial Growth Factor Receptor; FGFR: Fibroblast Growth Factor Receptor; KIT: c-Kit Receptor aka CD117.

Sorafenib (Nexavar®) is a multi-kinase small molecule inhibitor able to block CRAF, BRAF, VEGFR2, PDGFRβ, KIT and FLT3; is used in clinical trials as monotherapy or in combination with standard therapy (Wilhelm et al., 2006; Liu et al., 2006). Brivanib, a dual tyrosine kinase inhibitor of VEGFR and FGFR signaling, was active that in phase I clinical trials against metastatic solid tumors refractory to standard therapy (Park et al., 2011).

Imatinib mesilate (Gleevec®) binds to the inactive form of the BCR-ABL fusion protein inhibiting its activity and is used for the treatment of chronic myeloid leukemia. It also functions as a multi-target inhibitor of KIT and PDGFRβ. Due to this specificity it is also used in clinical trials for the treatment of metastatic GISTs and glioblastoma.

Other anti-VEGF therapeutic approaches are under pre-clinical and clinical trials (Roskoski, Jr., 2007; Kowanetz & Ferrara, 2006).

*Anti-EGFR therapy* - EGFR receptor was one of the first tyrosine kinase to be linked to tumor development and the dysregulation of one or more components of its pathway are a common trait of several tumor types. For this reason many molecules have been developed to try to inhibit the EGFR aberrant activity at different levels. Many of the mAbs and small molecules directly target the EGF receptor and some are currently used in clinical practice.

Gefitinib (Iressa®) was the first EGFR small molecule inhibitor to enter clinical trials (Schiller, 2003). In combination with standard therapy its activity has been evaluated in several tumor types such as non-small cell lung cancer and squamous cell carcinoma of the head and neck although no improvement in overall survival and response rate has been reported yet.

Cetuximab (Erbitux®), a human-mouse chimeric antibody able to bind and inhibit EGF receptor is used for the treatment of metastatic colorectal cancer (Goldberg, 2005). A higher response rate to the therapy was observed in combination with irinotecan, oxaliplatin or radiotherapy in different tumor types, highlighting the importance of acting on different cellular activities to inhibit tumor growth.

Panitumumab (Vectibix®) is another anti-EGFR antibody (Giusti et al., 2007) that has shown efficacy in chemotherapy refractory colorectal cancers and is being used in clinical trials for the treatment of esophageal, head and neck and lung tumors. Trastuzumab (Herceptin®) is a mAb approved in 1998 for the treatment of HER2-positive breast cancer patients in combination with paclitaxel and doxorubicin. This molecule is able to bind to the extracellular domain of ERBB2 preventing receptor dimerization and the subsequent signaling cascade.

Most of the failures with the use of some of these drugs may be due to a wrong selection of the patients. Indeed the utility of a personalized therapy derived from a patient selection based on tumor molecular profile has been demonstrated for several of these targeted therapeutics, including cetuximab and trastuzumab. The presence of a specific genomic and/or proteomic profile in fact correlates with the response to the therapy. Finally, other molecules that target multiple members of the EGF receptor family are currently under investigation (Reid et al., 2007) and some of them such as XL647 and AEE788 have shown to be active *in vitro* and are in different phases of clinical trials.

Considering the complexity of the mechanisms regulating tumor progression, the most effective approach in impairing tumor development is to simultaneously target different pathways. The increasing knowledge about the crosstalk between cancer cells and tumor microenvironment will allow the development of new drugs in order to block different players of the signaling cascades. The goal is that with the use of therapies involving complementary and synergistic combinations will increase drug efficacy and reduce toxicity as well as the risk of development of resistance to the treatment.

### 3.2 Apoptotic molecules

The ability of tumor cells to evade apoptosis is one of the hallmarks of cancer progression and can play a significant role in their resistance to conventional therapeutic regimens. To overcome resistance to apoptosis through the development of therapeutic drugs tackling the single components of the pathway is one of the efforts that is being attempted to potentiate the anti-tumoral therapy (Reed & Pellecchia, 2005). Researchers have also focused the attention on different agents able to indirectly modulate apoptosis (Fig. 3). Histone deacetylase (HDAC) inhibitors, for example, can reduce transcription of anti-apoptotic molecules of the Bcl2 family and are currently under investigation in clinical trials. Small-molecule drugs and mAbs directed against various RTKs analyzed in the previous section also affect this pathway and induce tumor cells to become more sensitive to apoptosis. Personalized treatments can be achieved given that the tumor-specific genetic lesions that affect sensitivity or resistance to apoptosis are well known (Zivny et al., 2010). In addition, different therapeutic strategies have been hypothesized or are currently under evaluation taking into account all the microenvironment molecules found to affect apoptosis. For instance, the *in vitro* anti-proliferative effect of exogenous SPARC could be exploited therapeutically by administering recombinant SPARC or one of its derivate peptides to patients. Pre-clinical studies are encouraging and demonstrate that subcutaneously administered SPARC can inhibit the growth of neuroblastoma xenografts in mice (Chlenski et al., 2002). Moreover, exogenous SPARC can reverse the acquired resistance to chemotherapeutic agents (Tai et al., 2005). As previously explained, integrins are involved in anchorage independent growth, anoikis resistance and metastasis formation, which are all characteristics of malignant tumor cells. For this reason small molecule antagonists able to block the integrin binding to the ECM molecules are currently under evaluation. As an example RGD-mimetic peptides have been extensively used in pre-clinical studies (Eble & Haier, 2006). Cilengitide, a cyclic peptidic antagonist of $\alpha_v\beta_3$ and $\alpha_v\beta_5$, to block also RGD-independent effects and to achieve a more efficacious anti-tumoral effect, for example (Paolillo et al., 2009). Furthermore, thanks to the capacity of the HS side chains of HSPGs to bind a multitude of growth factors, chemochines, cytochines and enzymes, neutralizing antibodies or antisense oligonucleotides have been demonstrated to enhance apoptosis in a number of tumor cells and may represent promising therapeutic approaches (Fukumoto et al., 2000). The abnormal PG expression in cancer and stromal cells may serve as a biomarker for tumor progression and patient survival. In this context, the better understanding of role of PGs in cancer progression may represent a novel approach in directly targeting the tumor microenvironment (Theocharis et al., 2010).

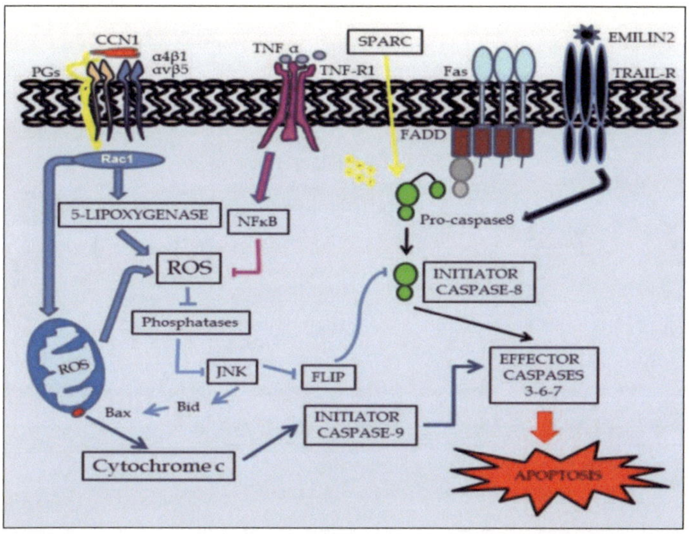


Fig. 3. Schematic representation of the therapeutic strategies targeting apoptosis. PGs: Proteoglycans; $\alpha_4\beta_1$ and $\alpha_v\beta_5$: integrin receptors; CCN1, SPARC and EMILIN2: extracellular matrix molecules; TNF α: Tumor Necrosis Factor α; TNF-R1: Tumor Necrosis Factor Receptor 1; Fas and TRAIL-R (TNF-Related Apoptosis Inducing Ligand Receptor) death receptors; FADD (Fas-Associated protein with Death Domain): adapter molecule of the extrinsic apoptotic pathway; ROS: Reactive Oxygen Species; FLIP: FLICE-like inhibitory protein.

Finally, also the ECM molecule EMILIN2 may represent a good target in this context and increasing its levels at the tumor site may suggest a therapeutic use since EMILIN2 exerts pro-apoptotic effects for tumor cells enhancing the extrinsic apoptotic pathway but leaves normal cells unharmed. This hypothesis is well supported by pre-clinical studies (Mongiat et al., 2007; Mongiat et al., 2010).

### 3.3 Cells of the microenvironment

*Targeting CAFs* - CAFs are the primary cells within the tumor stroma that determine the tumor dynamics. Despite their frequent genomic instability, they are more sensitive to chemotherapeutic drugs than tumor cells and thus are considered potential innovative therapeutic targets (Fig. 4). Many epithelial tumor cells secrete PDGF but lack PDGFR that is expressed by CAFs and its activation is frequently associated with metastases in colon carcinomas (Pietras et al., 2001; Bouzin & Feron, 2007; Haubeiss et al., 2010). In a recent study, the activity of four different FDA approved PDGF inhibitors such as Dasatinib, Imatinib, Nilotinib and Sorafenib has been compared and all were found to reduce CAFs' viability. Dasatinib resulted the most efficacious and inhibited not only CAFs' viability, but also induced a quiescent state and partially reverting their phenotype to normal. In addition, the incubation of cancer cells with conditioned media from CAFs pre-incubated with Dasatinib resulted in a significant reduction of tumor cell proliferation (Haubeiss et al., 2010). PDGF inhibitors also reduced the contractility of myofibroblasts in the tumor, thereby reducing interstitial fluid pressure and increasing chemotherapeutic drugs uptake. Encouraging results in inhibiting PDGFβ-R were also obtained using CDP860, a Fab' fragment-polyethylene glycol conjugate (Bouzin & Feron, 2007).

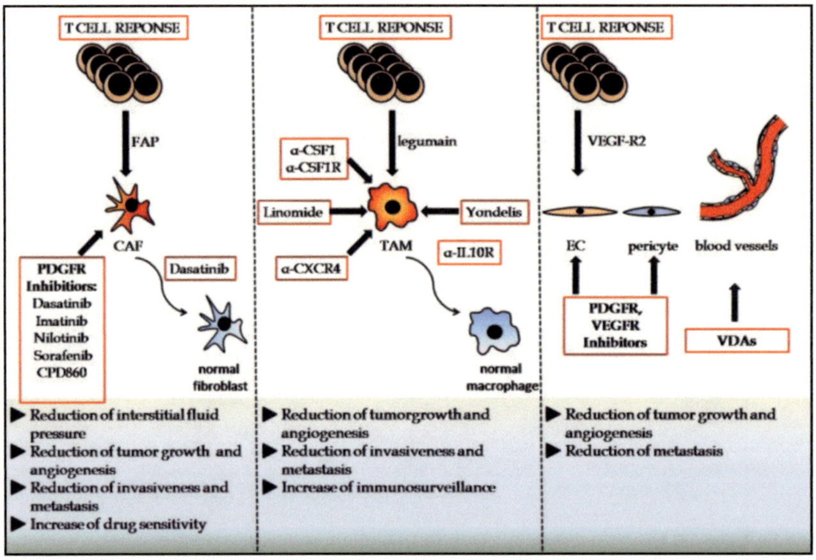


Fig. 4. Schematic representation of the therapeutic strategies targeting tumor associated cells FAP: Fibroblast Activating Protein; CAF: Cancer Associated Fibroblasts; PDGFR: Platelet-Derived Growth Factor Receptor; α-CSF1 and α-CSF1R: antibodies against the Colony Stimulating Factor 1 and its receptor; α-CXCR4: antibodies against the C-X-C chemockine receptor type 4; α-IL10R: antibodies against the Interleukin 10 Receptor ; VEGFR2: Vascular Endothelial Growth Factor 2; VDAs: Vascular Disrupting Agents.

Another potential therapeutic target is the Fibroblast Activating Protein (FAP), a serine protease actively implicated in ECM remodeling and over-expressed in different tumors. Several studies underline its involvement in immunosuppression, promotion of tumor growth and increased metastatic potential (Bouzin & Feron, 2007; Loeffler et al., 2006; Kraman et al., 2010). Apart from a FAP-antibody an oral DNA vaccine against FAP is also under evaluation. Through a specific CD8+ T cell-mediated killing of CAFs, this vaccine successfully affected both primary tumor growth and metastases of multidrug-resistant murine colon and breast carcinomas. Accordingly, FAP vaccinated mice display a reduction of intra-tumoral collagen I and thus an increased doxorubicin uptake leading in many cases to tumor rejection and increased lifespan (Loeffler et al., 2006).

*Targeting TAMs* - Possible therapeutic strategies targeting TAMs are aimed at reducing the number and the function of these cells and/or increasing their antitumor activity. Different groups reported that TAM are committed to produce high levels of the inhibitory cytokine IL10, which mediates defective IL12 production and NF-kB activation in TAMs, an event which is very important in determining TAMs activity and that is frequently correlated with poor prognosis. It has been demonstrated that the employment of anti-IL10 receptor antibodies and Toll-like receptor 9 ligand CpG can restore NF-kB activity and revert the macrophages phenotype from M2 to M1 status, thus activating an innate response against tumor (Guiducci et al., 2005).

Another way to reduce the number of TAMs is to target molecules that are involved in the recruitment of macrophages. In this perspective, the employment of antibodies against chemokines or chemokines receptors such as CFS1/CSF-1R could have important therapeutic effects.

Given the important role of TAMs in supporting angiogenesis, antiangiogenic drugs also represent a therapeutic tool against TAMs. Tumor infiltrating macrophages are a significant source of VEGF that act as a loop by recruiting other macrophages. Thus targeting this growth factor could reduce the number of TAMs in the tumor stroma. Linomide is an interesting antiangiogenic drug that is effective in the reduction of tumor growth in a murine prostate cancer model. Its activity includes the inhibition of macrophages recruitment and the increase of antiangiogenic molecules in TAMs such as IL12, IL18, CXCL10 and CXCL9. Hypoxia induces HIF, and hence VEGF expression in TAMs and HIF could represent another interesting target. Hypoxia signaling also leads to an increase in CXCR4 expression both on TAMs and ECs and CXCR4 antibodies such as AMD3100 inhibit tumor angiogenesis *in vivo* (Mantovani et al., 2004; Mantovani et al., 2006).

Anti-tumor agents with selective cytotoxic activity on monocyte-macrophages would be ideal therapeutic tools for their combined action on tumor cells and TAMs. Yondelis (Trabectedin), a natural product derived from the marine organism *Ecteinascidia turbinate* displays a potent anti-tumor activity and is specifically cytotoxic to macrophages and TAMs, while sparing the lymphocyte sub-set (Sessa et al., 2005). In addition, Yondelis inhibits the production of CCL2 and IL6 by TAMs which in turn contribute to growth suppression of inflammation-associated human tumors (Allavena et al., 2005).

A legumain-based vaccine represents another strategy aimed at inducing the host to contrast the infiltration of TAMs in the tumor. In fact, legumain, a member of the endopeptidase family, is highly over-expressed by TAMs in murine and human breast tumor tissues, and hence provides an ideal strategy for breast tumor targeting (Lewen et al., 2008; Xiang et al., 2008). The vaccination of mice against legumain provides a robust CD8+ T cell response against TAMs, significantly reducing tumor growth. Moreover, a dramatic reduction in TGFβ, TNFα, MMP9 and VEGF expression is induced, with a consequent reduction of both angiogenesis and metastatic rate (Luo et al., 2006).

*Targeting ECs and pericytes* - Besides targeting pro-angiogenetic growth factors and cytokines as mentioned above it is also possible to specifically target ECs and pericytes. The selective disruption of tumor vessels through the employment of the so called vascular disrupting agents (VDAs) is a potentially useful alternative strategy. These compounds that predominantly affect the tumor periphery and small tumor masses have a different mechanism of action and tolerability profile compared with conventional antiangiogenic drugs and thus may provide an additional clinical benefit for a wide patient population. VDAs act to disrupt the established tumor vasculature in order to create an extensive necrosis in the tumor core. On the basis of their mechanism of action, VDAs are divided into 2 groups. The first includes the tubulin-binding agents that selectively target tumor ECs by disrupting their cytoskeleton. The second VDAs group includes compounds related to flavone acetic acid and they act in two ways; they induce ECs apoptosis and indirectly increase the intra-tumoral concentrations of TNFα and other cytokines, as well as nitric oxide, leading to an inhibition of tumor flow (Boehm et al., 2010; McKeage & Baguley, 2010).

### 3.4 ECM and angiogenesis

As previously mentioned, anti-angiogenic therapy represent a promising strategy for cancer therapy and offers the chance to avoid resistance to chemotherapeutic treatments. J. Folkman's long-standing vision of angiogenesis as a therapeutic target has been increasingly validated in both traditional transplant tumor models and genetically engineered mouse models of cancer (Szentirmai et al., 2008). Important targets in this context are ECM molecules (Fig. 5) which can exert both pro-angiogenic or anti-angiogenic effects (Tabruyn & Griffioen, 2007).

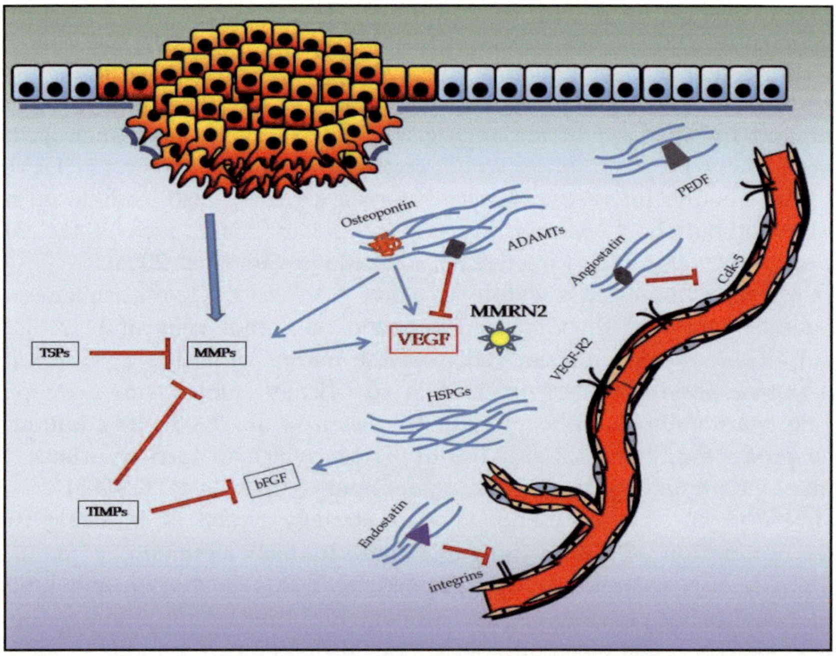


Fig. 5. Schematic representation of the therapeutic strategies targeting angiogenesis hinging on ECM molecules; TSPs: thrombospondins; MMPs: metalloproteinases; bFGF: basic Fibroblast Growth Factor; HSPGs: Heparan Sulfate Proteoglycans; VEGF and VEGFR2: Vascular Endothelial Growth Factor and one of its receptors; MMRN2: MULTIMERIN2; ADAMTS: A Disintegrin And Metalloproteinase with Thrombospondin Motifs; PEDF: Pigment Epithelial-Derived Factor; cdk-5: cyclin dependent kinase 5.

*Pro-angiogenic ECM proteins* - Many ECM proteins surrounding the vasculature including collagens, laminins, and fibronectins are pro-angiogenic promoting EC survival, proliferation, migration and tube formation. Pro-angiogenic factors such as VEGF, bFGF and TGF-β are bound and sequestered by the ECM via the heparan-like glycosaminoglycans. Fibronectin, a fairly ubiquitous and abundant ECM protein that becomes assembled into fibrils at the cell surface, is necessary for vasculogenesis, in fact if this gene is knocked out mice die before birth due among others, to vascular bed defects. An alternatively-spliced form of fibronectin that contains an extra B domain has been found in fetal and neoplastic tissues but not in normal adult tissues; this isoform was found to be synthesized by the vascular cells in malignant astrocytoma (Castellani et al., 2002) and its expression appears to be a precise diagnostic marker of the highest grade of glioma or glioblastoma. Also other studies demonstrate that this isoform may be a good marker of angiogenesis (Santimaria et al., 2003) and could also be a therapeutic target.

Osteopontin, a secreted cell attachment protein, seems to be over-expressed in association with increased tumor angiogenesis (Hirama et al., 2003). The proangiogenic function of osteopontin can be attributed to its ability to promote VEGF-directed dermal microvascular EC migration (Senger et al., 1996) and to increase MMP-2 levels in an RGD-dependent manner (Teti et al., 1998). Additionally, osteopontin-bound integrin $\alpha_v\beta_3$ inhibits NF-kB-dependent EC apoptosis (Cooper et al., 2002).

Tenascin-C is a glycoprotein composed of six subunits covalently associated by disulfide bonds. Different human Tenascin-C isoforms are generated by alternative splicing with aberrantly regulation in neoplastic tissues (Jones & Jones, 2000). It is expressed around angiogenic vessels in many tumors and there is evidence that it promotes and regulates angiogenesis *in vitro* and *in vivo*. Indeed the antibodies directed against Tenascin-C in glioma patients induced a significant inhibition of tumor angiogenesis.

HSPGs are necessary for stable binding of the proangiogenic growth factor bFGF to its receptor (Ornitz et al., 1992) and alterations in HS glycosamminoglycan in breast carcinoma have been shown to result in an increase in bFGF binding and receptor complex assembly.

Perlecan deposited along blood vessels basement membrane is thought to mediate structural and functional interactions with different molecules (Iozzo, 2005; Mongiat et al., 2003a). Intact perlecan is thought to be a pro-angiogenic HSPG as: *i)* its expression is altered during embryonic vasculogenesis and in neoplasia (Tapanadechopone et al., 2001; Zhou et al., 2004) perlecan-null mice show severe and sometimes fatal vascular and chondrogenic defects (Costell et al., 1999); *iii)* antisense targeting of perlecan blocks tumor growth and angiogenesis *in vivo* (Sharma et al., 1998); and *iv)* increased perlecan expression stimulates angiogenesis (Jiang & Couchman, 2003). Tumor cell secreted perlecan is thought to promote EC sprouting and proliferation, thereby promoting angiogenesis (Jiang et al., 2004). Interestingly a degradation product of perlecan (endorepellin) exerts an opposite effect (Mongiat et al., 2003b).

Transmembrane chondroitin sulphate proteoglycan NG2 is another protein involved in tumor angiogenesis and has been shown to promote EC spreading perycite function (Ozerdem & Stallcup, 2003). An additional proangiogenic mechanism by which NG2 promotes angiogenesis includes its ability to bind and sequester angiostatin, thus blocking its antiangiogenic function (Chekenya et al., 2002). All these molecules may represent important tools for the development of drugs able to counteract blood vessel formation.

*Anti-angiogenic ECM proteins* - Among the molecules that counteract blood vessel formation thrombospondin-1 (TSP-1) and thrombospondin-2 (TSP-2) are the best studied and their expression in tumor tissues is often inversely correlated with angiogenesis (Adams, 2001; Adams & Lawler, 2004; Armstrong & Bornstein, 2003). The mechanisms by which they can inhibit angiogenesis include: *i)* the induction of EC apoptosis by the binding of TSP-1, and potentially TSP-2, to CD36, thereby inducing Fas ligand expression (Jimenez et al., 2000; Nor et al., 2000); *ii)* the clearance of MMP-2 following lysosomal degradation of the TSP-2/MMP-2 complex (Armstrong et al., 2002; Rodriguez-Manzaneque et al., 2001) and *iii)* inhibition of EC proliferation (Armstrong et al., 2002).

Another extensively studied molecule is angiostatin, the cleavage product of plasminogen, the only not ECM antiangiogenic protein among the molecules described above. Angiostatin was shown to inhibit EC proliferation and motility and to down-regulate the protein level of cyclin-dependent kinase 5 (cdk5), a cdk absent in quiescent EC and induced by bFGF (Sharma et al., 2004). Angiostatin also acts by upregulating the mRNA levels of FasL and reducing the level of c-Flip which activates the extrinsic apoptotic pathway.

Other endogenous angiogenesis inhibitors include cryptic fragments from ECM molecules such as endostatin, a specific and potent anti-angiogenic factor generated from the proteolytic cleavage of collagen XVIII by matrix metalloproteinases, elastases or cathepsins (Kim et al., 2009). Endostatin inhibits EC proliferation and migration and causes EC G1 arrest and apoptotic cell death (Dhanabal et al., 1999). These properties have provided clues for development of an anti-tumor strategy with proven therapeutic effectiveness in numerous models of neoplasia.

Pigment epithelial-derived factor (PEDF) was initially identified as an antiangiogenic protein. Its high expression has been linked to decreased microvessel density and suppression of tumor growth in a number of tumors including glioma as well as prostate carcinoma and melanoma (Abe et al., 2004). In support of a role for PEDF in inhibiting angiogenesis, increased microvessel density is found in PEDF deficient mouse tissues (Doll et al., 2003), in addition PEDF inhibits cornea neovascularisation. The mechanism whereby PEDF acts to inhibit angiogenesis likely resides on its ability to bind collagen and to potentially interfere with the adhesion of cells to the collagen (Meyer et al., 2002) as well as triggering Fas up-regulation and down-regulation of the VEGF mRNA levels (Takenaka et al., 2005).

MULTIMERIN2 (MMRN2), also known as EndoGlyx-1, is an ECM glycoprotein exclusively expressed in the blood vessel in close proximity with the endothelium. In neoplastic tissues, MMRN2 is consistently found to be deposited along tumor capillaries and, in certain tumors, in the "hot spots" of neoangiogenesis (Belien et al., 1999). This protein is characterized by a short cluster of charged amino acids (10 out of 27 residues) located between the coiled-coil region and the C1q-like domain. The basic amino acids are arranged in a sequence similar to that of the consensus motifs responsible for the ionic interactions with glucosaminoglycans, such as heparin and heparan sulfate (Hileman et al., 1998) and are also found in heparin binding proteins such as the von Willebrand factor (Sobel et al., 1992). Given its deposition in tight contact with the EC surface, we have hypothesized the involvement of this protein in the regulation of angiogenesis and demonstrated that MMRN2 functions as a homeostatic molecule for ECs preventing their sprouting to form new vessels (unpublished results). This strong anti-angiogenic effect is reflected in a potent *in vivo* anti-tumor activity effect following treatment with MMRN2. For these reasons we are confident that this molecule represents a promising tool for the development of novel approaches to impair angiogenesis and tumor growth.

### 3.5 ECM molecules involved in invasion and metastasis.

The targeting of ECM components and ECM-remodeling enzymes that would prevent changes of the stroma homeostasis promoting cancer progression has received much attention and is becoming an increasingly attractive therapeutic approach for preventing cancer progression and metastasis (Fig. 6).

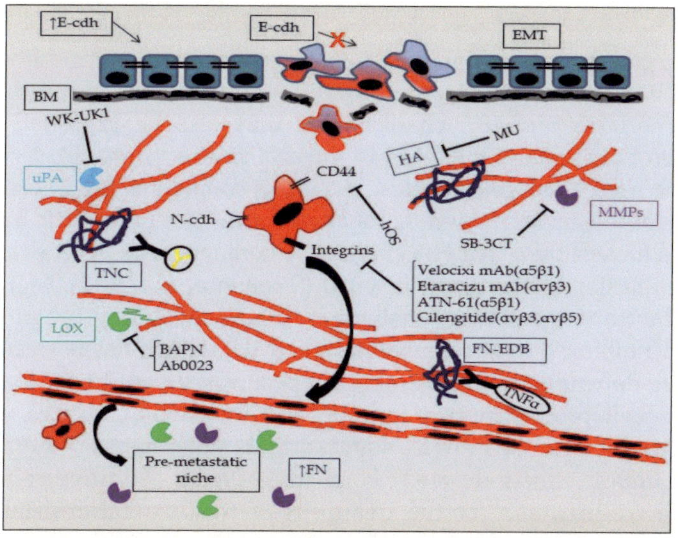


Fig. 6. Schematic representation of the therapeutic strategies targeting the metastatic processes. E-cdh: E-cadherin; EMT: Epithelial-Mesenchymal Transition; BM: Basement Membrane; WK-UT1: uPA (urokinase-type Plasminogen Activator) inhibitor; TNC: Tenascin-c; LOX: lysil oxidase activity; BAPN: β-aminoproprionitrile LOX inhibitor; Ab0023 inhibitory monoclonal antibody specific for the LOX family member LOXL2; N-cdh: N-cadherin; hOS: hyaluronan oligosaccharides; HA: Hyaluronan; MU: HA syntetase inhibitor 4-methylumbelliferone; MMPs: metalloproteinases; SB-3CT: MMP-2 and -9 inhibitor; FN: fibronectin; FN-EDB: oncofetal form of fibronectin; TNFα: Tumor Necrosis Factor α.

*ECM components* - The peculiar expression of tumor-associated ECM components may offer the opportunity to develop new strategies for cancer treatment, either targeting their function associated to tumor progression or by exploiting their specific localization to delivery bioactive molecules to the tumors. The ECM components are highly abundant in tumors and are often more stable than cell surface antigens. One example of this type of approach is offered by tenascin-C (TNC), which exerts different effects both on tumor cells and also on the many cell types within the tumor, thus affecting cancer progression. The effects on tumor and stromal cells are exerted very early in tumorigenesis and persist during tumor progression. Currently, the most promising approach is to target TNC with a specific mAb (81C6) coupled to radioactive molecules. This strategy has been successful in patients with recurrent primary and metastatic brain tumors, and is currently in clinical trials (Xing et al., 2010). A similar approach targeting the oncofetal form of fibronectin (FN-EDB) containing an extra-domain, and often up-regulated in tumors was particularly successful. Anti-FN-EDB antibodies show specific localization to a range of tumors, including brain, lung and colorectal cancers. This antibody has been used as a vehicle for TNFα and has been shown to induce necrosis in tumors (Allen & Louise, 2011).

*Cell-cell and cell-ECM interactions* - Integrin-targeted therapeutics have recently been proved beneficial in delivering chemotherapeutics, oncolytic viruses, proapoptotic peptides and redionucleotides to both tumor cells and the supporting vasculature. Recent studies showed that delivery of targeted nanoparticles loaded with doxorubicin to integrin $\alpha_V\beta_3$-positive tumor vasculature inhibited metastases while eliminating the toxicity and patients' weight loss associated with the systemic administration of this drug (Desgrosellier & Cheresh, 2010).

HA contributes to cancer progression in many types of carcinomas and it is up-regulated in tumor stroma; its activated CD44 receptor is over-expressed in solid tumors unlike the non-tumorigenic counterparts and this characteristic may also be exploited to develop new therapies. The membrane receptor CD44 can internalize HA, thus, HA-carrying drugs have the potential to be used as targeted drugs. HA–drug conjugates are internalized via CD44, and the drug is released and activated mainly by intracellular enzymatic hydrolysis. Several preclinical studies have shown that HA chemically conjugated to cytotoxic agents improves the anticancer properties of the agent in vitro (Sironen et al., 2011). Manipulation of HA synthesis alters the tumorigenicity of malignant tumors, including breast cancer. Recently, the HA syntetase inhibitor 4-methylumbelliferone (MU), which has been reported to inhibit HA synthesis dose-dependently in several cell types, was shown to exert anti-tumor effects inhibiting *in vitro* cell proliferation, migration and invasion (Urakawa et al., 2011). MU suppresses intra-osseous tumor growth, suggesting its potential as a therapeutic candidate for established breast cancer-derived bone metastasis. Additive effects of MU in combination with trastuzumab for the treatment of trastuzumab-resistant breast cancers have also been reported both in *in vitro* and *in vivo* experiments.

The expression of integrins by various cell types involved in tumor progression and their ability to crosstalk with growth factor receptors has made them appealing therapeutic targets. Integrin inhibitors have been extensively studied as anti-cancer agents because integrins play a dual function: they are involved in invasion of tumor cells out of the primary tumor site to the metastatic sites, but they also regulate ECs migration into the tumor mass during angiogenesis (Veiseh et al., 2011). Velociximab, a chimeric mAb that inhibits integrin $\alpha_5\beta_1$, has been used in clinical phase II trials for renal cell carcinoma, metastatic melanoma and pancreatic cancer. The rationale of using velociximab in cancer therapy is based on the fact that this specific integrin is expressed by endothelial cells and up-regulated in tumor vasculature (Jarvelainen et al., 2009). The use of etaracizumab, a blocking antibody for $\alpha_V\beta_3$ integrin, directly affects not only cancer cell growth and angiogenesis, but also osteoclast attachment, suggesting a possible efficacy in reducing bone metastasis (Desgrosellier & Cheresh, 2010).

Another strategy is based on the development of small-molecules compounds or peptide mimetics in order to block the integrin signaling pathways activated by ECM remodeling. A successful example of this strategy is cilengitide, a cyclic RGD peptide that inhibits integrins $\alpha_V\beta_3$ and $\alpha_V\beta_5$, that has been proven promising in lung and prostate cancer patients and for the treatment of glioblastoma (Allen & Louise, 2011). ATN-61 is a non-RGD-based peptide inhibitor of integrin $\alpha_5\beta_1$ blocking breast cancer growth and metastasis and, in combination with fluorouracil, significantly reduces liver metastasis in mouse models of colon cancer (Desgrosellier & Cheresh, 2010). Targeting other types of ECM receptors has also been attempted. For example the administration of hyaluronan oligosaccharides (hOS), which interfere with the CD44-hyaluronan interaction are effective inhibitors of the progression of several tumor types, including mammary and lung carcinoma.

Likewise, increasing the cadherins expression could inhibit cell invasion by strengthening cell-cell adhesions, thus preventing the cell from escaping the primary tumor. Indeed, forcing the overexpression of cadherins has been the focus of some anti-invasion therapy studies (Junxia et al., 2010).

*Modification enzymes* – The inhibition of LOX activity reduces primary tumor growth and mechanotransduction in the mammary epithelium. LOX inhibition prevents the invasion of tumor cells *in vivo* and abrogates bone marrow derived cells recruitment and the establishment of metastasis. It also destabilizes already-formed metastases reducing their growth and improves patients' survival (Cox & Erler, 2011). LOX inhibitors are currently in development for clinical use. For example, a small-molecule lysyl oxidase inhibitor called β-aminoproprionitrile (BAPN) is available for clinical studies and it prevents the invasion of metastatic breast cancer and melanoma cell lines *in vitro* (Baker et al., 2011). More recently the efficacy of BAPN was outperformed by the use of an inhibitory mAb (AB0023) specific for LOXL2, a member of the LOX family, that was efficacious in both primary and metastatic xenograft models of cancer, as well as in liver and lung fibrosis models (Barry-Hamilton et al., 2010).

*Proteases* - On the basis of the pivotal roles that MMPs play in several steps of cancer progression, many efforts have been spent with the aim of developing safe and effective agents targeting MMPs. Several generations of MMPs inhibitors have been tested in phase II clinical trials, including peptidomimetics, non-peptidomimetics and tetracycline derivates (Gialeli et al., 2011). Unfortunately so far the results have been disappointing; all the clinical trials involving the use of MMPs inhibitors have failed to show significant efficacy and to increase the rates of patients' survival (Cox & Erler, 2011). The poor success of this approach largely depended on the toxicity of the compounds for normal tissues, to the conflicting roles of MMPs in both promoting and reducing metastatic dissemination, and to the functional redundancy between the family members. Nevertheless, the ongoing challenge is the development of a new generation of highly specific MMPs inhibitors, as for example SB-3CT that binds to the active site of MMP-2 and -9 and re-establishes the pro-enzyme structure. These new compounds aim at targeting the enzymes involved in ECM remodeling avoiding unwanted side effects. To increase the specificity of MMPs inhibitors, the future of drug development comprises the use of molecules targeting specific exo-sites, specific binding sites outside the active domain of the metalloprotease involved in substrate selection (Gialeli et al., 2011).

Finally, also the uPA system (uPAS), due its involvement in many steps of cancer progression, including angiogenesis, cell proliferation, invasion and growth at the metastatic site, represents a suitable source for the development of new anti-cancer drugs. Several therapeutical approaches aimed at inhibiting the uPA/uPAR functions lead to anti-tumor effects in xenograft models, including selective inhibitors of uPA activity such as WK-UK1, antagonist peptides, mAbs able to prevent uPA/uPAR binding and gene therapy techniques aimed at silencing uPA/uPAR expression. However, although promising, all these strategies need definitive confirmation in humans as, up to now, only few uPA inhibitors have been used in clinical trial (Ulisse et al., 2009).

## 4. Conclusions

The cells and molecules of the tumor microenvironment hold the potential for the development of innovative therapeutic approaches. Many of the molecules and approaches that we have taken into account in this chapter are currently in clinical trials, while some have only been suggested based on preliminary results and require further investigations. To avoid problems of toxicity and resistance to the treatments the future of cancer therapy is likely to involve the use of combinatorial treatments that will include conventional chemotherapeutic agents at lower doses and novel molecules able to halt tumor development with little or no toxicity for the patient.

## 5. References

Abe, R., Shimizu, T., Yamagishi, S., Shibaki, A., Amano, S., Inagaki, Y., Watanabe, H., Sugawara, H., Nakamura, H., Takeuchi, M., Imaizumi, T. & Shimizu, H. (2004). Overexpression of pigment epithelium-derived factor decreases angiogenesis and inhibits the growth of human malignant melanoma cells in vivo, *Am J Pathol* 164, 1225-1232

Abrams, T.J., Lee, L.B., Murray, L.J., Pryer, N.K. & Cherrington, J.M. (2003). SU11248 inhibits KIT and platelet-derived growth factor receptor beta in preclinical models of human small cell lung cancer, *Mol. Cancer Ther.* 2, 471-478

Adams, J.C. (2001). Thrombospondins: multifunctional regulators of cell interactions, *Annu. Rev Cell Dev. Biol* 17, 25-51

Adams, J.C. & Lawler, J. (2004). The thrombospondins, *Int. J Biochem. Cell Biol* 36, 961-968

Adderley, S.R. & Fitzgerald, D.J. (2000). Glycoprotein IIb/IIIa antagonists induce apoptosis in rat cardiomyocytes by caspase-3 activation, *J Biol Chem.* 275, 5760-5766

Allavena, P., Sica, A., Garlanda, C. & Mantovani, A. (2008). The Yin-Yang of tumor-associated macrophages in neoplastic progression and immune surveillance, *Immunol. Rev* 222, 155-161

Allavena, P., Signorelli, M., Chieppa, M., Erba, E., Bianchi, G., Marchesi, F., Olimpio, C.O., Bonardi, C., Garbi, A., Lissoni, A., de, B.F., Jimeno, J. & D'Incalci, M. (2005). Anti-inflammatory properties of the novel antitumor agent yondelis (trabectedin): inhibition of macrophage differentiation and cytokine production, *Cancer Res* 65, 2964-2971

Allen, M. & Louise, J.J. (2011). Jekyll and Hyde: the role of the microenvironment on the progression of cancer, *J Pathol* 223, 162-176

Armstrong, L.C., Bjorkblom, B., Hankenson, K.D., Siadak, A.W., Stiles, C.E. & Bornstein, P. (2002). Thrombospondin 2 inhibits microvascular endothelial cell proliferation by a caspase-independent mechanism, *Mol. Biol Cell* 13, 1893-1905

Armstrong, L.C. & Bornstein, P. (2003). Thrombospondins 1 and 2 function as inhibitors of angiogenesis, *Matrix Biol* 22, 63-71

Augsten, M., Hagglof, C., Pena, C. & Ostman, A. (2010). A digest on the role of the tumor microenvironment in gastrointestinal cancers, *Cancer Microenviron.* 3, 167-176

Baker, A.M., Cox, T.R., Bird, D., Lang, G., Murray, G.I., Sun, X.F., Southall, S.M., Wilson, J.R. & Erler, J.T. (2011). The role of lysyl oxidase in SRC-dependent proliferation and metastasis of colorectal cancer, *J Natl. Cancer Inst.* 103, 407-424

Barry-Hamilton, V., Spangler, R., Marshall, D., McCauley, S., Rodriguez, H.M., Oyasu, M., Mikels, A., Vaysberg, M., Ghermazien, H., Wai, C., Garcia, C.A., Velayo, A.C., Jorgensen, B., Biermann, D., Tsai, D., Green, J., Zaffryar-Eilot, S., Holzer, A., Ogg, S., Thai, D., Neufeld, G., Van, V.P. & Smith, V. (2010). Allosteric inhibition of lysyl oxidase-like-2 impedes the development of a pathologic microenvironment, *Nat Med.* 16, 1009-1017

Belien, J.A., Somi, S., de Jong, J.S., van Diest, P.J. & Baak, J.P. (1999). Fully automated microvessel counting and hot spot selection by image processing of whole tumour sections in invasive breast cancer, *J Clin Pathol* 52, 184-192

Bishop, J.R., Schuksz, M. & Esko, J.D. (2007). Heparan sulphate proteoglycans fine-tune mammalian physiology, *Nature* 446, 1030-1037

Boehm, S., Rothermundt, C., Hess, D. & Joerger, M. (2010). Antiangiogenic drugs in oncology: a focus on drug safety and the elderly - a mini-review, *Gerontology* 56, 303-309

Bouzin, C. & Feron, O. (2007). Targeting tumor stroma and exploiting mature tumor vasculature to improve anti-cancer drug delivery, *Drug Resist. Updat.* 10, 109-120

Brooks, S.A., Lomax-Browne, H.J., Carter, T.M., Kinch, C.E. & Hall, D.M. (2010). Molecular interactions in cancer cell metastasis, *Acta Histochem.* 112, 3-25

Campbell, N.E., Kellenberger, L., Greenaway, J., Moorehead, R.A., Linnerth-Petrik, N.M. & Petrik, J. (2010). Extracellular matrix proteins and tumor angiogenesis, *J Oncol.* 2010, 586905

Carmeliet, P., Lampugnani, M.G., Moons, L., Breviario, F., Compernolle, V., Bono, F., Balconi, G., Spagnuolo, R., Oosthuyse, B., Dewerchin, M., Zanetti, A., Angellilo, A., Mattot, V., Nuyens, D., Lutgens, E., Clotman, F., de Ruiter, M.C., Gittenberger-de, G.A., Poelmann, R., Lupu, F., Herbert, J.M., Collen, D. & Dejana, E. (1999). Targeted deficiency or cytosolic truncation of the VE-cadherin gene in mice impairs VEGF-mediated endothelial survival and angiogenesis, *Cell* 98, 147-157

Castellani, P., Borsi, L., Carnemolla, B., Biro, A., Dorcaratto, A., Viale, G.L., Neri, D. & Zardi, L. (2002). Differentiation between high- and low-grade astrocytoma using a human recombinant antibody to the extra domain-B of fibronectin, *Am J Pathol* 161, 1695-1700

Chekenya, M., Hjelstuen, M., Enger, P.O., Thorsen, F., Jacob, A.L., Probst, B., Haraldseth, O., Pilkington, G., Butt, A., Levine, J.M. & Bjerkvig, R. (2002). NG2 proteoglycan promotes angiogenesis-dependent tumor growth in CNS by sequestering angiostatin, *FASEB J* 16, 586-588

Chetty, C., Lakka, S.S., Bhoopathi, P., Kunigal, S., Geiss, R. & Rao, J.S. (2008). Tissue inhibitor of metalloproteinase 3 suppresses tumor angiogenesis in matrix metalloproteinase 2-down-regulated lung cancer, *Cancer Res* 68, 4736-4745

Chlenski, A., Liu, S., Crawford, S.E., Volpert, O.V., DeVries, G.H., Evangelista, A., Yang, Q., Salwen, H.R., Farrer, R., Bray, J. & Cohn, S.L. (2002). SPARC is a key Schwannian-derived inhibitor controlling neuroblastoma tumor angiogenesis, *Cancer Res* 62, 7357-7363

Chua, C.C., Rahimi, N., Forsten-Williams, K. & Nugent, M.A. (2004). Heparan sulfate proteoglycans function as receptors for fibroblast growth factor-2 activation of extracellular signal-regulated kinases 1 and 2, *Circ Res* 94, 316-323

Coghlin, C. & Murray, G.I. (2010). Current and emerging concepts in tumour metastasis, *J Pathol* 222, 1-15

Cooper, C.R., Chay, C.H. & Pienta, K.J. (2002). The role of alpha(v)beta(3) in prostate cancer progression, *Neoplasia.* 4, 191-194

Costell, M., Gustafsson, E., Aszodi, A., Morgelin, M., Bloch, W., Hunziker, E., Addicks, K., Timpl, R. & Fassler, R. (1999). Perlecan maintains the integrity of cartilage and some basement membranes, *J Cell Biol* 147, 1109-1122

Cox, T.R. & Erler, J.T. (2011). Remodeling and homeostasis of the extracellular matrix: implications for fibrotic diseases and cancer, *Dis. Model. Mech.* 4, 165-178

Dancey, J. & Sausville, E.A. (2003). Issues and progress with protein kinase inhibitors for cancer treatment, *Nat Rev Drug Discov.* 2, 296-313

Deckers, M.M., van Bezooijen, R.L., van der Horst, G., Hoogendam, J., van Der, B.C., Papapoulos, S.E. & Lowik, C.W. (2002). Bone morphogenetic proteins stimulate angiogenesis through osteoblast-derived vascular endothelial growth factor A, *Endocrinology* 143, 1545-1553

Desgrosellier, J.S. & Cheresh, D.A. (2010). Integrins in cancer: biological implications and therapeutic opportunities, *Nat Rev Cancer* 10, 9-22

Dhanabal, M., Volk, R., Ramchandran, R., Simons, M. & Sukhatme, V.P. (1999). Cloning, expression, and in vitro activity of human endostatin, *Biochem. Biophys. Res Commun.* 258, 345-352

Doliana, R., Bot, S., Bonaldo, P. & Colombatti, A. (2000). EMI, a novel cysteine-rich domain of EMILINs and other extracellular proteins, interacts with the gC1q domains and participates in multimerization, *FEBS Lett.* 484, 164-168

Doll, J.A., Stellmach, V.M., Bouck, N.P., Bergh, A.R., Lee, C., Abramson, L.P., Cornwell, M.L., Pins, M.R., Borensztajn, J. & Crawford, S.E. (2003). Pigment epithelium-derived factor regulates the vasculature and mass of the prostate and pancreas, *Nat Med.* 9, 774-780

Dunn, J.R., Reed, J.E., du Plessis, D.G., Shaw, E.J., Reeves, P., Gee, A.L., Warnke, P. & Walker, C. (2006). Expression of ADAMTS-8, a secreted protease with antiangiogenic properties, is downregulated in brain tumours, *Br. J Cancer* 94, 1186-1193

Eble, J.A. & Haier, J. (2006). Integrins in cancer treatment, *Curr. Cancer Drug Targets.* 6, 89-105

Elbauomy, E.S., Green, A.R., Lambros, M.B., Turner, N.C., Grainge, M.J., Powe, D., Ellis, I.O. & Reis-Filho, J.S. (2007). FGFR1 amplification in breast carcinomas: a chromogenic in situ hybridisation analysis, *Breast Cancer Res* 9, R23

Erez, N., Truitt, M., Olson, P., Arron, S.T. & Hanahan, D. (2010). Cancer-Associated Fibroblasts Are Activated in Incipient Neoplasia to Orchestrate Tumor-Promoting Inflammation in an NF-kappaB-Dependent Manner, *Cancer Cell* 17, 135-147

Erler, J.T., Bennewith, K.L., Cox, T.R., Lang, G., Bird, D., Koong, A., Le, Q.T. & Giaccia, A.J. (2009). Hypoxia-induced lysyl oxidase is a critical mediator of bone marrow cell recruitment to form the premetastatic niche, *Cancer Cell* 15, 35-44

Erler, J.T. & Giaccia, A.J. (2006). Lysyl oxidase mediates hypoxic control of metastasis, *Cancer Res* 66, 10238-10241

Ferrara, N., Hillan, K.J. & Novotny, W. (2005). Bevacizumab (Avastin), a humanized anti-VEGF monoclonal antibody for cancer therapy, *Biochem. Biophys. Res Commun.* 333, 328-335

Folkman, J. (1971). Tumor angiogenesis: therapeutic implications, *N. Engl. J. Med.* 285, 1182-1186

Folkman, J. (2006). Angiogenesis, *Annu. Rev Med.* 57, 1-18

Folkman, J. & Klagsbrun, M. (1987). Angiogenic factors, *Science* 235, 442-447

Fridlender, Z.G., Sun, J., Kim, S., Kapoor, V., Cheng, G., Ling, L., Worthen, G.S. & Albelda, S.M. (2009). Polarization of tumor-associated neutrophil phenotype by TGF-beta: "N1" versus "N2" TAN, *Cancer Cell* 16, 183-194

Frisch, S.M. & Screaton, R.A. (2001). Anoikis mechanisms, *Curr. Opin. Cell Biol* 13, 555-562

Fukumoto, M., Takahashi, J.A., Murai, N., Ueba, T., Kono, K. & Nakatsu, S. (2000). Induction of apoptosis in glioma cells: an approach to control tumor growth by blocking basic fibroblast growth factor autocrine loop, *Anticancer Res* 20, 4059-4065

Geho, D.H., Bandle, R.W., Clair, T. & Liotta, L.A. (2005). Physiological mechanisms of tumor-cell invasion and migration, *Physiology (Bethesda. )* 20, 194-200

Gialeli, C., Theocharis, A.D. & Karamanos, N.K. (2011). Roles of matrix metalloproteinases in cancer progression and their pharmacological targeting, *FEBS J* 278, 16-27

Giatromanolaki, A., Sivridis, E. & Koukourakis, M.I. (2006). Angiogenesis in colorectal cancer: prognostic and therapeutic implications, *Am J Clin Oncol.* 29, 408-417

Gilmore, A.P. (2005). Anoikis, *Cell Death. Differ.* 12 Suppl 2, 1473-1477

Ginath, S., Menczer, J., Friedmann, Y., Aingorn, H., Aviv, A., Tajima, K., Dantes, A., Glezerman, M., Vlodavsky, I. & Amsterdam, A. (2001). Expression of heparanase, Mdm2, and erbB2 in ovarian cancer, *Int. J Oncol.* 18, 1133-1144

Giralt, J., Navalpotro, B., Hermosilla, E., de, T., I, Espin, E., Reyes, V., Cerezo, L., de las, H.M., Cajal, S., Armengol, M. & Benavente, S. (2006). Prognostic significance of vascular endothelial growth factor and cyclooxygenase-2 in patients with rectal cancer treated with preoperative radiotherapy, *Oncology* 71, 312-319

Giusti, R.M., Shastri, K.A., Cohen, M.H., Keegan, P. & Pazdur, R. (2007). FDA drug approval summary: panitumumab (Vectibix), *Oncologist.* 12, 577-583

Goldberg, R.M. (2005). Cetuximab, *Nat Rev Drug Discov.* Suppl, S10-S11

Gorringe, K.L., Jacobs, S., Thompson, E.R., Sridhar, A., Qiu, W., Choong, D.Y. & Campbell, I.G. (2007). High-resolution single nucleotide polymorphism array analysis of epithelial ovarian cancer reveals numerous microdeletions and amplifications, *Clin Cancer Res* 13, 4731-4739

Gregory, A.D. & Houghton, A.M. (2011). Tumor-Associated Neutrophils: New Targets for Cancer Therapy, *Cancer Res*

Guiducci, C., Vicari, A.P., Sangaletti, S., Trinchieri, G. & Colombo, M.P. (2005). Redirecting in vivo elicited tumor infiltrating macrophages and dendritic cells towards tumor rejection, *Cancer Res* 65, 3437-3446

Guruvayoorappan, C. (2008). Tumor versus tumor-associated macrophages: how hot is the link?, *Integr. Cancer Ther.* 7, 90-95

Guttery, D.S., Shaw, J.A., Lloyd, K., Pringle, J.H. & Walker, R.A. (2010). Expression of tenascin-C and its isoforms in the breast, *Cancer Metastasis Rev* 29, 595-606

Han, S., Sidell, N., Roser-Page, S. & Roman, J. (2004). Fibronectin stimulates human lung carcinoma cell growth by inducing cyclooxygenase-2 (COX-2) expression, *Int. J. Cancer* 111, 322-331

Haubeiss, S., Schmid, J.O., Murdter, T.E., Sonnenberg, M., Friedel, G., van der Kuip, H. & Aulitzky, W.E. (2010). Dasatinib reverses cancer-associated fibroblasts (CAFs) from primary lung carcinomas to a phenotype comparable to that of normal fibroblasts, *Mol. Cancer* 9, 168

Hawinkels, L.J., Zuidwijk, K., Verspaget, H.W., de Jonge-Muller, E.S., van, D.W., Ferreira, V., Fontijn, R.D., David, G., Hommes, D.W., Lamers, C.B. & Sier, C.F. (2008). VEGF release by MMP-9 mediated heparan sulphate cleavage induces colorectal cancer angiogenesis, *Eur. J Cancer* 44, 1904-1913

Hazan, R.B., Qiao, R., Keren, R., Badano, I. & Suyama, K. (2004). Cadherin switch in tumor progression, *Ann. N. Y. Acad. Sci.* 1014, 155-163

Herbst, R.S. (2004). Review of epidermal growth factor receptor biology, *Int. J Radiat. Oncol. Biol Phys.* 59, 21-26

Hermiston, M.L. & Gordon, J.I. (1995). In vivo analysis of cadherin function in the mouse intestinal epithelium: essential roles in adhesion, maintenance of differentiation, and regulation of programmed cell death, *J Cell Biol* 129, 489-506

Hileman, R.E., Fromm, J.R., Weiler, J.M. & Linhardt, R.J. (1998). Glycosaminoglycan-protein interactions: definition of consensus sites in glycosaminoglycan binding proteins, *Bioessays* 20, 156-167

Hinoda, Y., Sasaki, S., Ishida, T. & Imai, K. (2004). Monoclonal antibodies as effective therapeutic agents for solid tumors, *Cancer Sci.* 95, 621-625

Hirama, M., Takahashi, F., Takahashi, K., Akutagawa, S., Shimizu, K., Soma, S., Shimanuki, Y., Nishio, K. & Fukuchi, Y. (2003). Osteopontin overproduced by tumor cells acts as a potent angiogenic factor contributing to tumor growth, *Cancer Lett.* 198, 107-117

Houghton, A.M. (2010). The paradox of tumor-associated neutrophils: fueling tumor growth with cytotoxic substances, *Cell Cycle* 9, 1732-1737

Hu, M. & Polyak, K. (2008). Microenvironmental regulation of cancer development, *Curr. Opin. Genet. Dev.* 18, 27-34

Hubbard, S.R. & Miller, W.T. (2007). Receptor tyrosine kinases: mechanisms of activation and signaling, *Curr. Opin. Cell Biol* 19, 117-123

Hunter, T. (1995). Protein kinases and phosphatases: the yin and yang of protein phosphorylation and signaling, *Cell* 80, 225-236

Ikeguchi, M., Fukuda, K., Yamaguchi, K., Kondo, A., Tsujitani, S. & Kaibara, N. (2003a). Quantitative analysis of heparanase gene expression in esophageal squamous cell carcinoma, *Ann. Surg. Oncol.* 10, 297-304

Ikeguchi, M., Hirooka, Y. & Kaibara, N. (2003b). Heparanase gene expression and its correlation with spontaneous apoptosis in hepatocytes of cirrhotic liver and carcinoma, *Eur. J Cancer* 39, 86-90

Imai, K. & Takaoka, A. (2006). Comparing antibody and small-molecule therapies for cancer, *Nat Rev Cancer* 6, 714-727

Iozzo, R.V. (2005). Basement membrane proteoglycans: from cellar to ceiling, *Nat Rev Mol. Cell Biol* 6, 646-656

Iozzo, R.V. & San Antonio, J.D. (2001). Heparan sulfate proteoglycans: heavy hitters in the angiogenesis arena, *J Clin Invest* 108, 349-355

Ishizuka, T., Tanabe, C., Sakamoto, H., Aoyagi, K., Maekawa, M., Matsukura, N., Tokunaga, A., Tajiri, T., Yoshida, T., Terada, M. & Sasaki, H. (2002). Gene amplification profiling of esophageal squamous cell carcinomas by DNA array CGH, *Biochem. Biophys. Res Commun.* 296, 152-155

Jarvelainen, H., Sainio, A., Koulu, M., Wight, T.N. & Penttinen, R. (2009). Extracellular matrix molecules: potential targets in pharmacotherapy, *Pharmacol. Rev* 61, 198-223

Jiang, X. & Couchman, J.R. (2003). Perlecan and tumor angiogenesis, *J Histochem. Cytochem.* 51, 1393-1410

Jiang, X., Multhaupt, H., Chan, E., Schaefer, L., Schaefer, R.M. & Couchman, J.R. (2004). Essential contribution of tumor-derived perlecan to epidermal tumor growth and angiogenesis, *J Histochem. Cytochem.* 52, 1575-1590

Jimenez, B., Volpert, O.V., Crawford, S.E., Febbraio, M., Silverstein, R.L. & Bouck, N. (2000). Signals leading to apoptosis-dependent inhibition of neovascularization by thrombospondin-1, *Nat. Med.* 6, 41-48

Jin, Z. & El-Deiry, W.S. (2005). Overview of cell death signaling pathways, *Cancer Biol Ther.* 4, 139-163

Jones, P.L. & Jones, F.S. (2000). Tenascin-C in development and disease: gene regulation and cell function, *Matrix Biol* 19, 581-596

Junxia, W., Ping, G., Yuan, H., Lijun, Z., Jihong, R., Fang, L., Min, L., Xi, W., Ting, H., Ke, D. & Huizhong, Z. (2010). Double strand RNA-guided endogeneous E-cadherin up-regulation induces the apoptosis and inhibits proliferation of breast carcinoma cells in vitro and in vivo, *Cancer Sci.* 101, 1790-1796

Kalluri, R. (2003). Basement membranes: structure, assembly and role in tumour angiogenesis, *Nat. Rev. Cancer* 3, 422-433

Kalluri, R. & Zeisberg, M. (2006). Fibroblasts in cancer, *Nat. Rev. Cancer* 6, 392-401

Kim, H.S., Lim, S.J. & Park, Y.K. (2009). Anti-angiogenic factor endostatin in osteosarcoma, *APMIS* 117, 716-723

Kowanetz, M. & Ferrara, N. (2006). Vascular endothelial growth factor signaling pathways: therapeutic perspective, *Clin Cancer Res* 12, 5018-5022

Kraman, M., Bambrough, P.J., Arnold, J.N., Roberts, E.W., Magiera, L., Jones, J.O., Gopinathan, A., Tuveson, D.A. & Fearon, D.T. (2010). Suppression of antitumor immunity by stromal cells expressing fibroblast activation protein-alpha, *Science* 330, 827-830

Kuperwasser, C., Chavarria, T., Wu, M., Magrane, G., Gray, J.W., Carey, L., Richardson, A. & Weinberg, R.A. (2004). Reconstruction of functionally normal and malignant human breast tissues in mice, *Proc. Natl. Acad. Sci. U. S. A* 101, 4966-4971

Lee, S., Jilani, S.M., Nikolova, G.V., Carpizo, D. & Iruela-Arispe, M.L. (2005). Processing of VEGF-A by matrix metalloproteinases regulates bioavailability and vascular patterning in tumors, *J Cell Biol* 169, 681-691

Lewen, S., Zhou, H., Hu, H.D., Cheng, T., Markowitz, D., Reisfeld, R.A., Xiang, R. & Luo, Y. (2008). A Legumain-based minigene vaccine targets the tumor stroma and suppresses breast cancer growth and angiogenesis, *Cancer Immunol. Immunother.* 57, 507-515

Lewis, C.E. & Pollard, J.W. (2006). Distinct Role of Macrophages in Different Tumor Microenvironments, *Cancer Res.* 66, 605-612

Li, H., Fan, X. & Houghton, J. (2007). Tumor microenvironment: the role of the tumor stroma in cancer, *J. Cell Biochem.* 101, 805-815

Liu, L., Cao, Y., Chen, C., Zhang, X., McNabola, A., Wilkie, D., Wilhelm, S., Lynch, M. & Carter, C. (2006). Sorafenib blocks the RAF/MEK/ERK pathway, inhibits tumor angiogenesis, and induces tumor cell apoptosis in hepatocellular carcinoma model PLC/PRF/5, *Cancer Res* 66, 11851-11858

Loeffler, M., Kruger, J.A., Niethammer, A.G. & Reisfeld, R.A. (2006). Targeting tumor-associated fibroblasts improves cancer chemotherapy by increasing intratumoral drug uptake, *J Clin Invest* 116, 1955-1962

Luo, Y., Zhou, H., Krueger, J., Kaplan, C., Lee, S.H., Dolman, C., Markowitz, D., Wu, W., Liu, C., Reisfeld, R.A. & Xiang, R. (2006). Targeting tumor-associated macrophages as a novel strategy against breast cancer, *J Clin Invest* 116, 2132-2141

Malinda, K.M., Nomizu, M., Chung, M., Delgado, M., Kuratomi, Y., Yamada, Y., Kleinman, H.K. & Ponce, M.L. (1999). Identification of laminin alpha1 and beta1 chain peptides active for endothelial cell adhesion, tube formation, and aortic sprouting, *FASEB J* 13, 53-62

Mantovani, A., Allavena, P. & Sica, A. (2004). Tumour-associated macrophages as a prototypic type II polarised phagocyte population: role in tumour progression, *Eur. J Cancer* 40, 1660-1667

Mantovani, A., Sozzani, S., Locati, M., Allavena, P. & Sica, A. (2002). Macrophage polarization: tumor-associated macrophages as a paradigm for polarized M2 mononuclear phagocytes, *Trends Immunol.* 23, 549-555

Mantovani, A., Porta, C., Rubino, L., Allavena, P. & Sica, A. (2006). Tumor-associated macrophages (TAMs) as new target in anticancer therapy, *Drug Discovery Today: Therapeutic Strategies* 3, 361-366

Marastoni, S., Ligresti, G., Lorenzon, E., Colombatti, A. & Mongiat, M. (2008). Extracellular matrix: a matter of life and death, *Connect. Tissue Res.* 49, 203-206

McKeage, M.J. & Baguley, B.C. (2010). Disrupting established tumor blood vessels: an emerging therapeutic strategy for cancer, *Cancer* 116, 1859-1871

Mendel, D.B., Laird, A.D., Xin, X., Louie, S.G., Christensen, J.G., Li, G., Schreck, R.E., Abrams, T.J., Ngai, T.J., Lee, L.B., Murray, L.J., Carver, J., Chan, E., Moss, K.G., Haznedar, J.O., Sukbuntherng, J., Blake, R.A., Sun, L., Tang, C., Miller, T., Shirazian, S., McMahon, G. & Cherrington, J.M. (2003). In vivo antitumor activity of SU11248, a novel tyrosine kinase inhibitor targeting vascular endothelial growth factor and platelet-derived growth factor receptors: determination of a pharmacokinetic/pharmacodynamic relationship, *Clin Cancer Res* 9, 327-337

Meredith, J.E., Jr., Fazeli, B. & Schwartz, M.A. (1993). The extracellular matrix as a cell survival factor, *Mol. Biol Cell* 4, 953-961

Meyer, C., Notari, L. & Becerra, S.P. (2002). Mapping the type I collagen-binding site on pigment epithelium-derived factor. Implications for its antiangiogenic activity, *J Biol Chem.* 277, 45400-45407

Misra, S., Heldin, P., Hascall, V.C., Karamanos, N.K., Skandalis, S.S., Markwald, R.R. & Ghatak, S. (2011). Hyaluronan-CD44 interactions as potential targets for cancer therapy, *FEBS J*

Mongiat, M., Fu, J., Oldershaw, R., Greenhalgh, R., Gown, A.M. & Iozzo, R.V. (2003a). Perlecan protein core interacts with extracellular matrix protein 1 (ECM1), a glycoprotein involved in bone formation and angiogenesis, *J. Biol. Chem.* 278, 17491-17499

Mongiat, M., Ligresti, G., Marastoni, S., Lorenzon, E., Doliana, R. & Colombatti, A. (2007). Regulation of the extrinsic apoptotic pathway by the extracellular matrix glycoprotein EMILIN2, *Mol. Cell Biol.* 27, 7176-7187

Mongiat, M., Marastoni, S., Ligresti, G., Lorenzon, E., Schiappacassi, M., Perris, R., Frustaci, S. & Colombatti, A. (2010). The extracellular matrix glycoprotein elastin microfibril interface located protein 2: a dual role in the tumor microenvironment, *Neoplasia.* 12, 294-304

Mongiat, M., Mungiguerra, G., Bot, S., Mucignat, M.T., Giacomello, E., Doliana, R. & Colombatti, A. (2000). Self-assembly and supramolecular organization of EMILIN, *J. Biol. Chem.* 275, 25471-25480

Mongiat, M., Sweeney, S.M., San Antonio, J.D., Fu, J. & Iozzo, R.V. (2003b). Endorepellin, a novel inhibitor of angiogenesis derived from the C terminus of perlecan, *J. Biol. Chem.* 278, 4238-4249

Motzer, R.J. & Bukowski, R.M. (2006). Targeted therapy for metastatic renal cell carcinoma, *J Clin Oncol.* 24, 5601-5608

Motzer, R.J., Rini, B.I., Bukowski, R.M., Curti, B.D., George, D.J., Hudes, G.R., Redman, B.G., Margolin, K.A., Merchan, J.R., Wilding, G., Ginsberg, M.S., Bacik, J., Kim, S.T., Baum, C.M. & Michaelson, M.D. (2006). Sunitinib in patients with metastatic renal cell carcinoma, *JAMA* 295, 2516-2524

Murdoch, C., Muthana, M., Coffelt, S.B. & Lewis, C.E. (2008). The role of myeloid cells in the promotion of tumour angiogenesis, *Nat Rev Cancer* 8, 618-631

Nor, J.E., Mitra, R.S., Sutorik, M.M., Mooney, D.J., Castle, V.P. & Polverini, P.J. (2000). Thrombospondin-1 induces endothelial cell apoptosis and inhibits angiogenesis by activating the caspase death pathway, *J Vasc Res* 37, 209-218

Nozue, M., Isaka, N. & Fukao, K. (2001). Over-expression of vascular endothelial growth factor after preoperative radiation therapy for rectal cancer, *Oncol. Rep.* 8, 1247-1249

Ogasawara, S., Yano, H., Iemura, A., Hisaka, T. & Kojiro, M. (1996). Expressions of basic fibroblast growth factor and its receptors and their relationship to proliferation of human hepatocellular carcinoma cell lines, *Hepatology* 24, 198-205

Orimo, A., Gupta, P.B., Sgroi, D.C., Arenzana-Seisdedos, F., Delaunay, T., Naeem, R., Carey, V.J., Richardson, A.L. & Weinberg, R.A. (2005). Stromal fibroblasts present in invasive human breast carcinomas promote tumor growth and angiogenesis through elevated SDF-1/CXCL12 secretion, *Cell* 121, 335-348

Ornitz, D.M., Yayon, A., Flanagan, J.G., Svahn, C.M., Levi, E. & Leder, P. (1992). Heparin is required for cell-free binding of basic fibroblast growth factor to a soluble receptor and for mitogenesis in whole cells, *Mol. Cell Biol* 12, 240-247

Ozerdem, U. & Stallcup, W.B. (2003). Early contribution of pericytes to angiogenic sprouting and tube formation, *Angiogenesis.* 6, 241-249

Pang, R. & Poon, R.T. (2006). Angiogenesis and antiangiogenic therapy in hepatocellular carcinoma, *Cancer Lett.* 242, 151-167

Paolillo, M., Russo, M.A., Serra, M., Colombo, L. & Schinelli, S. (2009). Small molecule integrin antagonists in cancer therapy, *Mini. Rev Med. Chem.* 9, 1439-1446

Park, J.W., Finn, R.S., Kim, J.S., Karwal, M., Li, R.K., Ismail, F., Thomas, M., Harris, R., Baudelet, C., Walters, I. & Raoul, J.L. (2011). Phase II, Open-Label Study of Brivanib as First-Line Therapy in Patients with Advanced Hepatocellular Carcinoma, *Clin Cancer Res* 17, 1973-1983

Pepper, M.S. (2001). Role of the matrix metalloproteinase and plasminogen activator-plasmin systems in angiogenesis, *Arterioscler Thromb Vasc Biol* 21, 1104-1117

Pietras, K. & Ostman, A. (2010). Hallmarks of cancer: interactions with the tumor stroma, *Exp. Cell Res* 316, 1324-1331

Pietras, K., Ostman, A., Sjoquist, M., Buchdunger, E., Reed, R.K., Heldin, C.H. & Rubin, K. (2001). Inhibition of platelet-derived growth factor receptors reduces interstitial hypertension and increases transcapillary transport in tumors, *Cancer Res* 61, 2929-2934

Pollard, J.W. (2004). Tumour-educated macrophages promote tumour progression and metastasis, *Nat Rev Cancer* 4, 71-78

Rasanen, K. & Vaheri, A. (2010). Activation of fibroblasts in cancer stroma, *Exp. Cell Res* 316, 2713-2722

Reed, J.C. & Pellecchia, M. (2005). Apoptosis-based therapies for hematologic malignancies, *Blood* 106, 408-418

Reichert, J.M., Rosensweig, C.J., Faden, L.B. & Dewitz, M.C. (2005). Monoclonal antibody successes in the clinic, *Nat Biotechnol.* 23, 1073-1078

Reid, A., Vidal, L., Shaw, H. & de, B.J. (2007). Dual inhibition of ErbB1 (EGFR/HER1) and ErbB2 (HER2/neu), *Eur. J Cancer* 43, 481-489

Rodriguez-Manzaneque, J.C., Lane, T.F., Ortega, M.A., Hynes, R.O., Lawler, J. & Iruela-Arispe, M.L. (2001). Thrombospondin-1 suppresses spontaneous tumor growth and inhibits activation of matrix metalloproteinase-9 and mobilization of vascular endothelial growth factor, *Proc. Natl. Acad. Sci. U. S. A* 98, 12485-12490

Roskoski, R., Jr. (2007). Vascular endothelial growth factor (VEGF) signaling in tumor progression, *Crit Rev Oncol. Hematol.* 62, 179-213

Rothhammer, T., Bataille, F., Spruss, T., Eissner, G. & Bosserhoff, A.K. (2007). Functional implication of BMP4 expression on angiogenesis in malignant melanoma, *Oncogene* 26, 4158-4170

Rouet, V., Hamma-Kourbali, Y., Petit, E., Panagopoulou, P., Katsoris, P., Barritault, D., Caruelle, J.P. & Courty, J. (2005). A synthetic glycosaminoglycan mimetic binds vascular endothelial growth factor and modulates angiogenesis, *J Biol Chem.* 280, 32792-32800

Sahadevan, K., Darby, S., Leung, H.Y., Mathers, M.E., Robson, C.N. & Gnanapragasam, V.J. (2007). Selective over-expression of fibroblast growth factor receptors 1 and 4 in clinical prostate cancer, *J Pathol* 213, 82-90

Santimaria, M., Moscatelli, G., Viale, G.L., Giovannoni, L., Neri, G., Viti, F., Leprini, A., Borsi, L., Castellani, P., Zardi, L., Neri, D. & Riva, P. (2003). Immunoscintigraphic detection of the ED-B domain of fibronectin, a marker of angiogenesis, in patients with cancer, *Clin Cancer Res* 9, 571-579

Sasisekharan, R., Shriver, Z., Venkataraman, G. & Narayanasami, U. (2002). Roles of heparan-sulphate glycosaminoglycans in cancer, *Nat Rev Cancer* 2, 521-528

Sato, S., Kigawa, J., Minagawa, Y., Okada, M., Shimada, M., Takahashi, M., Kamazawa, S. & Terakawa, N. (1999). Chemosensitivity and p53-dependent apoptosis in epithelial ovarian carcinoma, *Cancer* 86, 1307-1313

Sattler, M. & Salgia, R. (2004). Targeting c-Kit mutations: basic science to novel therapies, *Leuk. Res* 28 Suppl 1, S11-S20

Scatena, M., Almeida, M., Chaisson, M.L., Fausto, N., Nicosia, R.F. & Giachelli, C.M. (1998). NF-kappaB mediates alphavbeta3 integrin-induced endothelial cell survival, *J Cell Biol* 141, 1083-1093

Schiller, J.H. (2003). New directions for ZD1839 in the treatment of solid tumors, *Semin. Oncol.* 30, 49-55

Seidler, D.G., Goldoni, S., Agnew, C., Cardi, C., Thakur, M.L., Owens, R.T., McQuillan, D.J. & Iozzo, R.V. (2006). Decorin protein core inhibits in vivo cancer growth and metabolism by hindering epidermal growth factor receptor function and triggering apoptosis via caspase-3 activation, *J. Biol. Chem.* 281, 26408-26418

Senger, D.R., Ledbetter, S.R., Claffey, K.P., Papadopoulos-Sergiou, A., Peruzzi, C.A. & Detmar, M. (1996). Stimulation of endothelial cell migration by vascular permeability factor/vascular endothelial growth factor through cooperative mechanisms involving the alphavbeta3 integrin, osteopontin, and thrombin, *Am J Pathol* 149, 293-305

Seo, D.W., Li, H., Guedez, L., Wingfield, P.T., Diaz, T., Salloum, R., Wei, B.Y. & Stetler-Stevenson, W.G. (2003). TIMP-2 mediated inhibition of angiogenesis: an MMP-independent mechanism, *Cell* 114, 171-180

Sessa, C., de, B.F., Perotti, A., Bauer, J., Curigliano, G., Noberasco, C., Zanaboni, F., Gianni, L., Marsoni, S., Jimeno, J., D'Incalci, M., Dall'o, E. & Colombo, N. (2005). Trabectedin for women with ovarian carcinoma after treatment with platinum and taxanes fails, *J Clin Oncol.* 23, 1867-1874

Sharma, B., Handler, M., Eichstetter, I., Whitelock, J.M., Nugent, M.A. & Iozzo, R.V. (1998). Antisense targeting of perlecan blocks tumor growth and angiogenesis in vivo, *J Clin Invest* 102, 1599-1608

Sharma, M.R., Tuszynski, G.P. & Sharma, M.C. (2004). Angiostatin-induced inhibition of endothelial cell proliferation/apoptosis is associated with the down-regulation of cell cycle regulatory protein cdk5, *J Cell Biochem.* 91, 398-409

Simon, R., Richter, J., Wagner, U., Fijan, A., Bruderer, J., Schmid, U., Ackermann, D., Maurer, R., Alund, G., Knonagel, H., Rist, M., Wilber, K., Anabitarte, M., Hering, F., Hardmeier, T., Schonenberger, A., Flury, R., Jager, P., Fehr, J.L., Schraml, P., Moch, H., Mihatsch, M.J., Gasser, T. & Sauter, G. (2001). High-throughput tissue microarray analysis of 3p25 (RAF1) and 8p12 (FGFR1) copy number alterations in urinary bladder cancer, *Cancer Res* 61, 4514-4519

Sironen, R.K., Tammi, M., Tammi, R., Auvinen, P.K., Anttila, M. & Kosma, V.M. (2011). Hyaluronan in human malignancies, *Exp. Cell Res* 317, 383-391

Sobel, M., Soler, D.F., Kermode, J.C. & Harris, R.B. (1992). Localization and characterization of a heparin binding domain peptide of human von Willebrand factor, *J Biol Chem.* 267, 8857-8862

Sottile, J. (2004). Regulation of angiogenesis by extracellular matrix, *Biochim. Biophys. Acta* 1654, 13-22

Steeg, P.S. (2006). Tumor metastasis: mechanistic insights and clinical challenges, *Nat Med.* 12, 895-904

Szentirmai, O., Baker, C.H., Bullain, S.S., Lin, N., Takahashi, M., Folkman, J., Mulligan, R.C. & Carter, B.S. (2008). Successful inhibition of intracranial human glioblastoma multiforme xenograft growth via systemic adenoviral delivery of soluble endostatin and soluble vascular endothelial growth factor receptor-2: laboratory investigation, *J Neurosurg.* 108, 979-988

Tabruyn, S.P. & Griffioen, A.W. (2007). Molecular pathways of angiogenesis inhibition, *Biochem. Biophys. Res Commun.* 355, 1-5

Tai, I.T., Dai, M., Owen, D.A. & Chen, L.B. (2005). Genome-wide expression analysis of therapy-resistant tumors reveals SPARC as a novel target for cancer therapy, *J Clin Invest* 115, 1492-1502

Takenaka, K., Yamagishi, S., Jinnouchi, Y., Nakamura, K., Matsui, T. & Imaizumi, T. (2005). Pigment epithelium-derived factor (PEDF)-induced apoptosis and inhibition of vascular endothelial growth factor (VEGF) expression in MG63 human osteosarcoma cells, *Life Sci.* 77, 3231-3241

Tang, M.J. & Tai, I.T. (2007). A novel interaction between procaspase 8 and SPARC enhances apoptosis and potentiates chemotherapy sensitivity in colorectal cancers, *J. Biol. Chem.* 282, 34457-34467

Tapanadechopone, P., Tumova, S., Jiang, X. & Couchman, J.R. (2001). Epidermal transformation leads to increased perlecan synthesis with heparin-binding-growth-factor affinity, *Biochem. J* 355, 517-527

Teti, A., Farina, A.R., Villanova, I., Tiberio, A., Tacconelli, A., Sciortino, G., Chambers, A.F., Gulino, A. & Mackay, A.R. (1998). Activation of MMP-2 by human GCT23 giant cell tumour cells induced by osteopontin, bone sialoprotein and GRGDSP peptides is RGD and cell shape change dependent, *Int. J Cancer* 77, 82-93

Theocharis, A.D., Skandalis, S.S., Tzanakakis, G.N. & Karamanos, N.K. (2010). Proteoglycans in health and disease: novel roles for proteoglycans in malignancy and their pharmacological targeting, *FEBS J* 277, 3904-3923

Tilghman, R.W., Cowan, C.R., Mih, J.D., Koryakina, Y., Gioeli, D., Slack-Davis, J.K., Blackman, B.R., Tschumperlin, D.J. & Parsons, J.T. (2010). Matrix rigidity regulates cancer cell growth and cellular phenotype, *PLoS ONE* 5, e12905

Todorovicc, V., Chen, C.C., Hay, N. & Lau, L.F. (2005). The matrix protein CCN1 (CYR61) induces apoptosis in fibroblasts, *J. Cell Biol.* 171, 559-568

Trimboli, A.J., Cantemir-Stone, C.Z., Li, F., Wallace, J.A., Merchant, A., Creasap, N., Thompson, J.C., Caserta, E., Wang, H., Chong, J.L., Naidu, S., Wei, G., Sharma, S.M., Stephens, J.A., Fernandez, S.A., Gurcan, M.N., Weinstein, M.B., Barsky, S.H., Yee, L., Rosol, T.J., Stromberg, P.C., Robinson, M.L., Pepin, F., Hallett, M., Park, M., Ostrowski, M.C. & Leone, G. (2009). Pten in stromal fibroblasts suppresses mammary epithelial tumours, *Nature* 461, 1084-1091

Ulisse, S., Baldini, E., Sorrenti, S. & D'Armiento, M. (2009). The urokinase plasminogen activator system: a target for anti-cancer therapy, *Curr. Cancer Drug Targets.* 9, 32-71

Urakawa, H., Nishida, Y., Wasa, J., Arai, E., Zhuo, L., Kimata, K., Kozawa, E., Futamura, N. & Ishiguro, N. (2011). Inhibition of hyaluronan synthesis in breast cancer cells by 4-Methylumbelliferone suppresses tumorigenicity in vitro and metastatic lesions of bone in vivo, *Int. J Cancer*

Vazquez, F., Hastings, G., Ortega, M.A., Lane, T.F., Oikemus, S., Lombardo, M. & Iruela-Arispe, M.L. (1999). METH-1, a human ortholog of ADAMTS-1, and METH-2 are members of a new family of proteins with angio-inhibitory activity, *J Biol Chem.* 274, 23349-23357

Veiseh, O., Kievit, F.M., Ellenbogen, R.G. & Zhang, M. (2011). Cancer Cell Invasion: Treatment and Monitoring Opportunities in Nanomedicine, *Adv. Drug Deliv. Rev*

Walker, A., Turnbull, J.E. & Gallagher, J.T. (1994). Specific heparan sulfate saccharides mediate the activity of basic fibroblast growth factor, *J Biol Chem.* 269, 931-935

Wernert, N. (1997). The multiple roles of tumour stroma, *Virchows Arch.* 430, 433-443

Whiteside, T.L. (2007). The role of death receptor ligands in shaping tumor microenvironment, *Immunol. Invest* 36, 25-46

Wilhelm, S., Carter, C., Lynch, M., Lowinger, T., Dumas, J., Smith, R.A., Schwartz, B., Simantov, R. & Kelley, S. (2006). Discovery and development of sorafenib: a multikinase inhibitor for treating cancer, *Nat Rev Drug Discov.* 5, 835-844

Wilkins-Port, C.E. & Higgins, P.J. (2007). Regulation of extracellular matrix remodeling following transforming growth factor-beta1/epidermal growth factor-stimulated epithelial-mesenchymal transition in human premalignant keratinocytes, *Cells Tissues. Organs* 185, 116-122

Xiang, R., Luo, Y., Niethammer, A.G. & Reisfeld, R.A. (2008). Oral DNA vaccines target the tumor vasculature and microenvironment and suppress tumor growth and metastasis, *Immunol. Rev* 222, 117-128

Xing, F., Saidou, J. & Watabe, K. (2010). Cancer associated fibroblasts (CAFs) in tumor microenvironment, *Front Biosci.* 15, 166-179

Zhou, Z., Wang, J., Cao, R., Morita, H., Soininen, R., Chan, K.M., Liu, B., Cao, Y. & Tryggvason, K. (2004). Impaired angiogenesis, delayed wound healing and retarded tumor growth in perlecan heparan sulfate-deficient mice, *Cancer Res* 64, 4699-4702

Zivny, J., Klener, P., Jr., Pytlik, R. & Andera, L. (2010). The role of apoptosis in cancer development and treatment: focusing on the development and treatment of hematologic malignancies, *Curr. Pharm. Des* 16, 11-33

Zlobec, I., Steele, R. & Compton, C.C. (2005). VEGF as a predictive marker of rectal tumor response to preoperative radiotherapy, *Cancer* 104, 2517-2521

Zwick, E., Bange, J. & Ullrich, A. (2002). Receptor tyrosine kinases as targets for anticancer drugs, *Trends Mol. Med.* 8, 17-23

# 12

# Cyclin-Dependent Kinases (Cdk) as Targets for Cancer Therapy and Imaging

Franziska Graf[1], Frank Wuest[2] and Jens Pietzsch[1]
[1]*Institute of Radiopharmacy, Helmholtz-Zentrum Dresden-Rossendorf*
[2]*Department of Oncology, University of Alberta*
[1]*Germany*
[2]*Canada*

## 1. Introduction

Aberration in proliferation and consequently in cell cycle control is a common aspect in carcinogenesis. As master cell cycle regulating proteins in all eukaryotic cells the Cyclin-dependent kinases (Cdk) were identified by Leland Hartwell, Paul Nurse, and Timothy Hunt in the 1970s and 1980s. Chronological activation of respective Cdk according to respective cell cycle phase $G_1$, S, $G_2$ or M is mediated through association with a regulatory Cyclin subunit, phosphorylation of Cdk and binding of endogenous activators and inhibitors, as well as subcellular localization (Shapiro, 2006).

In human cells four Cdk are essential components of the cell cycle machinery with key functions also in human cancer cells: Cdk1, Cdk2, Cdk4, and Cdk6 (Fig. 1) (Malumbres & Barbacid, 2009). First, Cyclin D-dependent kinases Cdk4 and Cdk6 are activated in human cell cycle in response to mitogenic signals to initiate $G_1$ phase progression and prepare DNA duplication in S phase (Malumbres & Barbacid, 2005). Cdk4-Cyclin D or Cdk6-Cyclin D and later also Cdk2-Cyclin E complexes sequentially phosphorylate retinoblastoma proteins (Rb) on different serine and threonine residues. Resulting Rb protein inactivation is required for the transcriptional activation of genes in $G_1$/S phase (Harbour & Dean, 2000). In $G_1$ phase endogenous inhibitors of monomeric Cdk4 and Cdk6 like INK4 and inhibitors of Cdk2/Cdk4/Cdk6-Cyclin complexes like Cip and Kip proteins exert important influence on Cdk catalytic activity (Blain, 2008; Sherr & Roberts, 1999). Once the cell irreversibly passed restriction point R at the end of $G_1$ phase, Cdk2-Cyclin A complex is formed, facilitating orderly execution of S phase events like DNA replication and centrosome cycle through phosphorylation of various proteins (Malumbres & Barbacid, 2005). Activation of Cdk1 by Cyclin A is required for DNA damage checkpoint control, later Cdk1-Cyclin B for $G_2$/ M phase transition and initiation of mitosis, especially chromosome condensation and microtubule dynamics (Malumbres & Barbacid, 2009). Therefore, active Cdk1-Cyclin complexes mediate phosphorylation of about 70 substrates, e. g., minichromosome maintenance (MCM), p53, lamins, and dyneins.

Initiation of cell re-entrance from $G_0$ to $G_1$ phase and early inactivation of Rb is assigned to Cdk3-Cyclin C (Ren & Rollins, 2004). Another Cyclin-dependent kinase, Cdk5, is involved in the regulation of neuronal function (Cruz & Tsai, 2004).

The second group of proteins belonging to Cdk family – Cdk7 to Cdk13 – are involved in the activation of cell cycle kinases and transcriptional regulation (Akoulitchev et al., 2000; Chen et al., 2006; Chen et al., 2007; Garriga & Grana, 2004; Hu et al., 2007; Kasten & Giordano, 2001). Cdk7 in complex with Cyclin H is given a special importance since it is the only Cdk activating kinase (CAK) in mammalian cells phosphorylating a threonine residue in the conserved T-loop of Cdk (Lolli & Johnson, 2005).

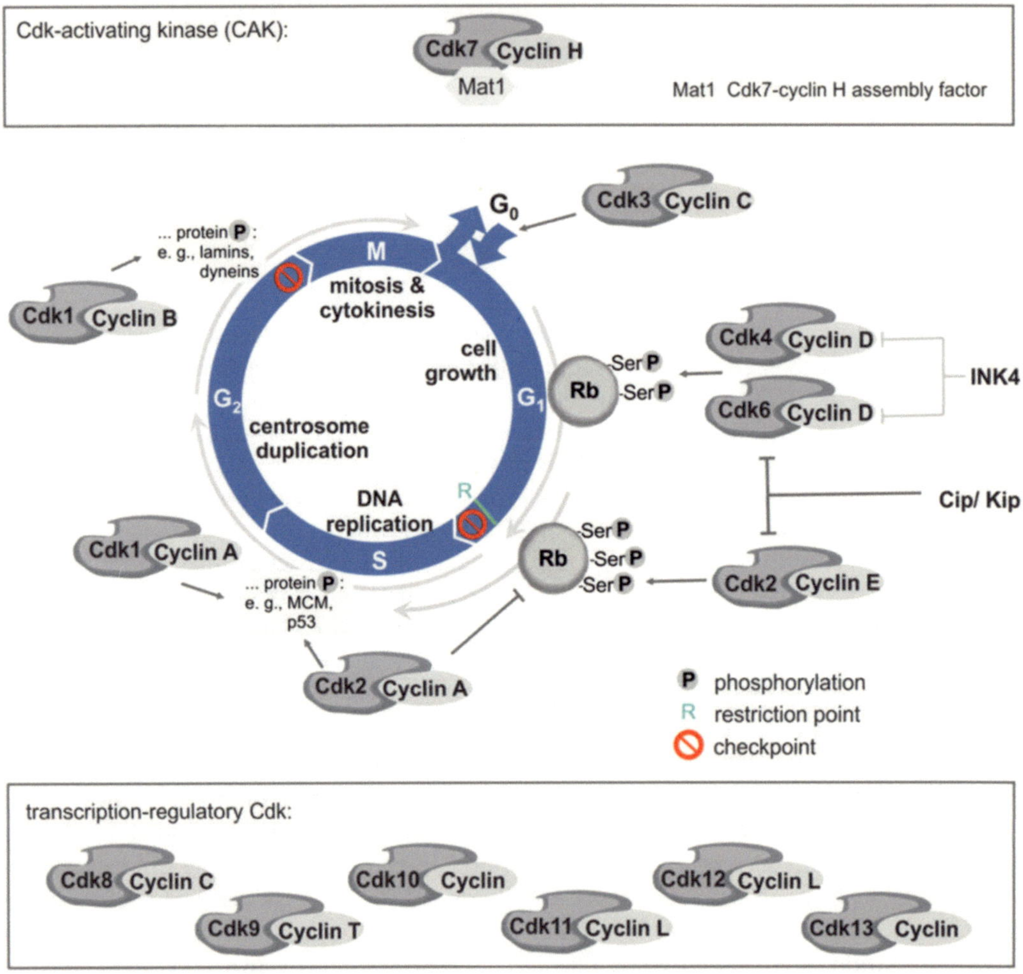


Fig. 1. Overview of human cell cycle activation and transcriptional regulation through Cdk-Cyclin complexes

## 2. Role of cyclin-dependent kinases in carcinogenesis

As important components of cell cycle activation and control the Cyclin-dependent kinase protein family contributes to tumor development and, in fact, an universal abnormal regulation of Cdk pathways has been described in human tumors induced by multiple mechanisms (Malumbres & Barbacid, 2009). Various genetic and epigenetic alterations in

human cancer including mutations and amplification of Cdk and positive regulatory Cyclin subunits, mutations or silencing of substrates (Rb) and endogenous Cdk inhibitors (INK4, Cip/ Kip proteins) lead to a hyperactivation of Cdk regulatory pathways (Table 1) (Deshpande et al., 2005; Malumbres & Barbacid, 2005). In consequence, critical cell cycle checkpoints are ignored resulting in abnormal cell proliferation and tumor progression.
Although tumor cells exhibit rather infrequent mutations of *cdk* genes – with the exception of $G_1$ kinases Cdk4 and Cdk6 – amplification, overexpression or hyperactivation of basic cell cycle regulators is a general feature of human tumors (Easton et al., 1998; Kim et al., 1999; Sotillo et al., 2001; Wolfel et al., 1995). Cdk hyperactivation is often affected by mutations of Cdk regulatory subunits. In consequence, overexpression of Cyclin A, Cyclin B, Cyclin E, and Cyclin D were reported in a wide spectrum of tumors, like leukemia or carcinomas and were associated with poor prognosis (Johansson & Persson, 2008; Ko et al., 2009). A common alteration in human tumors was demonstrated for tumor suppressor gene *rb*. Altered Rb proteins, momentous for transcriptional control, are insensitive to Cdk regulation and accelerate cell cycle progression (Nevins, 2001). Finally, abnormal regulation or inactivation of Cdk endogenous inhibitors p15$^{INK4B}$, p16$^{INK4A}$ and p27$^{Kip1}$ was described in numerous human tumors leading to enhanced Cdk activity (Ruas & Peters, 1998; Tsihlias et al., 1999).

| | alteration | occurrence in cancer type |
|---|---|---|
| **Cdk1** | upregulation/ overexpression | hepatoma, carcinoma, leukemia |
| **Cdk2** | upregulation/ overexpression | hepatoma, carcinoma, leukemia |
| **Cdk4** | point mutation R24C<br>amplification/ overexpression | melanoma, insulinoma, sarcoma<br>carcinoma, glioma, sarcoma, … |
| **Cdk6** | analogous R24C mutation<br>chromosomal translocations<br>amplification/ overexpression | neuroblastoma<br>lymphoma, leukemia<br>carcinoma, glioma, sarcoma, … |
| **Cyclins (A, B, E, D)** | amplification/ overexpression<br>chromosomal translocations | carcinoma, leukemia, …<br>lymphoma, adenoma |
| **Rb** | mutation<br>promoter methylation<br>sequestration | retinoblastoma, osteosarcoma, carcinoma<br>brain tumors<br>carcinoma, melanoma, neuroblastoma |
| **p15INK4B, p16INK4A** | deletion<br>promoter methylation | carcinoma, lymphoma, melanoma, …<br>melanoma |
| **p27Kip1** | decreased transcription<br>increased degradation | glioblastoma, carcinoma, melanoma, …<br>carcinoma, lymphoma |

Table 1. Genetic and epigenetic alterations of Cdk pathway components in human cancer (Graf et al., 2010; Ortega et al., 2002; Weinberg, 2007)

Universal abnormal regulation of Cdk pathways especially in $G_1$/ S phase suggests involvement and importance of these kinases in carcinogenesis, despite of uncertain results concerning dependence of Cdk2, Cdk4 and Cdk6 on cell cycle progression in embryogenesis (Malumbres & Barbacid, 2009; Santamaria et al., 2007).

In consequence, cell cycle regulating Cdks are attractive molecular targets for new (radio)pharmaceutical strategies in both cancer therapy and diagnosis, considering the heterogeneity of Cdk activity in different human tumor types. Compounds directly inhibiting the cell cycle machinery hold promise in restoring missing cellular Cdk regulators and arrest of proliferating cells, thus providing a non-genotoxic therapy modality. Conspicuous amplification of Cdk in tumor cells provides an opportunity for visualization of tumors by means of positron emission tomography (PET).

## 3. Overview of small molecule Cdk inhibitors: Selectivity and mode of action

In the last decade, numerous of structurally diverse small molecules inhibitors of Cdk activity have been developed and evaluated *in vitro* and *in vivo*. Thereby, structural information of different Cdk, in complex with corresponding regulatory Cyclin subunits, and in association with inhibitors facilitated the development of new potent compounds with high specificity for Cdk versus other protein kinases (De Bondt et al., 1993; Jeffrey et al., 1995; Sridhar et al., 2006). Motivation of Cdk specific targeting was attributed to high cytotoxicities of first generation of unspecific kinase inhibitors, e. g., staurosporine targeting several protein kinase families, which limited clinical application (Sielecki et al., 2000). In addition, effort to the identification of Cdk-subtype selective inhibitors has been made to optimize therapeutic success and minimize side effects for cancer patients. In first preclinical and clinical trials of potent, pharmacological Cdk inhibitors only misleading results for tumor treatment were revealed due to non-specific and/or non-selective targeting (Shapiro, 2006). According to this, Cdk inhibitors were classified to their effects on Cdk family members as pan-Cdk or highly selective Cdk inhibitors. Nevertheless, the classification of Cdk inhibitors often reveals the subjective view of the authors, not least because of different experimental setup of Cdk affinity measurements, missing data of the selectivities to many kinases and diffuse boundaries between Cdk inhibitors with broad and narrow activity profile.

The major targets of pharmacological Cdk inhibitors are key enzymes regulating interphase (Cdk2, Cdk4, Cdk6) and mitotic Cdk1. But often also Cdk activating kinase Cdk7 and transcriptional Cdk, e. g., Cdk9 are affected.

All potent small molecule Cdk inhibitors interact with the catalytic active site of Cdk and compete with ATP or block ATP binding. Several review articles of the last decade well document the development and evaluation of dozens of Cdk inhibitors representing different chemical classes (Galons et al., 2010; Rizzolio et al., 2010; Senderowicz & Sausville, 2000; Sharma et al., 2008; Sridhar, 2006). About 25 of them reached clinical trials. However, several studies with Cdk inhibitors showing promising preclinical results – for example AG-024322, AZD5438, R547, SNS-032, and ZK 304709 – had to be terminated or were discontinued after phase I (Lapenna & Giordano, 2009) (www.clinical trials.gov).

This book chapter will focus on 9 promising compounds tested in clinical trials at the time: AT7519, BAY 1000394, flavopiridol, P1446A-05, P276-00, PD 0332991, PHA-848125, R-roscovitine, and SCH 727965 (Fig. 2, Table 2).

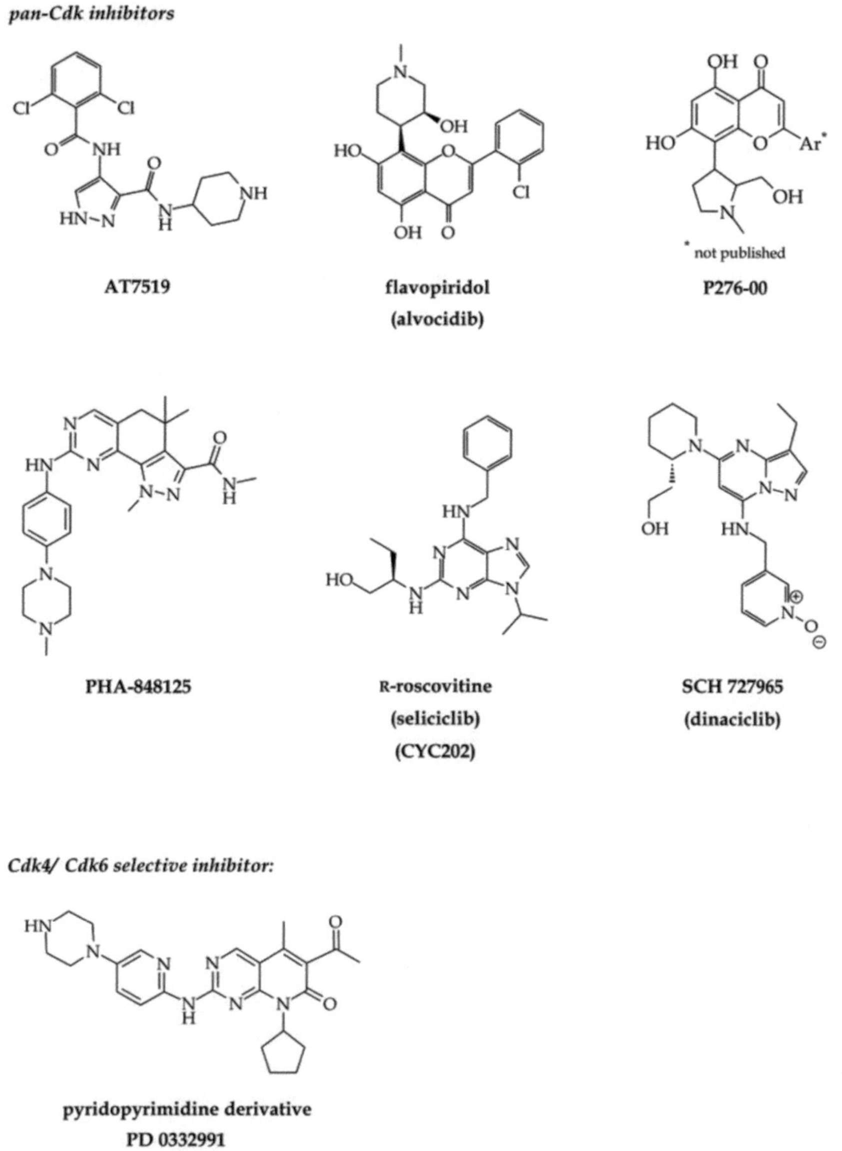


*pan-Cdk inhibitors*

Fig. 2. Molecular structures of selected Cdk inhibitors tested in clinical trials at the time

Most of the Cdk inhibitors are less selective and affect several Cdk family members, not only resulting in cell cycle arrest via blocking of Cdk1, Cdk2, and Cdk4, but also in manipulation of RNA synthesis through targeting of transcriptional kinases Cdk7 and Cdk9. Combination of cell cycle kinase inactivation and Cdk9 inhibition has been shown to trigger cell death via promotion of apoptosis in tumor cells (Cai et al., 2006). Otherwise, toxic effects of transcriptional manipulation in non-tumor cells via inhibition of Cdk7 and Cdk9 could be crucial for therapeutic application of single agent Cdk inhibitors. In addition, it has to be considered, that unselective targeting of transcriptional Cdk, e. g., Cdk10 and Cdk11 would diminish therapeutic effects, due to their relevance for tumor suppression and apoptosis (Chandramouli et al., 2007; Iorns et al., 2008).

Among the first compounds described with Cdk specificity flavopiridol and R-roscovitine as derivatives of natural products were developed. All other Cdk inhibitors are mainly synthetic compounds.

**Flavopiridol**, an alkaloid derivative and member of the flavone group, displayed antiproliferative and cytotoxic effects on tumor cells at nanomolar concentrations (Sedlacek et al., 1996). This observation was associated with cell cycle arrest through inhibition of Cdk and induction of apoptosis in human hematopoietic cell lines, breast, lung, as well as head and neck squamous cell carcinoma (Kaur et al., 1992; Konig et al., 1997; Parker et al., 1998; Patel et al., 1998). In spite of inconsistent data of $IC_{50}$ and $K_d$ values for different Cdk, flavopiridol showed high affinity to all Cdk with $IC_{50}$ values below 400 nM and exhibit higher selectivity to Cdk9 ($IC_{50}$ < 10 nM) (Chao et al., 2000; Sedlacek, 2001; Sedlacek, 1996). Cdk9, as well as Cdk7 inhibition lead to profound influence on cellular transcription, e. g., on mRNA transcripts for cell cycle regulators Cyclin D, antiapoptotic proteins Bcl-2 and Mcl-2, and NFκB as well as p53 pathway (Lam et al., 2001; Lu et al., 2004). Independent from good antitumorigenic effects in preclinical studies, in 2008 only low specificity of flavopiridol for Cdk has been demonstrated due to nanomolar affinity to also 25 other protein kinases, like GSK3β and ERK (Karaman et al., 2008), maybe leading to discouraging results in some clinical trials (see next section).

Screening of about hundred compounds structurally related to flavopiridol identified **P276-00** as potent Cdk specific inhibitor with moderate selectivity for Cdk1, Cdk4, and Cdk9 (Joshi et al., 2007a). Similar to flavopiridol, P276-00 showed antiproliferative and proapoptotic activity in human breast, colon, lung, prostate carcinoma, and promyelocytic leukemia cell lines *in vitro* (Joshi et al., 2007b). Decreased Rb phosphorylation, $G_1$/ $G_2$ phase arrest, and caspase-dependent apoptosis could be observed in preclinical studies with multiple myeloma cells *in vitro* and *in vivo* (Manohar et al., 2011; Raje et al., 2009).

The purine derivative **R-roscovitine** inhibits Cdk1, Cdk2, Cdk5, Cdk7, and Cdk9 with selectivity to Cdk4 and Cdk6 (Meijer et al., 1997). In consequence, R-roscovitine lead to arrest of tumor cells in almost all cell cycle phases and affected cell proliferation, as it was demonstrated for over 60 human tumor cell lines (e. g., melanoma, lung, breast, colon carcinoma, leukemia). *In vivo* activity in mice bearing colorectal carcinoma xenografts, but also in hematopoietic progenitors (Mcclue et al., 2002; Raynaud et al., 2005; Song et al., 2007) and enhancement of antitumor effects of radiation and doxorubicin in combination with R-roscovitine was reported (Appleyard et al., 2009; Maggiorella et al., 2003). Like flavopiridol and other Cdk inhibitors with broad spectrum, several additional effects have been described for R-roscovitine *in vitro*: interruption of transcriptional elongation, interference with survival-associated pathways (IκB kinase inhibition), induction of p53 phosphorylation and apoptosis (Alvi et al., 2005; Dey et al., 2008; Hahntow et al., 2004).

A novel potent Cdk inhibitor with striking similarity to R-roscovitine regarding both chemical structure and cytotoxic properties is pyrazolo[1,5-*a*]pyrimidine derivative **SCH 727965** (Parry et al., 2010). SCH 727965 inhibits Cdk1, Cdk2, Cdk5 and Cdk9 activity *in vitro* in low nanomolar concentrations ($IC_{50}$ < 5 nM) and exhibited antiproliferative effects due to complete suppression of Rb phosphorylation and apoptosis induction, respectively.

Fragment-based screening techniques identified pyrazole-3-carboxamide **AT7519** as potent Cdk2 inhibitor and antiproliferative agent (Wyatt et al., 2008). AT7519 caused cell cycle arrest, growth inhibition, and apoptosis in a large spectrum of human solid tumor cells and colon carcinoma xenograft models (Squires et al., 2009). Influence on transcriptional regulating Cdk, as well as GSK3β, resulting in induction of apoptotic pathways was observed in multiple myeloma and leukemia cell lines (Santo et al., 2010; Squires et al., 2010).

Optimization of selectivity and physicochemical properties of pyrazolo[4,3-*h*]quinazoline-3-carboxamide derivatives identified **PHA-848125** as potent Cdk inhibitor ($IC_{50} < 400$ nM) with inhibitory effects on cell cycle progression and Rb phosphorylation *in vitro* in a wide range of tumor cell lines (Brasca et al., 2009; Caporali et al., 2010). Among a panel of 43 other serine-threonine and tyrosine kinases only tropomyosin receptor kinase A (TRKA), linked to cancer cell survival, was inhibited by PHA-848125 in the same nanomolar range ($IC_{50}$ 53 nM). *In vivo* characterization of oral active compound PHA-848125 showed a dose-dependent inhibition of human A2780 ovarian carcinoma xenograft tumor growth on mice up to 91%. Significant tumor growth inhibition was also observed in a K-Ras mutant lung adenocarcinoma transgenic mouse model, carcinogen-induced tumors, and in disseminated primary leukemia models (Albanese et al., 2010; Degrassi et al., 2010).

Only a few details have been published for pan-Cdk inhibitor **BAY 1000394** with unknown structure targeting Cdk1, Cdk2, Cdk4 and Cdk9 with high affinity ($IC_{50} < 10$ nM) (Siemeister et al., 2010). Inhibition of cell proliferation was amongst others depicted for breast, cervical, and colorectal human tumor cell lines and described to be independent of Rb, p53 and tumor suppressor gene status. Suppression of Rb phosphorylation and growth inhibition after treatment with BAY 1000394 was observed in preclinical studies in a broad range of tumor xenografts.

*Cdk4/ Cdk6 selective inhibitors*

Several compounds, particularly, members of chemical classes of benzothiadiazines, diarylureas, indolocarbazoles, oxindoles, pyrido[2,3-*d*]pyrimidines, thienopyrimidinhy drazones, thioacridones, and triaminopyrimidines were developed in the last decade and described with preferential selectivity to Cdk4 and Cdk6 (Graf, 2010; Lee & Sicinski, 2006). Cdk4 and Cdk6 reveal due to their high homology and identical substrate specificities comprehensive activities in the cell cycle. According to the occurrence in different tissues Cdk4 and Cdk6 compensate each other in function (Ciemerych & Sicinski, 2005; Meyerson & Harlow, 1994). **P1446A-05** and pyrido[2,3-*d*]pyrimidine **PD 0332991** seem to be the most promising compounds due to their inclusion in clinical evaluation. Unfortunately, no information about chemical structure and mechanism of Cdk4 selective inhibition is provided in the literature for P1446A-05. However, potency of PD 0332991 to inhibit Cdk4 and Cdk6 pathway and tumor cell progression has been extensively studied *in vitro*, as well as *in vivo* in mouse xenograft models (Baughn et al., 2006; Fry et al., 2004; Menu et al., 2008; Saab et al., 2006). In all studies an antiproliferative response to PD 0332991 treatment as a result of $G_1$ phase arrest after inhibition of Cdk4- and Cdk6-mediated Rb phosphorylation was observed in lymphoma, myeloma, sarcoma, breast, lung, and colon carcinoma. Though, treatment efficiency of Cdk4/ Cdk6 selective inhibitors like PD 0332991 is limited to tumors with wild-type *rb* gene status. Furthermore, PD 0332991 does not induce apoptosis and seems to be ineffective in the majority of quiescent $G_0$/ $G_1$ arrested leukemic cells with primarily defects in apoptosis pathway, as it was demonstrated for chronic lymphocytic leukemia (Wesierska-Gadek et al., 2011).

## 4. Cdk inhibitors for cancer therapy

Despite of promising preclinical data and numerous potent Cdk inhibitors in clinical trials, none of these molecules has already been approved as drug for cancer therapy. Nevertheless, evaluation of various Cdk inhibitors contributed to important information about bioavailability, pharmacokinetics, as well as, competing toxicities and lead to alterations in dosing schedule to reach a maximum in response. To date, monotherapy did not demonstrate convincing utility of a certain Cdk inhibitor for cancer treatment, although clinical trials of several hematologic malignancies have shown stable disease. Encouraging results depicting antitumor activity of Cdk inhibitors also in solid tumors have been obtained in various combination studies with cytostatic or cytotoxic agents. However, beneficial effects of Cdk inhibition alone and in combination with other chemotherapeutic agents to tumor treatment must be demonstrated in randomized clinical trials in the future.

Information about current clinical trials of Cdk inhibitors were achieved from the webpage *www.clinicaltrials.gov* and a summary is given in Table 2.

**Flavopiridol** was the first Cdk inhibitor entering clinical trials. Since the early 1990s flavopiridol was extensively studied in patients with refractory neoplasms, a variety of solid tumors and hematopoietic malignancies. Clinical trials with single flavopiridol were completed for, e. g., advanced gastric cancer, endometrial adenocarcinoma, metastatic melanoma, multiple myeloma, and non-small cell lung cancer in phase II, but only unsatisfying results concerning antitumor activity and toxicities like myelosuppression, diarrhea as well as thromboses were observed (Burdette-Radoux et al., 2004; Dispenzieri et al., 2006; Grendys et al., 2005; Schwartz et al., 2001; Shapiro et al., 2001). Also, no response to flavopiridol administered as 24 hour continuous infusion in chronic lymphocytic leukemia patients was observed (Flinn et al., 2005). Detection of high serum protein binding of flavopiridol and collection of pharmacokinetic data contributed to the adjustment of treatment-schedule of flavopiridol. In consequence, hematopoietic malignancies showed encouraging responses to flavopiridol. Weekly application of flavopiridol as a single agent for 6 weeks in a phase I study of chronic lymphocytic leukemia patients achieved a median progression-free survival of 12 month (Byrd et al., 2007; Phelps et al., 2009). Addition of prophylactic corticosteroid dexamethasone to flavopiridol treatment improved tolerability in chronic lymphocytic leukemia patients (Lin et al., 2009). In combination with cytostatic drugs cytosine arabinoside and mitoxantrone in phase II clinical trials a 75% response rate of patients with acute myelogenous leukemia was observed (Karp et al., 2007). Combined treatment of flavopiridol with chemotherapeutic agents cisplatin, carboplatin, docetaxel, gemcitabine, irinotecan or paclitaxel, respectively, have shown response or at least stable disease in phase I trials (Bible et al., 2005; Fekrazad et al., 2010; Fornier et al., 2007; George et al., 2008). However, subsequent phase II clinical trial with flavopiridol in combination with docetaxel resulted again in disappointing activity and significant toxicity in patients with metastatic pancreatic adenocarcinoma (Carvajal et al., 2009). Currently ongoing and recruiting clinical studies focus on evaluation of flavopiridol (combined with chemotherapeutic agents like bortezomib, oxaliplatin, or respectively, lenalidomide) in patients with B-cell neoplasms, lymphoma, multiple myeloma, and germ cell tumors.

**P276-00** is currently in phase I/II clinical trials to determine anticancer activity in patients with advanced Cyclin D1 positive malignant melanoma, mantle cell lymphoma, squamous cell head and neck carcinoma, and multiple myeloma. A phase I study in patients with advanced refractory neoplasms has already been completed. No results have been provided in the literature yet. Combination studies currently recruiting patients are initiated for

P276-00 administered along with radiation in head and neck squamous cell carcinoma patients, and in combination with gemcitabine in patients with advanced pancreatic cancer.

A phase I clinical trial of **R-roscovitine** has been performed in 22 patients with advanced cancer utilizing several schedules resulting in only minor therapeutical success with hypokalemia, rash and fatigue as dose limiting side-effects (Benson et al., 2007). Further evaluation of R-roscovitine in patients with non-small cell lung cancer was described: R-roscovitine in combination with cisplatin and gemcitabine in phase I showed similar adverse events, e. g., hypokalemia, liver γ-glutamyltranspeptidase elevation, vomiting, and a 42.9% response rate in 14 patients (Siegel-Lakhai et al., 2005). A phase II study of oral R-roscovitine to treat non-small cell lung cancer has been terminated without any reports on available data. Antitumor activity and pharmacodynamic effects of R-roscovitine sequentially administered with sapacitabine was initiated in 2009 in patients with advanced solid tumors.

Safety and tolerability of **SCH 727965** was demonstrated in phase I clinical trials for multiple malignant indications including solid tumors, non-Hodgkin's lymphoma, multiple myeloma, and chronic lymphocytic leukemia (Shapiro et al., 2008). The drug was administered once every 21 days as a 2 hour intravenous infusion and dose limiting toxicity was neutropenia. To improve treatment success a phase I study currently recruiting patients is initiated in patients with advanced cancer for schedule adjustment (3 infusions ever 7 days in a 28 day cycle). First results in previously treated patients with chronic lymphocytic leukemia showed common toxicities, like fatigue, nausea, and diarrhea, but also evidence of therapeutic benefit of SCH 727965 (Flynn et al., 2009). In an active phase II clinical trial activity of SCH 727965 in patients with advanced breast cancer, non-small cell lung cancer, mantle cell lymphoma, or B-cell chronic lymphocytic leukemia each in comparison to standard treatment (capecitabine, erlotinib, bortezomib, or alemtuzumab) is determined. Furthermore, phase I/II studies including patients with malignant melanoma and multiple myeloma, as well as plasma cell neoplasms will be performed.

Two phase I/II studies with **AT7519**, currently recruiting patients are under evaluation. Single AT7519 treatment of patients with advanced/metastatic solid tumors or refractory non-Hodgkin's lymphoma will provide data to applicable dose, pharmacokinetics, pharmacodynamics and side effects. First results of this study suggested evidence of clinical activity of AT7519, due to reduction of PCNA, a protein required for DNA replication, as a result of Cdk inhibition and an increase of apoptosis markers (Mahadevan et al., 2011). Mucositis, neutropenia, and reversible thrombocytopenia were identified as dose limiting toxicities. In another ongoing clinical trial, efficacy of either AT7519 alone or AT7519 in combination with proteasome inhibitor bortezomib is determined in patients with previously treated multiple myeloma.

**PHA-848125** was first evaluated in a multi center phase I study to investigate the safety and pharmacokinetics in patients with advanced/ metastatic solid tumors. Oral administration of PHA-848125 in different treatment schedules showed good tolerability with ataxia and tremors as dose-limiting side-effects and occasional hematological toxicities (Benouaich-Amiel et al., 2010; Cresta et al., 2010; Tibes et al., 2008). Similar results were found in a phase I study of PHA-848125 in combination with gemcitabine (Bahleda et al., 2010). Antitumor activity of PHA-848125 is currently assessed in phase II clinical trials in patients with recurrent or metastatic thymic carcinoma previously treated with chemotherapeutic agents.

Clinical studies of pan-Cdk inhibitor **BAY 1000394** and Cdk4 selective inhibitor **P1446A-05** are in the beginning and thus less well documented. Both compounds are tested in first clinical trials at the moment to identify tolerated dose of the drug and to determine both limiting side effects and efficacy in patients with advanced solid tumors. Evaluation of P1446A-05 includes also hematologic malignancies.

**PD 0332991** was first tested in a phase I dose escalation trial in 57 patients with Rb positive advanced cancer (e. g., breast, colorectal cancer, melanoma) (O'dwyer et al., 2007). Doses from 25 mg to 150 mg of single agent PD 0332991 were administered orally for 21 days in a 28 days cycle. Stable disease was manifested for 9 patients and dose limiting toxicity was myelosuppression. Another phase I study assessing mechanism of action, safety, and pharmacodynamic effects of PD 0332991 was performed in patients with mantle cell lymphoma using fluorine-18-labeled fluorodeoxyglucose ([$^{18}$F]FDG) and fluorothymidine ([$^{18}$F]FLT) positron emission tomography imaging (Leonard et al., 2008). Numerous phase II clinical trials of PD 0332991 are ongoing and currently recruiting patients: with advanced non-small cell lung cancer, with refractory solid tumors, with recurrent Rb positive glioblastoma, and with metastatic liposarcoma. Evaluation of PD 0332991 in combination with letrozole for treatment of hormone-receptor positive advanced breast cancer, in combination with bortezomib for mantle cell lymphoma, as well as in combination with velcade and dexamethasone in patients with multiple myeloma is ongoing after encouraging antitumor activity was revealed in phase I clinical trials (Niesvizky et al., 2009; Niesvizky et al., 2010; Slamon et al., 2010).

## 5. Specific aspects regarding kinase inhibitor resistance

An important problem for new approaches in cancer therapy, also resulting in significant limitations of the potential use of kinase inhibitors, is the resistance of tumor cells to cytotoxic anticancer drugs acquired during therapy. As a relevant example, resistance to kinase inhibitor imatinib selective for Bcl-Abl was observed in chronic myelogeneous leukemia and gastrointestinal stromal tumor patients (Bixby & Talpaz, 2011; Wang et al., 2011). Development of kinase inhibitor resistance is accomplished by increased expression and even more common by specific point mutations of Bcl-Abl oncogene. In consequence, association of inhibitor with kinase is prevented without rigorous effects on enzyme activity. Despite of no reported appearance of Cdk inhibitor resistance in clinical trials so far, essential side chains for Cdk inhibitor specificity and selectivity, but not for ATP binding were predicted. An aromatic amino acid in the conserved Cdk domain, e. g., phenylalanine-80 in Cdk2, provides a hydrophobic site for essential *van der Waals* contacts with the Cdk inhibitor (for example isopropyl of R-roscovitine and acetyl of PD 0332991) (Krystof & Uldrijan, 2010). In parallel to mutation-based steric hindrance of a aurora B inhibitor causing kinase resistance (Girdler et al., 2008), histidine residues in Cdk4 and Cdk6 have been predicted to contribute to selectivity of PD 0332991 and discriminate Cdk1 and Cdk2 (Lu & Schulze-Gahmen, 2006). Point mutations modifying these side chains could directly result in the loss of Cdk inhibitor binding. However, findings of sufficiency of Cdk1 to drive the mammalian cell cycle in mouse embryogenesis raise the questions if Cdk1 could substitute all the other interphase Cdks in human tumor cells anyway and whether a point mutation is likely to cause resistance to a pharmacological Cdk inhibitor (Santamaria, 2007).

| inhibitor | targets (IC50) | clinical trials in patients with |
|---|---|---|
| AT7519 | Cdk2, Cdk5, Cdk9 (< 50 nM)<br>Cdk1, Cdk4, Cdk6 (≤ 210 nM)<br>GSK3β (89 nM)<br>(Squires, 2009) | - advanced, metastatic solid tumors, non-Hodgkin's lymphoma (phase I)<br>- multiple myeloma (alone and in combination with bortezomib (phase I) |
| BAY 1000394 | Cdk1, Cdk2, Cdk4, Cdk9 (≤ 11 nM)<br>(Siemeister, 2010) | - advanced solid tumors (phase I) |
| flavopiridol (alvocidib) | Cdk4, Cdk9 (< 50 nM)<br>Cdk1, Cdk2, Cdk6, Cdk7 (≤ 400 nM)<br>GSK3β (450 nM)<br>(Sedlacek, 2001) | - lymphoma, multiple myeloma, leukemia, sarcoma, various advanced solid tumors (alone and in combination with cytotoxic agents) (phase I, II) |
| P1446A-05 | Cdk4 (n. a.)<br>(www.piramallifesciences.com) | - advanced refractory malignancies (hematologic or solid tumors) (phase I) |
| P276-00 | Cdk1, Cdk4, Cdk9 (< 100 nM)<br>Cdk2, Cdk6 (≤ 400 nM)<br>Cdk7, GSK3β (2.8 μM)<br>other protein kinases (> 10 μM)<br>(Joshi, 2007a) | - head and neck squamous cell carcinoma, multiple myeloma, mantle cell lymphoma, melanoma (phase I, II)<br>- head and neck squamous cell carcinoma (in combination with radiation) (phase I, II)<br>- advanced pancreatic cancer (in combination with gemcitabine) (phase I, II) |
| PD 0332991 | Cdk4, Cdk6 (≤ 15 nM)<br>Cdk1, Cdk2, Cdk5, other protein kinases (> 10 μM)<br>(Fry, 2004) | - mantle cell lymphoma (alone and in combination with bortezomib) (phase I)<br>- advanced cancer (phase I)<br>- refractory solid tumors, non-small cell lung cancer, glioblastoma, liposarcoma (phase II)<br>- hormone-receptor positive breast cancer (alone and in combination with letrozole) (phase I, II)<br>- multiple myeloma (in combination with velcade and dexamethasone) (phase I, II) |
| PHA-848125 | Cdk2 (45/363 nM)<br>Cdk1, Cdk4, Cdk5, Cdk7 (< 400 nM)<br>TRKA (53 nM)<br>(Brasca, 2009) | - advanced/ metastatic solid tumors (phase I)<br>- thymic carcinoma (phase II) |
| R-roscovitine (seliciclib) (CYC202) | Cdk1, Cdk2, Cdk5, Cdk7, Cdk9 (≤ 800 nM)<br>Cdk4, Cdk6, other protein kinases (≥ 14 μM)<br>(Meijer, 1997; Popowycz et al., 2009) | - non-small cell lung cancer (phase II)<br>- advanced solid tumors (in combination with sapacitabine) (phase I) |
| SCH 727965 (dinaciclib) | Cdk1, Cdk2, Cdk5, Cdk9 (< 5 nM)<br>(Parry, 2010) | - advanced solid tumors, lymphoma, leukemia (phase I)<br>- melanoma, multiple myeloma (phase I, II)<br>- advanced breast and lung cancer (phase II)<br>- lymphoma, leukemia (phase II) |

Table 2. Cdk inhibitors currently under clinical evaluation. Information to clinical trials were obtained from *www.clinical trials.gov.* (GSK3β: glycogen synthase kinase 3β; TRKA: tropomyosin receptor kinase A)

Referring to this, a critical view on the advantages and disadvantages of Cdk inhibitor selectivity for the success of therapeutic approaches should be given. Is development of exclusively selective Cdk inhibitors challenging tumor therapy?

First of all, due to high homology in Cdk active sites development of monospecific Cdk inhibitor is nearly impossible. This prediction becomes apparent by the given $IC_{50}$ values in the list of potent Cdk inhibitors in clinical trials (Table 2). Only PD 0332991 exhibits high selectivity to Cdk4 and Cdk6 *in vitro*. But at certain pharmacological concentrations, there is no exclusion of influence on various members of Cdk family.

Cdk inhibitors with improved selectivity promise minimization of undesired side effects, since no effects on global transcriptional machinery (Cdk7, Cdk9) would be expected in healthy cells as it was described for pan-Cdk inhibitors. Certainly, selective inactivation of any Cdk would not be as efficient as inhibition of multiple Cdk, including Cdk1, and involves the risk of easy development of Cdk inhibitor resistance, especially by alterations in the primarily targeted pathway. The response on Cdk4 and Cdk6 selective inhibitor PD 0332991 is significantly linked to functional Rb, transcriptional repression through E2F and the ability to attenuate Cdk2 activity, otherwise resistance to PD 0332991 acquired in tumor cell lines (Dean et al., 2010). In contrast, high efficiency of treatment in Cdk4/ Cdk6-dependent tumors and even reversal of resistance to estrogen receptor pathway targeting with tamoxifen by combined therapy with PD 0332991 could be achieved (Finn et al., 2009).

Pan-Cdk inhibitors affect multiple pathways in tumor cells and attack heterogeneous malignant cells (e. g., chronic lymphocytic leukemia, multiple myeloma), hindering Cdk inhibitor resistance. But, one has to consider the consequences of pan-Cdk inhibitors on healthy proliferating cells, like hematopoietic and dermal cells *in vivo,* which are much more sensitive to blockage of global cell cycle machinery and regulators.

To emulate and characterize Cdk inhibitor resistance *in vitro,* ambitions to generate cellular models were described. An increased activity due to increased protein synthesis of Cyclin E and simple overexpression of Cdk1 was observed in ovarian and colorectal carcinoma cell lines with acquired resistance to flavopiridol (Bible et al., 2000; Smith et al., 2001). But overexpression of Cyclin E in the cells is not mandatory associated with decreased sensitivity to flavopiridol (Smith, 2001). Also no evidence to mutational modification of Cdk was given in the studies. In fact, resistance to flavopiridol and another Cdk inhibitor was related to increased expression or activity of ATP-binding cassette transporter ABCG2 minimizing accumulation of the inhibitors and responsible for multidrug resistance in certain cancer cells (Robey et al., 2001; Seamon et al., 2006). Thus, mechanisms of resistance to Cdk inhibitors described to date seem to be inconsistent in dependence of the genetic status of different cell lines. Decreased sensitivity to a certain drug is often a result of multiple alterations in the tumor cells and further studies will elucidate the appearance of Cdk-associated genetic changes as a consequence of long-term treatment with Cdk inhibitor.

A hopeful therapeutic strategy to overcome development of inhibitor resistance is the combination of Cdk inhibitors with common chemotherapeutic agents for fast and effective elimination of malignant cells. Recent clinical studies with combined therapeutic regimes will clarify the benefit for the patients.

## 6. Cdk inhibitors as molecular probes for cancer imaging

The development of potent radiolabeled Cdk inhibitors, as radiotracers for tumor visualization using positron emission tomography (PET) is a novel approach allowing functional, non-invasive characterization and imaging of Cdk in human tumors. Particularly, radiolabeled Cdk4/Cdk6 inhibitors are of interest for the assessment of Cdk4/Cdk6 protein status and activity in human tumors in current translational cancer research. PET affords the opportunity of three-dimensional imaging and quantitation of physiological processes *in vivo*. Additionally, PET provides pharmacological data of radiolabeled Cdk4/Cdk6 inhibitors, which may help to understand mechanism of action *in vivo* and estimate the applicability of the compounds for tumor therapy.

In this regard, new Cdk4/Cdk6 inhibitors derived from pyrido[2,3-*d*]pyrimidine lead structure (Vanderwel et al., 2005) were designed, synthesized and characterized in our institute for the first time. Evaluation of five compounds - CKIA, CKIB, CKIC, CKID, and CKIE - showed specific and selective inhibition of Cdk4/ Cdk6-mediated pathway, induction of $G_1$ phase arrest and blocking of tumor cell proliferation in pharmacological concentrations (Graf et al., 2009; Graf, 2010). Most potent Cdk4/ Cdk6 inhibitors CKIA, CKIB, and CKIE were radiolabeled with positron-emitters iodine-124 [$^{124}$I] or fluorine-18 [$^{18}$F], respectively, and characterized concerning their radiopharmacological properties in cellular radiotracer uptake studies, biodistribution and, small animal PET studies (Graf, 2009; Graf, 2010; Koehler et al., 2010). Iodine-124 with a half-life of 4.18 days allows extended radiopharmacological evaluation. Nevertheless, minor positron emission (26%) and high positron energy are disadvantages leading to low resolution PET images. Most frequently used PET nuclide fluorine-18 exhibits nearly 97% positron emission with a half-life of 109.8 minutes.

*In vitro* radiotracer uptake studies using [$^{124}$I]CKIA, [$^{124}$I]CKIB, and [$^{18}$F]CKIE demonstrated substantial tumor cell uptake, an important prerequisite for PET studies, in NMRI nu/nu mice bearing the human squamous cell carcinoma tumor FaDu. Dynamic small animal PET studies demonstrated rapid clearance of [$^{124}$I]CKIA, [$^{124}$I]CKIB, and [$^{18}$F]CKIE from the blood and fast hepatobiliary excretion. The half-life of radiotracer elimination from the blood was calculated to between 7.2 and 7.9 min. Only marginal tumor uptake of radiotracers [$^{124}$I]CKIA and [$^{124}$I]CKIB was observed. In the case of [$^{18}$F]CKIE higher uptake was detected in the peripheral cell-cycle active region of the tumor one hour after intravenous injection (Fig. 3). However, the constant tumor-to-muscle ratio of 1.5 suggests a non-Cdk4- or non-Cdk6-mediated association of [$^{18}$F]CKIE in human tumor xenografts in mice.

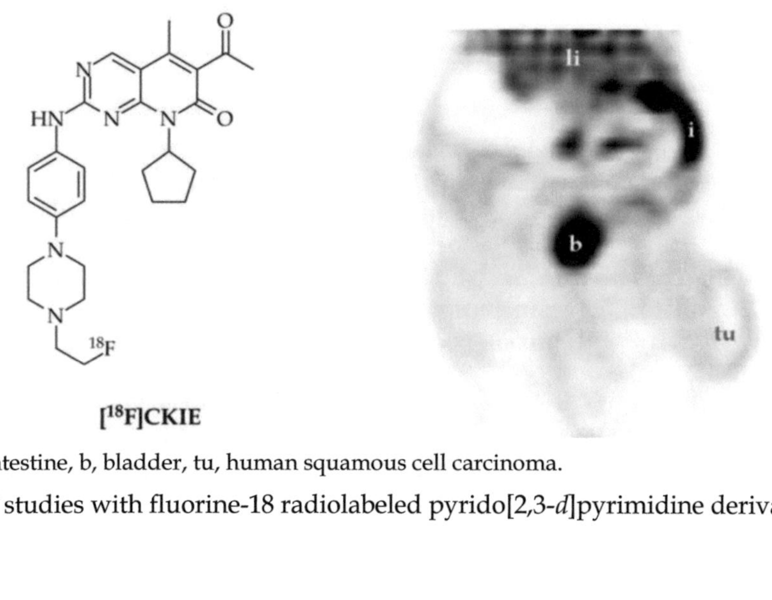


**[$^{18}$F]CKIE**

li, liver, i, intestine, b, bladder, tu, human squamous cell carcinoma.

Fig. 3. PET studies with fluorine-18 radiolabeled pyrido[2,3-*d*]pyrimidine derivative CKIE

In conclusion, the short biological half-life in the blood and low tumor uptake of the studied radiolabeled pyrido[2,3-*d*]pyrimidines limit the clinical application of these Cdk4/ Cdk6 inhibitors as radiotracers for the characterization of Cdk4/Cdk6 in tumors by means of PET. Nevertheless, further development and evaluation of suitable radiolabeled Cdk inhibitors with optimized properties *in vivo* are still of outstanding interest for the prospective functional characterization of Cdk in tumors by means of PET.

## 7. Conclusion

Critical contribution of cell cycle regulating kinases Cdk to carcinogenesis provides a promising target for diagnostic characterization of malignancies and development of novel therapeutic interventions. Numerous compounds directly inhibiting Cdk and, as a consequence, cell proliferation have been developed, and 9 of them are currently under clinical evaluation (phase I and II) as antitumor agents. Most of the candidates are pan-Cdk inhibitors affecting several Cdk family members with advantages in efficiency of tumor treatment due to not only inhibition of cell proliferation but also apoptosis induction. Only one inhibitor - pyrido[2,3-*d*]pyrimidine PD 0332991 - has been comprehensible described with preferential selectivity for Cdk4 and Cdk6 applicable for Rb positive tumors with primarily defects in Cdk4/ Cdk6 pathway. Application of Cdk inhibitors to patients with advanced cancers resulted in stabilization of disease. Combination with classical chemotherapeutic agents and adjustment of therapeutic schedules may also cause tumor regression and contribute to prevention of drug resistance. More detailed preclinical evaluation using suitable tumor models and focused clinical trials will give valuable implications for new mechanism-based approaches and Cdk drug developments as well as tumor specific treatment.

## 8. Acknowledgment

The authors are grateful to Mareike Barth, Catharina Heinig, Regina Herrlich, and Andrea Suhr for their excellent technical assistance. The authors thank Birgit Mosch, Ph.D., Ralf Bergmann, Ph.D., Torsten Kniess, Ph.D., and Lena Koehler, Ph.D., for many stimulating discussions.

## 9. References

Akoulitchev, S.; Chuikov, S. & Reinberg, D. (2000). TFIIH is negatively regulated by cdk8-containing mediator complexes. *Nature,* Vol.407, No.6800, pp. 102-6

Albanese, C.; Alzani, R.; Amboldi, N.; Avanzi, N.; Ballinari, D.; Brasca, M. G.; Festuccia, C.; Fiorentini, F.; Locatelli, G.; Pastori, W.; Patton, V.; Roletto, F.; Colotta, F.; Galvani, A.; Isacchi, A.; Moll, J.; Pesenti, E.; Mercurio, C. & Ciomei, M. (2010). Dual targeting of CDK and tropomyosin receptor kinase families by the oral inhibitor PHA-848125, an agent with broad-spectrum antitumor efficacy. *Mol Cancer Ther,* Vol.9, No.8, pp. 2243-54

Alvi, A. J.; Austen, B.; Weston, V. J.; Fegan, C.; MacCallum, D.; Gianella-Borradori, A.; Lane, D. P.; Hubank, M.; Powell, J. E.; Wei, W.; Taylor, A. M.; Moss, P. A. & Stankovic, T. (2005). A novel CDK inhibitor, CYC202 (R-roscovitine), overcomes the defect in p53-dependent apoptosis in B-CLL by down-regulation of genes involved in transcription regulation and survival. *Blood,* Vol.105, No.11, pp. 4484-91

Appleyard, M. V.; O'Neill, M. A.; Murray, K. E.; Paulin, F. E.; Bray, S. E.; Kernohan, N. M.; Levison, D. A.; Lane, D. P. & Thompson, A. M. (2009). Seliciclib (CYC202, R-roscovitine) enhances the antitumor effect of doxorubicin in vivo in a breast cancer xenograft model. *Int J Cancer,* Vol.124, No.2, pp. 465-72

Bahleda, R.; Spreafico, A.; Soria, J.; Moldovan, C.; Belli, C.; Fiorentini, F.; Scaburri, A.; Pacciarini, M. A.; Laffranchi, B. & Reni, M. (2010). Phase I study of the oral CDK-TRKA inhibitor PHA-848125 in combination with gemcitabine in advanced solid tumors. *J Clin Oncol,* Vol.28, 15s (Suppl.), abstract 3063

Baughn, L. B.; Di Liberto, M.; Wu, K.; Toogood, P. L.; Louie, T.; Gottschalk, R.; Niesvizky, R.; Cho, H.; Ely, S.; Moore, M. A. & Chen-Kiang, S. (2006). A novel orally active small molecule potently induces G1 arrest in primary myeloma cells and prevents tumor growth by specific inhibition of cyclin-dependent kinase 4/6. *Cancer Res,* Vol.66, No.15, pp. 7661-7

Benouaich-Amiel, A.; Mazza, E.; Massard, C.; Gaviani, P.; Fiorentini, F.; Scaburri, A.; Pacciarini, M. A. & Calvo, E. (2010). Phase I study of the oral CDK-TRKA inhibitor PHA-848125 in recurrent malignant glioma (MG). *J Clin Oncol,* Vol.28, 15s (Suppl.), abstract 2087

Benson, C.; White, J.; De Bono, J.; O'Donnell, A.; Raynaud, F.; Cruickshank, C.; McGrath, H.; Walton, M.; Workman, P.; Kaye, S.; Cassidy, J.; Gianella-Borradori, A.; Judson, I. & Twelves, C. (2007). A phase I trial of the selective oral cyclin-dependent kinase inhibitor seliciclib (CYC202; R-Roscovitine), administered twice daily for 7 days every 21 days. *Br J Cancer,* Vol.96, No.1, pp. 29-37

Bible, K. C.; Boerner, S. A.; Kirkland, K.; Anderl, K. L.; Bartelt, D., Jr.; Svingen, P. A.; Kottke, T. J.; Lee, Y. K.; Eckdahl, S.; Stalboerger, P. G.; Jenkins, R. B. & Kaufmann, S. H. (2000). Characterization of an ovarian carcinoma cell line resistant to cisplatin and flavopiridol. *Clin Cancer Res,* Vol.6, No.2, pp. 661-70

Bible, K. C.; Lensing, J. L.; Nelson, S. A.; Lee, Y. K.; Reid, J. M.; Ames, M. M.; Isham, C. R.; Piens, J.; Rubin, S. L.; Rubin, J.; Kaufmann, S. H.; Atherton, P. J.; Sloan, J. A.; Daiss, M. K.; Adjei, A. A. & Erlichman, C. (2005). Phase 1 trial of flavopiridol combined with cisplatin or carboplatin in patients with advanced malignancies with the assessment of pharmacokinetic and pharmacodynamic end points. *Clin Cancer Res,* Vol.11, No.16, pp. 5935-41

Bixby, D. & Talpaz, M. (2011). Seeking the causes and solutions to imatinib-resistance in chronic myeloid leukemia. *Leukemia,* Vol.25, No.1, pp. 7-22

Blain, S. W. (2008). Switching cyclin D-Cdk4 kinase activity on and off. *Cell Cycle,* Vol.7, No.7, pp. 892-8

Brasca, M. G.; Amboldi, N.; Ballinari, D.; Cameron, A.; Casale, E.; Cervi, G.; Colombo, M.; Colotta, F.; Croci, V.; D'Alessio, R.; Fiorentini, F.; Isacchi, A.; Mercurio, C.; Moretti, W.; Panzeri, A.; Pastori, W.; Pevarello, P.; Quartieri, F.; Roletto, F.; Traquandi, G.; Vianello, P.; Vulpetti, A. & Ciomei, M. (2009). Identification of N,1,4,4-tetramethyl-8-{[4-(4-methylpiperazin-1-yl)phenyl]amino}-4,5-dihydro-1H-pyrazolo[4,3-h]quinazoline-3-carboxamide (PHA-848125), a potent, orally available cyclin dependent kinase inhibitor. *J Med Chem,* Vol.52, No.16, pp. 5152-63

Burdette-Radoux, S.; Tozer, R. G.; Lohmann, R. C.; Quirt, I.; Ernst, D. S.; Walsh, W.; Wainman, N.; Colevas, A. D. & Eisenhauer, E. A. (2004). Phase II trial of flavopiridol, a cyclin dependent kinase inhibitor, in untreated metastatic malignant melanoma. *Invest New Drugs,* Vol.22, No.3, pp. 315-22

Byrd, J. C.; Lin, T. S.; Dalton, J. T.; Wu, D.; Phelps, M. A.; Fischer, B.; Moran, M.; Blum, K. A.; Rovin, B.; Brooker-McEldowney, M.; Broering, S.; Schaaf, L. J.; Johnson, A. J.; Lucas, D. M.; Heerema, N. A.; Lozanski, G.; Young, D. C.; Suarez, J. R.; Colevas, A. D. & Grever, M. R. (2007). Flavopiridol administered using a pharmacologically derived schedule is associated with marked clinical efficacy in refractory, genetically high-risk chronic lymphocytic leukemia. *Blood,* Vol.109, No.2, pp. 399-404

Cai, D.; Latham, V. M., Jr.; Zhang, X. & Shapiro, G. I. (2006). Combined depletion of cell cycle and transcriptional cyclin-dependent kinase activities induces apoptosis in cancer cells. *Cancer Res,* Vol.66, No.18, pp. 9270-80

Caporali, S.; Alvino, E.; Starace, G.; Ciomei, M.; Brasca, M. G.; Levati, L.; Garbin, A.; Castiglia, D.; Covaciu, C.; Bonmassar, E. & D'Atri, S. (2010). The cyclin-dependent kinase inhibitor PHA-848125 suppresses the in vitro growth of human melanomas sensitive or resistant to temozolomide, and shows synergistic effects in combination with this triazene compound. *Pharmacol Res,* Vol.61, No.5, pp. 437-48

Carvajal, R. D.; Tse, A.; Shah, M. A.; Lefkowitz, R. A.; Gonen, M.; Gilman-Rosen, L.; Kortmansky, J.; Kelsen, D. P.; Schwartz, G. K. & O'Reilly, E. M. (2009). A phase II study of flavopiridol (Alvocidib) in combination with docetaxel in refractory, metastatic pancreatic cancer. *Pancreatology,* Vol.9, No.4, pp. 404-9

Chandramouli, A.; Shi, J.; Feng, Y.; Holubec, H.; Shanas, R. M.; Bhattacharyya, A. K.; Zheng, W. & Nelson, M. A. (2007). Haploinsufficiency of the cdc2l gene contributes to skin cancer development in mice. *Carcinogenesis,* Vol.28, No.9, pp. 2028-35

Chao, S. H.; Fujinaga, K.; Marion, J. E.; Taube, R.; Sausville, E. A.; Senderowicz, A. M.; Peterlin, B. M. & Price, D. H. (2000). Flavopiridol inhibits P-TEFb and blocks HIV-1 replication. *J Biol Chem,* Vol.275, No.37, pp. 28345-8

Chen, H. H.; Wang, Y. C. & Fann, M. J. (2006). Identification and characterization of the CDK12/cyclin L1 complex involved in alternative splicing regulation. *Mol Cell Biol,* Vol.26, No.7, pp. 2736-45

Chen, H. H.; Wong, Y. H.; Geneviere, A. M. & Fann, M. J. (2007). CDK13/CDC2L5 interacts with L-type cyclins and regulates alternative splicing. *Biochem Biophys Res Commun,* Vol.354, No.3, pp. 735-40

Ciemerych, M. A. & Sicinski, P. (2005). Cell cycle in mouse development. *Oncogene,* Vol.24, No.17, pp. 2877-98

Cresta, S.; Sessa, C.; Del Conte, G.; Locatelli, A.; Gallerani, E.; Fiorentini, F.; Scaburri, A.; Pacciarini, M. A.; Alzani, R. & Gianni, L. (2010). Phase I study of the oral CDK-TRKA inhibitor PHA-848125 administered with prolonged schedules of administration. *J Clin Oncol,* Vol.28, 15s (Suppl.), abstract 3065

Cruz, J. C. & Tsai, L. H. (2004). A Jekyll and Hyde kinase: roles for Cdk5 in brain development and disease. *Curr Opin Neurobiol,* Vol.14, No.3, pp. 390-4

De Bondt, H. L.; Rosenblatt, J.; Jancarik, J.; Jones, H. D.; Morgan, D. O. & Kim, S. H. (1993). Crystal structure of cyclin-dependent kinase 2. *Nature,* Vol.363, No.6430, pp. 595-602

Dean, J. L.; Thangavel, C.; McClendon, A. K.; Reed, C. A. & Knudsen, E. S. (2010). Therapeutic CDK4/6 inhibition in breast cancer: key mechanisms of response and failure. *Oncogene,* Vol.29, No.28, pp. 4018-32

Degrassi, A.; Russo, M.; Nanni, C.; Patton, V.; Alzani, R.; Giusti, A. M.; Fanti, S.; Ciomei, M.; Pesenti, E. & Texido, G. (2010). Efficacy of PHA-848125, a cyclin-dependent kinase inhibitor, on the K-Ras(G12D)LA2 lung adenocarcinoma transgenic mouse model: evaluation by multimodality imaging. *Mol Cancer Ther,* Vol.9, No.3, pp. 673-81

Deshpande, A.; Sicinski, P. & Hinds, P. W. (2005). Cyclins and cdks in development and cancer: a perspective. *Oncogene,* Vol.24, No.17, pp. 2909-15

Dey, A.; Wong, E. T.; Cheok, C. F.; Tergaonkar, V. & Lane, D. P. (2008). R-Roscovitine simultaneously targets both the p53 and NF-kappaB pathways and causes potentiation of apoptosis: implications in cancer therapy. *Cell Death Differ,* Vol.15, No.2, pp. 263-73

Dispenzieri, A.; Gertz, M. A.; Lacy, M. Q.; Geyer, S. M.; Fitch, T. R.; Fenton, R. G.; Fonseca, R.; Isham, C. R.; Ziesmer, S. C.; Erlichman, C. & Bible, K. C. (2006). Flavopiridol in patients with relapsed or refractory multiple myeloma: a phase 2 trial with clinical and pharmacodynamic end-points. *Haematologica,* Vol.91, No.3, pp. 390-3

Easton, J.; Wei, T.; Lahti, J. M. & Kidd, V. J. (1998). Disruption of the cyclin D/cyclin-dependent kinase/INK4/retinoblastoma protein regulatory pathway in human neuroblastoma. *Cancer Res,* Vol.58, No.12, pp. 2624-32

Fekrazad, H. M.; Verschraegen, C. F.; Royce, M.; Smith, H. O.; Chyi Lee, F. & Rabinowitz, I. (2010). A phase I study of flavopiridol in combination with gemcitabine and irinotecan in patients with metastatic cancer. *Am J Clin Oncol,* Vol.33, No.4, pp. 393-7

Finn, R. S.; Dering, J.; Conklin, D.; Kalous, O.; Cohen, D. J.; Desai, A. J.; Ginther, C.; Atefi, M.; Chen, I.; Fowst, C.; Los, G. & Slamon, D. J. (2009). PD 0332991, a selective cyclin D kinase 4/6 inhibitor, preferentially inhibits proliferation of luminal estrogen receptor-positive human breast cancer cell lines in vitro. *Breast Cancer Res,* Vol.11, No.5, pp. R77

Flinn, I. W.; Byrd, J. C.; Bartlett, N.; Kipps, T.; Gribben, J.; Thomas, D.; Larson, R. A.; Rai, K.; Petric, R.; Ramon-Suerez, J.; Gabrilove, J. & Grever, M. R. (2005). Flavopiridol administered as a 24-hour continuous infusion in chronic lymphocytic leukemia lacks clinical activity. *Leuk Res,* Vol.29, No.11, pp. 1253-7

Flynn, J. M.; Johnson, A. J.; Andritsos, L.; Blum, K. A.; Jones, J. A.; Wiley, E. A.; Hu, W.; Hessler, J.; Smith, L. L.; Lucas, D. M.; Small, K.; Statkevich, P.; Grever, M. R.; Bannerji, R. & Byrd, J. C. (2009). The Cyclin Dependent Kinase Inhibitor SCH 727965 Demonstrates Promising Pre-Clinical and Early Clinical Activity in Chronic Lymphocytic Leukemia. *Blood (ASH Annual Meeting Abstracts),* Vol.114, abstract 886

Fornier, M. N.; Rathkopf, D.; Shah, M.; Patil, S.; O'Reilly, E.; Tse, A. N.; Hudis, C.; Lefkowitz, R.; Kelsen, D. P. & Schwartz, G. K. (2007). Phase I dose-finding study of weekly docetaxel followed by flavopiridol for patients with advanced solid tumors. *Clin Cancer Res,* Vol.13, No.19, pp. 5841-6

Fry, D. W.; Harvey, P. J.; Keller, P. R.; Elliott, W. L.; Meade, M.; Trachet, E.; Albassam, M.; Zheng, X.; Leopold, W. R.; Pryer, N. K. & Toogood, P. L. (2004). Specific inhibition of cyclin-dependent kinase 4/6 by PD 0332991 and associated antitumor activity in human tumor xenografts. *Mol Cancer Ther,* Vol.3, No.11, pp. 1427-38

Galons, H.; Oumata, N. & Meijer, L. (2010). Cyclin-dependent kinase inhibitors: a survey of recent patent literature. *Expert Opin Ther Pat,* Vol.20, No.3, pp. 377-404

Garriga, J. & Grana, X. (2004). Cellular control of gene expression by T-type cyclin/CDK9 complexes. *Gene,* Vol.337, pp. 15-23

George, S.; Kasimis, B. S.; Cogswell, J.; Schwarzenberger, P.; Shapiro, G. I.; Fidias, P. & Bukowski, R. M. (2008). Phase I study of flavopiridol in combination with Paclitaxel and Carboplatin in patients with non-small-cell lung cancer. *Clin Lung Cancer,* Vol.9, No.3, pp. 160-5

Girdler, F.; Sessa, F.; Patercoli, S.; Villa, F.; Musacchio, A. & Taylor, S. (2008). Molecular basis of drug resistance in aurora kinases. *Chem Biol,* Vol.15, No.6, pp. 552-62

Graf, F.; Koehler, L.; Kniess, T.; Wuest, F.; Mosch, B. & Pietzsch, J. (2009). Cell Cycle Regulating Kinase Cdk4 as a Potential Target for Tumor Cell Treatment and Tumor Imaging. *J Oncol,* Vol.2009, pp. 106378

Graf, F.; Mosch, B.; Koehler, L.; Bergmann, R.; Wuest, F. & Pietzsch, J. (2010). Cyclin-dependent kinase 4/6 (cdk4/6) inhibitors: perspectives in cancer therapy and imaging. *Mini Rev Med Chem,* Vol.10, No.6, pp. 527-39

Grendys, E. C., Jr.; Blessing, J. A.; Burger, R. & Hoffman, J. (2005). A phase II evaluation of flavopiridol as second-line chemotherapy of endometrial carcinoma: a Gynecologic Oncology Group study. *Gynecol Oncol,* Vol.98, No.2, pp. 249-53

Hahntow, I. N.; Schneller, F.; Oelsner, M.; Weick, K.; Ringshausen, I.; Fend, F.; Peschel, C. & Decker, T. (2004). Cyclin-dependent kinase inhibitor Roscovitine induces apoptosis in chronic lymphocytic leukemia cells. *Leukemia,* Vol.18, No.4, pp. 747-55

Harbour, J. W. & Dean, D. C. (2000). The Rb/E2F pathway: expanding roles and emerging paradigms. *Genes Dev,* Vol.14, No.19, pp. 2393-409

Hu, D.; Valentine, M.; Kidd, V. J. & Lahti, J. M. (2007). CDK11(p58) is required for the maintenance of sister chromatid cohesion. *J Cell Sci,* Vol.120, No.Pt 14, pp. 2424-34

Iorns, E.; Turner, N. C.; Elliott, R.; Syed, N.; Garrone, O.; Gasco, M.; Tutt, A. N.; Crook, T.; Lord, C. J. & Ashworth, A. (2008). Identification of CDK10 as an important determinant of resistance to endocrine therapy for breast cancer. *Cancer Cell,* Vol.13, No.2, pp. 91-104

Jeffrey, P. D.; Russo, A. A.; Polyak, K.; Gibbs, E.; Hurwitz, J.; Massague, J. & Pavletich, N. P. (1995). Mechanism of CDK activation revealed by the structure of a cyclinA-CDK2 complex. *Nature,* Vol.376, No.6538, pp. 313-20

Johansson, M. & Persson, J. L. (2008). Cancer therapy: targeting cell cycle regulators. *Anticancer Agents Med Chem,* Vol.8, No.7, pp. 723-31

Joshi, K. S.; Rathos, M. J.; Joshi, R. D.; Sivakumar, M.; Mascarenhas, M.; Kamble, S.; Lal, B. & Sharma, S. (2007a). In vitro antitumor properties of a novel cyclin-dependent kinase inhibitor, P276-00. *Mol Cancer Ther,* Vol.6, No.3, pp. 918-25

Joshi, K. S.; Rathos, M. J.; Mahajan, P.; Wagh, V.; Shenoy, S.; Bhatia, D.; Chile, S.; Sivakumar, M.; Maier, A.; Fiebig, H. H. & Sharma, S. (2007b). P276-00, a novel cyclin-dependent inhibitor induces G1-G2 arrest, shows antitumor activity on cisplatin-resistant cells and significant in vivo efficacy in tumor models. *Mol Cancer Ther,* Vol.6, No.3, pp. 926-34

Karaman, M. W.; Herrgard, S.; Treiber, D. K.; Gallant, P.; Atteridge, C. E.; Campbell, B. T.; Chan, K. W.; Ciceri, P.; Davis, M. I.; Edeen, P. T.; Faraoni, R.; Floyd, M.; Hunt, J. P.; Lockhart, D. J.; Milanov, Z. V.; Morrison, M. J.; Pallares, G.; Patel, H. K.; Pritchard, S.; Wodicka, L. M. & Zarrinkar, P. P. (2008). A quantitative analysis of kinase inhibitor selectivity. *Nat Biotechnol,* Vol.26, No.1, pp. 127-32

Karp, J. E.; Smith, B. D.; Levis, M. J.; Gore, S. D.; Greer, J.; Hattenburg, C.; Briel, J.; Jones, R. J.; Wright, J. J. & Colevas, A. D. (2007). Sequential flavopiridol, cytosine arabinoside, and mitoxantrone: a phase II trial in adults with poor-risk acute myelogenous leukemia. *Clin Cancer Res,* Vol.13, No.15 Pt 1, pp. 4467-73

Kasten, M. & Giordano, A. (2001). Cdk10, a Cdc2-related kinase, associates with the Ets2 transcription factor and modulates its transactivation activity. *Oncogene,* Vol.20, No.15, pp. 1832-8

Kaur, G.; Stetler-Stevenson, M.; Sebers, S.; Worland, P.; Sedlacek, H.; Myers, C.; Czech, J.; Naik, R. & Sausville, E. (1992). Growth inhibition with reversible cell cycle arrest of carcinoma cells by flavone L86-8275. *J Natl Cancer Inst,* Vol.84, No.22, pp. 1736-40

Kim, J. H.; Kang, M. J.; Park, C. U.; Kwak, H. J.; Hwang, Y. & Koh, G. Y. (1999). Amplified CDK2 and cdc2 activities in primary colorectal carcinoma. *Cancer,* Vol.85, No.3, pp. 546-53

Ko, M. T.; Su, C. Y.; Huang, S. C.; Chen, C. H. & Hwang, C. F. (2009). Overexpression of cyclin E messenger ribonucleic acid in nasopharyngeal carcinoma correlates with poor prognosis. *J Laryngol Otol,* Vol.123, No.9, pp. 1021-6

Koehler, L.; Graf, F.; Bergmann, R.; Steinbach, J.; Pietzsch, J. & Wuest, F. (2010). Radiosynthesis and radiopharmacological evaluation of cyclin-dependent kinase 4 (Cdk4) inhibitors. *Eur J Med Chem,* Vol.45, No.2, pp. 727-37

Konig, A.; Schwartz, G. K.; Mohammad, R. M.; Al-Katib, A. & Gabrilove, J. L. (1997). The novel cyclin-dependent kinase inhibitor flavopiridol downregulates Bcl-2 and induces growth arrest and apoptosis in chronic B-cell leukemia lines. *Blood,* Vol.90, No.11, pp. 4307-12

Krystof, V. & Uldrijan, S. (2010). Cyclin-dependent kinase inhibitors as anticancer drugs. *Curr Drug Targets,* Vol.11, No.3, pp. 291-302

Lam, L. T.; Pickeral, O. K.; Peng, A. C.; Rosenwald, A.; Hurt, E. M.; Giltnane, J. M.; Averett, L. M.; Zhao, H.; Davis, R. E.; Sathyamoorthy, M.; Wahl, L. M.; Harris, E. D.; Mikovits, J. A.; Monks, A. P.; Hollingshead, M. G.; Sausville, E. A. & Staudt, L. M. (2001). Genomic-scale measurement of mRNA turnover and the mechanisms of action of the anti-cancer drug flavopiridol. *Genome Biol,* Vol.2, No.10, pp. 0041.1-0041.11

Lapenna, S. & Giordano, A. (2009). Cell cycle kinases as therapeutic targets for cancer. *Nat Rev Drug Discov,* Vol.8, No.7, pp. 547-66

Lee, Y. M. & Sicinski, P. (2006). Targeting cyclins and cyclin-dependent kinases in cancer: lessons from mice, hopes for therapeutic applications in human. *Cell Cycle,* Vol.5, No.18, pp. 2110-4

Leonard, J. P.; LaCasce, A.; Smith, M. R.; Ariela Noy, A.; Yap, J. T.; Van den Abbeele, A. D.; Yu, J. Q.; Chen-Kiang, S.; Ely, S. A.; Vallabhajosula, S.; Chirieac, L. R.; Larson, S. M.; Shapiro, G. I. & Schoder, H. (2008). Cdk4/6 Inhibitor PD 0332991 Demonstrates Cell Cycle Inhibition Via FLT-PET Imaging and Tissue Analysis in Patients with Recurrent Mantle Cell Lymphoma *Blood (ASH Annual Meeting Abstracts),* Vol.112, abstract 264

Lin, T. S.; Ruppert, A. S.; Johnson, A. J.; Fischer, B.; Heerema, N. A.; Andritsos, L. A.; Blum, K. A.; Flynn, J. M.; Jones, J. A.; Hu, W.; Moran, M. E.; Mitchell, S. M.; Smith, L. L.; Wagner, A. J.; Raymond, C. A.; Schaaf, L. J.; Phelps, M. A.; Villalona-Calero, M. A.; Grever, M. R. & Byrd, J. C. (2009). Phase II study of flavopiridol in relapsed chronic lymphocytic leukemia demonstrating high response rates in genetically high-risk disease. *J Clin Oncol,* Vol.27, No.35, pp. 6012-8

Lolli, G. & Johnson, L. N. (2005). CAK-Cyclin-dependent Activating Kinase: a key kinase in cell cycle control and a target for drugs? *Cell Cycle,* Vol.4, No.4, pp. 572-7

Lu, H. & Schulze-Gahmen, U. (2006). Toward understanding the structural basis of cyclin-dependent kinase 6 specific inhibition. *J Med Chem,* Vol.49, No.13, pp. 3826-31

Lu, X.; Burgan, W. E.; Cerra, M. A.; Chuang, E. Y.; Tsai, M. H.; Tofilon, P. J. & Camphausen, K. (2004). Transcriptional signature of flavopiridol-induced tumor cell death. *Mol Cancer Ther,* Vol.3, No.7, pp. 861-72

Maggiorella, L.; Deutsch, E.; Frascogna, V.; Chavaudra, N.; Jeanson, L.; Milliat, F.; Eschwege, F. & Bourhis, J. (2003). Enhancement of radiation response by roscovitine in human breast carcinoma in vitro and in vivo. *Cancer Res,* Vol.63, No.10, pp. 2513-7

Mahadevan, D.; Plummer, R.; Squires, M. S.; Rensvold, D.; Kurtin, S.; Pretzinger, C.; Dragovich, T.; Adams, J.; Lock, V.; Smith, D. M.; Von Hoff, D. & Calvert, H. (2011). A phase I pharmacokinetic and pharmacodynamic study of AT7519, a cyclin-dependent kinase inhibitor in patients with refractory solid tumors. *Ann Oncol,* pp.

Malumbres, M. & Barbacid, M. (2005). Mammalian cyclin-dependent kinases. *Trends Biochem Sci,* Vol.30, No.11, pp. 630-41

Malumbres, M. & Barbacid, M. (2009). Cell cycle, CDKs and cancer: a changing paradigm. *Nat Rev Cancer,* Vol.9, No.3, pp. 153-66

Manohar, S. M.; Rathos, M. J.; Sonawane, V.; Rao, S. V. & Joshi, K. S. (2011). Cyclin-dependent kinase inhibitor, P276-00 induces apoptosis in multiple myeloma cells by inhibition of Cdk9-T1 and RNA polymerase II-dependent transcription. *Leuk Res,* in press.

McClue, S. J.; Blake, D.; Clarke, R.; Cowan, A.; Cummings, L.; Fischer, P. M.; MacKenzie, M.; Melville, J.; Stewart, K.; Wang, S.; Zhelev, N.; Zheleva, D. & Lane, D. P. (2002). In vitro and in vivo antitumor properties of the cyclin dependent kinase inhibitor CYC202 (R-roscovitine). *Int J Cancer,* Vol.102, No.5, pp. 463-8

Meijer, L.; Borgne, A.; Mulner, O.; Chong, J. P.; Blow, J. J.; Inagaki, N.; Inagaki, M.; Delcros, J. G. & Moulinoux, J. P. (1997). Biochemical and cellular effects of roscovitine, a potent and selective inhibitor of the cyclin-dependent kinases cdc2, cdk2 and cdk5. *Eur J Biochem,* Vol.243, No.1-2, pp. 527-36

Menu, E.; Garcia, J.; Huang, X.; Di Liberto, M.; Toogood, P. L.; Chen, I.; Vanderkerken, K. & Chen-Kiang, S. (2008). A novel therapeutic combination using PD 0332991 and bortezomib: study in the 5T33MM myeloma model. *Cancer Res,* Vol.68, No.14, pp. 5519-23

Meyerson, M. & Harlow, E. (1994). Identification of G1 kinase activity for cdk6, a novel cyclin D partner. *Mol Cell Biol,* Vol.14, No.3, pp. 2077-86

Nevins, J. R. (2001). The Rb/E2F pathway and cancer. *Hum Mol Genet,* Vol.10, No.7, pp. 699-703

Niesvizky, R.; Ely, S.; Jayabalan, D. S.; Manco, M. C.; Singhal, S.; Crann, M.; Courtney, R.; DuFresne, C.; Wilner, K. D.; Chen, I.; Mark, T.; Leonard, J. P.; Coleman, M.; DiLiberto, M.; Huang, X. & Chen-Kiang, S. (2009). A Phase I Trial of PD 0332991, a Novel, Orally-Bioavailable CDK4/6-Specific Inhibitor Administered in Combination with Bortezomib and Dexamethasone to Patients with Relapsed and Refractory Multiple Myeloma. *Blood (ASH Annual Meeting Abstracts),* Vol.114, abstract 1877

Niesvizky, R.; Lentzsch, S.; Badros, A. Z.; Chanan-Khan, A. A.; Singhal, S. B.; Zonder, J. A.; Vij, R.; Huang, X.; DiLiberto, M.; Courtney, R.; Shaik, M. N.; Kim, S. T.; Randolph,

S.; Ely, S. A. & Chen-Kiang, S. (2010). A Phase I Study of PD 0332991: Complete CDK4/6 Inhibition and Tumor Response In Sequential Combination with Bortezomib and Dexamethasone for Relapsed and Refractory Multiple Myeloma. *Blood (ASH Annual Meeting Abstracts)*, Vol.116, abstract 860

O'Dwyer, P. J.; LoRusso, P.; DeMichele, A.; Gupta, V.; Barbi, A.; Dials, H. J.; Chen, I.; Courtney, R.; Wilner, K. & Schwartz, G. K. (2007). A phase I dose escalation trial of a daily oral CDK 4/6 inhibitor PD-0332991. *J Clin Oncol (ASCO Annual Meeting Proceedings Part I)*, Vol.25, 18S (June 20 Suppl.), abstract 3550

Ortega, S.; Malumbres, M. & Barbacid, M. (2002). Cyclin D-dependent kinases, INK4 inhibitors and cancer. *Biochim Biophys Acta*, Vol.1602, No.1, pp. 73-87

Parker, B. W.; Kaur, G.; Nieves-Neira, W.; Taimi, M.; Kohlhagen, G.; Shimizu, T.; Losiewicz, M. D.; Pommier, Y.; Sausville, E. A. & Senderowicz, A. M. (1998). Early induction of apoptosis in hematopoietic cell lines after exposure to flavopiridol. *Blood*, Vol.91, No.2, pp. 458-65

Parry, D.; Guzi, T.; Shanahan, F.; Davis, N.; Prabhavalkar, D.; Wiswell, D.; Seghezzi, W.; Paruch, K.; Dwyer, M. P.; Doll, R.; Nomeir, A.; Windsor, W.; Fischmann, T.; Wang, Y.; Oft, M.; Chen, T.; Kirschmeier, P. & Lees, E. M. (2010). Dinaciclib (SCH 727965), a novel and potent cyclin-dependent kinase inhibitor. *Mol Cancer Ther*, Vol.9, No.8, pp. 2344-53

Patel, V.; Senderowicz, A. M.; Pinto, D., Jr.; Igishi, T.; Raffeld, M.; Quintanilla-Martinez, L.; Ensley, J. F.; Sausville, E. A. & Gutkind, J. S. (1998). Flavopiridol, a novel cyclin-dependent kinase inhibitor, suppresses the growth of head and neck squamous cell carcinomas by inducing apoptosis. *J Clin Invest*, Vol.102, No.9, pp. 1674-81

Phelps, M. A.; Lin, T. S.; Johnson, A. J.; Hurh, E.; Rozewski, D. M.; Farley, K. L.; Wu, D.; Blum, K. A.; Fischer, B.; Mitchell, S. M.; Moran, M. E.; Brooker-McEldowney, M.; Heerema, N. A.; Jarjoura, D.; Schaaf, L. J.; Byrd, J. C.; Grever, M. R. & Dalton, J. T. (2009). Clinical response and pharmacokinetics from a phase 1 study of an active dosing schedule of flavopiridol in relapsed chronic lymphocytic leukemia. *Blood*, Vol.113, No.12, pp. 2637-45

Popowycz, F.; Fournet, G.; Schneider, C.; Bettayeb, K.; Ferandin, Y.; Lamigeon, C.; Tirado, O. M.; Mateo-Lozano, S.; Notario, V.; Colas, P.; Bernard, P.; Meijer, L. & Joseph, B. (2009). Pyrazolo[1,5-a]-1,3,5-triazine as a purine bioisostere: access to potent cyclin-dependent kinase inhibitor (R)-roscovitine analogue. *J Med Chem*, Vol.52, No.3, pp. 655-63

Raje, N.; Hideshima, T.; Mukherjee, S.; Raab, M.; Vallet, S.; Chhetri, S.; Cirstea, D.; Pozzi, S.; Mitsiades, C.; Rooney, M.; Kiziltepe, T.; Podar, K.; Okawa, Y.; Ikeda, H.; Carrasco, R.; Richardson, P. G.; Chauhan, D.; Munshi, N. C.; Sharma, S.; Parikh, H.; Chabner, B.; Scadden, D. & Anderson, K. C. (2009). Preclinical activity of P276-00, a novel small-molecule cyclin-dependent kinase inhibitor in the therapy of multiple myeloma. *Leukemia*, Vol.23, No.5, pp. 961-70

Raynaud, F. I.; Whittaker, S. R.; Fischer, P. M.; McClue, S.; Walton, M. I.; Barrie, S. E.; Garrett, M. D.; Rogers, P.; Clarke, S. J.; Kelland, L. R.; Valenti, M.; Brunton, L.; Eccles, S.; Lane, D. P. & Workman, P. (2005). In vitro and in vivo pharmacokinetic-pharmacodynamic relationships for the trisubstituted aminopurine cyclin-dependent kinase inhibitors olomoucine, bohemine and CYC202. *Clin Cancer Res*, Vol.11, No.13, pp. 4875-87

Ren, S. & Rollins, B. J. (2004). Cyclin C/cdk3 promotes Rb-dependent G0 exit. *Cell,* Vol.117, No.2, pp. 239-51

Rizzolio, F.; Tuccinardi, T.; Caligiuri, I.; Lucchetti, C. & Giordano, A. (2010). CDK inhibitors: from the bench to clinical trials. *Curr Drug Targets,* Vol.11, No.3, pp. 279-90

Robey, R. W.; Medina-Perez, W. Y.; Nishiyama, K.; Lahusen, T.; Miyake, K.; Litman, T.; Senderowicz, A. M.; Ross, D. D. & Bates, S. E. (2001). Overexpression of the ATP-binding cassette half-transporter, ABCG2 (Mxr/BCrp/ABCP1), in flavopiridol-resistant human breast cancer cells. *Clin Cancer Res,* Vol.7, No.1, pp. 145-52

Ruas, M. & Peters, G. (1998). The p16INK4a/CDKN2A tumor suppressor and its relatives. *Biochim Biophys Acta,* Vol.1378, No.2, pp. F115-77

Saab, R.; Bills, J. L.; Miceli, A. P.; Anderson, C. M.; Khoury, J. D.; Fry, D. W.; Navid, F.; Houghton, P. J. & Skapek, S. X. (2006). Pharmacologic inhibition of cyclin-dependent kinase 4/6 activity arrests proliferation in myoblasts and rhabdomyosarcoma-derived cells. *Mol Cancer Ther,* Vol.5, No.5, pp. 1299-308

Santamaria, D.; Barriere, C.; Cerqueira, A.; Hunt, S.; Tardy, C.; Newton, K.; Caceres, J. F.; Dubus, P.; Malumbres, M. & Barbacid, M. (2007). Cdk1 is sufficient to drive the mammalian cell cycle. *Nature,* Vol.448, No.7155, pp. 811-5

Santo, L.; Vallet, S.; Hideshima, T.; Cirstea, D.; Ikeda, H.; Pozzi, S.; Patel, K.; Okawa, Y.; Gorgun, G.; Perrone, G.; Calabrese, E.; Yule, M.; Squires, M.; Ladetto, M.; Boccadoro, M.; Richardson, P. G.; Munshi, N. C.; Anderson, K. C. & Raje, N. (2010). AT7519, A novel small molecule multi-cyclin-dependent kinase inhibitor, induces apoptosis in multiple myeloma via GSK-3beta activation and RNA polymerase II inhibition. *Oncogene,* Vol.29, No.16, pp. 2325-36

Schwartz, G. K.; Ilson, D.; Saltz, L.; O'Reilly, E.; Tong, W.; Maslak, P.; Werner, J.; Perkins, P.; Stoltz, M. & Kelsen, D. (2001). Phase II study of the cyclin-dependent kinase inhibitor flavopiridol administered to patients with advanced gastric carcinoma. *J Clin Oncol,* Vol.19, No.7, pp. 1985-92

Seamon, J. A.; Rugg, C. A.; Emanuel, S.; Calcagno, A. M.; Ambudkar, S. V.; Middleton, S. A.; Butler, J.; Borowski, V. & Greenberger, L. M. (2006). Role of the ABCG2 drug transporter in the resistance and oral bioavailability of a potent cyclin-dependent kinase/Aurora kinase inhibitor. *Mol Cancer Ther,* Vol.5, No.10, pp. 2459-67

Sedlacek, H. H. (2001). Mechanisms of action of flavopiridol. *Crit Rev Oncol Hematol,* Vol.38, No.2, pp. 139-70

Sedlacek, H. H.; Czech, J.; Naik, R.; Kaur, G.; Worland, P.; Losiewicz, M.; Parker, B.; Carlson, B.; Smith, A.; Senderowicz, A. & Sausville, E. (1996). Flavopiridol (L86 8275; NSC 649890), a new kinase inhibitor for tumor therapy. *International Journal of Oncology,* Vol.9, No.6, pp. 1143-1168

Senderowicz, A. M. & Sausville, E. A. (2000). Preclinical and clinical development of cyclin-dependent kinase modulators. *J Natl Cancer Inst,* Vol.92, No.5, pp. 376-87

Shapiro, G. I. (2006). Cyclin-dependent kinase pathways as targets for cancer treatment. *J Clin Oncol,* Vol.24, No.11, pp. 1770-83

Shapiro, G. I.; Bannerji, R.; Small, K.; Black, S.; Statkevich, P.; Abutarif, M.; Moseley, J.; Yao, S.; Takimoto, C. H. & Mita, M. M. (2008). A phase I dose-escalation study of the safety, pharmacokinetics (PK) and pharmacodynamics (PD) of the novel cyclin-dependent kinase inhibitor SCH 727965 administered every 3 weeks in subjects with advanced malignancies. *J Clin Oncol,* Vol.26, (May 20 Suppl.), abstract 3532

Shapiro, G. I.; Supko, J. G.; Patterson, A.; Lynch, C.; Lucca, J.; Zacarola, P. F.; Muzikansky, A.; Wright, J. J.; Lynch, T. J., Jr. & Rollins, B. J. (2001). A phase II trial of the cyclin-dependent kinase inhibitor flavopiridol in patients with previously untreated stage IV non-small cell lung cancer. *Clin Cancer Res,* Vol.7, No.6, pp. 1590-9

Sharma, P. S.; Sharma, R. & Tyagi, R. (2008). Inhibitors of cyclin dependent kinases: useful targets for cancer treatment. *Curr Cancer Drug Targets,* Vol.8, No.1, pp. 53-75

Sherr, C. J. & Roberts, J. M. (1999). CDK inhibitors: positive and negative regulators of G1-phase progression. *Genes Dev,* Vol.13, No.12, pp. 1501-12

Siegel-Lakhai, W. S.; Rodenstein, D. O.; Beijnen, J. H.; Gianella-Borradori, A.; Schellens, J. H. & Talbot, D. C. (2005). Phase I study of seliciclib (CYC202 or R-roscovitine) in combination with gemcitabine (gem)/cisplatin (cis) in patients with advanced Non-Small Cell Lung Cancer (NSCLC). *J Clin Oncol (ASCO Annual Meeting Proceedings),* Vol.23, 16S, Part I of II (June 1 Suppl.), abstract 2060

Sielecki, T. M.; Boylan, J. F.; Benfield, P. A. & Trainor, G. L. (2000). Cyclin-dependent kinase inhibitors: useful targets in cell cycle regulation. *J Med Chem,* Vol.43, No.1, pp. 1-18

Siemeister, G.; Lücking, U.; Wengner, A.; Lienau, P.; Schatz, C.; Mumberg, D. & Ziegelbauer, K. (2010). Pharmacologic profile of the oral novel pan-CDK inhibitor BAY 1000394 in chemosensitive and chemorefractory tumor models. *Proceedings of the 101st Annual Meeting of the American Association for Cancer Research (AACR),* Abstract number 3883, Washington, DC. Philadelphia (PA), Apr 17-21, 2010

Slamon, D. J.; Hurvitz, S. A.; Applebaum, S.; Glaspy, J. A.; Allison, M. K.; DiCarlo, B. A.; Courtney, R. D.; Kim, S. T.; Randolph, S. & Finn, R. S. (2010). Phase I study of PD 0332991, cyclin-D kinase (CDK) 4/6 inhibitor in combination with letrozole for first-line treatment of patients with ER-positive, HER2-negative breast cancer. *J Clin Oncol,* Vol.28, 15s (Suppl.) abstract 3060

Smith, V.; Raynaud, F.; Workman, P. & Kelland, L. R. (2001). Characterization of a human colorectal carcinoma cell line with acquired resistance to flavopiridol. *Mol Pharmacol,* Vol.60, No.5, pp. 885-93

Song, H.; Vita, M.; Sallam, H.; Tehranchi, R.; Nilsson, C.; Siden, A. & Hassan, Z. (2007). Effect of the Cdk-inhibitor roscovitine on mouse hematopoietic progenitors in vivo and in vitro. *Cancer Chemother Pharmacol,* Vol.60, No.6, pp. 841-9

Sotillo, R.; Dubus, P.; Martin, J.; de la Cueva, E.; Ortega, S.; Malumbres, M. & Barbacid, M. (2001). Wide spectrum of tumors in knock-in mice carrying a Cdk4 protein insensitive to INK4 inhibitors. *EMBO J,* Vol.20, No.23, pp. 6637-47

Squires, M. S.; Cooke, L.; Lock, V.; Qi, W.; Lewis, E. J.; Thompson, N. T.; Lyons, J. F. & Mahadevan, D. (2010). AT7519, a cyclin-dependent kinase inhibitor, exerts its effects by transcriptional inhibition in leukemia cell lines and patient samples. *Mol Cancer Ther,* Vol.9, No.4, pp. 920-8

Squires, M. S.; Feltell, R. E.; Wallis, N. G.; Lewis, E. J.; Smith, D. M.; Cross, D. M.; Lyons, J. F. & Thompson, N. T. (2009). Biological characterization of AT7519, a small-molecule inhibitor of cyclin-dependent kinases, in human tumor cell lines. *Mol Cancer Ther,* Vol.8, No.2, pp. 324-32

Sridhar, J.; Akula, N. & Pattabiraman, N. (2006). Selectivity and potency of cyclin-dependent kinase inhibitors. *AAPS J,* Vol.8, No.1, pp. E204-21

Tibes, R.; Jimeno, A.; Von Hoff, D. D.; Walker, R.; Pacciarini, M. A.; Scaburri, A.; Fiorentini, F.; Borad, M. J.; Jameson, G. S. & Hidalgo, M. (2008). Phase I dose escalation study of the oral multi-CDK inhibitor PHA-848125. *J Clin Oncol,* Vol.26, (May 20 Suppl.), abstract 3531

Tsihlias, J.; Kapusta, L. & Slingerland, J. (1999). The prognostic significance of altered cyclin-dependent kinase inhibitors in human cancer. *Annu Rev Med,* Vol.50, pp. 401-23

VanderWel, S. N.; Harvey, P. J.; McNamara, D. J.; Repine, J. T.; Keller, P. R.; Quin, J., 3rd; Booth, R. J.; Elliott, W. L.; Dobrusin, E. M.; Fry, D. W. & Toogood, P. L. (2005). Pyrido[2,3-d]pyrimidin-7-ones as specific inhibitors of cyclin-dependent kinase 4. *J Med Chem,* Vol.48, No.7, pp. 2371-87

Wang, W. L.; Conley, A.; Reynoso, D.; Nolden, L.; Lazar, A. J.; George, S. & Trent, J. C. (2011). Mechanisms of resistance to imatinib and sunitinib in gastrointestinal stromal tumor. *Cancer Chemother Pharmacol,* Vol.67 Suppl. 1, pp. S15-24

Weinberg, R. A. (2007). *The biology of cancer,* Garland Science, ISBN 0-8153-4078-8, New York, USA

Wesierska-Gadek, J.; Maurer, M.; Zulehner, N. & Komina, O. (2011). Whether to target single or multiple CDKs for therapy? That is the question. *J Cell Physiol,* Vol.226, No.2, pp. 341-9

Wolfel, T.; Hauer, M.; Schneider, J.; Serrano, M.; Wolfel, C.; Klehmann-Hieb, E.; De Plaen, E.; Hankeln, T.; Meyer zum Buschenfelde, K. H. & Beach, D. (1995). A p16INK4a-insensitive CDK4 mutant targeted by cytolytic T lymphocytes in a human melanoma. *Science,* Vol.269, No.5228, pp. 1281-4

Wyatt, P. G.; Woodhead, A. J.; Berdini, V.; Boulstridge, J. A.; Carr, M. G.; Cross, D. M.; Davis, D. J.; Devine, L. A.; Early, T. R.; Feltell, R. E.; Lewis, E. J.; McMenamin, R. L.; Navarro, E. F.; O'Brien, M. A.; O'Reilly, M.; Reule, M.; Saxty, G.; Seavers, L. C.; Smith, D. M.; Squires, M. S.; Trewartha, G.; Walker, M. T. & Woolford, A. J. (2008). Identification of N-(4-piperidinyl)-4-(2,6-dichlorobenzoylamino)-1H-pyrazole-3-carboxamide (AT7519), a novel cyclin dependent kinase inhibitor using fragment-based X-ray crystallography and structure based drug design. *J Med Chem,* Vol.51, No.16, pp. 4986-99

13

# Targeting Tumor Perfusion and Oxygenation Modulates Hypoxia and Cancer Sensitivity to Radiotherapy and Systemic Therapies

Bénédicte F. Jordan[1] and Pierre Sonveaux[2]
[1]*Biomedical Magnetic Resonance Group*
[2]*Pole of Pharmacology (FATH5349), University of Louvain (UCL) Medical School*
*Belgium*

## 1. Introduction

Hypoxia, a partial pressure of oxygen ($pO_2$) below physiological needs, is a limiting factor affecting the efficiency of radiotherapy. Indeed, the reaction of reactive oxygen species (ROS, produced by water radiolysis) with DNA is readily reversible unless oxygen stabilizes the DNA lesion. While normal tissue oxygenation is around 40 mm Hg, both rodent and human tumors possess regions of tissue oxygenation below 10 mm Hg, at which tumor cells become increasingly resistant to radiation damage (radiobiological hypoxia) (Gray, 1953). Because of this so-called "oxygen enhancement effect", the radiation dose required to achieve the same biologic effect is about three times higher in the absence of oxygen than in the presence of normal levels of oxygen (Gray et al., 1953; Horsman & van der Kogel, 2009). Hypoxic tumor cells, which are therefore more resistant to radiotherapy than well oxygenated ones, remain clonogenic and contribute to the therapeutic outcome of fractionated radiotherapy (Rojas et al., 1992).

Tumor hypoxia results from the imbalance between oxygen delivery by poorly efficient blood vessels and oxygen consumption by tumor cells with high metabolic activities. On the one hand, oxygen delivery is impaired by structural abnormalities present in the tumor vasculature (Munn, 2003). They include caliber variations with dilated and narrowed single branches of tumor vessels, non-hierarchical vascular networks, disturbed precapillary architecture, and incomplete vascular walls. These structural abnormalities cause numerous functional impairments, i.e. increased transcapillary permeability, increased vascular permeability, interstitial hypertension, and increased flow resistance (Boucher et al., 1996; McDonald & Baluk, 2002). It is however important to note that, although hastily formed immature tumor microvessels lack smooth muscle layer(s) and are therefore unable to provide autoregulation, it is not uncommon to find mature blood vessels with smooth muscle layers and neural junctions inside slow-growing tumors (e.g. most human tumors) (Feron, 2004). On the other hand, the altered tumor cell metabolism with elevated metabolic rates also contributes to the occurrence of hypoxic regions in tumors and further causes extracellular acidification. Tumor hypoxia occurs in two ways: chronic hypoxia (or diffusion-limited hypoxia), and acute hypoxia (or perfusion-limited or fluctuating hypoxia). Chronic hypoxia has classically been thought to result from long diffusion distances between tumor vessels as the consequence of the more rapid expansion of tumors cells than that of the supporting vasculature (Vaupel et al., 1989). It is now well established that steep longitudinal gradients of $pO_2$ along the vascular tree, as opposed to radial diffusion of oxygen, can largely contribute to deficiencies in tumor oxygen supply (Dewhirst et al., 1999). The origin of acute hypoxia in tumors is not firmly established. The commonly held view has been that acute hypoxia results primarily from vascular stasis, which stems from one of three causes: 1) vascular collapse in regions of high tumor interstitial pressure, 2) vessel plugging by leukocytes, and 3) impingement of tumor cells on the vascular lumen. It has been demonstrated that temporal instability in tumor red blood cell flux could lead to transient hypoxia (Kimura et al., 1996), and Dewhirst linked temporal changes in microvessel red blood cell flux to changes in the oxygen content in the same vessel (Dewhirst et al., 1996). Factors that may contribute to flow fluctuations include arteriolar vasomotion and rapid vascular modeling (Baudelet et al., 2004, 2006; Dewhirst et al., 1996; Patan et al., 1996). More recent studies indicate a widespread presence of fluctuating hypoxia in solid tumors (Cardena-Navia et al., 2008).

The effect of tumor hypoxia on the response to treatment by ionizing radiation has been demonstrated in a multitude of experimental studies. In a series of clinical studies in the early nineties, Vaupel and others showed definitively that measurements of $pO_2$ by polarographic microelectrodes provided useful criteria for predicting the response of tumors to radiation therapy (Gatenby et al., 1988; Hockel et al., 1993; Okunieff et al., 1993; Stone et al., 1993; Thomas et al., 1994). These results stimulated considerable efforts in defining and evaluating therapeutic approaches designed to overcome tumor hypoxia as source of resistance (Horsman & van der Kogel, 2009). A particular area under focus is thus to combine radiotherapy with treatments that increase tumor $pO_2$. Other approaches consist to chemically radiosensitize hypoxic cells or alternatively to exploit hypoxia as a mean to selectively kill the resistant population of hypoxic cells. Before the advent of imaging methods able to provide non-invasively oxygen estimation, animal and clinical studies were generally designed to evaluate the effect of a given treatment on tumor $pO_2$ as measured by Eppendorf or histological markers of tumor hypoxia. The clinical end points were generally locoregional control and survival. Modifiers of oxygen delivery tested in clinical trials included hyperbaric oxygen therapy (HBO), oxygen and carbogen breathing. Hypoxic cell radiosensitizers (possessing a selective toxicity for the radioresistant hypoxic cells) tested in clinical trials included metronidazole, misonidazole, nimorazole, and tirapazamine. In a systematic review, J. Overgaard (2007) identified 10,108 patients in 86 randomized trials designed to modify tumor hypoxia in patients treated with curative attempted primary radiation therapy alone. Overall modification of tumor hypoxia significantly improved the effect of radiotherapy for the outcome of locoregional control and with an associated significant overall survival benefit. No significant influence was found on the incidence of distant metastases or on the risk of radiation-related complications. From this meta-analysis, the authors concluded in 2007 that "Ample data exist to support a high level of evidence for the benefit of hypoxic modification. However, hypoxic modification still has no impact on general clinical practice".

Currently, the most advanced therapeutic interventions used in the clinic to target tumor hypoxia are either the DAHANCA (Danish head and neck cancer) trial, the application of the ARCON (Accelerated radiotherapy, carbogen and nicotinamide) protocol, and phase III studies with Tirapazamine. In the DAHANCA phase III study, nimorazole has been used as hypoxic radiosensitizer on 422 patients, and it was shown that this compound improves the effect of radiotherapeutic management in head and neck cancer (Overgaard et al., 1998). Since these results, nimorazole administration became part of the standard irradiation protocol for Head and Neck cancer in Denmark. However, these findings have had no impact on general clinical practice except for Denmark because earlier generations of these agents induced rather severe peripheral neuropathy and because nearly all of the individual phase III trials yielded negative or inconclusive results (Ang, 2010). The ARCON protocol consists in the combination of accelerated radiotherapy to overcome tumor cell proliferation, carbogen breathing to overcome diffusion-limited hypoxia, and nicotinamide to minimize capillary bed shutdown and thereby reduce perfusion-related acute hypoxia. Phase I and II clinical trials have shown the feasibility and tolerability of the treatment and have produced promising results in term of tumor control, in particular in cancer of the head and neck and bladder (Kaanders et al., 2002). A large improvement in survival was demonstrated using this approach during radiotherapy for bladder cancer. The randomized multicentre phase III trial, designed and coordinated at Mount Vernon Cancer Centre, demonstrated a 13% benefit in overall survival when radiotherapy was combined with carbogen and nicotinamide compared to radiotherapy alone (ASTRO, 2009). Results from a large phase III trial launched to test this regimen will become available within the next 2 years. Finally, Tirapazamine (TPZ) has attracted interest after preclinical studies showing that in addition to augmenting the cytotoxicity of both radiation and cisplatin, this compound selectively kills hypoxic cells (Rischin et al., 2001; 2005). Phase I and II studies of the combination of TPZ with radiation and cisplatin were performed on patients with locally advanced head and neck carcinoma. On the basis of the phase II data, a large international phase III trial was launched (Peters et al., 2010). Surprisingly, the combination did not show any evidence of improvement in overall survival. Nevertheless, patients were not previously screened for tumor hypoxia, the study was multicentric with some centers enrolling fewer than five patients and a consequent decrease in the quality of radiotherapy planning and delivery which can have dramatic consequences on outcome (Ang, 2010).

This chapter will explore 2 strategies to radiosensitize tumors to X-rays: to increase oxygen delivery by exploiting the reactivity of mature tumor vessels (the so-called 'provascular' approach) and to decrease oxygen consumption by tumor cells. The goal of the provascular approach is to temporarily increase tumor perfusion and oxygenation through pharmacological interventions. Accordingly, radiotherapy could benefit from tumor reoxygenation whereas a decrease in interstitial pressure could facilitate tumor accessibility to circulating drugs. Alternatively, a second approach is to decrease the oxygen consumption by tumor cells since theoretical modeling studies demonstrated that reducing $O_2$ consumption was far more efficient at reducing tumor hypoxia than increasing blood $pO_2$ or flow (Secomb et al., 1995). We will also describe attempts to combine both approaches that can be considered as complementary strategies. The evaluation and validation of these adjuvant therapies require imaging techniques capable to accurately monitor tumor perfusion and oxygenation.

From the clinical analyses cited above, it also appeared that the variation in the results among the trials reflects a considerable heterogeneity among tumors and that patient individualization would be mandatory for the success of such therapeutic approach. There is therefore an essential need to predict individually the presence of hypoxic regions in tumors. Based on individual tumor characteristics and/or the ability to alleviate tumor hypoxia, it will become possible to adapt the individual treatment either by delivering optimal radiation doses into the resistant areas or by delivering an associated treatment for potentiating the efficacy of radiation treatments. In the early nineties, invasive techniques such as polarographic electrodes have been used in clinical studies to definitely establish the value of hypoxia as a predictive marker of the response of tumors to irradiation. Although this method was successful in demonstrating the central role played by tumor hypoxia in the clinical response to radiation therapy, it has never been used in standard clinical practice because of its invasiveness and the difficulty to systematically carry out longitudinal studies in individual patients. Fortunately, it is now possible to estimate tumor oxygenation by using minimally or non invasive techniques. This will be the purpose of the last part of this chapter.

## 2. Improving oxygen delivery to the tumor: The provascular approach

Tumors are highly heterogeneous and this heterogeneity extends to the tumor vasculature (see introduction). Beside neovessels that are the target of anti-angiogenic agents, human and rodent tumors also contain blood vessels that are structurally mature (Mattson et al., 1978; Peterson & Mattson, 1984). These vessels possess the minimal contractile features (such as pericytes or vascular smooth muscle cells) endowing them with vasocontractile properties. The intrinsic reactivity of tumor-feeding vessels modulates oxygen delivery and the accessibility of circulating drugs to the tumor. A selective and transient dilation of these vessels should thus improve the tumor response to radiotherapy (which depends on tumor oxygenation) and chemotherapy (which depends on perfusion and on the vascular exchange area). We termed this approach 'provascular' to contrast with antivascular and anti-angiogenic approaches that are destructive by nature (Sonveaux, 2008). The net effect of systemic vasodilation on tumor $pO_2$ is unpredictable because it primarily depends on the arrangement of vessels (in series or in parallel) between the tumor and surrounding host tissues (Zlotecki et al., 1995). The key issue to resolve is thus to identify tumor-selective vasodilators. Treatment optimization would also require to monitor on individual bases the tumor response to treatment, preferentially using early surrogate, predictive and non-invasive markers.

### 2.1 Nitric Oxide (NO) and endothelin-1 (ET1) related strategies

Physiologically, the vascular tone is determined by the balance between nitric oxide (NO, a potent vasodilator) and endothelin-1 (ET1, a potent vasoconstrictor) (Sonveaux & Feron, 2005a). A number of studies have explored the functionality and the provascular exploitability of these 2 systems, as described below.

#### 2.1.1 Exogenous and endogenous NO

NO was initially investigated for its vasodilatory activity and NO-donors were anticipated to improve the therapeutic efficacy of chemo- and radiotherapy upon combinational delivery (Sonveaux et al., 2009). We first considered the effect of the application of exogenous NO on tumor hemodynamic parameters and radiation response. This was performed by systemic administration of NO donor compounds, including isosorbide dinitrate (Jordan et al., 2000), Xanthinol Nicotinate (Segers et al., 2010), and S-nitroso-captopril (Jordan et al., 2010a). The stimulation of the production of endogenous NO was also achieved by administration of insulin (Jordan et al., 2002). All treatments resulted in a transient acute improvement of experimental tumor oxygenation with a consecutive increase in tumor radiosensitivity upon sequential administration of X-rays during the reoxygenation window identified for each tumor model (Jordan et al., 2010a). The reoxygenation effect was shown to be due to an increase in tumor blood flow for Isosorbide Dinitrate, Xanthinol Nicotinate and S-nitrosocaptopril, using either dynamic contrast-enhanced magnetic resonance imaging (DCE-MRI), where the number of perfused voxels and/or Ktrans, Kep, or Vp parameters was increased (see 5.2.1) , or patent blue staining (Jordan & Gallez, 2010b). Importantly, for some co-treatments, the increase in blood flow occurred concomitantly with a decrease in the rate of oxygen consumption by tumor cells. Inhibition of tumor cell respiration is the main mechanism accounting for insulin-induced tumor reoxygenation (see below).

Endogenous NO is produced by a series of enzymes collectively termed NO-synthases (NOS). The endothelial isoform, eNOS, is adapted for the local stimulation of vasodilation following a response to stimuli that release calcium from intracellular stores and promote a calcium-calmodulin-dependent release of eNOS from its inhibitory complex with caveolin-1 (Cav-1) (Arnold et al., 1977; Michel et al., 1997). This mode of activation allows the transient production of micromolar amounts of NO responsible for vasodilatation. Using myography, we showed that this system is insensitive to classical eNOS stimulators (such as acetylcholine) selectively in tumor arterioles, thus suggesting that strategies able to restore eNOS activity would selectively target tumor vessels (Sonveaux et al., 2002). Among different treatments, we have found that ionizing radiations themselves were able to restore the normal vasodilatory properties of tumor vessels. X-rays, through the production of reactive oxygen species (ROS), indeed induce an increase in eNOS expression concomitantly with a decrease in Cav-1 expression, which removes a functional brake promoting eNOS activation (Sonveaux et al., 2002, 2009). Irradiations further stimulate NO production through the ROS-dependent activation of the PI3 kinase pathway, a well described pathway supporting Akt-mediated eNOS phosphorylation (on Ser1177, human sequence) and activation (Sonveaux et al., 2003, 2007a). We documented that radiation-induced vasodilation takes an active part in the antitumor effects of X-rays by showing that eNOS inhibition between the first and second irradiation of a clinical regimen of fractionated radiotherapy results in the total loss of the antitumor efficacy of the second dose, whereas eNOS inhibition before a single dose does not preclude cytotoxic effects (Sonveaux et al., 2002). Active vasodilation after each of the consecutive doses of fractionated radiotherapy is associated with a window of tumor reoxygenation that offers a scientific rationale for the clinical use of radiotherapy in its fractionated mode.

### 2.1.2 *S*-nitrosylated hemoglobin and nitrites

A smart delivery of exogenous NO would help to resolve the Steal Effect, a process through which systemic vasodilation may in fact reduce tumor perfusion and oxygenation by redirecting blood to normal blood vessels that are generally more sensitive to vasoactive treatments and constitute a denser network (Zlotecki et al., 1995). Using hemoglobin (Hb) is an interesting approach because Hb is a physiological NO carrier (in the form of S-nitrosothiol) poised to deliver NO selectively in hypoxic tissues such as tumors (Sonveaux et al., 2005b). NO delivery, indeed, is possible only after the conformational change associated with Hb deoxygenation (Jia et al., 1996; McMahon et al., 2002; Stamler et al., 1997). Using cell-free human S-nitrosylated Hb (SNO-Hb) in rats, we documented a transient increase in tumor perfusion, but only when SNO-Hb was delivered in oxygenated blood (i.e., intra-arteriolar injection or intravenous injection concomitantly with carbogen breathing) (Sonveaux et al., 2005b). In deoxygenated blood, SNO-Hb would otherwise readily deoxygenate and release NO at the site of delivery. While increased tumor perfusion at low dose SNO-Hb is primarily attributable to central effects (i.e., baroreceptor inhibition), SNO-Hb at higher doses could act as a tumor-selective vasodilator and could therefore be used as a radiosensitizing treatment. Inhalation of the NO-donor gas ethyl nitrite, which promotes the S-nitrosylation of intra-erythrocytic Hb in the lungs, could have the same effects while minimizing toxic side effects associated with the administration of naked Hb (Moya et al., 2002; Sonveaux et al., 2007b).

While the use of SNO-Hb exploits hypoxia as a mean to selectively deliver NO to tumors, one can also take advantage of the low pH coupled to the high metabolic activities of many solid tumors. Nitrites for example can be reduced to NO either by enzymatic catalysis (nitrite reductase activities of xanthine oxidase, eNOS and Hb) or by non enzymatic disproportionation, and these processes are facilitated in an acidic microenvironment (Angelo et al., 2006; Godber et al., 2000; Modin et al., 2001; Vanin et al., 2007; Zweier et al., 1999). They have been used clinically as an antidote for cyanide poisoning (Holland & Kozlowski, 1986), which also indicates that they can be safely administrated to humans. We therefore tested whether the low pH of tumors (on average pH 6.7) could be exploited to generate NO from nitrites selectively in tumors. We observed *ex vivo* that nitrite-induced vasodilation was more pronounced at pH 6.7 compared to pH 7.4 (Frerart et al., 2008). We also found that the bioactivity of nitrites at low pH encompassed NO-mediated inhibition of tumor cell respiration, which indicates that the robust and transient increase in tumor $pO_2$ after nitrite delivery to mice is the result of the combination of vasoactive and metabolic responses. When administered to reach a plasma concentration of 100 μM in mice, nitrites sensitized tumors to radiotherapy (Frerart et al., 2008). Further clinical applications are however confronted to financial issues: clinical trials are now warranted whereas nitrites or their use in cancer therapy can not be patented.

### 2.1.3 Endothelin-1 inhibitors

Endothelin-1 (ET-1) is a strong vasoconstrictor and an autocrine growth factor produced by tumor cells (Haynes & Webb, 1994; Shichiri et al., 1991). It has a key role in the accommodation of vasoactive blood vessels to variations in intraluminal pressure: ET-1 mediates the myogenic tone, a vasoconstriction that buffers perfusion changes when the blood pressure increases (Huang & Koller, 1997). In tumors, the constant exposure of arterioles to ET-1 *in vivo* results in an increased myogenic tone that can be detected *ex vivo* (Sonveaux et al., 2004). We reasoned that it constituted a reserve for vasorelaxation that could be exploited to sensitize tumors to radio- and chemotherapy. ET-1 induces vasoconstriction when binding to $ET_A$ receptors expressed by contractile vascular cells (Maguire & Davenport, 1995). Using the $ET_A$ antagonist BQ123, we observed *ex vivo* a vasodilation selectively in tumor vessels (compared to size-matched vessels from nonmalignant tissues) that translated *in vivo* into increased tumor perfusion and oxygenation (Sonveaux et al., 2004). Both responses were tumor-selective and transient. BQ123 as a pretreatment therefore improved the antitumor effects of X-ray radiotherapy and cyclophosphamide (after systemic delivery) (Martinive et al., 2006; Sonveaux et al., 2004).

## 2.2 Normalization effect of anti-angiogenic agents

Given that anti-angiogenic agents will likely be combined with radiation therapy, it is critical to understand alterations in tumor oxygenation and perfusion, as well as to define optimal time points for the delivery of radiation. Our group previously studied the modifications in the tumor environment early after treatment with the anti-angiogenic agent thalidomide, with a special focus on a possible normalization of the tumor vasculature (Jain, 2001; Tong et al., 2004) that could be beneficial for radiotherapy. Our results showed an increase in tumor $pO_2$ during the first 2 days of thalidomide treatment, which was likely the result of the ability of thalidomide to modify tumor microenvironmental parameters such as the vascular supply and tumor perfusion, as shown by DCE-MRI (see 5.2.1) and histological analysis using the endothelial marker CD31 (Ansiaux et al., 2005). Indeed, the histological analysis revealed profound modifications in the vascular supply: a reduction in the number of tumor microvessels after thalidomide treatment together with a dilation of the remaining vessels with no decrease in the tumor vascular density. The perfusion measured by DCE-MRI showed an increased plasma volume fraction (see 5.2.1), which could be explained by the shift to larger blood vessel diameters as observed in histology analysis, perhaps due to compensation for the loss of small vessels. Interestingly, similar observations were not obtained using more specific anti-angiogenic agents such as SU-5416 or ZD-6474 (Ansiaux et al., 2006; 2009). For these compounds, tumor reoxygenation was rather due to a decrease in the rate of oxygen consumption by tumor cell and no normalization effect was observed in the tumor models under study (see below). We hypothesized that specific inhibition of vascular endothelial growth factor (VEGF) signaling via VEGFR2 by SU-5416 or ZD-6474 may have been compensated by another angiogenic pathway such as basic fibroblast growth factor (bFGF), platelet-derived growth factor (PDGF), transforming growth factor (TGF)-β, or Tie-2 signaling (Folkman et al., 2001; Stratmann et al., 1998); contrary to thalidomide which acts on different angiogenic pathways. It is nevertheless important to note that these findings are specific to the tumor models under study, since ZD-6474 was described earlier to be able to decrease both flow and permeability in human colon tumors (Bradley et al., 2008) and was able to induce transient normalization of the vasculature in gliomas (Claes et al., 2008).

## 3. Decreasing oxygen consumption by tumor cells

Tumor oxygenation is a matter of supply and demand. Whereas the provascular strategy intends to improve oxygen supply, several strategies are aimed at decreasing oxygen consumption by tumor cells rendering molecular $O_2$ available for the stabilization of radiation-induced DNA damage. Indeed, theoretical modeling studies demonstrated that reducing $O_2$ consumption could be more efficient at reducing tumor hypoxia than increasing blood $pO_2$ or flow (Secomb, 1995). Two main targets can be considered for inhibiting oxygen consumption: (i) direct interference with the mitochondrial respiratory chain (at different levels), and (ii) modulation of the redox status to change the mitochondrial membrane potential (Pilkington et al., 2008); the final aim being a subsequent increase in tumor $pO_2$ and enhancement of the efficacy of radiotherapy.
In contrast to provascular strategies, Laser Doppler flowmetry, DCE-MRI and electron paramagnetic resonance (EPR) oximetry have revealed that the radiosensitizing effects of these treatments are primarily caused by a decrease in the rate of oxygen consumption by tumor cells, thus allowing oxygen to be redirected from a metabolic fate to the stabilization of DNA lesions. Indeed, apart from NO donors, all the treatments described below did not show any significant increase in tumor blood flow concomitant to the increase in tumor oxygenation. Some of them even showed a decrease in tumor blood flow that was

counteracted by the dramatic decrease in oxygen consumption by tumor cells (i.e. insulin and NS-398). In addition, regarding NO-mediated treatments, our models showed that the radiotherapeutic response not only depended on the tumor $pO_2$ but also on the net level of NO achieved at the time of irradiation, NO itself being able to stabilize irradiation-induced DNA lesions *in vivo* (Jordan et al., 2004).

The first drug that was described to inhibit oxygen consumption in tumors was meta-iodobenzylguanidine (MIBG), which causes an inhibition of the mitochondrial site I electron transfer, inhibition of NAD(P)H oxidation, and is described to alter tumor glycolysis by inhibiting oxygen consumption (Biaglow et al., 1998). We consecutively focused on different innovative treatments that may alter oxygen consumption by tumor cells, as listed below.

### 3.1 Insulin

This hormone was known to increase blood flow in human skeletal muscle and was postulated to be an important modulator of tumor oxygenation (Jordan et al., 2002). Indeed, we showed that insulin had a profound effect on tumor oxygenation that was not due to an increase in tumor blood flow but to a decrease in tumor cell oxygen consumption. The increase in tumor oxygenation resulted in an important enhancement in the sensitivity of tumors to irradiation. The likely scenario involves a stimulation of eNOS and a consequent increase in NO release. As NO regulates mitochondrial respiration by virtue of reversible interactions with cytochrome c oxidase (complex IV), an increase in NO release consequently decreased cell respiration (Jordan et al., 2002). A preclinical study confirmed the dose-dependant increase in tumor oxygenation and radiation sensitivity by insulin, without any increase in the radiation toxicity for normal tissues (Jordan et al., 2006a).

### 3.2 Glucocorticoids

Earlier work had demonstrated that the administration of cortisone to rats resulted in both the inhibition of oxygen consumption and the uncoupling of oxidative phosphorylation in liver mitochondria (Kimberg et al., 1968). Glucocorticoids seemed to decrease the cytochrome c oxidase (complex IV) activity of isolated rat kidney mitochondria by a direct mechanism (Simon et al., 1998). Our group showed an important increase in tumor oxygenation induced by an effect on oxygen consumption. Decreased oxygen consumption could be explained by the capacity of glucocorticoids to inhibit cytochrome c oxidase of the mitochondrial respiratory chain. The result of this increase in tumor oxygenation was an improvement of the radiation efficacy by a factor of 1.7 (Crokart et al., 2007).

### 3.3 Anti-inflammatory drugs

Several reports indicated that many non-steroidal anti-inflammatory drugs (NSAIDs) uncouple mitochondrial oxidative phosphorylation with important consequences on cell oxygen consumption. However, it was suggested that the response was dependent on the dose as well as on the type of NSAIDs. For the first time, our group reported that the administration of NSAIDs induced a dramatic increase in tumor oxygenation explained by reduced oxygen consumption. An increase in the tumor response was observed when the irradiation was applied at the time of maximal reoxygenation (Crokart et al., 2005).

### 3.4 Thyroid hormones

Chronic alteration in the thyroid status has been shown to affect mitochondrial oxygen consumption in skeletal muscle (Gredilla et al., 2001). Also, studies have demonstrated that hypothyroidism slows down the neoplastic process, whereas administration of a thyroid hormone preparation restores tumor growth rates (Mishkin et al., 1981; Shoemaker & Dagher, 1979; Theodossiou et al., 1999). In humans, several case reports have indicated a prolonged survival in the presence of hypothyroidism (Cristofanilli et al., 2005; Hercbergs & Leith, 1993). Moreover, a decrease in the thyroid function may also serve to favorably influence the response to treatment. Finally, patients presented an enhanced response rate to chemotherapy and survived significantly longer under hypothyroidism (Hercbergs et al., 2003). Our group recently demonstrated that the thyroid status is associated with a significant change in tumor radiosensitivity since the regrowth delay was increased in hypothyroid mice compared to euthyroid mice. Mechanistically, we demonstrated that the higher level of tumor oxygenation in hypothyroid mice results from a significant reduction in the oxygen consumption rate of tumors (Jordan et al., 2007).

### 3.5 NO donors

We recently tested whether *S*-nitrosocaptopril, a molecule combining a NO donor and an angiotensin converting enzyme inhibitor (ACE inhibitor), could temporarily improve the hemodynamic status of experimental tumors. We identified a time window during which tumor oxygenation was improved, as a result of a combined effect on tumor blood flow and oxygen consumption. Consequently, the administration of *S*-nitrosocaptopril contributed to the increase in efficacy of radiation therapy, an effect that was not observed with captopril alone (Jordan et al., 2010a).

### 3.6 Anti-angiogenic agents

As stated earlier, two anti-angiogenic agents, SU-5416 and ZD-6474, have also been identified as potent inhibitors of oxygen consumption (Ansiaux et al., 2007, 2009). Our major findings regarding those specific anti-angiogenic agents were the following: (a) SU-5416 and ZD-67474 both induce an increase in tumor oxygenation at an early phase of treatment (after 2 days of daily injections); (b) this tumor reoxygenation can be exploited to increase the efficacy of combined radiotherapy; (c) the mechanism of increase in tumor oxygenation does not involve a "normalization" of the tumor vasculature as described previously for thalidomide in the same tumor model (Ansiaux et al., 2005) but is consistent with the decrease in the rate of oxygen consumption by the tumor cells. Indeed, at this early stage of the treatment, no apparent remodeling of the tumor vasculature and no changes in tumor perfusion and permeability parameters were observed, using histological and DCE-MRI analysis, respectively. We however demonstrated a reduction in tumor oxygen consumption after those treatments. The reduction factor in oxygen consumption observed was sufficient to abolish tumor hypoxia, as we reported previously using the treatments listed above.

## 4. Hyperthermia: Combining provascular and oxygen consumption effects in a single treatment

Hyperthermia is a potent adjuvant therapy with radiotherapy and chemotherapy, and the perfect illustration of a strategy combining transient, local vasodilatation with the inhibition of tumor cell respiration. The heat treatment consists of elevating the temperature of tumors to a supra-physiological range of 40°C to 45°C at which tumor reoxygneation occurs with limited skin toxicity. Hyperthermia induces a graded response in tissues characterized by decreased oxygen consumption at temperatures ≥ 40°C, vasodilatation between 41°C and 41.5°C, and vascular damage above 42°C. Although direct tumor cell killing was demonstrated *in vitro* at higher temperatures, long-term tumor control has never been demonstrated using hyperthermia as the sole treatment modality. Vasodilation only modestly contributes to tumor reoxygenation at the low thermal doses. Increased $pO_2$ rather primarily results from changes in oxygen consumption in the target cells, and at least two different processes have been identified to contribute to this response. It is now well demonstrated that an important target of heat is proteins among which enzymes of the respiratory chain are more sensitive to heat inactivation/denaturation than glycolytic enzymes (Lepock et al., 1987; Kelleher et al., 1995). But the inhibition of mitochondrial respiration by heat lasts longer than the turnover time of respiratory enzymes, suggesting the existence of an additional mechanism. Dewhirst in collaboration with our group (Moon et al., 2010) recently demonstrated that mild hyperthermia activates the transcription factor hypoxia-inducible factor 1 (HIF-1) through an hypoxia-independent mechanism involving the sequential activation of Extracellular signal-Regulated Kinases (ERK) by heat shock, ERK-induced upregulation of the expression of the Nox1 subunit of NAD(P)H oxidase, increased ROS production by NAD(P)H oxidase, ROS-induced HIF-1$\alpha$ protein stabilization, and, ultimately, HIF-1 activation. HIF-1 target genes include most glycolytic enzymes and transporters as well as major pro-angiogenic molecules such as VEGF. Among these genes, we showed that pyruvate dehydrogenase kinase 1 (PDK1) largely mediates the inhibition of mitochondrial respiration by heat in tumor cells through inhibiting pyruvate dehydrogenase (PDH), i.e., the enzyme coupling glycolysis to the tricarboxylic acid (TCA) cycle (Moon et al., 2010). Furthermore, consistent with the increase in VEGF expression that we also observed in heat-treated tumors, we documented an increased vascular density in perfused tumor areas where oxygen is extracted from the blood. Tumor reoxygenation by mild hyperthermia is thus a multifaceted process involving the combination of decreased $O_2$ consumption by tumor cells and increased $O_2$ delivery by blood vessels. This and the fact that reoxygenation occurs at thermal doses lower than those inducing vascular damage justifies the use of mild hyperthermia as a combination treatment notably with radiotherapy. Although several clinical trials have confirmed that combining heat and radiotherapy is indeed associated with better patient treatment outcome (Brizel et al., 1996; Jones et al., 2003, 2005; Vujaskovic et al., 2003), the future clinical development of hyperthermia strongly relies on designing tools allowing for homogeneous thermal dose distribution and improving imaging techniques able to correlate thermal maps of tumors to the clinical outcome of patients (Dewhirst et al., 2010).

## 5. Non invasive imaging of tumor oxygenation and perfusion

The study of magnetic resonance (MR) markers over the past decade has provided evidence that the tumor microenvironment and hemodynamics play a major role in determining therapy outcome. Therefore, the identification of relevant non-invasive imaging endpoints is of crucial importance in the management of cancer patients. Improvement of the therapeutic index was evidenced in numerous preclinical studies that used multimodal imaging. The impact of non-invasive imaging in oncology extends from guiding preclinical development of targeted biomarkers and therapeutic agents, to assisting in the diagnosis and staging of tumors in the clinic, as well as monitoring the therapeutic response.

### 5.1 Tumor oxygenation measurements

There is a critical need for developing dynamic, non-invasive methods for direct oxygen mapping in the clinical practice. Although hypoxia is recognized as a crucial issue in many disorders and in treatment response, the lack of easy-to-use and efficient methods to quantify oxygen deprivation hampers further pathophysiological understanding and restricts the clinical implementation of oxygen mapping techniques resulting in the absence of gold standard for measuring hypoxia in the day-to-day practice (Tatum et al., 2006). Below is a non exhaustive review of the most relevant non invasive methods able to assess tumor hemodynamic parameters. Methods to measure absolute $pO_2$ mostly encompass EPR oximetry and $^{19}F$ relaxometry whereas indirect methods include Blood Oxygen Level-Dependent (BOLD) MRI, Oxygen enhanced relaxation MRI, Oxygen enhanced longitudinal relaxation MRI and positron emission tomography (PET) tracers retained in hypoxic regions. Of note, our group has also developed innovative methods to assess tumor oxygen consumption *in vitro* and *in vivo*, which have been reviewed elsewhere (Jordan & Gallez, 2011).

### 5.1.1 Electron Paramagnetic Resonance (EPR) oximetry

EPR is a MR method that detects only species containing unpaired electrons (Gallez & Swartz, 2004a). One of the numerous applications of EPR is *in vivo* oximetry. Molecular oxygen is a triplet radical that possesses two unpaired electrons which are responsible for its paramagnetism. However, EPR is not able to detect oxygen itself when dissolved in fluids near room temperature: in biological systems, the output signal lines are so broadened as to be undetectable. Indirect methods exist. Most of these methods rely on the paramagnetic properties of molecular oxygen, which acts as an efficient relaxer for other paramagnetic species (Gallez et al., 2004b). The enhancement of relaxation rates scales linearly with the concentration of oxygen over a wide range of oxygen tensions. The lack of detectable levels of endogenous paramagnetic species makes it necessary to use exogenous paramagnetic materials. Variations in $pO_2$ of less than 1mmHg can be detected using particulate materials. While EPR spectroscopy provides local measurements, EPR imaging techniques provide spatially resolved measurements of these materials. The spatial distribution of free radicals can be performed utilizing magnetic field gradients in a manner similar to that of MRI. Spectral–spatial EPR imaging encodes both the spatial distribution of the spin probe and the spectral information, which allows the mapping of molecular oxygen (Kuppusamy et al., 2003). For this purpose, the use of soluble EPR materials such as trityl radicals is more convenient as they can diffuse in the whole tissue.

EPR oximetry was compared with other methods that provide direct or indirect measurements of tumor oxygenation: with polarographic electrodes, the distribution of nitroimidazoles, the BOLD effect in MRI, and $pO_2$ recordings using OxyLite (reviewed in Gallez et al., 2004b). Two major challenges are now considered for moving this technology into the clinic: (i) assuring biocompatibility of the oxygen sensors in humans and (ii) modifying the instruments so that they can be used for humans instead of small animals (Swartz et al., 2004).

### 5.1.2 $^{19}F$ relaxometry

$^{19}F$ NMR spectroscopy and imaging of perfluorocarbon (PFC) emulsions (hydrocarbons with protons having been replaced with fluorine nuclei) has been extensively exploited to measure the oxygen tension of biological systems in preclinical studies. The $^{19}F$ MR signal of the PFC is sensitive to the $pO_2$ of the surrounding tumor tissue, and acts as an oximeter. The principle behind $^{19}F$ MR oximetry relies on the linear increase of the NMR spin-lattice relaxation rate $R_1$ ($=1/T_1$) of PFC emulsions with increasing oxygen tension (Mason et al.

1996). $^{19}F$ MR oximetry provides a sensitive measure of tissue oxygen tension and is a powerful approach for monitoring tumor hypoxia. Several PFCs have been used for NMR oximetry, but hexafluorobenzene (HFB) is preferred (Mason et al., 1996; Zhao, et al., 2004) because it has a six-fold symmetry with a single $^{19}F$ NMR resonance, and a low sensitivity to temperature. Its spin lattice relaxation rate is highly sensitive to $pO_2$ and exhibits a linear relationship across the entire range of tissue oxygenation.

Mason and colleagues have been successfully developing fluorocarbon relaxometry using echo planar imaging for dynamic oxygen mapping (FREDOM) MRI following direct intratumoral injection of the oxygen reporter molecule HFB. Our group further developed an MRI fluorocarbon oximetry technique using snapshot inversion recovery with an improved temporal resolution of 1.5 minutes (vs. 6.5 minutes for FREDOM) (Jordan et al., 2009). Our method therefore provides a rapid way to map tumor oxygenation and is particularly suitable to monitor acute changes of $pO_2$ in tumors, including spontaneous fluctuations (Jordan et al., 2009; Magat et al., 2010). The translation to the clinic is currently limited by the lack of development of coils in the clinical setting, and the lack of characterization of PFCs in humans.

#### 5.1.3 Blood Oxygen Level Dependent (BOLD) MRI

Functional MRI (fMRI) was first developed as an indirect method of imaging brain activity at high temporal resolution (Ogawa et al., 1990). The relative decrease in deoxyhemoglobin concentration, which has a paramagnetic effect, can be detected by MRI as a weak transient rise in the $T_2$* weighted signal. This is the BOLD contrast principle. Apart from its very large application in neuroscience, the use of BOLD contrast in tumors brought with it new challenges of understanding and interpretation. Since then, BOLD MRI has become a useful tool for addressing important questions regarding the pathophysiology of tumors. However, it has both advantages and disadvantages. One advantage of BOLD MRI is that it is noninvasive and can be used to monitor real time changes of tumor oxygenation during pharmacological treatments or to monitor spontaneous fluctuations in experimental tumors (Baudelet & Gallez 2002; Baudelet et al., 2004). It does not require externally administered contrast medium or radioactive isotopes, it can be repeated as necessary, and flow dependence can be decoupled. BOLD MRI, in combination with hypercapnia and hyperoxia, is also an attractive method for assessing maturation and the functional state of tumor blood vessels (Baudelet et al., 2006). As for disadvantages, BOLD MRI is unfortunately a non-quantitative method for monitoring tumor $pO_2$. This is the result of the extreme sensitivity of changes in $R_2$* to the basal state of tumor oxygenation and blood volume fraction. The intra and intertumoral distribution of these parameters may be greatly heterogeneous, making it very difficult to compare estimated $pO_2$ changes between two regions or individuals. Even more problematic is the fact that the change in $R_2$* is not always indicative of the change in $pO_2$. Concomitant changes in blood volume, blood pH and metabolic status can lead to smaller-than-expected or even negative changes in $R_2$* (Baudelet & Gallez, 2002). Similarly, changes in oxygen consumption rate has been described to result in a lack of change in $R_2$* even though absolute $pO_2$ is increased (Jordan et al., 2006b).

#### 5.1.4 Oxygen enhanced longitudinal relaxation MRI

An alternative MRI technique for evaluating change in tumor oxygenation using endogenous contrast relies in the increase of the proton longitudinal relaxation rate ($R_1$) of water containing oxygen, due to the paramagnetic properties of oxygen. The measured change in $R_1$ is, in theory, proportional to the change in tissue oxygen concentration (O'Connor et al., 2007, 2009). Studies have indeed demonstrated that oxygen-enhanced MRI produces measurable signal changes in normal tissues in patients and is feasible on conventional clinical scanners. Therefore, oxygen-induced increase in $R_1$ has the potential to provide noninvasive measurements of change in tumor oxygen concentration, distinct from BOLD imaging. Nevertheless, the technique still lacks in sensitivity and the measured delta $R_1$ may include errors resulting from changes independent of tissue oxygen content, such as alteration in blood flow or tissue $H_2O$ content (O'Connor et al., 2009).

### 5.1.5 Hypoxia assessed by Positron Emission Tomography (PET)

$^{18}$F-labeled fluoromisonidazole ($^{18}$F-MISO) is probably the most widely used PET imaging agent for hypoxia. $^{18}$F-MISO accumulates in tissues by binding to intracellular macromolecules when $pO_2$ < 10 mm Hg. Retention within tissues is dependent on nitroreductase activity (that is, on the reduction status of a $NO_2$ group on the imidazole ring) and accumulation in hypoxic tissues over a range of blood flows has been observed (Tatum et al., 2006). $^{18}$F-MISO is only sensitive to the presence of hypoxia in viable cells: $^{18}$F-MISO is not retained in necrosis because the electron transport chain that reduces the nitroimidazole to a bioreductive alkylating agent is no longer active (Padhani et al., 2007). Nevertheless, $^{18}$F-MISO PET is able to monitor the changing hypoxia status of lung tumors during radiotherapy (Koh et al., 1995). Studies in sarcoma (Rajendran et al., 2003) and head and neck cancer (Rajendran et al., 2004) have demonstrated a correlation of $^{18}$F-MISO uptake with poor outcome to radiation and chemotherapy. Other $^{18}$F labeled nitroimidazoles are currently evaluated, including EF3 and fluoroazomycin arabinoside (FAZA), for example (Tatum et al., 2006).

## 5.2 Tumor perfusion measurements

Microvascular parameters such as permeability and perfusion are of particular interest in the context of the abnormal tumor microvascular network. Useful imaging systems have been developed to monitor angiogenesis and the microvasculature *in vivo*, including DCE-MRI (Choyke, et al. 2003), PET and Single Photon Emission Computed Tomography (SPECT), CT, Doppler ultrasound, and optical imaging methods (see Jennings, et al., 2008).

### 5.2.1 Dynamic Contrast Enhanced MRI

DCE-MRI consists in the acquisition of serial MR images before, during, and after the administration of an intravenous contrast agent (CA) to produce time series images that enable pixel-by-pixel analysis of contrast kinetics within a tumor. Pharmacokinetic models provide a means of summarizing contrast enhancement data in terms of parameters that relate to the underlying vascular anatomy and physiology. As described by Tofts et al. (1999), the essential features of a variety of models are covered by the generalized kinetic model. Most methods of analyzing dynamic contrast-enhanced $T_1$-weighted data acquired with low molecular contrast medium use a compartmental analysis to obtain some combination of the three principal parameters: the transfer constant Ktrans in $min^{-1}$ (volume transfer constant between blood plasma and ESS), the rate constant Kep in $min^{-1}$ (rate constant between blood plasma and extravascular extracellular space [ESS]) and the volume of ESS per unit volume of tissue space, Vp (no unit). DCE-MRI has evolved from an experimental technique to a clinically feasible adjunct procedure that can be integrated into a standard morphologic imaging protocol. It does provide unique non-invasive functional information on the properties of tumors related to microcirculation (distribution volume, permeability, and perfusion). This information can improve diagnostic characterization, the follow-up of therapy, and tumor staging; and it provides tools to facilitate advanced molecular imaging. Preclinical and clinical studies suggest that a successful antivascular treatment results in a decrease in the rate of enhancement along with a decreased amplitude and a slower washout, and that poor response can result in persistent abnormal enhancement (Gillies et al., 2002).

### 5.2.2 Positron emission tomography

Generally, PET measures of tumor perfusion have used ($^{15}O$)-labeled radiotracers. The so-called steady state method requires inhalation of $^{15}O$-$CO_2$ and the dynamic method requires an intravenous bolus injection of $^{15}O$-$H_2O$ (Jennings et al., 2008). A requirement for quantification of perfusion using dynamic methods is an accurate determination of an arterial input function, which can be obtained non-invasively in a purely arterial region of interest, such as the aorta.

### 5.2.3 Computed tomography

In X-ray CT, the tissue contrast is based on variable attenuation coefficients of the object absorbing the X-rays. Hemodynamic parameters may be extracted from dynamic changes in X-ray attenuation caused by the intravenous injection of an iodinated contrast agent. Perfusion CT data can deliver quantitative hemodynamic information, such as blood volume, blood flow, permeability surface-area product and mean transit time (MTT) (Jennings et al., 2008).

### 5.2.4 Doppler ulstrasound

There are several different ultrasonic approaches designed specifically to measure blood flow including transit time, continuous-wave Doppler, pulsed and color Doppler, and power Doppler flowmeters, requiring the use of microbubbles (filled with air, perfluorocarbon, sulfur hexafluoride or nitrogen), which expand and contract because of pressure from the acoustical transmit pulse, and the primary mode of echogenicity is the impedance mismatch between the microbubble–blood interface, making them significantly more echogenic than normal tissue. Typical parameters that are estimated using Doppler ultrasound include: percent intratumor contrast agent uptake, enhancement timing and pattern, percent blood volume fraction, red blood cell velocity, and perfusion; depending on the type of study and tracer used (Jennings et al., 2008).

## 6. Conclusions

Heterogeneities in blood flow and oxygenation are key characteristics of solid tumors and constitute a therapeutic challenge when these tumors are treated with radiotherapy or systemic therapies. Because oxygen stabilizes DNA lesions, tumors become increasingly resistant to radiotherapy and to several forms of chemotherapy when the tumor $pO_2$ decreases below a threshold of 10 mmHg. In the past decades, basic and preclinical researches have identified several adjuvant treatments aimed at transiently increasing tumor oxygenation at the time of radiotherapy. Their identification was based on an increasing understanding of the origins of tumor hypoxia, which logically opened two main avenues: co-treatments designed to (1) improve the oxygen supply from blood vessels at the time of radiotherapy (with different strategies such as increasing the $O_2$ content of blood, inducing tumor-specific vasodilation, or normalizing vascular structures), and (2) reduce the rate of $O_2$ consumption by tumor cells through metabolic interventions. Theoretical models now validated preclinically have revealed that the metabolic strategy has the highest impact on tumor radiosensitivity, but the best opportunity still resides in treatments combining both vascular and metabolic effects, as perfectly illustrated with hyperthermia. Most systemic anticancer treatments are also confronted to the difficulty to reach a target often located at distance from blood vessels, thus indicating that in this case increased tumor perfusion (i.e., decreased resistance to flow) could improve tumor bioavailability. NO-donors, ET-1 inhibitors, radiotherapy or heat as adjuvant provascular treatments, or anti-angiogenic therapies and chemotherapy used in a 'vascular normalization' mode, have all demonstrated their capacity to chemosensitize tumors in preclinical settings. Most of the adjuvant treatments described here could theoretically be exploited therapeutically by the off-label use of existing FDA-approved drugs, but it has also become evident that a given tumor in a given patient would respond differently than the tumor of the patient next-door. It is therefore urgent to develop and implement in the clinics imaging techniques able not only to provide predictive markers but also biological markers of the response to such combinational interventions. The MR and PET techniques that we reviewed here are among the most-sensitive non-invasive techniques having proved their highly valuable power as to measure changes in tumor perfusion and oxygenation preclinically. Current challenges include the FDA approval of exogenous tracers and sensors when needed, scaling-up tools initially dedicated for small laboratory animals and adapting imaging protocols to the clinical situation, the transfer to the clinics of the expertise needed for protocol design and data interpretation and, as importantly, a careful consideration of societal cost issues.

## 7. Acknowledgements

Works at the authors' labs are supported by grants from the European Research Council (FP7/2007-2013 ERC Independent Researcher Starting Grant 243188 TUMETABO to P.S.), the Belgian *Fonds National de la Recherche Scientifique* (F.R.S.-FNRS), the *Communauté Française de Belgique* (ARC 09/14-020), the *Fondation Belge Contre le Cancer* (200-2008), the *Fonds Joseph Maisin*, the Saint-Luc Foundation, and the *Pôle d'Attraction Interuniversitaire* PAI VI (P6/38). B.F.J. and P.S. are F.R.S.-FNRS Research Associates. For any correspondence contact P.S.; email: pierre.sonveaux@uclouvain.be.

## 8. References

Ang, KK. (2010). More lessons learned from the suffocation of hypoxia. *J Clin Oncol.*, Vol.28, No.18, pp. 2941-2943.

Angelo, M.; Singel, D.J. & Stamler, J.S. (2006). An S-nitrosothiol (SNO) synthase function of hemoglobin that utilizes nitrite as a substrate. *P Natl Acad Sci USA*, Vol.103, pp. 8366-8371.

Ansiaux, R.; Baudelet, C.; Jordan, BF.; Beghein, N.; Sonveaux, P.; De Wever, J.; Martinive, P.; Gregoire, V.; Feron, O. & Gallez, B. (2005). Thalidomide radiosensitizes tumors through early changes in the tumor microenvironment. *Clin Cancer Res.*, Vol.11, pp. 743-750.

Ansiaux R.; Baudelet C.; Jordan BF.; Crokart N.; Martinive P.; DeWever J.; Grégoire V.; Feron O. & Gallez B. (2006). Mechanism of reoxygenation after antiangiogenic therapy using SU5416 and its importance for guiding combined antitumor therapy. *Cancer Res.*, Vol.66, No.19, pp.9698-9704.

Ansiaux, R.; Dewever, J.; Gregoire, V.; Feron, O.; Jordan, B.F. & Gallez, B. (2009). Decrease in tumor cell oxygen consumption after treatment with vandetanib (ZACTIMA; ZD6474) and its effect on response to radiotherapy. *Radiat Res.*, Vol.172, No.5, pp. 584-591.

Arnold, W.P.; Mittal, C.K.; Katsuki, S.& Murad, F. (1977). Nitric oxide activates guanylate cyclase and increases guanosine 3':5'-cyclic monophosphate levels in various tissue preparations. *P Natl Acad Sci USA*, Vol.74, pp. 3203-3207.

Baudelet, C. & Gallez, B. (2002). How does blood oxygen level-dependent (BOLD) contrast correlate with oxygen partial pressure (pO2) inside tumors? *Magn Reson Med.*, Vol.48, pp. 980-986.

Baudelet, C.; Ansiaux, R.; Jordan, B.F.; Havaux, X.; Macq, B. & Gallez, B. (2004). Physiological noise in murine solid tumours using $T_2$*-weighted gradient-echo imaging: a marker of tumour acute hypoxia? *Phys Med Biol.*, Vol.49, pp. 3389-3411.

Baudelet, C.; Cron, G.O.; Ansiaux, R.; Crokart, N.; DeWever, J.; Feron, O. & Gallez, B. (2006). The role of vessel maturation and vessel functionality in spontaneous fluctuations of T2*-weighted GRE signal within tumors. *NMR Biomed.*, Vol.19, pp. 69-76.

Biaglow, J.E.; Manevich, Y.; Leeper, D.; Chance, B.; Dewhirst, M.W.; Jenkins, W.T.; Tuttle, S.W.; Wroblewski, K.; Glickson, J.D.; Stevens, C. & Evans, S.M. (1998). MIBG inhibits respiration: potential for radio- and hyperthermic sensitization. *Int J Radiat Oncol.*, Vol.42, No.4, pp. 871-876.

Boucher, Y.; Leunig, M. & Jain, R.K. (1996). Tumor angiogenesis and interstitial hypertension. *Cancer Res.*, Vol.56, pp. 4264-4266.

Bradley, D.P.; Tessier, J.L.; Checkley, D. & Kuribayashi, H. (2008). Effects of AZD2171 and vandetanib (ZD6474, Zactima) on haemodynamic variables in an SW620 human colon tumour model: an investigation using dynamic contrast-enhanced MRI and the rapid clearance blood pool contrast agent, P792. *NMR Biomed.*, Vol.21, pp. 42-52.

Brizel, D.M.; Scully, S.P.; Harrelson, J.M.; Layfield, L.J.; Dodge, R.K.; Charles, H.C.; Samulski, T.V.; Prosnitz, L.R. & Dewhirst, M.W. (1996). Radiation therapy and hyperthermia improve the oxygenation of human soft tissue sarcomas. *Cancer Res.*, Vol.56, pp. 5347-5350.

Cárdenas-Navia, L.I.; Mace; D.; Richardson, R.A.; Wilson, D.F.; Shan S. & Dewhirst, M.W. (2008). The pervasive presence of fluctuating oxygenation in tumors. *Cancer Res.*, Vol.68, pp. 5812-5819.

Choyke, P.L.; Dwyer, A.J. & Knopp, M.V. (2003). Functional tumor imaging with dynamic contrast-enhanced magnetic resonance imaging. *J Magn Reson Imaging*, Vol.17, pp. 509-520.

Claes, A., Wesseling, P., Jeuken, J., Maass, C., Heerschap A. & Leenders, W.P. (2008). Antiangiogenic compounds interfere with chemotherapy of brain tumors due to vessel normalization. *Mol Cancer Ther.*, Vol.7, pp. 71-78.

Cristofanilli, M.; Yamamura, Y.; Kau S.W.; Bevers, T., Strom S.; Patangan M.; Hsu L.; Krishnamurthy S.; Theriault R.L. & Hortobagyi G.N. (2005). Thyroid hormone and breast carcinoma. Primary hypothyroidism is associated with a reduced incidence of primary breast carcinoma. *Cancer,* Vol.103, pp.1122-1128.

Crokart, N.; Radermacher, K.; Jordan, B.F.; Baudelet, C.; Cron, G.O.; Gregoire, V.; Beghein, N.; Bouzin, C.; Feron, O. & Gallez, B. (2005). Tumor radiosensitization by antiinflammatory drugs: evidence for a new mechanism involving the oxygen effect. *Cancer Res.*, Vol.65, No.17, pp.7911-7916.

Crokart, N.; Jordan, B.F.; Baudelet, C.; Cron, G.O.; Hotton, J.; Radermacher, K.; Gregoire, V.; Beghein, N.; Martinive, P.; Bouzin, C.; Feron, O. & Gallez B. (2007). Glucocorticoids modulate tumor radiation response through a decrease in tumor oxygen consumption. *Clin Cancer Res.*, Vol.13, pp. 630-635.

Dewhirst, M.W.; Kimura, H.; Rehmus, S.W.; Braun, R.D.; Papahadjopoulos, D.; Hong, K. & Secomb, T.W. (1996). Microvascular studies on the origins of perfusion-limited hypoxia. *Brit J Cancer,* Vol.27, pp. S247-S251.

Dewhirst, M.W.; Ong, E.T.; Braun, R.D.; Smith, B.; Klitzman, B.; Evans, S.M. & Wilson, D. (1999). Quantification of longitudinal tissue pO2 gradients in window chamber tumours: impact on tumour hypoxia. *Brit J Cancer,* Vol.79, pp. 1717-1722.

Dewhirst, M.W.; Thrall, D.E.; Palmer, G.; Schroeder, T.; Vujaskovic, Z.; Cecil, C.H.; Macfall, J. & Wong, T. (2010). Utility of functional imaging in prediction or assessment of treatment response and prognosis following thermotherapy. *Int J Hyperther.*, Vol.26, pp. 283-293.

Feron, O. (2004). Targeting the tumor vascular compartment to improve conventional cancer therapy. *Trends Pharmacol Sci.*, Vol.25, No.10, pp. 536-542.

Frerart, F.; Sonveaux, P.; Rath, G.; Smoos, A.; Meqor, A.; Charlier, N.; Jordan, B.F.; Saliez, J.; Noel, A.; Dessy, C.; Gallez, B. & Feron, O. (2008). The acidic tumor microenvironment promotes the reconversion of nitrite into nitric oxide: towards a new and safe radiosensitizing strategy. *Clin Cancer Res.*, Vol.14, pp. 2768-2774.

Folkman, J.; Browder, T. & Palmblad, J. (2001). Angiogenesis research: guidelines for translation to clinical application. *Thromb Haemostasis,* Vol.86, pp. 23–33.

Gallez, B. & Swartz, H.M. (2004a). In vivo EPR: when, how and why? *NMR Biomed.*, Vol.17, pp. 223-225.

Gallez, B.; Baudelet, C. & Jordan, B.F. (2004b). Assessment of tumor oxygenation by electron paramagnetic resonance: principles and applications. *NMR Biomed.*, Vol.17, pp. 240-262.

Gatenby, R.A.; Kessler, H.B.; Rosenblum, J.S.; Coia, L.R.; Moldofsky, P.J.; Hartz, W.H. & Broder, G.J. (1988). Oxygen distribution in squamous cell carcinoma metastases and its relationship to outcome of radiation therapy. *Int J Radiat Oncol.*, Vol.14, pp. 831-838.

Gillies, R.J.; Raghunand, N.; Karczmar, G.S. & Bhujwalla, Z.M. (2002). MRI of the tumor microenvironment. *J Magn Reson Imaging,* Vol.16, No.4, pp. 430-450.

Godber, B.L.; Doel, J.J.; Sapkota, G.P.; Blake, D.R.; Stevens, C.R.; Eisenthal, R. & Harrison, R. (2000). Reduction of nitrite to nitric oxide catalyzed by xanthine oxidoreductase. *J Biol Chem.*, Vol.275, pp. 7757-7763.

Gray, L.H.; Conger, A.D.; Ebert, M.; Hornszy, S. & Scott, O.C. (1953). The concentration of oxygen dissolved in tissues at the time of irradiation as a factor in radiotherapy. *Brit J Radiol.*, Vol.26, pp. 638-648.

Gredilla, R.; Lopez, T.M.; Portero-Otin, M.; Pamplona, R. & Barja, G. (2001). Influence of hyper- and hypothyroidism on lipid peroxidation, unsaturation of phospholipids, glutathione system and oxidative damage to nuclear and mitochondrial DNA in mice skeletal muscle. *Mol Cell Biochem.*, Vol.221, pp. 41-48.

Haynes, W.G. & Webb, D.J. (1994). Contribution of endogenous generation of endothelin-1 to basal vascular tone. *Lancet*, Vol.344, pp. 852-854.

Hercbergs A.A. & Leith J.T. (1993). Spontaneous remission of metastatic lung cancer following myxedema coma - an apoptosis-related phenomenon? *J Natl Cancer I.*, Vol.85, pp. 1342-1343.

Hercbergs, A.A.; Goyal, L.K.; Suh, J.H.; Lee, S.; Reddy, C.A.; Cohen, B.H.; Stevens, G.H.; Reddy, S.K.; Peereboom, D.M. & Barnett, G.H. (2003). Propylthiouracil-induced chemical hypothyroidism with high-dose tamoxifen prolongs survival in recurrent high grade glioma: a phase I/II study. *Anticancer Res.*, Vol.23, pp. 617-626.

Hockel, M.; Vorndran, B.; Schlenger, K.; Baussmann, E. & Knapstein, P.G. (1993). Tumor oxygenation: a new predictive parameter in locally advanced cancer of the uterine cervix. *Gynecol Oncol.*, Vol.51, pp. 141-149.

Holland, M.A. & Kozlowski, L.M. (1986). Clinical features and management of cyanide poisoning. *ClinPharm.*, Vol.5, pp. 737-741.

Horsman, M.R. & van der Kogel, A.J. (2009). Therapeutic approaches to tumor hypoxia, In: *Basic Clinical Radiobiology (4th edition)*, Joiner, M. & van der Kogel, A., pp. 233-245, H. Arnold, London (UK).

Huang, A. & Koller, A. (1997). Endothelin and prostaglandin H2 enhance arteriolar myogenic tone in hypertension. *Hypertension*, Vol.30, pp. 1210-1215.

Jain, R.K. (2001). Normalizing tumor vasculature with anti-angiogenic therapy: a new paradigm for combination therapy. *Nat Med.*, Vol.7, pp. 987-989.

Jennings, D.; Raghunand, N. & Gillies, R.J. (2008). Imaging hemodynamics. *Cancer Metast Rev.*, Vol.27, pp. 589-613.

Jia, L.; Bonaventura, C.; Bonaventura, J. & Stamler, J.S. (1996). S-nitrosohaemoglobin: a dynamic activity of blood involved in vascular control. *Nature*, Vol.380, pp. 221-226.

Jones, E.L.; Samulski, T.V.; Dewhirst, M.W.; Alvarez-Secord, A.; Berchuck, A.; Clarke-Pearson, D.; Havrilesky, L.J.; Soper, J. & Prosnitz, L.R. (2003). A pilot Phase II trial of concurrent radiotherapy, chemotherapy, and hyperthermia for locally advanced cervical carcinoma. *Cancer*, Vol.98, pp. 277-282.

Jones, E.L.; Oleson, J.R.; Prosnitz, L.R.; Samulski, T.V.; Vujaskovic, Z.; Yu, D.; Sanders, L.L. & Dewhirst, M.W. (2005). Randomized trial of hyperthermia and radiation for superficial tumors. *J Clin Oncol.*, Vol.23, pp. 3079-3085.

Jordan, B.F.; Misson, P.; Demeure, R.; Baudelet, C.; Beghein, N. & Gallez, B. (2000). Changes in tumor oxygenation/perfusion induced by the no donor, isosorbide dinitrate, in comparison with carbogen: monitoring by EPR and MRI. *Int J Radiat Oncol.*, Vol.48, No.2, pp. 565-570.

Jordan, B.F.; Gregoire, V.; Demeure, R.J.; Sonveaux, P.; Feron, O.; O'Hara, J.; Vanhulle, V.P.; Delzenne, N. & Gallez, B. (2002). Insulin increases the sensitivity of tumors to irradiation: involvement of an increase in tumor oxygenation mediated by a nitric oxide-dependent decrease of the tumor cells oxygen consumption. *Cancer Res.*, Vol.62, pp. 3555-3561.

Jordan, B.F.; Sonveaux, P.; Feron, O.; Gregoire, V.; Beghein, N.; Dessy, C. & Gallez, B. (2004). Nitric oxide as a radiosensitizer: evidence for an intrinsic role in addition to its effect on oxygen delivery and consumption. *Int J Cancer*, Vol.109, No.5, pp. 768-773.

Jordan, B.F.; Beghein, N.; Crokart, N.; Baudelet, C.; Gregoire, V. & Gallez, B. (2006a). Preclinical safety and antitumor efficacy of insulin combined with irradiation. *Radiother Oncol.*, Vol.81, No.1, pp. 112-117.

Jordan, B.F.; Crokart, N.; Baudelet, C.; Cron, G.O.; Ansiaux, R. & Gallez, B. (2006b). Complex relationship between changes in oxygenation status and changes in $R^*_2$: the case of insulin and NS-398, two inhibitors of oxygen consumption. *Magn Reson Med.*, Vol.56, pp. 637-643.

Jordan, B.F.; Christian, N.; Crokart, N.; Gregoire, V.; Feron, O. & Gallez B. (2007). Thyroid status is a key modulator of tumor oxygenation: implication for radiation therapy. *Radiat Res.*, Vol.168, No.4, pp. 428-432.

Jordan, B.F.; Cron, G.O. & Gallez, B. (2009) Rapid monitoring of oxygenation by 19F magnetic resonance imaging: simultaneous comparison with fluorescence quenching. *Magn Reson Med.*, Vol.61, pp. 634-638.

Jordan, B.F.; Peeterbroeck, J.; Karroum, O.; Diepart, C.; Magat, J.; Gregoire, V. & Gallez, B. (2010a). Captopril and S-nitrosocaptopril as potent radiosensitizers: Comparative study and underlying mechanisms. *Cancer Lett.*, Vol.293, No.2, pp. 213-219.

Jordan, B.F. & Gallez, B. (2010b). Surrogate MR markers of response to chemo- or radiotherapy in association with co-treatments: a retrospective analysis of multi-modal studies. *Contrast Media Mol I.*, Vol.5, No.6, pp. 323-332.

Jordan, B.F. & Gallez, B. (2011). Non-invasive imaging of the tumor microenvironment, In: *Tumor microenvironement*, Siemann, D.W., pp. 229-270, John Wiley & Sons Inc., Oxford (UK).

Kaanders, J.H.; Bussink, J. & Van der Kogel, A.J. (2002). ARCON: a novel biology-based approach in radiotherapy. *Lancet Oncol.*, Vol.3, pp. 728-737.

Kelleher, D.K.; Engel, T. & Vaupel, P.W. (1995). Changes in microregional perfusion, oxygenation, ATP and lactate distribution in subcutaneous rat tumours upon water-filtered IR-A hyperthermia. *Int J Hyperther.*, Vol.11, pp. 241-255.

Kimberg, D.V.; Loud, A.V. & Wiener, J. (1968). Cortisone-induced alterations in mitochondrial function and structure. *J Cell Biol.*, Vol.37, No.1, pp. 63-79.

Kimura, H.; Braun, R.D.; Ong, E.T.; Hsu, R.; Secomb, T.W.; Papahadjopoulos, D.; Hong, K. & Dewhirst, M.W. (1996). Fluctuations in red cell flux in tumor microvessels can lead to transient hypoxia and reoxygenation in tumor parenchyma. *Cancer Res.*, Vol.56, pp. 5522-5528.

Koh, W.J.; Bergman, K.S.; Rasey, J.S.; Peterson, L.M.; Evans, M.L.; Graham, M.M.; Grierson, J.R.; Lindsley, K.L.; Lewellen, T.K.; Krohn, K.A. & Griffin T.W. (1995). Evaluation of oxygenation status during fractionated radiotherapy in human nonsmall cell lung cancers using [F18]fluoromisonidazole positron emission tomography. *Int J Radiat Oncol.*, Vol.33, pp. 391–398.

Kuppusamy, P.; Chzhan, M. & Zweier, J.L. (2003). Principles of imaging in vivo EPR (ESR), In: *Theory and applications: biological magnetic resonance volume 18*, Berliner L.J., pp. 99-152, Kluwer Academic/Plenum, New York (USA).

Lepock, J.R.; Cheng, K.H.; Al Qysi, H.; Sim, I.; Koch, C.J. & Kruuv, J. (1987). Hyperthermia-induced inhibition of respiration and mitochondrial protein denaturation in CHL cells. *Int J Hyperther.*, Vol.3, pp. 123-132.

Magat, J.; Jordan, B.F.; Cron, G.O. & Gallez, B. (2010). Noninvasive mapping of spontaneous fluctuations in tumor oxygenation using 19F MRI. *Med Phys.*, Vol.37, No.10, pp. 5434-5441.

Maguire, J.J. & Davenport, A.P. (1995). ETA receptor-mediated constrictor responses to endothelin peptides in human blood vessels in vitro. *Brit J Pharmacol.*, Vol.115, pp. 191-197.

Martinive, P.; De Wever, J.; Bouzin, C.; Baudelet, C.; Sonveaux, P.; Gregoire, V.; Gallez, B. & Feron, O. (2006). Reversal of temporal and spatial heterogeneities in tumor perfusion identifies the tumor vascular tone as a tunable variable to improve drug delivery. *Mol Cancer Ther.*, Vol.5, pp. 1620-1627.

Mason, R.P.; Rodbumrung, W. & Antich, P.P. (1996). Hexafluorobenzene: a sensitive 19F NMR indicator of tumor oxygenation. *NMR Biomed.*, Vol.9, pp. 125–134.

Mattson, J.; Appelgren, L.; Karlsson, L. & Peterson, H.I. (1978). Influence of vasoactive drugs and ischaemia on intra-tumour blood flow distribution. *Eur J Cancer.*, Vol.14, No.7, pp. 761-764.

McDonald, D.M. & Baluk, P. (2002). Significance of blood vessel leakiness in cancer. *Cancer Res.*, Vol.62, pp. 5381-5385.

McMahon, T.J.; Moon, R.E.; Luschinger, B.P.; Carraway, M.S.; Stone, A.E.; Stolp, B.W.; Gow, A.J.; Pawloski, J.R.; Watke, P.; Singel, D.J.; Piantadosi, C.A. & Stamler, J.S. (2002). Nitric oxide in the human respiratory cycle. *Nat Med.*, Vol.8, pp. 711-717.

Michel, J.B.; Feron, O.; Sase, K.; Prabhakar, P. & Michel, T. (1997). Caveolin versus calmodulin. Counterbalancing allosteric modulators of endothelial nitric oxide synthase. *J Biol Chem.*, Vol.272, pp. 25907-25912.

Mishkin, S.Y.; Pollack, R.; Yalovsky, M.A.; Morris, H.P. & Mishkin S. (1981). Inhibition of local and metastatic hepatoma growth and prolongation of survival after induction of hypothyroidism. *Cancer Res.*, Vol.41, pp. 3040-3045.

Modin, A.; Bjorne, H.; Herulf, M.; Alving, K.; Weitzberg, E. & Lundberg, J. O. (2001). Nitrite-derived nitric oxide: a possible mediator of 'acidic-metabolic' vasodilation. *Acta Physiol Scand.*, Vol.171, pp. 9-16.

Moon, E.J.; Sonveaux, P.; Porporato, P.E.; Danhier, P.; Gallez, B.; Batinic-Haberle, I.; Nien, Y.C.; Schroeder, T. & Dewhirst, M.W. (2010). NADPH oxidase-mediated reactive oxygen species production activates hypoxia-inducible factor-1 (HIF-1) via the ERK pathway after hyperthermia treatment. *P Natl Acad Sci USA*, Vol.107, pp. 20477-20482.

Moya, M.P.; Gow, A.J.; Califf, R.M.; Goldberg, R.N. & Stamler, J.S. (2002). Inhaled ethyl nitrite gas for persistent pulmonary hypertension of the newborn. *Lancet*, Vol.360, pp. 141-143.

Munn, L.L. (2003). Aberrant vascular architecture in tumors and its importance in drug-based therapies. *Drug Discov Today*, Vol.8, pp. 396-403.

O'Connor, J.P.; Jackson, A.; Buonaccorsi, G.A.; Buckley, D.L.; Roberts, C.; Watson, Y.; Cheung, S.; McGrath, D.M.; Naish, J.H.; Rose, C.J.; Dark, P.M.; Jayson, G.C. & Parker, G.J. (2007). Organ-specific effects of oxygen and carbogen gas inhalation on tissue longitudinal relaxation times. *Magn Reson Med.*, Vol.58, No.3, pp. 490-496.

O'Connor, J.P.; Naish, J.H.; Jackson, A.; Waterton , J.C.; Watson, Y.; Cheung, S.; Buckley, D.L.; McGrath, D.M.; Buonaccorsi, G.A.; Mills, S.J.; Roberts, C.; Jayson, G.C. & Parker, G.J. (2009). Comparison of normal tissue R1 and R*2 modulation by oxygen and carbogen. *Magn Reson Med.*, Vol.61, No.1, pp. 75-83.

Ogawa, S.; Lee, T.M.; Kay, A.R. & Tank, D.W. (1990). Brain magnetic resonance imaging with contrast dependent on blood oxygenation. *P Natl Acad Sci USA*, Vol.87, pp. 9868-9872.

Okunieff, P.; Hoeckel, M.; Dunphy, E.P.; Schlenger, K.; Knoop, C. & Vaupel, P. (1993). Oxygen tension distributions are sufficient to explain the local response of human breast tumors treated with radiation alone. *Int J Radiat Oncol.*, Vol.26, pp. 631-636.

Overgaard, J.; Hansen, H.S.; Overgaard, M.; Bastholt, L.; Berthelsen, A.; Specht, L.; Lindeløv, B. & Jorgensen, K. (1998). A randomized double-blind phase III study of nimorazole as a hypoxic radiosensitizer of primary radiotherapy in supraglottic larynx and pharynx carcinoma. Results of the Danish Head and Neck Cancer Study (DAHANCA) Protocol 5-85. *Radiother Oncol.*, Vol.46, pp. 135-146.

Overgaard, J. (2007). Hypoxic radiosensitization: adored and ignored. *J Clin Oncol.*, Vol.25, pp. 4066-4074.

Padhani, A.R.; Krohn, K.A.; Lewis, J.S. & Alber, M. (2007). Imaging oxygenation of human tumours. *Eur Radiol.*, Vol.17, No.4, pp. 861–872.

Patan, S.; Munn, L.L. & Jain, R.K. (1996). Intussusceptive microvascular growth in a human colon adenocarcinoma xenograft: a novel mechanism of tumor angiogenesis. *Microvasc Res.*, Vol.51, pp. 260-272.

Peters, L.J.; O'Sullivan, B.; Giralt, J.; Fitzgerald, T.J.; Trotti, A.; Bernier, J.; Bourhis, J.; Yuen, K.; Fisher, R. & Rischin, D. (2010). Critical impact of radiotherapy protocol compliance and quality in the treatment of advanced head and neck cancer: results from TROG 02.02. *J Clin Oncol.*, Vol.28,No.18, pp. 2996-3001.

Peterson, H.I. & Mattson, J. Vasoactive drugs and tumor blood flow. (1984). *Biorheology*, Vol.21, No.4, pp. 503-508.

Pilkington, G.J.; Parker, K. & Murray, S.A. (2008). Approaches to mitochondrially mediated cancer therapy. *Semin Cancer Biol.*, Vol.18, No.3, pp. 226-235.

Rajendran, J.G.; Wilson, D.C.; Conrad, E.U.; Peterson, L.M.; Bruckner, J.D.; Rasey, J.S.; Chin, L.K.; Hofstrand, P.D.; Grierson, J.R.; Eary, J.F. & Krohn, K.A. (2003). [(18)F] FMISO and [(18)F]FDG PET imaging in soft tissue sarcomas: correlation of hypoxia, metabolism and VEGF expression. *Eur J Nucl Med Mol I.*, Vol.30, pp. 695-704.

Rischin, D.; Peters, L.; Hicks, R.; Hughes, P.; Fisher, R.; Hart, R.; Sexton, M.; D'Costa, I. & von Roemeling, R. (2001). Phase I trial of concurrent tirapazamine, cisplatin, and radiotherapy in patients with advanced head and neck cancer. *J Clin Oncol.*, Vol.19, No.2, pp. 535-542.

Rischin, D.; Peters, L.; Fisher, R.; Macann, A.; Denham, J.; Poulsen, M.; Jackson, M.; Kenny, L.; Penniment, M.; Corry, J.; Lamb, D. & McClure, B. (2005). Tirapazamine, Cisplatin, and Radiation versus Fluorouracil, Cisplatin, and Radiation in patients with locally advanced head and neck cancer: a randomized phase II trial of the Trans-Tasman Radiation Oncology Group (TROG 98.02). *J Clin Oncol.*, Vol.23, No.1, pp. 79-87.

Rojas, A.; Joiner, M.C.; Hodgkiss, R.J.; Carl, U.; Kjellen, E. & Wilson, G.D. (1992). Enhancement of tumor radiosensitivity and reduced hypoxia-dependent binding of a 2-nitroimidazole with normobaric oxygen and carbogen: a therapeutic comparison with skin and kidneys. *Int J Radiat Oncol.*, Vol.23, No.2, pp. 361-366.

Secomb, T.W.; Hsu, R.; Ong, E.T.; Gross, J.F. & Dewhirst, M.W. (1995). Analysis of the effects of oxygen supply and demand on hypoxic fraction in tumors. *Acta Oncol.*, Vol.34, No.3, pp. 313-316.

Segers, J.; Crokart, N.; Danhier, P.; Gregoire, V.; Jordan, B.F. & Gallez, B. (2010). Use of Xanthinol Nicotinate as a co-treatment for radio- and chemo-therapy in experimental tumors. *Int J Cancer.*, Vol.126, No.2, pp. 583-588.

Shichiri, M.; Hirata, Y.; Nakajima, T.; Ando, K.; Imai, T.; Yanagisawa, M.; Masaki, T. & Marumo, F. (1991). Endothelin-1 is an autocrine/paracrine growth factor for human cancer cell lines. *J Clin Invest.*, Vol.87, pp. 1867-1871.

Shoemaker, J.P. & Dagher R.K. (1979). Remissions of mammary adenocarcinoma in hypothyroid mice given 5-fluorouracil and chloroquine phosphate. *J Natl Cancer I.*, Vol.62, pp. 1575-1578.

Simon, N.; Jolliet, P.; Morin, C.; Zini, P.; Urien, S. & Tillement, J.P. (1998). Glucocorticoids decrease cytochrome c oxidase activity of isolated rat kidney mitochondria. *FEBS Lett.*, Vol.435, pp. 25-28.

Sonveaux, P.; Dessy, C.; Brouet, A.; Jordan, B.F.; Gregoire, V.; Gallez, B.; Balligand, J.L. & Feron, O. (2002). Modulation of the tumor vasculature functionality by ionizing radiation accounts for tumor radiosensitization and promotes gene delivery. *FASEB J.*, Vol.16, pp. 1979-1981.

Sonveaux, P.; Brouet, A.; Havaux, X.; Gregoire, V.; Dessy, C.; Balligand, J.L. & Feron, O. (2003). Irradiation-induced angiogenesis through the up-regulation of the nitric oxide pathway: implications for tumor radiotherapy. *Cancer Res.*, Vol.63, pp. 1012-1019.

Sonveaux, P.; Dessy, C.; Martinive, P.; Havaux, X.; Jordan, B.F.; Gallez, B.; Gregoire, V.; Balligand, J.L. & Feron, O. (2004). Endothelin-1 is a critical mediator of myogenic tone in tumor arterioles: implications for cancer treatment. *Cancer Res.*, Vol.64, pp. 3209-3214.

Sonveaux, P. & Feron, O. (2005a). Nitric oxide and tumor biology, In: *Nitric Oxide, Cell Signaling, and Gene Expression*. Lamas, S. & Cadenas, E., pp. 393-418, CRC press, Boca Raton (USA).

Sonveaux, P.; Kaz, A.M.; Snyder, S.A.; Richardson, R.A.; Cardenas-Navia, L.I.; Braun, R.D.; Pawloski, J.R.; Tozer, G.M.; Bonaventura, J.; McMahon, T.J.; Stamler, J.S. & Dewhirst, M.W. (2005b). Oxygen regulation of tumor perfusion by S-nitrosohemoglobin reveals a pressor activity of nitric oxide. *Circ Res.*, Vol.96, pp. 1119-1126.

Sonveaux, P.; Frerart, F.; Bouzin, C.; Brouet, A.; DeWever, J.; Jordan, B.F.; Gallez, B. & Feron, O. (2007a). Irradiation promotes Akt-targeting therapeutic gene delivery to the tumor vasculature. *Int J Radiat Oncol.*, Vol.67, pp. 1155-1162.

Sonveaux, P.; Lobysheva, I.I.; Feron, O. & McMahon, T.J. (2007b). Transport and peripheral bioactivities of nitrogen oxides carried by red blood cell hemoglobin: role in oxygen delivery. *Physiology*, Vol.22, pp. 97-112.

Sonveaux, P. (2008). Provascular strategy: targeting functional adaptations of mature blood vessels in tumors to selectively influence the tumor vascular reactivity and improve cancer treatment. *Radiother Oncol.*, Vol.86, No.3, pp. 300-313.

Sonveaux, P.; Jordan, B.F.; Gallez, B. & Feron O. (2009). Nitric oxide delivery to cancer: why and how? *Eur J Cancer*, Vol.45, No.8, pp. 1352-1369.

Stamler, J.S.; Jia, L.; Eu, J.P.; McMahon, T.J.; Demchenko, I.T.; Bonaventura, J.; Gernert, K. & Piantadosi, C.A. (1997). Blood flow regulation by S-nitrosohemoglobin in the physiological oxygen gradient. *Science*, Vol.276, pp. 2034-2037.

Stone, H.B.; Brown, J.M.; Phillips, T.L. & Sutherland, R.M. (1993). Oxygen in human tumors: correlations between methods of measurement and response to therapy. Summary of a workshop held November 19-20, 1992, at the National Cancer Institute, Bethesda, Maryland. *Radiat Res.*, Vol.136, pp. 422-434.

Stratmann, A.; Risau, W. & Plate, K.H. (1998). Cell type-specific expression of angiopoietin-1 and angiopoietin-2 suggests a role in glioblastoma angiogenesis. *Am J Pathol.*, Vol.153, pp. 1459-1466.

Swartz, H.M.; Khan, N.; Buckey, J.; Comi, R.; Gould, L.; Grinberg, O.; Hartford, A.; Hopf, H.; Hou, H.; Hug, E.; Iwasaki, A.; Lesniewski, P.; Salikhov, I. & Walczak, T. (2004). Clinical applications of EPR: overview and perspectives. *NMR Biomed.*, Vol.17, pp. 335–351.

Tatum, J.L.; Kelloff, G.J.; Gillies, R.J.; Arbeit, J.M.; Brown, J.M.; Chao, K.S.; Chapman, J.D.; Eckelman, W.C.; Fyles, A.W.; Giaccia, A.J.; Hill, R.P.; Koch, C.J.; Krishna, M.C.; Krohn, K.A.; Lewis, J.S.; Mason, R.P.; Melillo, G.; Padhani, A.R.; Powis, G.; Rajendran, J.G.; Reba, R.; Robinson, S.P.; Semenza, G.L.; Swartz, H.M.; Vaupel, P.; Yang, D.; Croft, B.; Hoffman, J.; Liu, G.; Stone, H. & Sullivan, D. (2006). Hypoxia: importance in tumor biology, noninvasive measurement by imaging, and value of its measurement in the management of cancer therapy. *Int J Radiat Biol.*, Vol.82, pp. 699-757.

Theodossiou, C., Skrepnik, N.; Robert, E.G.; Prasad, C.; Axelrad, T.W.; Schapira D.V. & Hunt, D.V. (1999). Propylthiouracil-induced hypothyroidism reduces xenograft tumor growth in athymic nude mice. *Cancer*, Vol.86, pp. 1596-1601.

Thomas, C.D.; Chavaudra, N.; Martin, L. & Guichard, M. (1994). Correlation between radiosensitivity, percentage hypoxic cells and pO2 measurements in one rodent and two human tumor xenografts. *Radiat Res.*, Vol.139, pp. 1-8.

Tofts, P.S.; Brix, G.; Buckley, D.L.; Evelhoch, J.L.; Henderson, E.; Knopp, M.V.; Larsson, H.B.; Lee, T.Y.; Mayr, N.A.; Parker, G.J.; Port, R.E.; Taylor, J. & Weisskoff, R.M. (1999). Estimating kinetic parameters from dynamic contrast-enhanced T(1)-weighted MRI of a diffusable tracer: standardized quantities and symbols. *J Magn Reson Imaging*, Vol.10, pp. 223-232.

Tong, R.T.; Boucher, Y.; Kozin, S.V.; Winkler, F.; Hicklin, D.J. & Jain, R.K. (2004). Vascular normalization by vascular endothelial growth factor receptor 2 blockade induces a pressure gradient across the vasculature and improves drug penetration in tumors. *Cancer Res.*, Vol.64, pp. 3731-3736.

Vanin, A.F.; Bevers, L.M.; Slama-Schwok, A. & van Faassen, E.E. (2007). Nitric oxide synthase reduces nitrite to NO under anoxia. *Cell Mol Life Sci.*, Vol.64, pp. 96-103.

Vaupel, P.; Okunieff, P. & Neuringer, L.J. (1989). Blood flow, tissue oxygenation, pH distribution, and energy metabolism of murine mammary adenocarcinomas during growth. *Adv Exp Med Biol.*, Vol.248, pp. 835-845.

Vujaskovic, Z.; Rosen, E.L.; Blackwell, K.L.; Jones, E.L.; Brizel, D.M.; Prosnitz, L.R.; Samulski, T.V. & Dewhirst, M.W. (2003). Ultrasound guided pO2 measurement of breast cancer reoxygenation after neoadjuvant chemotherapy and hyperthermia treatment. *Int J Hyperther.*, Vol.19, pp. 498-506.

Zhao, D.; Jiang, L. & Mason, R.P. (2004). Measuring changes in tumor oxygenation. *Method Enzymol.*, Vol.386, pp. 378-418.

Zlotecki, R.A.; Baxter, L.T.; Boucher, Y. & Jain, R.K. (1995). Pharmacologic modification of tumor blood flow and interstitial fluid pressure in a human tumor xenograft: network analysis and mechanistic interpretation. *Microvasc Res.*, Vol.50, No.3, pp. 429-43.

Zweier, J.L.; Samouilov, A.; & Kuppusamy, P. (1999). Non-enzymatic nitric oxide synthesis in biological systems. *Biochim Biophys Acta*, Vol.1411, pp. 250-262.

# 14

# Significance, Mechanisms, and Progress of Anticancer Drugs Targeting HGF-Met

Katsuya Sakai, Takahiro Nakamura,
Yoshinori Suzuki and Kunio Matsumoto
*Division of Tumor Dynamics and Regulation*
*Cancer Research Institute, Kanazawa University, Kakuma, Kanazawa*
*Japan*

## 1. Introduction

Because growth factors and their receptors play critical roles in cancer development and progression, they are potential target molecules in molecular-targeted cancer therapy. Hepatocyte growth factor (HGF) was discovered and cloned as a mitogenic protein for hepatocytes (Nakamura et al., 1984; Nakamura et al., 1989; Miyazawa et al., 1989). These early studies implicated an important role for HGF in regeneration of the liver. The receptor for HGF was identified as the Met transmembrane receptor tyrosine kinase in 1991 (Bottaro et al., 1991; Naldini et al., 1991). The Met oncogene was first isolated as a fused transforming gene from a human osteosarcoma-derived cell line, wherein sequences from the TPR (translocated promoter region) were fused to the Met sequence (Tpr-Met) (Cooper et al., 1984). In 1991, the scatter factor, originally identified as a fibroblast-derived cell motility factor for epithelial cells (Stoker et al., 1987), was shown to be an identical molecule to HGF (Weidner et al., 1990). These findings implicated further biological and pathophysiological roles for HGF in epithelial wound healing, epithelial-mesenchymal interaction, and cancer development and invasion. Based on its close involvement – not only in tumor development, invasion, and metastasis but also in resistance to anticancer therapies – the HGF-Met pathway has become a hot target in anticancer drug development (Comoglio et al., 2008; Sattler & Salgia, 2009; Hanahan & Weinberg, 2011). In most cases in the relationship between growth factors and their receptor tyrosine kinases, a single growth factor activates multiple receptors that have structural similarities, while a single growth factor receptor has multiple ligands with structural and functional similarities. By contrast, the sole receptor of HGF is Met, while the sole ligand of Met is HGF; the relationship between HGF and Met is a "one-to-one relationship." This unique biochemical characteristic in the HGF-Met pathway promotes drug development by targeting HGF-Met through either the activation or the inhibition of the HGF-Met pathway.

## 2. Biochemical and biological characteristics

Biologically active HGF, a protein composed of 697 or 692 amino acids, is a heterodimeric molecule composed of an α-chain and a β-chain (Fig. 1A). The α-chain contains 4 kringle domains, while the β-chain contains a serine protease-like structure (Nakamura et al., 1989; Miyazawa et al., 1989). HGF has a structural similarity to plasminogen, which is a heterodimeric serine protease containing 5 kringle domains. HGF is biosynthesized as a prepro-form of 728 amino acids, including a signal sequence and both α- and β-chains. After cleavage of a signal peptide of the first 31 amino acids, a single-chain HGF is further cleaved between Arg494 and Val495, and this processing is coupled to the conversion of biologically inactive pro-HGF to active HGF (Fig. 1A). Several proteases in the serum or cell membranes are involved in the activation of single-chain HGF, including HGF activator, urokinase-type plasminogen activator, plasma kallikrein, coagulation factors XII and XI, matriptase, and hepsin (Kataoka & Kawaguchi, 2010).

The Met receptor is composed of structural domains that include the extracellular Sema (the domain found in semaphorin receptors), PSI (the domain found in plexins, semaphorins and integrins) and IPT (the domain found in immunoglobulins, plexins, and transcription factors) domains, the transmembrane domain, and the intracellular juxtamembrane and tyrosine kinase domains (Fig. 1B) (Park et al., 1987). The Sema domain serves as a key element for ligand binding (Gherardi et al., 2006), while an involvement of IPT-3 and IPT-4 in the binding to HGF was demonstrated by another approach (Basilico et al., 2008).

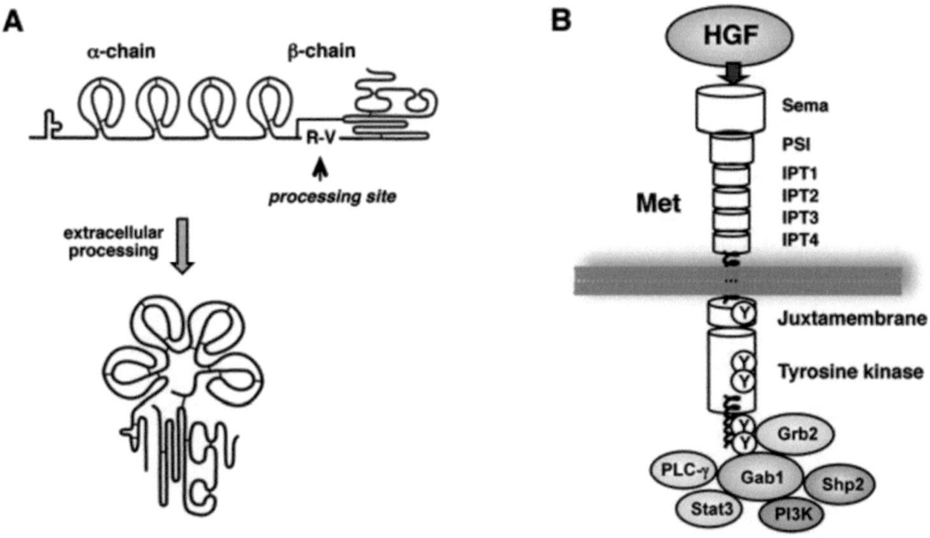


Fig. 1. (**A**) Processing and structure of single-chain proHGF and mature HGF. (**B**) Domain structures of the Met receptor and representative signaling molecules that associate with Met.

HGF and Met genes are widely expressed, and HGF is expressed in mesenchymal/stromal cells, predominantly rather than exclusively. Deletion of either the HGF or Met gene in mice lethally disrupts embryogenesis, including impairing development of the placenta and liver, and disabling dynamic migration of myogenic precursor cells (Schmidt et al., 1995; Uehara et al., 1995; Bladt et al., 1995; Birchmeier et al., 2003). In adulthood, HGF and Met play important roles in protection and regeneration of various tissues following injuries and pathology (Nakamura et al., 2011). Tissue-specific deletion of the Met gene revealed that the HGF-Met pathway plays a critical role in regeneration of the liver, kidney, and skin (Huh et al., 2004; Borowiak et al., 2004; Chmielowiec et al., 2007; Ma et al., 2009). Met-deficient epidermal keratinocytes were unable to contribute to re-epithelialization in skin wound healing, because of a disability in keratinocyte migration (Chmielowiec et al., 2007). HGF induces 3-dimensional (3-D) tubulogenesis in epithelial cells such as renal and mammary grand epithelial cells (Fig. 2) (Montesano et al., 1991). These approaches emphasize a particular role of the HGF-Met pathway in the migration of cells during development, morphogenesis, and regeneration. However, the dynamic actions of HGF in wound healing and tissue reconstruction – even in a 3-D spatial scaffold – remind us of the malignant behavior of tumors, i.e., invasion and metastasis (Fig. 2). Aberrant activation of the Met receptor in tumor cells participates in the malignant progression of tumor cells.

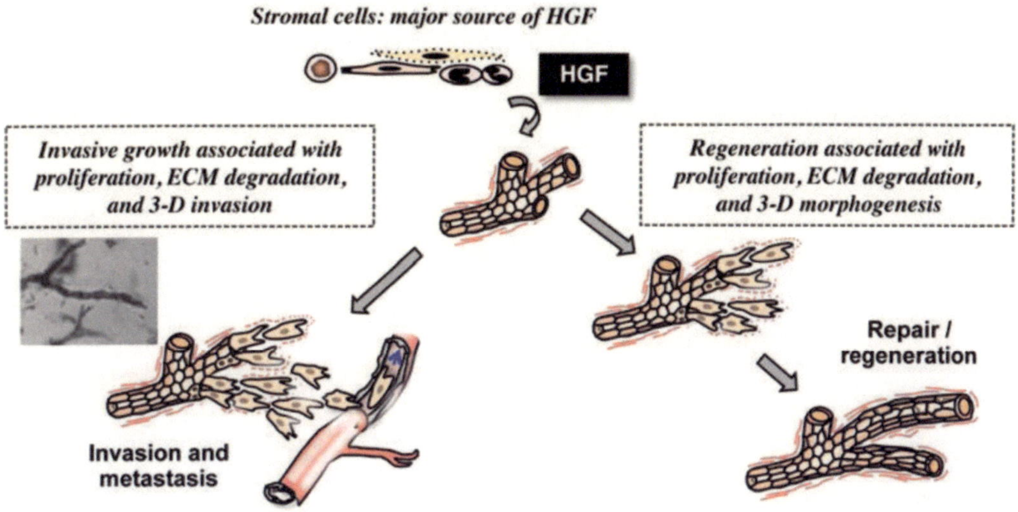


Fig. 2. Outline for biological actions of HGF in tumor invasion-metastasis and tissue regeneration.

## 3. Met receptor activation

HGF binds to Met through 2 different mechanisms: the α-chain binds with high affinity while the β-chain binds with low affinity. Among the α-chain, NK1 (the N-terminal and first kringle domains) in the α-chain of HGF provides a high-affinity binding site for Met. The α-chain alone exhibits high-affinity binding to Met, whereas the binding of the α-chain does not activate Met (Matsumoto et al., 1998). When Met is occupied by the α-chain, the low-affinity binding of the β-chain induces activation of Met and biological responses. Hence, the α-chain is a high-affinity binding module to Met, while the β-chain is an activation module for Met. The structure of the complex of HGF β-chain and Sema was revealed by crystallographic analysis (Fig. 3A) (Stamos et al., 2004). The HGF β-chain binds to a series of protruding polar side chains from Met, which originate from 3 separate loops: residues 124–128, residues 190–192, and residues 218–223. Although the α-chain of HGF binds to Met with much higher affinity than that of the HGF β-chain, the crystalline structure for the interaction between the HGF α-chain and the extracellular region of Met is yet to be determined.

The Met tyrosine kinase domain follows a conserved bilobal protein kinase architecture mainly with an N-terminal, β-sheet-containing domain linked through a hinge segment mainly to the α-helical C lobe (Fig. 3B) (Schiering et al., 2003; Wang et al., 2006). The characteristic feature of Met is the presence of the C-terminal tail that contains tyrosine residues ($^{1349}$YVHVNAT$^{1356}$YVNV). Binding of HGF to the extracellular region of Met results in receptor dimerization and phosphorylation of multiple tyrosine residues within the cytoplasmic region. Phosphorylation of Tyr1234 and Tyr1235 within the tyrosine kinase domain positively regulates the catalytic activity of tyrosine kinase (Fig. 3B). The staurosporine analog K-252a inhibits Met tyrosine kinase through its binding in the ATP pocket (Schiering et al., 2003). The phosphorylation of C-terminal tyrosine residues Tyr1349 and Tyr1356 recruits intracellular signaling molecules, including PI3K (phosphatidylinositol 3-kinase), Grb2 (growth-factor-receptor-bound protein 2), Gab1 (Grb2-associated binder 1), PLCγ (phospholipase Cγ), and Shp2 (SH2-domain-containing protein tyrosine phosphatase 2). Direct interaction of Gab1 with tyrosine phosphorylated Met is mediated by the Met-binding site in Gab1, and Gab1 is the most crucial substrate for the HGF-Met pathway (Ponzetto et al., 1994; Sachs et al., 2000).

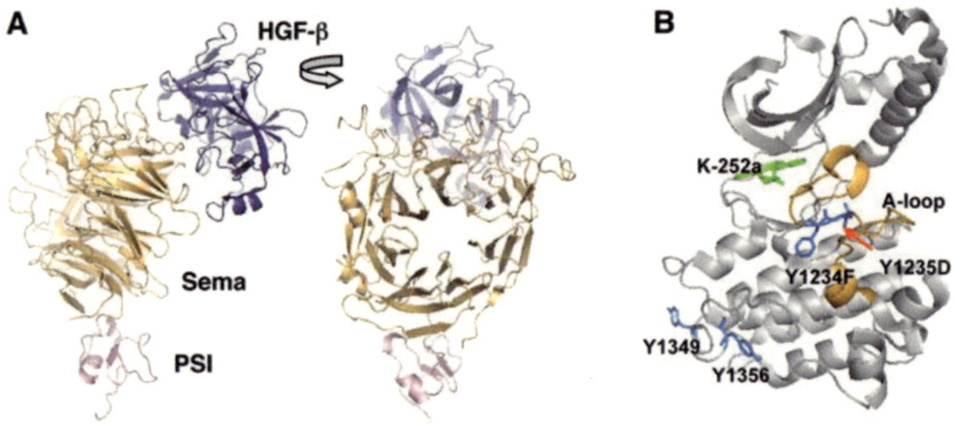


Fig. 3. Crystal structures for the complex of HGF β-chain and the Met Sema domain (**A**) and the Met tyrosine kinase domain (**B**). The crystal structures for the complex of HGF β-chain and the Met Sema domain were reported by Stamos et al. (2003) (PDB number: 1SHY). The crystal structure for Met tyrosine kinase was reported by Schiering et al. (2003) (PDB number 1ROP). In **B**, the activation loop (A-loop) is shown in yellow, K-252a in green, and selected tyrosine residues (Y1234F, Y1235D, Y1349, Y1356) are in blue.

The cytoplasmic juxtamembrane domain, which is composed of 47 highly conserved amino acids, acts as a negative regulator in terms of Met-dependent signal transduction. Cbl, an E3 ubiquitin ligase, binds phosphorylated Y1003 of Met, and this Cbl binding results in Met ubiquitination, endocytosis and transport to the endosomal compartment, then degradation (Peschard et al., 2001). Cbl-mediated degradation of the activated Met provides a mechanism that attenuates or terminates Met-mediated signaling. Phosphorylation of Ser985 in the juxtamembrane domain regulates the activation status of Met upon HGF stimulation. Ser985 is phosphorylated by protein kinase-C and is dephosphorylated by protein phosphatase-2A (Gandino et al., 1994; Hashigasako et al., 2004). In cells in which

Ser985 is phosphorylated, HGF-induced activation of Met is suppressed. Therefore, activation of protein kinase-C, which occurs by different types of extracellular stimuli, regulates HGF-dependent Met inactivation/activation.

## 4. HGF-Met in cancer development and progression

### 4.1 Cancer development

In normal tissues the activation of the Met receptor is tightly regulated, perhaps exclusively in a ligand-dependent manner. Aberrant activation of Met is associated with tumor development or progression to a tumor with malignant characteristics (Comoglio et al., 2004; Christensen et al., 2005; Matsumoto & Nakamura, 2006). Overexpression of Met through transcriptional upregulation has been noted in several cancers, including thyroid, ovarian, pancreatic, prostatic, renal, hepatocellular, breast, and colorectal cancers. Overexpression of Met through gene amplification was found in cancers with highly invasive and malignant characteristics, including gastric and esophageal carcinomas, medulloblastoma, and non-small-cell lung carcinomas (NSCLC) with acquired resistance to epidermal growth factor receptor (EGFR) tyrosine kinase inhibitors (see below). Autocrine and paracrine activation of Met through overexpression of HGF has been noted in breast cancer, glioblastoma, rhabdomyosarcoma, osteosarcoma, and in NSCLC with acquired and intrinsic resistance to EGFR tyrosine kinase inhibitors.

The missense mutations in the Met gene are the causative genetic disorders in inherited, and in some sporadic, papillary renal carcinomas (Schmidt et al., 1997). Mutations found in papillary renal carcinomas are located in the tyrosine kinase domain of the Met receptor, and these Met mutations are likely to be gain-of-function mutations (Jeffers et al., 1997; Michieli et al., 1999). In addition to papillary renal carcinoma, missense mutations in the Met gene have been found in different types of cancers, including lung cancer, hepatocellular carcinoma, and gastric cancer in the Sema, IPT, juxtamembrane, and tyrosine kinase domains (Christensen et al., 2005; Cipriani et al., 2009).

### 4.2 Cancer invasion and metastasis

The biological programs regulated by the HGF-Met pathway are adopted in cancer tissues, particularly for their invasive and metastatic behavior (Birchmeier et al., 2003; Matsumoto & Nakamura, 2006): 1) the dissociation of cancer cells at the primary site; 2) invasion, i.e., detachment from the primary site and migration through the basement membrane and stroma; and, 3) escape from apoptosis in anchorage-independent conditions during circulation. In a unique 3-D invasion in collagen gel, HGF was identified as a fibroblast-derived factor that definitively induces invasiveness of oral carcinoma cells (Matsumoto et al., 1989; Matsumoto et al., 1994). HGF increases extracellular protease expression coupled with the dissociation of cancer cells and their motility by which HGF promotes invasion in 3-D extracellular matrices and subsequent metastasis. HGF-Met signaling participates in the transition of epithelial to mesenchymal cell types (Birchmeier et al., 2003). Angiogenic and lymphangiogenic activities of HGF may facilitate cancer metastasis (Jiang et al., 2005). Collectively, the HGF-Met pathway has become a hot target in research and development of molecular targeted therapy for cancer, particularly to inhibit cancer invasion and metastasis (Hanahan & Weinberg, 2011).

### 4.3 Resistance to EGFR tyrosine kinase inhibitors

Gefitinib and erlotinib, selective inhibitors for EGFR tyrosine kinase, show favorable responses in NSCLC, especially those expressing activating mutations in EGFR (Lynch et al., 2004; Paez et al., 2004). Recent phase III clinical trials demonstrated that patients with EGFR mutant NSCLC had superior outcomes with gefitinib treatment, compared with standard first-line cytotoxic chemotherapy (Maemondo et al., 2010; Mitsudomi et al., 2010). However, almost without exception, the patients developed acquired resistance to EGFR tyrosine kinase inhibitors within several years (Morita et al., 2009). Furthermore, 20–25% of the patients with EGFR-activating mutations showed intrinsic resistance to EGFR tyrosine kinase inhibitors.

Three mechanisms have been noted to induce acquired resistance to EGFR tyrosine kinase inhibitors in NSCLC with activating EGFR mutants. One is the T790M second mutation in *EGFR* (Kobayashi et al., 2005). Second is the amplification of the Met gene (Engelman et al., 2007) (Fig. 4A, left). The T790M second mutation occurs in about half of all patients with acquired resistance to gefitinib or erlotinib. Recent studies showed that Met gene amplification was detected in ~20% of patients with acquired resistance to gefitinib or erlotinib (Bean et al., 2007; Turke et al., 2010). As the third mechanism, HGF-dependent Met activation has been noted (Yano et al., 2008). HGF induces resistance to EGFR tyrosine kinase inhibitors in EGFR mutant lung cancer (Yano et al., 2008) (Fig. 4, right). In clinical specimens, HGF overexpression was detected in a population of specimens from EGFR mutant lung cancer patients who showed intrinsic or acquired resistance to EGFR tyrosine kinase inhibitors indicating the clinical relevance of this resistance mechanism in lung cancer (Yano et al., 2008; Turke et al., 2010; Onitsuka et al., 2010). HGF can be produced by both cancer cells and host stromal cells such as fibroblasts (Matsumoto et al., 1994; Khoury et al., 2005; Matsumoto & Nakamura, 2006) (Fig. 4B). Tumor-associated fibroblasts expressed HGF at high levels in tumors from a population of NSCLC patients, and co-injection of HGF-producing human lung fibroblast cells with gefitinib-sensitive EGFR mutant lung cancer cells caused gefitinib resistance, which could be reversed by anti-HGF antibody and NK4, an antagonist against HGF (Wang et al., 2009). These results indicated that HGF derived from host stromal cells and/or HGF secreted from cancer cells induced resistance to EGFR tyrosine kinase inhibitors through paracrine and/or autocrine actions (Fig. 4B).

In some cases, a small fraction of cells with Met gene amplification pre-exists before exposure to EGFR tyrosine kinases, and HGF accelerates expansion of cells with Met gene amplification in the presence of EGFR tyrosine kinase inhibitors (Turke et al., 2010). HGF expression was higher in the drug-resistant specimens than in the pretreatment specimens (Turke et al., 2010). The results suggested that minor clones with Met gene amplification pre-existed before treatment with EGFR tyrosine kinase inhibitors, and that HGF accelerated expansion of a pre-existing minor population of tumor cells with Met gene amplification, which showed there is a relationship between HGF level and Met gene amplification. In recent studies, the EGFR-T790M second mutation and HGF expression were detected simultaneously in acquired resistant tumors in a considerable number of patients treated with gefitinib or erlotinib. EGFR-T790M second mutation was found in 7 of 10 NSCLC patients who acquired resistance to gefitinib, and 5 of 6 cases with EGFR-T790M second mutation showed high levels of HGF expression (Onitsuka et al., 2010). In 27 patients resistant to EGFR tyrosine kinase inhibitors, EGFR-T790M second mutation was seen in 15 of 27 cases, and 11 of these 15 tumors showed high-level HGF expression (Turke et al., 2010).

Collectively, expression of HGF in cancer cells and/or host stromal cells closely participated in the resistance to EGFR tyrosine kinase inhibitors in NSCLC, even in NSCLC with Met gene amplification.

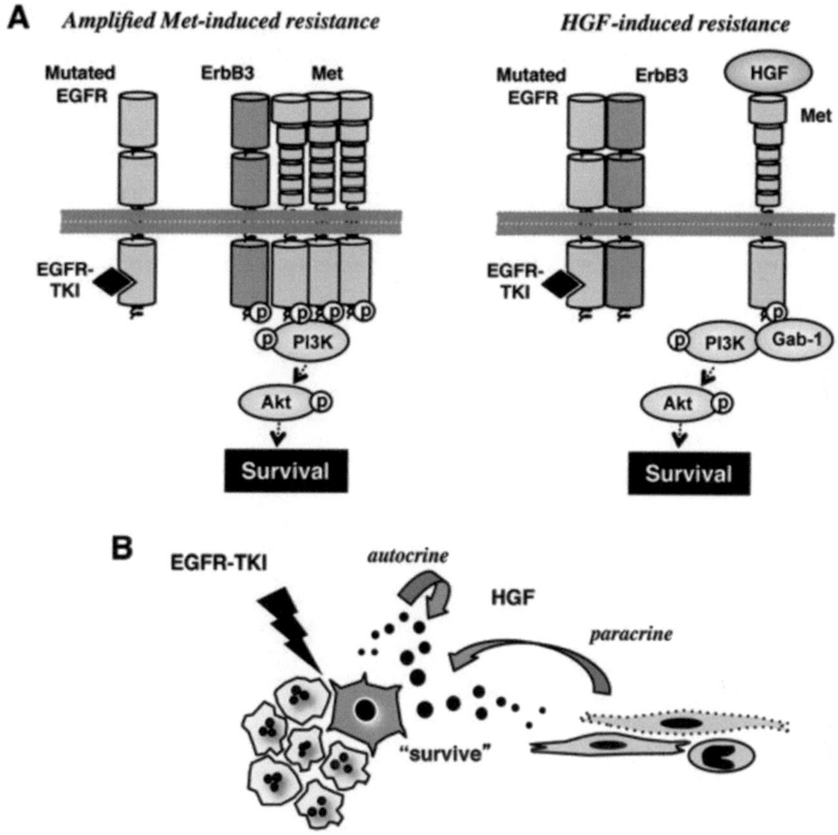


Fig. 4. Drug resistance of non-small-cell lung cancer (NSCLC) against EGFR tyrosine kinase inhibitors (EGFR-TKIs) through HGF-Met pathway. (**A**) Drug resistance through Met gene amplification (left) and HGF-dependent Met activation (right). Amplified Met associates with ErbB3 activates downstream signaling such as the PI3-Akt pathway, leading to the survival of cancer cells. HGF-dependent Met phosphorylation activates the PI3K-Akt pathway, independent of EGFR and ErbB3. (**B**) Outline for the resistance of NSCLC against EGFR-TKI by an HGF-dependent mechanism. HGF acts through an autocrine and/or paracrine manner.

### 4.4 Resistance to antiangiogenic therapy

Clinical results of antiangiogenic therapy in human patients have not been as promising as expected earlier (Schmidt, 2009). Until recently there had been a question as to why tumors become resistant to antiangiogenic therapy. Experimental studies have suggested that hypoxia generated by angiogenesis inhibitor or the blockage of new blood vessels triggers signaling molecules that make tumors more aggressive and metastatic (Schmidt, 2009).

In a model of pancreatic neuroendocrine cancer, inhibition of vascular endothelial cell growth factor receptor (VEGFR) tyrosine kinase shrank the primary tumor, but it also made the surviving cancer more aggressive with more metastatic behavior (Casanovas et al., 2005). Pathological and clinical studies indicate that the presence of hypoxic regions within neoplastic lesions correlates with poor prognosis and an increased risk of the development of distant metastases (Höckel & Vaupel, 2001). Importantly, a hypoxic condition induced the transcriptional activation of the Met receptor gene and subsequent amplification of HGF-Met signaling, thereby increasing the invasiveness of cancer cells (Penancchietti et al., 2004). A connection between hypoxia and the Met receptor seems to explain why hypoxia often correlates with invasive and metastatic behavior. Angiogenesis inhibition retards tumor growth by oxygen deprivation, at least in part. However, hypoxia caused by the inhibition of angiogenesis enhances HGF-Met signaling, thereby promoting tumor invasion and metastasis. The involvement of the HGF-Met pathway in the aggressive characteristics in the hypoxic regions of cancers, which includes tumors treated with antiangiogenic drugs, is considerable.

## 5. Drug discovery and development

Close involvement of aberrant HGF-Met signaling in tumorigenesis and progression to malignant disease has facilitated drug discovery and development. Several distinct lines of approach to the inhibition of the HGF-Met pathway have been demonstrated, including small synthetic inhibitors of Met tyrosine kinase, ribozymes, small-interfering RNA (siRNA), neutralizing monoclonal antibodies (mAbs), soluble forms of Met, antagonists composed of selected domains in HGF, and uncleavable single-chain HGF (Fig. 5). Among recombinant protein-based inhibitors, conventionally called biologics in drug development, mAbs targeting HGF or Met have been in clinical development earlier than the other biological inhibitors, predominantly because of their availability due to established technologies for manufacturing of recombinant mAbs.

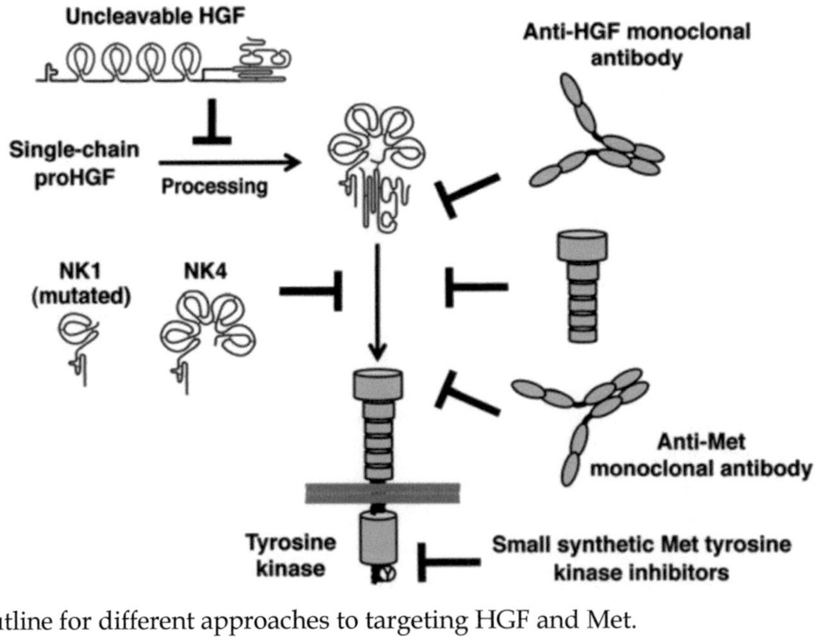


Fig. 5. Outline for different approaches to targeting HGF and Met.

## 5.1 Biologicals

Biological inhibitors against HGF-Met include the following: 1) selected domains in HGF (NK4 and engineered NK1); 2) engineered single-chain HGF forms that are resistant to proteolytic processing; 3) truncated soluble forms of the Met extracellular region; and, 4) humanized monoclonal antibodies (mAbs) against HGF or Met.

Among the α-chain of HGF, NK2 (the N-terminal, 1st kringle, and 2nd kringle domains), an alternative splicing variant, was first shown to competitively antagonize the growth stimulation by HGF (Chan et al., 1991). However, NK2 was later shown to stimulate cell motility and enhance HGF-driven metastasis in a mouse model (Stahl et al., 1997; Yu & Merlino, 2002).

NK4 is the first identified HGF-Met inhibitor devoid of biological activity through its Met binding. NK4 is composed of the N terminal and 4 kringle domains (Date et al., 1997; Matsumoto et al., 1998; Matsumoto et al., 2008). NK4 inhibits biological responses triggered by activation of HGF-Met signaling, including the spreading and invasion of cancer cells (Fig. 6). It should be emphasized that NK4 inhibits angiogenesis in addition to its antagonistic action against HGF, and this angioinhibitory action of NK4 is independent of its antagonist action against HGF. NK4 inhibited proliferation, migration, and tube formation of vascular endothelial cells induced by basic fibroblast growth factor and VEGF as well as by HGF (Kuba et al., 2001; Sakai et al., 2009). NK4 binds to perlecan and inhibits the cell-associated assembly of fibronectin, and the impaired fibronectin assembly suppresses integrin-dependent endothelial cell proliferation and migration. Having two different biological activities through completely different mechanisms is unique to NK4. Combination therapy of NK4 with antiangiogenic drugs is expected.

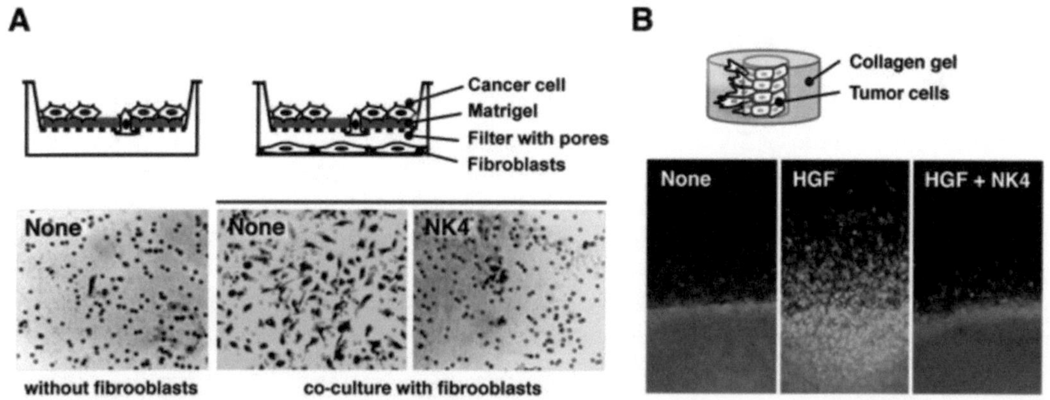


Fig. 6. Inhibition of tumor invasion by NK4. Invasion of human gallbladder cancer cells through the Matrigel basement membrane was induced by co-culture with stromal fibroblasts, and this aggressive invasion was inhibited by NK4 (**A**). 3-D invasion of human pleural malignant mesothelioma in collagen gel was enhanced by HGF, and was inhibited by NK4 (**B**).

The therapeutic effect of NK4 has been demonstrated in a variety of cancer models (Matsumoto et al., 2008). The inhibition of tumor growth by NK4 treatment was observed in a variety of tumors, and this inhibitory effect was associated with a reduction in blood vessels in tumor tissues. NK4 treatment inhibited *in situ* Met tyrosine phosphorylation, and this was associated with an inhibition of the spread and invasive growth of cancer cells (Matsumoto et al., 2008). NK4 treatment inhibited metastasis in different types of models, including breast, colon, gastric, lung, ovarian, and pancreatic carcinomas, and malignant melanoma. These results provided the base for proof-of-concept; inhibition of the HGF-Met pathway is a way to inhibit the invasive and metastatic growth of cancer. Moreover, the combination therapy of NK4 and gefitinib overcame HGF-induced gefitinib resistance of lung cancer in a mouse model (Wang et al., 2009).

NK1 was identified as a product of an alternative spliced variant of HGF, similar to NK2, that consists of the N-terminal and first kringle (K1) domains (Cioce et al., 1996). NK1 binds Met and acts as a partial agonist in cell-based assays and transgenic mice (Lokker et al., 1994; Schwall et al., 1996). Biochemical and structural analysis indicated the following two points: 1) NK1 is responsible for the high affinity binding of HGF to the Met-Sema domain; and, 2) Met dimerization may be mediated by the NK1-NK1 dimer interface (Watanabe et al., 2002; Gherardi et al., 2006). Based on structural analysis, mutations designed to alter the NK1 dimer interface (Y124A, K85A, K85A/D123A, and K85A/N127A) abolish its ability to promote Met dimerization, but these mutated NK1s retain Met-binding activity (Rubin et al., 2001; Tolbert et al., 2007). These NK1 mutants act as Met antagonists by inhibiting HGF-mediated cell scattering, proliferation, and invasion (Gherardi et al., 2006; Rubin et al., 2001; Tolbert et al., 2007). Although it is yet to be determined if NK1 acts as an angiogenesis inhibitor, NK1 can be expected to exert anti-cancer action by inhibiting the HGF-Met pathway.

Single-chain HGF variants that are resistant to proteolytic activation exploit the requirement for processing machinery that converts pro-HGF to mature HGF. Indeed, uncleavable forms of HGF have been engineered by substituting single amino acids in the proteolytic site, and these engineered uncleavable HGFs suppress Met-driven tumor growth, metastasis, and angiogenesis in murine tumor models (Mazzone et al., 2004). Related antagonists consisting of two-chain HGF mutants exploit the mechanism by which proteolytic conversion allosterically stabilizes HGF–Met binding to promote kinase activation (Kirchhofer et al., 2007). Insertion of the newly formed N-terminus of the HGF β chain into the activation pocket stabilizes the interaction between the HGF β chain and Met. Full-length 2-chain HGF mutants engineered to interrupt these interactions efficiently inhibited HGF-mediated Met activation. Studies on the structure-function relationship of Met extracellular domains provided the development of Met-based biological HGF-Met inhibitor. A soluble Met-Sema domain is not only necessary for Met receptor association but is also essential for HGF binding, whereby the Sema domain inhibits HGF-dependent and -independent receptor phosphorylation and functional receptor activation (Kong-Beltran et al., 2004). In a mouse model, soluble Met Sema domain suppressed tumor growth and metastasis (Michieli et al., 2004).

Among different types of mAbs against HGF or Met, one anti-Met mAb decreases Met activation by inducing ectodomain shedding and degradation (Petrelli et al., 2006), while the others inhibit the binding of HGF to Met. Neutralizing mAb against human HGF, such as L2G7, AMG102 and SCH900105 (formerly AV299) inhibited HGF-dependent Met activation and the growth of tumor xenografts in mice (Petrelli et al., 2006; Kim et al., 2006; Jun et al., 2007). AMG102 is currently in phase I and II clinical trials (HYPERLINK "http://www.clinicaltrials.gov" www.clinicaltrials.gov) (Table 1). AMG 102 was well tolerated in humans and adverse events were predominantly low grade (Cecchi et al., 2011). SCH900105 was also well tolerated by patients in phase I trials. In its first completed trial, SCH900105 treatment was associated with a stabilizing of disease in half of the patients (Cecchi et al., 2011).

| Classification and name | Target(s) | Stage | Clinical application |
|---|---|---|---|
| *Small synthetic* | | | |
| AMG 208 | Met | Phase-I | advanced solid tumors |
| ARQ197 | Met | Phase-I | advanced or metastatic solid tumors, healthy volunteers |
| | | Phase-II | advanced pancreatic cancer, non-small cell lung cancer, unresectable hepatocellular carcinoma, advanced pancreatic cancer |
| BMS-777607 | Met | Phase-I/II | advanced or metastatic solid tumors |
| E7050 | Met, VEGFR2 | Phase I | advanced solid tumors |
| GSK089 (GSK363089/XL880) | Met, Ron, VEGFR1-3, PDGFR, Kit, Flt-3, Tie-2 | Phase-I | solid tumors, papillary renal carcinoma, liver cancer |
| | | Phase-II | advanced or metastatic gastric cancer, papillary renal cancer, esophageal adenocarcinoma |
| JNJ38877605 | Met | Phase-I | advanced or refractory solid tumors |
| MGCD265 | | Phase-I/II | advanced malignancies, non-small cell lung cancer |
| MK-2461 | Met, Tie-2, Ron | Phase-I/II | advanced solid tumors |
| MK-8033 | Met | Phase-I | advanced solid tumors |
| MP470 | Met, Ret, Kit, PDGFR, Flt-3 | Phase-I | solid tumors, metastatic solid tumors, lymphoma |
| PF-02341066 | Met, Alk | Phase-I | advanced cancer, healthy volunteers |
| | | Phase-II | carcinoma, non-small cell lung cancer |
| | | Phase-III | carcinoma, non-small cell lung cancer |
| PF-04217903 | Met | Phase-I | advanced cancer, neoplasms |
| SGX 523 | Met | Phase-I | solid tumors, advanced cancer |
| XL184 | Met, VEGFR1-3, Ret, Kit, Flt-3, Tie-2 | Phase I | glioblastoma, advanced malignancies, solid tumors, lymphoma, thyroid cancer |
| | | Phase-II | glioblastoma multiforme, non-small cell lung cancer |
| | | Phase-III | medullary thyroid cancer |
| *Antibody* | | | |
| AMG102 (Anti-HGF) | HGF | Phase-I/II | advanced malignant glioma, prostate cancer, metastatic gastric and esophageal adenocarcinoma |
| | | Phase-II | renal cell cancer, advanced malignant glioma |
| MetMab (Anti-Met) | Met | Phase-II | non-small cell lung cancer |
| SCH900105 | HGF | Phase-I | advanced solid tumors, lymphomas, multiple myeloma |

Table 1. HGF-Met inhibitors in clinical development.

mAbs against Met with different characteristics have been developed (Martens et al., 2006; Jin et al., 2008; van der Horst et al., 2009; Pacchiana et al., 2010). Anti-Met mAb, MetMab (formerly OA5D5), is a monovalent mAb that blocked binding of HGF to the Met (Martens et al., 2006). Anti-Met mAb R13 and R28 synergistically inhibited HGF binding to MET and elicited antibody-dependent cellular cytotoxicity (van der Horst et al., 2009). The combination of R13/28 inhibited tumor growth in various colon tumor xenograft models. MetMab reduced Met phosphorylation, and this was associated with inhibition of orthotopic tumor growth and improvement of survival in a pancreatic xenograft model (Jin et al., 2008). MetMab is currently in phase I/II human clinical trials in comparison with erlotinib for patients with NSCLC (HYPERLINK "http://www.clinicaltrials.gov" www.clinicaltrials.gov).

### 5.2 Small synthetic kinase inhibitors

As small synthetic Met tyrosine kinase inhibitors, SU11274 and PHA665752 provided the basic notion that small synthetic Met tyrosine kinase inhibitors selectively inhibit Met activation and suppress tumor growth (Christensen ; 2003; Sattler et al., 2003; Berthou et al; 2004; Ma et al., 2005; Smolen et al., 2006). Subsequent research and development led to the discovery of various types of synthetic tyrosine kinase inhibitors with different structures, chemical properties, and target specificity. Based on the wealth of accumulated knowledge gained from the success of preclinical and clinical development of small synthetic tyrosine kinase inhibitors, more than 10 small synthetic Met tyrosine kinase inhibitors have been entered into clinical trials (Table 1).

PF-02341066 targets Met as well as anaplastic lymphoma kinase (ALK) (Sattler & Salgia, 2009). MP470 inhibits PDGFR, Kit, and Met tyrosine kinases. In combination with erlotinib, MP470 inhibited prostate cancer cell proliferation and tumor xenograft growth (Qi et al., 2009). E7050 targets both Met and VEGFR2 (Nakagawa et al., 2009). JNJ-38877605 shows a >1,000-fold selectivity for the Met kinase, compared to a >200-fold selectivity for related receptor tyrosine kinases (Eder et al., 2009). AMG 208 selectively inhibits both ligand-dependent and ligand-independent Met activation. BMS777607 has completed a phase I/II study in metastatic cancer patients (Schroeder et al., 2009). Phase I clinical trials were discontinued for SGX523 after renal toxicity was observed in patients receiving relatively low doses ( HYPERLINK "http://www.sgxpharma.com" www.sgxpharma.com).

PF02341066 and XL184 have progressed the furthest of all Met inhibitors in clinical development. PF-02341066 has greater Met selectivity compared with PF-04217903 (Timofeevski et al., 2009). Preclinical studies indicate PF-02341066 is highly effective against the product of the EML4-ALK translocation found in a subset of NSCLC patients (Shaw et al., 2009). PF-02341066t is currently in phase I, II, and III clinical trials ( HYPERLINK "http://www.clinicaltrials.gov" www.clinicaltrials.gov). XL184 targets Met, VEGFR2, and Ret. A current phase III trial is investigating the efficacy of XL184 as a first-line treatment, compared to a placebo, in patients with medullary thyroid cancer ( HYPERLINK "http://www.clinicaltrials.gov" www.clinicaltrials.gov).

## 6. Conclusion and perspective

Breakdown of the extracellular matrix scaffold and the concomitant cellular migration, mitogenesis, and morphogenesis that is driven by the HGF-Met system makes way for the construction and reconstruction of tissues during development and wound healing. Perhaps because of this, tumor cells use the HGF-Met pathway as a machine particularly for their spreading, metastasis, and evasion of microenvironmental predicaments. Therefore, activation and inhibition of the HGF-Met pathway are likely to be therapeutic approaches for the treatment of non-neoplastic diseases with tissue damage and for malignant diseases, respectively. HGF exhibits therapeutic effects for the protection and healing of tissues against tissue damage and pathology. Clinical trials using recombinant HGF or HGF gene drugs have been approved for the treatment of diseases with unmet needs.

Based on the basic knowledge of the significance of the HGF-Met pathway in tumor biology and pathology, during the last several years the one-to-one relationship between HGF and Met has facilitated the discovery and development of drug candidates that selectively inhibit HGF-Met in different ways. Preclinical and clinical development of drugs targeting HGF-Met will move into practice in the near future as new anticancer drugs. However, although drug discoveries in molecular-targeted cancer therapy have been beneficial for patients with malignancies, the appearance of persistent characteristics of malignant tumors in regard to resistance to anticancer therapies and drugs remains an obstacle to disease-free survival. The choice of the better, or best, way to inhibit HGF-Met signaling, i.e., ligand inhibition, receptor inhibition, biologics, mAb, or small synthetic, would gradually become clearer following clinical experiences.

## 7. Acknowledgement

The studies from the authors' laboratories were supported by Grants from the Ministry of Education, Culture, Science, Sports, and Technology of Japan, the Program for Promotion of Fundamental Studies in Health Sciences of the National Institute of Biomedical Innovation, and the Hokkou Foundation for the Promotion of Cancer Research.

## 8. References

Bean, J., Brennan, C., Shih, J.Y., Riely, G., Viale, A., Wang, L., Chitale, D., Motoi, N., Szoke, J., Broderick, S., Balak, M., Chang, W.C., Yu, C.J., Gazdar, A., Pass, H., Rusch, V., Gerald, W., Huang, S.F., Yang, P.C., Miller, V., Ladanyi, M., Yang, C.H., & Pao, W. (2007) MET amplification occurs with or without T790M mutations in EGFR mutant lung tumors with acquired resistance to gefitinib or erlotinib. *Proceeding National Academy of Science USA*, 104: 20932-20937

Basilico, C., Arnesano, A., Galluzzo, M., Comoglio, P.M. & Michieli, P. (2008) A high affinity hepatocyte growth factor-binding site in the immunoglobulin-like region of Met. *Journal of Biological Chemistry*, 283: 21267-21277

Berthou, S., Aebersold, D.M., Schmidt, L.S., Stroka, D., Heigl, C., Streit, B., Stalder, D., Gruber, G., Liang, C., Howlett, A.R., Candinas, D., Greiner, R.H., Lipson, K.E. & Zimmer, Y. (2003) The Met kinase inhibitor SU11274 exhibits a selective inhibition pattern toward different receptor mutated variants. *Oncogene*, 23: 5387-5393, 2004.

Birchmeier, C., Birchmeier, W., Gherardi, E. & Vande Woude, G.F. (2003) Met, metastasis, motility and more. *Nature Review Molecular Cell Biology*, 4: 915-925

Bladt, F., Riethmacher, D., Isenmann, S., Aguzzi, A. & Birchmeier, C. (1995) Essential role for the c-met receptor in the migration of myogenic precursor cells into the limb bud. *Nature*, 376: 768-771

Borowiak, M., Garratt, A.N., Wustefeld, T., Strehle, M., Trautwein, C. & Birchmeier, C. (2004) Met provides essential signals for liver regeneration. *Proceeding National Academy of Science USA*, 101: 10608-10613

Bottaro, D.P., Rubin, J.S., Faletto, D.L., Chan, A.M-I., Kmiecik, T.E., Vande Woude, G.F. & Aaronson, S.A. (1991) Identification of the hepatocyte growth factor receptor as the c-met proto-oncogene product. *Science,* 251: 802-804

Casanovas, O., Hicklin, D.J., Bergers, G. & Hanahan, D. (2005) Drug resistance by evasion of antiangiogenic targeting of VEGF signaling in late-stage pancreatic islet tumors. *Cancer Cell,* 8: 299-309

Cecchi, F., Rabe, D.C. & Bottaro, D.P. (2010) Targeting the HGF/Met signalling pathway in cancer. *European Journal of Cancer,* 46: 1260-1270

Chan, A.M., Rubin, J.S., Bottaro, D.P., Hirschfield, D.W., Chedid, M. & Aaronson, S.A. (1991) Identification of a competitive HGF antagonist encoded by an alternative transcript. *Science,* 254: 1382-1385

Chmielowiec, J., Borowiak, M., Morkel, M., Stradal, T., Munz, B., Werner, S., Wehland, J., Birchmeier, C. & Birchmeier, W. (2007) c-Met is essential for wound healing in the skin. *Journal of Cell Biology,* 177: 151-162

Christensen, J.G., Schreck, R., Burrows, J., Kuruganti, P., Chan, E., Le, P., Chen, J., Wang, X., Ruslim, L., Blake, R., Lipson, K.E., Ramphal, J., Do, S., Cui, J.J., Cherrington, J.M. & Mendel, D.B. (2003) A selective small molecule inhibitor of c-Met kinase inhibits c-Met-dependent phenotypes in vitro and exhibits cytoreductive antitumor activity in vivo. *Cancer Research,* 63: 7345-7355

Christensen, J.G., Burrows, J. & Salgia, R. (2005) c-Met as a target for human cancer and characterization of inhibitors for therapeutic intervention. *Cancer Letters,* 225: 1-26

Cioce, V., Csaky, K.G., Chan, A.M.L., Bottaro, D.P., Taylor, W.G., Jensen, R., Aaronson, S. & Rubin, J.S. (1996) Hepatocyte growth factor (HGF)/NK1 is a naturally occurring HGF/scatter factor variant with partial agonist/antagonist activity. *Journal of Biological Chemistry,* 271: 13110-13115

Cipriani, N.A., Abidoye, O.O., Vokes, E. & Salgia, R. (2009) MET as a target for treatment of chest tumors. *Lung Cancer,* 63: 169-179

Cooper, C.S., Park, M., Blair, D.G., Tainsky, M.A., Huebner, K., Croce, C.M. & Vande Woude, G.F. (1984) Molecular cloning of a new transforming gene from a chemically transformed human cell line. *Nature,* 311: 29-33

Comoglio, P.M., Giordano, S. & Trusolino, L. (2008) Drug development of MET inhibitors: targeting oncogene addiction and expedience. *Nature Review Drug Discovery,* 7: 504-516

Date, K., Matsumoto, K., Shimura, H., Tanaka, M. & Nakamura, T. (1997) HGF/NK4 is a specific antagonist for pleiotrophic actions of hepatocyte growth factor. *FEBS Letters,* 420: 1-6

Eder, J.P., Vande Woude, G.F., Boerner, S.A. & LoRusso, P.M. (2009) Novel therapeutic inhibitors of the c-Met signaling pathway in cancer. *Clinical Cancer Research,* 15: 2207-2214

Engelman, J.A., Zejnullahu, K., Mitsudomi, T., Song, Y., Hyland, C., Park, J.O., Lindeman, N., Gale, C.M., Zhao, X., Christensen, J., Kosaka, T., Holmes, A.J., Rogers, A.M., Cappuzzo, F., Mok, T., Lee, C., Johnson, B.E., Cantley, L.C. & Jänne, P.A. (2007) MET amplification leads to gefitinib resistance in lung cancer by activating ERBB3 signaling. *Science,* 316, 1039-1043

Gandino, L., Longati, P., Medico, E., Prat, M. & Comoglio, P.M. (1994) Phosphorylation of serine 985 negatively regulates the hepatocyte growth factor receptor kinase. *Journal of Biological Chemistry,* 269: 1815-1820

Gherardi, E., Sandin, S., Petoukhov, M.V., Finch, J., Youles, M.E., Ofverstedt, L.G., Miguel, R.N., Blundell, T.L., Vande Woude, G.F., Skoglund, U. & Svergun, D.I. (2006)

Structural basis of hepatocyte growth factor/scatter factor and MET signalling. *Proceeding National Academy of Science USA*, 103: 4046-4051

Hanahan, D. & Weinberg, R. (2011) Hallmarks of cancer: The next generation. *Cell*, 144: 646-674

Hashigasako, A., Machide, M., Nakamura, T., Matsumoto, K. & Nakamura T. (2004) Bi-directional regulation of Ser-985 phosphorylation of c-met via protein kinase C and protein phosphatase 2A involves c-Met activation and cellular responsiveness to hepatocyte growth factor. *Journal of Biological Chemistry*, 279: 26445-26452

Höckel, M. & Vaupel, P. (2001) Tumor hypoxia: definitions and current clinical, biologic, and molecular aspects. *Journal of National Cancer Institute*, 93: 266-276

Huh, C.G., Factor, V.M., Sanchez, A., Uchida, K., Conner, E.A. & Thorgeirsson, S.S. (2004) Hepatocyte growth factor/c-met signaling pathway is required for efficient liver regeneration and repair. *Proceeding National Academy of Science USA*, 101: 4477-4482

Jeffers, M., Schmidt, L., Nakagawa, N., Webb, C.P., Weirich, G., Kishida, T., Zbar, B. & Vande Woude, G.F. (1997) Activating mutations for the Met tyrosine kinase receptor in human cancer. *Proceeding National Academy of Science USA*, 94: 11445-11450

Jiang, W.G., Martin, T.A., Parr, C., Davies, G., Matsumoto, K., & Nakamura, T. (2005) Hepatocyte growth factor, its receptor, and their potential value in cancer therapies *Critical Reveiws in Oncology Hematology*, 53: 35-69

Jin, H., Yang, R., Zheng, Z., Romero, M., Ross, J., Bou-Reslan, H., Carano, R.A., Kasman, I., Mai, E., Young, J., Zha, J., Zhang, Z., Ross, S., Schwall, R., Colbern, G. & Merchant, M. (2008) MetMAb, the one-armed 5D5 anti-c-Met antibody, inhibits orthotopic pancreatic tumor growth and improves survival. *Cancer Research*, 68: 4360-4368

Jun, H.T., Sun, J., Rex, K., Radinsky, R., Kendall, R., Coxon, A. & Burgess, T.L. (2007) AMG 102, a fully human anti-hepatocyte growth factor/scatter factor neutralizing antibody, enhances the efficacy of temozolomide or docetaxel in U-87 MG cells and xenografts. *Clinical Cancer Research*, 13: 6735-6742

Lynch, T.J., Bell, D.W., Sordella, R., Gurubhagavatula, S., Okimoto, R.A., Brannigan, B.W., Harris, P.L., Haserlat, S.M., Supko, J.G., Haluska, F.G., Louis, D.N., Christiani, D.C., Settleman, J. & Haber, D.A. (2004) Activating mutations in the epidermal growth factor receptor underlying responsiveness of non-small-cell lung cancer to gefitinib. *New England Journal of Medicine*, 350: 2129-2139

Kataoka, H. & Kawaguchi, M. (2010) Hepatocyte growth factor activator (HGFA): pathophysiological functions *in vivo*. *FEBS Journal*, 277: 2230-2237

Khoury, H., Naujokas, M.A., Zuo, D., Sangwan, V., Frigault, M.M., Petkiewicz, S., Dankort, D.L., Muller, W.J. & Park M. (2005) HGF converts ErbB2/Neu epithelial morphogenesis to cell invasion. *Molecular Biology of Cell*, 16: 550-561

Kim, K.J., Wang, L., Su, Y.C., Gillespie, G.Y., Salhotra, A., Lal, B. & Laterra, J. (2006) Systemic anti-hepatocyte growth factor monoclonal antibody therapy induces the regression of intracranial glioma xenografts. *Clinical Cancer Research*, 12: 1292-1298

Kirchhofer, D., Lipari, M.T., Santell, L., Billeci, K.L., Maun, H.R., Sandoval, W.N., Moran, P., Ridgway, J., Eigenbrot, C. & Lazarus, R.A. (2007) Utilizing the activation mechanism of serine proteases to engineer hepatocyte growth factor into a Met antagonist. *Proceeding National Academy of Science. USA*, 104: 5306-5311

Kobayashi, S., Boggon, T.J., Dayaram, T., Jänne, P.A., Kocher, O., Meyerson, M., Johnson, B.E., Eck, M.J., Tenen, D.G. & Halmos, B. (2005) EGFR mutation and resistance of non-small-cell lung cancer to gefitinib. *New England Journal of Medicine*, 352: 786-792

Kong-Beltran, M., Stamos, J. & Wickramasinghe, D. (2004) The Sema domain of Met is necessary for receptor dimerization and activation. *Cancer Cell*, 6: 75-84

Kuba, K., Matsumoto, K., Date, K., Shimura, H., Tanaka, M. & Nakamura T. (2000) HGF/NK4, a four-kringle antagonist of hepatocyte growth factor, is an angiogenesis inhibitor that suppresses tumor growth and metastasis in mice. *Cancer Research*, 60: 6737-6743

Lokker, N.A., Presta, L.G. & Godowski, P.J. (1994) Mutational analysis and molecular modeling of the N-terminal kringle-containing domain of hepatocyte growth factor identifies amino acid side chains important for interaction with the c-Met receptor. *Protein Engineering*, 7: 895-903

Ma, P.C., Jagadeeswaran, R., Jagadeesh, S., Tretiakova, M.S., Nallasura, V., Fox, E.A., Hansen, M., Schaefer, E., Naoki, K., Lader, A., Richards, W., Sugarbaker, D., Husain, A.N., Christensen, J.G. & Salgia, R. (2005) Functional expression and mutations of c-Met and its therapeutic inhibition with SU11274 and small interfering RNA in non-small cell lung cancer. *Cancer Research*, 65: 1479-1488

Ma, H., Saenko, M., Opuko, A., Togawa, A., Soda, K., Marlier, A., Moeckel, G.W., Cantley, L.G. & Ishibe, S. (2009) Deletion of the Met receptor in the collecting duct decreases renal repair following ureteral obstruction. *Kidney International*, 76: 868-876

Maemondo, M., Inoue, A., Kobayashi, K., Sugawara, S., Oizumi, S., Isobe, H., Gemma, A., Harada, M., Yoshizawa, H., Kinoshita, I., Fujita, Y., Okinaga, S., Hirano, H., Yoshimori, K., Harada, T., Ogura, T., Ando, M., Miyazawa, H., Tanaka, T., Saijo, Y., Hagiwara, K., Morita, S., Nukiwa, T.; & North-East Japan Study Group. (2010) Gefitinib or chemotherapy for non-small-cell lung cancer with mutated EGFR. *New England Journal of Medicine*, 362: 2380-2388

Martens, T., Schmidt, N.O., Eckerich, C., Fillbrandt, R., Merchant, M., Schwall, R., Westphal, M. & Lamszus, K. (2006) A novel one-armed anti-c-Met antibody inhibits glioblastoma growth in vivo. *Clinical Cancer Research*, 12: 6144-6152

Matsumoto, K., Horikoshi, M., Rikimaru, K. & Enomoto, S. (1989) A study of an in vitro model for invasion of oral squamous cell carcinoma. *Journal of Oral Pathology and Medicine*, 18: 498-501

Matsumoto, K., Matsumoto, K., Nakamura, T. & Kramer, R.H. (1994) Hepatocyte growth factor/scatter factor induces tyrosine phosphorylation of focal adhesion kinase (p125FAK) and promotes migration and invasion by oral squamous cell carcinoma cells. *Journal of Biological Chemistry*, 269: 31807-31813

Matsumoto, K., Kataoka, H., Date, K. & Nakamura, T. (1998) Cooperative interaction between α-chain and β-chain of HGF on c-Met receptor confers ligand-induced receptor tyrosine phosphorylation and multiple biological responses. *Journal of Biological Chemistry*, 273: 22913-22920

Matsumoto, K. & Nakamura, T. (2006) Hepatocyte growth factor and the Met system as a mediator of tumor-stromal interactions. *International Journal of Cancer*, 119: 477-483

Matsumoto, K., Nakamura, T., Sakai, K. & Nakamura, T. (2008) Hepatocyte growth factor and Met in tumor biology and therapeutic approach with NK4. *Proteomics*, 8: 3360-3370

Mazzone, M., Basilico, C., Cavassa, S., Pennacchietti, S., Risio, M., Naldini, L., Comoglio, P.M. & Michieli, P. (2004) An uncleavable form of pro-scatter factor suppresses tumor growth and dissemination in mice. *Journal of Clinical Investigation*, 114: 1418-1432

Michieli, P., Basilico, C., Pennacchietti, S., Maffè, A., Tamagnone, L., Giordano, S., Bardelli, A. & Comoglio, P.M. (1999) Mutant Met-mediated transformation is ligand-dependent and can be inhibited by HGF antagonists. *Oncogene*, 18: 5221-5231

Michieli, P., Mazzone, M., Basilico, C., Cavassa, S., Sottile, A., Naldini, L. & Comoglio, P.M. (2004) Targeting the tumor and its microenvironment by a dual-function decoy Met receptor. *Cancer Cell*, 6: 61-73

Mitsudomi, T., Morita, S., Yatabe, Y., Negoro, S., Okamoto, I., Tsurutani, J., Seto, T., Satouchi, M., Tada, H., Hirashima, T., Asami, K., Katakami, N., Takada, M., Yoshioka, H., Shibata, K., Kudoh, S., Shimizu, E., Saito, H., Toyooka, S., Nakagawa, K., Fukuoka, M.; & West Japan Oncology Group. (2010) Gefitinib versus cisplatin plus docetaxel in patients with non-small-cell lung cancer harbouring mutations of the epidermal growth factor receptor (WJTOG3405): an open label, randomised phase 3 trial. *Lancet Oncology*, 11: 121-128

Miyazawa, K., Tsubouchi, H., Naka, D., Takahashi, K., Okigaki, M., Arakaki, N., Nakayama, H., Hirono, S., Sakiyama, O., Takahashi, K., Gohda, E., Daikuhara, Y. & Kitamura, N. (1989) Molecular cloning and sequence analysis of cDNA for human hepatocyte growth factor. *Biochemical and Biophysical Research Communications*, 163: 967-973

Montesano, R., Matsumoto, K., Nakamura, T. & Orci, L. (1991) Identification of a fibroblast-derived epithelial morphogen as hepatocyte growth factor. *Cell*, 67: 901-908

Morita, S., Okamoto, I., Kobayashi, K., Yamazaki, K., Asahina, H., Inoue, A., Hagiwara, K., Sunaga, N., Yanagitani, N., Hida, T., Yoshida, K., Hirashima, T., Yasumoto, K., Sugio, K., Mitsudomi, T., Fukuoka, M. & Nukiwa, T. (2009) Combined survival analysis of prospective clinical trials of gefitinib for non-small-cell lung cancer with EGFR mutations. *Clinical Cancer Research*, 15: 4493-4498

Nakagawa, T., Tohyama, O., Yamaguchi, A., Matsushima, T., Takahashi, K., Funasaka, S., Shirotori, S., Asada, M. & Obaishi, H. (2009) E7050: A dual c-Met and VEGFR-2 tyrosine kinase inhibitor promotes tumor regression and prolongs survival in mouse xenograft models. *Cancer Science.*, 101: 210-215

Nakamura, T., Nawa, K. & Ichihara, A. (1984) Partial purification and characterization of hepatocyte growth factor from serum of hepatectomized rats. *Biochemical and Biophysical Research Communications*, 122: 1450-1459

Nakamura, T., Nishizawa, T., Hagiya, M., Seki, T., Shimonishi, M., Sugimura, A., Tashiro, K. & Shimizu, S. (1989) Molecular cloning and expression of human hepatocyte growth factor. *Nature*, 342: 440-443

Nakamura, T., Sakai, K., Nakamura, T., Matsumoto, K. (2011) Hepatocyte growth factor twenty years on: much more than a growth factor. *Journal of Gastroenterology and Hepatology*, 6: 188-202

Naldini, L., Vigna, E., Narcimham, R.P., Gaudino, G., Zarnegar, R., Michalopoulos, G.K. & Comoglio PM. (1991) Hepatocyte growth factor stimulates the tyrosine kinase activity of the receptor encoded by the proto-oncogene c-*MET*. *Oncogene*, 6: 501-504

Onitsuka, T., Uramoto, H., Nose, N., Takenoyama, M., Hanagiri, T., Sugio, K. & Yasumoto, K. (2010) Acquired resistance to gefitinib: the contribution of mechanisms other than the T790M, MET, and HGF status. *Lung Cancer*, 68: 198-203

Pacchiana, G., Chiriaco, C., Stella, M.C., Petronzelli, F., De Santis, R., Galluzzo, M., Carminati, P., Comoglio, P.M., Michieli, P. & Vigna, E. (2010) Monovalency unleashes the full therapeutic potential of the DN-30 anti-Met antibody. *Journal of Biological Chemistry*, 285: 36149-3657

Paez, J.G., Jänne, P.A., Lee, J.C., Tracy, S., Greulich, H., Gabriel, S., Herman, P., Kaye, F.J., Lindeman, N., Boggon, T.J., Naoki, K., Sasaki, H., Fujii, Y., Eck, M.J., Sellers, W.R.,

Johnson, B.E. & Meyerson, M. (2004) EGFR mutations in lung cancer: correlation with clinical response to gefitinib therapy. *Science*, 304: 1497-1500

Park, M., Dean, M., Kaul, K., Braun, M.J., Gonda, M.A. & Vande Woude, G. (1987) Sequence of MET protooncogene cDNA has features characteristic of the tyrosine kinase family of growth-factor receptors. *Proceeding National Academy of Science USA*, 84: 6379-6383

Pennacchietti, S., Michieli, P., Galluzzo, M., Mazzone, M., Giordano, S. & Comoglio, P.M. (2003) Hypoxia promotes invasive growth by transcriptional activation of the met protooncogene. *Cancer Cell*, 3: 347-361

Peschard, P., Fournier, T.M., Lamorte, L., Naujokas, M.A., Band, H., Langdon, W.Y. & Park, M. (2001) Mutation of the c-Cbl TKB domain binding site on the Met receptor tyrosine kinase converts it into a transforming protein. *Molecular Cell*, 8: 995-1004

Petrelli, A., Circosta, P., Granziero, L., Mazzone, M., Pisacane, A., Fenoglio, S., Comoglio, P.M. & Giordano, S. (2006) Ab-induced ectodomain shedding mediates hepatocyte growth factor receptor down-regulation and hampers biological activity. *Proceeding National Academy of Science USA*, 103: 5090-5095

Ponzetto, C., Bardelli, A., Zhen, Z., Maina, F., Zonca, P., Giordano, S., Graziani, A., Panayotou, G. & Comoglio, P.M. (1994) A multifunctional docking site mediates signaling and transformation by the hepatocyte growth factor/scatter factor receptor family. *Cell*, 77: 261-271

Qi, W., Cooke, L.S., Stejskal, A., Riley, C., Croce, K.D., Saldanha, J.W., Bearss, D. & Mahadevan, D. (2009) MP470, a novel receptor tyrosine kinase inhibitor, in combination with Erlotinib inhibits the HER family/PI3K/Akt pathway and tumor growth in prostate cancer. *BMC Cancer*, 9: 142

Rubin, J.S., Day, R.M., Breckenridge, D., Atabey, N., Taylor, W.G., Stahl, S.J., Wingfield, P.T., Kaufman, J.D., Schwall, R. & Bottaro, D.P. (2001) Dissociation of heparan sulfate and receptor binding domains of hepatocyte growth factor reveals that heparan sulfate-c-met interaction facilitates signaling. *Journal of Biological Chemistry*, 276: 32977-32983

Sachs, M., Brohmann, H., Zechner, D., Müller, T., Hülsken, J., Walther, I., Schaeper, U., Birchmeier, C. & Birchmeier, W. (2000) Essential role of Gab1 for signaling by the c-Met receptor *in vivo*. *Journal of Cell Biology*, 150: 1375-1384

Sakai, K., Nakamura, T., Matsumoto, K. & Nakamura, T. (2009) Angioinhibitory Action of NK4 Involves Impaired Extracellular Assembly of Fibronectin Mediated by Perlecan-NK4 Association. *Journal of Biological Chemistry*, 284: 22491-22499

Sattler, M., Pride, Y.B., Ma, P., Gramlich, J.L., Chu, S.C., Quinnan, L.A., Shirazian, S., Liang, C., Podar, K., Christensen, J.G. & Salgia, R. (2003) A novel small molecule met inhibitor induces apoptosis in cells transformed by the oncogenic TPR-MET tyrosine kinase. *Cancer Research*, 63: 5462-5469

Sattler, M. & Salgia, R. (2009) The MET axis as a therapeutic target. *Update Cancer Ther.*, 3: 109-118

Schiering, N., Knapp, S., Marconi, M., Flocco, M.M., Cui, J., Perego, R., Rusconi, L. & Cristiani, C. (2003) Crystal structure of the tyrosine kinase domain of the hepatocyte growth factor receptor c-Met and its complex with the microbial alkaloid K-252a. *Proceeding National Academy of Science USA*, 100: 12654-12659

Schmidt, C., Bladt, F., Goedecke, S., Brinkmann, V., Zschiesche, W., Sharpe, M., Gherardi, E. & Birchmeier, C. (1995) Scatter factor/hepatocyte growth factor is essential for liver development. *Nature*, 373: 699-702

Schmidt, L., Duh, F., Chan, F., Kishida, T., Glenn, G., Choyke, P., Scherer, S.W., Zhuang, Z., Lubensky, I., Dean, M., Allikmets, R., Chidambaram, A., Bergerheim, U.R., Feltis, J.T., Casadevall, C., Zamarron, A., Bernues, M., Richard, S., Lips, C.J.M., Walther, M.M., Tsui, L., Geil, L., Orcutt, M.L., Stackhouse, T., Lipan, J., Slife, L., Brauch, H., Decker, J., Niehans, G., Hughson, M.D., Moch, H., Storkel, S., Lerman, M.I., Linehan, W.M. & Zbar, B. (1997) Germline and somatic mutations in the tyrosine kinase domain of the MET proto-oncogene in papillary renal carcinomas. *Nature Genetics*, 16: 68-73

Schmidt, C. (2009) Why do tumors become resistant to antiangiogenesis drugs? *Journal of National Cancer Institute*, 101: 1530-1532

Schroeder, G.M., An, Y., Cai, Z.W., Chen, X.T., Clark, C., Cornelius, L.A., Dai, J., Gullo-Brown, J., Gupta, A., Henley, B., Hunt, J.T., Jeyaseelan, R., Kamath, A., Kim, K., Lippy, J., Lombardo, L.J., Manne, V., Oppenheimer, S., Sack, J.S., Schmidt, R.J., Shen, G., Stefanski, K., Tokarski, J.S., Trainor, G.L., Wautlet, B.S., Wei, D., Williams, D.K., Zhang, Y., Zhang, Y., Fargnoli, J. & Borzilleri, R.M. (2009) Discovery of N-(4-(2-Amino-3-chloropyridin-4-yloxy)-3-fluorophenyl)-4-ethoxy-1-(4-fluor ophenyl)-2-oxo-1,2-dihydropyridine-3-carboxamide (BMS-777607), a elective and orally efficacious inhibitor of the Met kinase superfamily. *Journal of Medicinal Chemistry*, 52: 1251-1254

Schwall, R.H., Chang, L.Y., Godowski, P.J., Kahn, D.W., Hillan, K.J., Bauer, K.D., Zioncheck, T.F. (1996) Heparin induces dimerization and confers proliferative activity onto the hepatocyte growth factor antagonists NK1 and NK2. *Journal of Cell Biology*, 133: 709-718

Shaw, A.T., Yeap, B.Y., Mino-Kenudson, M., Digumarthy, S.R., Costa, D.B., Heist, R.S., Solomon, B., Stubbs, H., Admane, S., McDermott, U., Settleman, J., Kobayashi, S., Mark, E.J., Rodig, S.J., Chirieac, L.R., Kwak, E.L., Lynch, T.J. & Iafrate, A.J. (2009) Clinical features and outcome of patients with non-small-cell lung cancer who harbor EML4-ALK. *Journal of Clinical Oncology*, 27: 4247-4253

Smolen, G.A., Sordella, R., Muir, B., Mohapatra, G., Barmettler, A., Archibald, H., Kim, W.J., Okimoto, R.A., Bell, D.W., Sgroi, D.C., Christensen, J.G., Settleman, J. & Haber, D.A. (2006) Amplification of MET may identify a subset of cancers with extreme sensitivity to the selective tyrosine kinase inhibitor PHA-665752. *Proceeding National Academy of Science USA*, 103: 2316- 2321

Stahl, S.J., Wingfield, P.T., Kaufman, J.D., Pannell, L.K., Cioce, V., Sakata, H., Taylor, W.G., Rubin, J.S. & Bottaro, D.P. (1997) Functional and biophysical characterization of recombinant human hepatocyte growth factor isoforms produced in Escherichia coli. *Biochemical Journal*, 326: 763-772

Stamos, J., Lazarus, R.A., Yao, X., Kirchhofer, D. & Wiesmann, C. (2004) Crystal structure of the HGF β-chain in complex with the Sema domain of the Met receptor. *EMBO Journal*, 23: 2325-2335

Stoker, M., Gherardi, E., Perryman, M. & Gray, J. (1987) Scatter factor is a fibroblast-derived modulator of epithelial cell mobility. *Nature*, 327: 239-242

Timofeevski, S.L., McTigue, M.A., Ryan, K., Cui, J., Zou, H.Y., Zhu, J.X., Chau, F., Alton, G., Karlicek, S., Christensen, J.G. & Murray, B.W. (2009) Enzymatic characterization of c-Met receptor tyrosine kinase oncogenic mutants and kinetic studies with aminopyridine and triazolopyrazine inhibitors. *Biochemistry*, 48: 5339-5349

Tolbert, W.D., Daugherty, J., Gao, C., Xie, Q., Miranti, C., Gherardi, E., Vande Woude, G. & Xu, H.E. (2007) A mechanistic basis for converting a receptor tyrosine kinase agonist to an antagonist. *Proceeding National Academy of Science USA,* 104: 14592-14597

Turke, A.B., Zejnullahu, K., Wu, Y.L., Song, Y., Dias-Santagata, D., Lifshits, E., Toschi, L., Rogers, A., Mok, T., Sequist, L., Lindeman, N.I., Murphy, C., Akhavanfard, S., Yeap, B.Y., Xiao, Y., Capelletti, M., Iafrate, A.J., Lee, C., Christensen, J.G., Engelman, J.A. & Jänne, P.A. (2010) Preexistence and clonal selection of MET amplification in EGFR mutant NSCLC. *Cancer Cell*, 17: 77-88

Uehara, Y., Minowa, O., Mori, C., Shiota, K., Kuno, J., Noda, T., Kitamura, N. (1995) Placental defect and embryonic lethality in mice lacking hepatocyte growth factor/scatter factor. *Nature,* 373: 702-705

Van der Horst, E.H., Chinn, L., Wang, M., Velilla, T., Tran, H., Madrona, Y., Lam, A., Ji, M., Hoey, T.C. & Sato, A.K. (2009) Discovery of fully human anti-MET monoclonal antibodies with antitumor activity against colon cancer tumor models in vivo. *Neoplasia*, 11: 355-364

Wang, W., Marimuthu, A., Tsai, J., Kumar, A., Krupka, H.I., Zhang, C., Powell, B., Suzuki, Y., Nguyen, H., Tabrizizad, M., Luu, C. & West, B.L. (2006) Structural characterization of autoinhibited c-Met kinase produced by coexpression in bacteria with phosphatase. *Proceeding National Academy of Science USA* 103: 3563-3568

Wang, W., Li, Q., Yamada, T., Matsumoto, K., Matsumoto, I., Oda, M., Watanabe, G., Nakamura, T., Nishioka, Y., Sone, S. & Yano, S. (2009) Crosstalk to stromal fibroblasts induces resistance of lung cancer to EGFR tyrosine kinase inhibitors. *Clinical Cancer Research*, 15; 6630-6638

Watanabe, K., Chirgadze, D.Y., Lietha, D., de Jonge, H., Blundell, T.L. & Gherardi, E. (2002) A new crystal form of the NK1 splice variant of HGF/SF demonstrates extensive hinge movement and suggests that the NK1 dimer originates by domain swapping. *Journal of Molecular Biology*, 319: 283-288

Weidner, K.M., Behrens, J., Vanderkerckhove, J. & Birchmeier, W. (1990) Scatter factor: molecular characteristics and effect on the invasiveness of epithelial cells. *Journal of Cell Biology*, 111: 2097-2108

Yano, S., Wang, W., Li, Q., Matsumoto, K., Sakurama, H., Nakamura, T., Ogino, H., Kakiuchi, S., Hanibuchi, M., Nishioka, Y., Uehara, H., Mitsudomi, T., Yatabe, Y., Nakamura, T. & Sone, S. (2008) Hepatocyte growth factor induces gefitinib resistance of lung adenocarcinoma with EGF Receptor activating mutations. *Cancer Research*, 68: 6479-6487

Yu, Y. & Merlino, G. (2002) Constitutive c-Met signaling through a nonautocrine mechanism promotes metastasis in a transgenic transplantation model. *Cancer Research*, 62: 2951-2956

15

# Nuclear Survivin: Cellular Consequences and Therapeutic Implications

Sally P. Wheatley
*School of Biomedical Sciences, University of Nottingham*
*UK*

## 1. Introduction

Survivin is a cancer associated protein that is present in all embryonic cells, but whose expression is normally limited to actively proliferating cells in adults. During mitosis it is part of a conserved complex of chromosomal passenger proteins (CPPs), which is essential for chromosome biorientation and cell division (Ruchaud et al., 2007). Defects in CPP function cause errors in mitosis and cytokinesis and can lead to genomic instability, or "aneuploidy", a status indicative of tumorigenesis. First discovered by Altieri and co-workers (Ambrosini et al., 1998), survivin is the fourth most upregulated mRNA in the cancer transcriptome (Velculescu et al., 1999), and in many tumours its expression is detected throughout the cell cycle. Importantly increased survivin abundance correlates with tumour resistance to conventional radiation and chemotherapies, a correlation recapitulated in cultured cells in the laboratory (Chakravarti et al., 2004; Colnaghi et al., 2006). While involvement in mitosis alone is a valid reason for considering a protein as a biomarker, or a target for cancer therapy, the oncotherapeutic potential of survivin is compounded by the fact that it is also an inhibitor of cell death (for review see Altieri, 2008). The principle aim of this article is to highlight the manifestations of survivin expression in the nucleus and to discuss how these might be exploited for oncotherapeutic gain.

## 2. Subcellular localisation of survivin as a prognostic marker in cancer

Numerous clinical studies have reported differential localisation of survivin in the cytoplasm, the nucleus, or both in tumours and have correlated this with disease severity and patient survival, with the aim to determine the prognostic value of its localisation retrospectively. However, despite the plethora of data collected, the prognostic significance of the subcellular distribution of survivin in cancer remains unclear. In 2005 a review of the subject returned a hung jury, revealing more opposing conclusions and contradictions than commonalities (Li et al., 2005); see also (Xie et al., 2006). As most of these clinical-based studies used histopathological samples, the lack of uniformity in sample collection and preservation between labs, together with differences in antibody protocols and the subjective nature of the analysis are likely to have contributed to the variation within these data (Li et al., 2005). Differences in data acquisition and interpretation aside, survivin localisation does vary between tumour types, and if one considers more detailed factors within specific types of cancer, such as its grade, stage of differentiation, and whether it is benign or malignant, this approach could yield fruitful predictions. Indeed, Gallagher, Duffy and co-workers have recently validated this approach in tumour microarrays of breast cancers, in which they have recorded not just the cytoplasmic and nuclear placement of survivin in tumours, but the ratio between their distributions. Their automated analysis clearly removes the subjectivity of the interpreter, and also permits its application to high through-put screening (Brennan et al., 2008; Rexhepaj et al., 2010). In summary, while survivin's subcellular localisation may have prognostic value across a wide spectrum of tumours, correlating its distribution, or the ratio of its distribution with disease outcome within specific tumour types may be more effective.

## 3. Active export keeps survivin out of the nucleus

In an attempt to determine the biological significance of cytoplasmic versus nuclear localisation of survivin, and prompted by the ongoing debate regarding its prognostic potential in cancer, we (Colnaghi et al., 2006), and others (Knauer et al., 2007) began to investigate and manipulate survivin distribution in controlled conditions in the lab. These data have led to the widely accepted view that survivin is predominantly cytoplasmic in interphase cells (Figure 1A), gaining access to the nucleus in G2, in readiness for mitosis. While this is consistent with the cell cycle regulation of survivin transcription, it is in fact an oversimplification. One notable exception is exemplified by Temme and coworkers (2005), who reported that in exponentially growing normal human lung fibroblasts endogenous survivin is predominantly nuclear throughout the cell cycle. Interestingly they found that survivin localisation was age dependent, with cells from an early passage exhibiting strong nuclear accumulation, while cells of late passage (>16) displaying mostly cytoplasmic survivin. In full corroboration with other reports, survivin expression was absent from confluent G0 monolayers of these cells (Temme et al., 2005). Moreover, other groups have indicated that survivin can enter the nucleus as early as S-phase (Beardmore et al., 2004; Suzuki et al., 2000). These observations highlight the fact that multiple parameters including cell type, senescence and growth conditions can impact on survivin localisation, and suggest that many pathways contribute to its whereabouts both spatially and temporally. Indeed many subcellular pools of survivin exist, including an important fraction within the mitochondria (Dohi et al., 2007; Fortugno et al., 2002), and several groups have hypothesised that these separate pools correspond to the distinct functions of this "nodal" protein, see review by Altieri, 2008.

The first evidence that survivin actively shuttles between cytoplasmic and nuclear compartments, came from the work of Rodgriguez and coworkers, who used the fungal toxin leptomycin B (LMB) to demonstrate that its cytoplasmic localisation was maintained by CRM1/exportin- mediated transport, stimulated by Ran-GTP (Rodriguez et al., 2002). Using site-directed mutagenesis we (Colnaghi et al., 2006), and others (Knauer et al., 2007), identified a leucine-rich region in the central "linker" region of survivin between the BIR (baculovirus inhibitor of apoptosis repeat) domain, and its alpha-helical C-terminus as a nuclear export sequence (NES). Although clearly positioned within the central linker domain, estimations of the precise residues involved, 89-98 and 96-106, did not fully agree. Within a classic NES hydrophobic leucines are key as they are responsible for interaction with the CRM1 (exportin) via Ran-GTP, and despite the difference between our proposed sequences, there was consensus that both encompassed L96 and L98, with the sequence

proposed by (Knauer et al., 2007), more efficient at binding CRM1. Given the variance in the above studies and the proximity of the proposed NES to its homodimerisation interface (Verdecia et al., 2000), Engelsma et al., (2007) investigated this region in more detail. They proposed that residues 84-109, shown in red on the crystal structures in Figure 2, constitute a more complete sequence for the central NES. Furthermore, by mutating F101 and L102 to inhibit homodimerisation, they found that survivin was more efficiently removed from the nucleus than the wild type form, suggesting that monomeric survivin is more efficiently exported than homodimeric survivin. These authors further reported a second, unconventional NES present in the C-terminus of survivin, depicted in orange in Figure 2, and spanning the alpha-helix from residue 119 to its end (Engelsma et al., 2007; Rodriguez et al., 2002). Presumably this second NES would be operative in both monomers and dimers, and would act to further ensure survivin removal from the nucleus.
Trafficking of survivin between the nucleus and cytoplasm is also susceptible to regulation by post-translational modifications, including acetylation and phosphorylation. Survivin acetylation, which occurs at K129, and is facilitated by the acetyl transferase CREB-binding protein (CBP), has been implicated in aiding survivin transit out of the nucleus (Wang et al., 2010), presumably by affecting the activity of the C-terminal NES (Engelsma et al., 2007). Glucogen synthase kinase 3β (GSK3β) facilitates translocation of survivin into the nucleus, but whether phosphorylation of survivin by GSK3β is involved is not yet known (Li et al., 2008). Work from my lab has recently provided two lines of evidence that suggest that casein kinase 2 (CK2) phosphorylation helps to maintain survivin within the cytoplasm, as treatment with the CK2 specific inhibitor, TBB (4,5,6,7-tetrabromobenzotriazole), or mutation of threonine 48 (T48), the unique site targeted by CK2 in survivin, causes its accumulation in the nucleus (Barrett et al., 2011). This latter observation is curious because T48 lies in the BIR domain of survivin, which is from distinct from either NES, and would not affect binding to CRM1. Perhaps CK2 affects survivin import or its stability?

## 4. Getting into the nucleus

The molecular weight cut off for passive import across the nuclear membrane is approximately 45kD, thus at 16.5 kD survivin is sufficiently small to access the nucleus by passive diffusion even as a homodimer, or as a monomer tagged with a large fluorescent moiety such as green fluorescent protein, GFP (27kD). Whether an active component contributes to its import is unclear, but is supported by the observation that transit from the cytoplasm to the nucleus is abrogated when cells are chilled (Rodriguez et al., 2002), and would have the potential for its regulation, as suggested above for CK2, which could be exploited under challenging or stressful conditions. As survivin itself has no recognisable nuclear localisation signal (NLS) of its own, to facilitate nuclear entry survivin would presumably require a chaperone. While its mitotic partners, borealin, inner centromeric protein (INCENP) and aurora-B all have one or more NLS, co-expression analysis demonstrated that none of them can coerce survivin into the nucleus, instead, when co-expressed with borealin, borealin no longer localises to the nucleoli but is forced to relocate to the cytoplasm (Rodriguez et al., 2006). This is somewhat surprising given that borealin interacts with survivin at its homodimerisation interface and could potentially mask part of the central NES (Figure 2B), nevertheless, it points to the subtleties lying within the structure of this tiny protein. As mentioned above redistribution of survivin into the nucleus is promoted by activation of GSK3B, and although it is not yet known whether survivin is a substrate of this kinase, GSK3B can bind survivin directly and has a bipartite NLS (Li et al., 2008).

## 5. Isoforms

In addition to "wild type" survivin, alias survivin-alpha/BIRC5, several splice variants exist. The two most extensively studied are alternatively spliced at the exon 2-intron border, which generates the variants, survivin 2B, with an additional 23 aa after exon 2, and delta exon 3 (DeX3) which incurs a frame shift that results in a completely distinct C-terminal sequence (Mahotka et al., 2002; Mahotka et al., 1999). We, and others, have shown that consistent with the central positioning of the NES, 2B retains this sequence and is predominantly cytoplasmic when ectopically expressed in cultured cells, while DeX3 is nuclear, not only because it lacks the two NES sequences, but because it has its own, functional NLS in its C-terminus (Mahotka et al., 2002; Noton et al., 2006; Rodriguez et al., 2002). As for the nuclear-cytoplasmic debate, the prognostic importance of the expression of these forms is also a matter of controversy, and there are many reports correlating the expression of transcripts of these variants and localisation of their gene products with disease severity, most recently (Antonacopoulou et al., 2011) and (Takeno et al., 2010).

## 6. Consequence of nuclear residence

To determine the consequences of expressing survivin in the nucleus we fused survivin cDNA to an NLS and transfected it into cultured human cells (Colnaghi et al., 2006; Connell et al., 2008a). Upon expression we noted the abundance of NLS-survivin was significantly reduced compared with wild type survivin, present in the cytoplasm. Moreover the levels of survivin-NLS in the nuclear fraction could be restored by treatment with the proteasome inhibitor, MG132, or siRNA mediated depletion of the APC/C activator cdh1. From our data we concluded that coercing survivin into the nucleus facilitated its removal from the cell in a 26S-proteasome/cdh1 dependent manner (Connell et al., 2008a). Hence, in addition to import-export dynamics, stability is another key determinant of intranuclear localisation of survivin.

But why is it so important to keep survivin out of the nucleus? From our data on the accelerated clearance of NLS-survivin, and the presence of two NES sequences, it is clear that the cell has put in place multiple measures to eliminate survivin from the nucleus, so what are the consequences of its presence should it become resident there? In an early study by Suzuki and co-workers (2000) it was noted that upon release from serum starvation ectopically expressed survivin accumulated in the nucleus of human hepatoma cells. Interestingly they found that translocation of survivin to the nucleus coincided with an S-phase shift. At the molecular level they explained this precocious entry into S-phase as a downstream consequence of a direct interaction between survivin and cdk4. In essence, upon binding to cdk4 survivin competitively inhibits the interaction between cdk4 and $p16^{INKa}$, cdk4's natural inhibitor, allowing cdk4 to activate cdk2/cyclin E, which in turn hyperphosphorylates pRB derepressing transcription, and promotes passage through the G1 restriction point (Suzuki et al., 2000). Survivin-induced S-phase promotion has also been noted in breast cancer cells, T-lymphocytes, and haemopoietic cells, reviewed in (Fukuda and Pelus, 2006). Thus one manifestation of nuclear residence is accelerated entry into the cell cycle.

A second consequence of nuclear residence of survivin is the loss of its cytoprotective activity. Converging data from analysis of NES mutants (Colnaghi et al., 2006), NLS fusions (Connell et al., 2008a), LMB treatment (Knauer et al., 2007), GSK3β-activated cells (Li et al., 2008), and the response of cells in which nuclear survivin naturally occurs (Temme et al., 2007), have clearly demonstrated that nuclear survivin can no longer inhibit cell death, invoked by either the intrinsic or extrinsic apoptotic pathways. An apparent paradox here is that while cytoplasmic localisation of survivin is a requirement for it to protect cells from irradiation (IR), irradiation itself induces translocation of survivin to the nucleus (Chakravarti et al., 2004). In our hands, IR induces nuclear foci of survivin, which form as early as 60 minutes post-IR and can persist for many hours (Figure 1B), although a more dynamic response has been noted by others (Capalbo et al., 2010). This paradox, however, may be explained in part by data from Chan et al., (2010) who recently reported that during early stages of cell death, the CRM1/exportin pathway collapses. Although in their case retention of survivin in the nucleus as a result of compromised export, resulted in its rapid Ub-proteasome dependent rapid clearance (Chan et al., 2010), it is formally possible that failed export contributes to an initial sequestration of survivin in the nucleus, which may be followed by an altered rate of turnover, and eventually focus formation. Another plausible explanation for these data may be that the cells are arresting in G2 in response to DNA damage and that this is a time when survivin normally enters the nucleus in preparation for mitosis. Whatever the means by which these foci form have been shown to colocalise with the DNA damage marker, gamma-H2AX, and the DNA repair proteins, DNA-PK and Ku70 (Capalbo et al., 2010). Moreover, survivin translocation may be effected by the downstream chk1 and chk2 effector kinases, which respond to the PIK-family of kinases, ATR and ATM respectively, both pivotal upstream kinases in the DNA damage-repair pathways, and DNA-PK knock out cells accumulate nuclear survivin after UV irradiation (Asumen et al., 2010). Consistent with this, we identified DNA-PK and Ku70 as potential partners by Mass Spec analysis of in survivin co-immunoprecipitating proteins post-X-irradiation (Connell and Wheatley, unpublished), and similar data was published by (Capalbo et al., 2010). Whether survivin then aids in DNA repair per se remains to be determined, but early work from (Chakravarti et al., 2004) reported fewer comet tails post-IR in glioblastoma cell lines expressing survivin compared with control cells, indicating either less damage sustained or more efficient repair of DNA strand breaks.

Finally, could expression of survivin in the nucleus interfere with the cell's transcriptional programme? Although survivin has a zinc finger in its BIR domain, this fold is distinct from zinc rich domains found in many TFs, and accordingly survivin itself cannot bind directly to DNA(Klein et al., 2006). However, it has been suggested that survivin suppresses the cytokine activated transcription factor, STAT3, and that this association may be regulated acetylation of survivin at lysine, K129, in the carboxyl alpha helix (Wang et al., 2010). Although the consequences of this interaction are not clear at present, it is nevertheless intriguing that this could be one reason to eliminate survivin from the nucleus. In this regard it is important to note that significant new insight in the mitosis field has revealed that survivin interacts directly with the $NH_2$ tail of histone H3, which protrudes from the nucleosome, and that this interaction is dependent upon phosphorylation of threonine 3 in histone H3's (Kelly et al., 2010; Wang et al., 2010). As this phosphorylation event is placed by the mitosis specific kinase, haspin, it is unclear whether such an interaction could occur in non-mitotic cells, however, indirect interactions in addition to direct binding between survivin and H2A also facilitates chromatin association (Kelly et al., 2010; Yamagishi et al., 2010), and borealin has been demonstrated to bind dsDNA directly in vitro (Klein et al., 2006). Hence, although not a transcription factor itself, it is indeed plausible that survivin could indirectly modulate transcription.

## 7. Clinical implications

Despite its clear importance in cancer, strategies targeting survivin for oncotherapeutic gain have been rather elusive. The question posed here is whether "nuclear survivin" offers a unique therapeutic window? Now that it has been established that nuclear export is essential for activity of survivin as a tumour promoter, one possibility proposed by Stauber and colleagues, is the development of molecular decoys that interfere with its export by antagonising the NES(s). Potentially this strategy could be used to eliminate survivin and (re)sensitise tumours to current cancer therapies (Knauer et al., 2007; Stauber et al., 2007). Intriguingly in 2005, Otto and co-workers used a HLA-A2 restricted survivin peptide to vaccinate patients with advanced, stage IV melanoma. Serendipitously, the epitope selected was a peptide within the central NES of survivin, 96-104 (Colnaghi et al., 2006). Whether this peptide interfered with nuclear exportation of survivin in vivo was not addressed, but the treatment was well tolerated by patients and importantly it enhanced tumour cell apoptosis and caused regression of metastatic lesions (Otto et al., 2005).

We have taken a different angle, endeavouring to exploit the ability of survivin to accelerate cells into S-phase for therapeutic gain (Suzuki et al., 2000). In brief we infected cells with oncolytic viruses engineered to reproduce only in cells with a defective pRB pathway, in this case ovarian cancer cells. As viruses reproduce in S-phase of the host cell cycle, when we compared efficacy of cell lysis post-infection between control and survivin-NLS expressing cells, a marked increase in cytotoxicity was observed, suggesting that nuclear survivin expression synergised with oncolytic virus potency, to effectively eliminate cancer cells (Connell et al., 2008b). These data from cultured cells are promising, and given that survivin is an essential protein it is likely that its oncotherapeutic potential will be realised in combination strategies like this, rather than as a target for a single agent.

## 8. Concluding remarks

Survivin is a prosurvival factor that can promote S-phase entry; is essential for mitosis; whose presence renders cells resistant to apoptosis; and that is expressed at high levels almost universally in tumours. As a disease of inappropriate cell growth, cancer may arise through deregulated proliferation or failure to die in response to death inducing stimuli, and the success of therapeutic interventions is likely to be a case of tipping the balance between prosurvival and proapoptotic factors. For all these reasons the case for survivin as a novel anti-cancer target is compelling. The ability to dissect the pleiotropic functions of the protein apart by changes in its subcellular distribution may provide opportunities for therapeutic intervention and tailored targeting strategies.

## 9. Acknowledgements

Molecular structures were drawn using the UCSF Chimera package (www.cgl. ucsf.edu/chimera, (Pettersen et al., 2004).

## 10. References

Ambrosini, G., C. Adida, G. Sirugo, and D.C. Altieri. 1998. Induction of apoptosis and inhibition of cell proliferation by survivin gene targeting. *J. Biological Chemistry.* 273:11177-11182.

Antonacopoulou, A.G., K. Floratou, V. Bravou, A. Kottorou, F.-I. Dimitrakopoulos, S. Marousi, M. Stavropoulos, A.K. Koutras, C.D. Scopa, and H.P. Kalofonos. 2011. The survivin -31 snp in human colorectal cancer correlates with survivin splice variant expression and improved overall survival. *Cell Oncology.* epub 3rd May 2011.

Asumen, M.G., T.V. Ifeacho, L. Cockerham, C. Pfandl, and N.R. Wall. 2010. Dynamic changes to survivin subcellular localization are initiated by DNA damage. *OncoTargets and Therapy.* 3:129-137.

Barrett, R.M.A., R. Colanghi, and S.P. Wheatley. 2011. Threonine 48 in the BIR domain of survivin is critical to its mitotic and anti-apoptotic activities and can be phosphorylated by CK2 in vitro. *Cell Cycle* 10:538-548.

Beardmore, V.A., L.J. Ahonen, G.J. Gorbsky, and M.J. Kallio. 2004. Survivin dynamics increases at centromeres during G2/M phase transition and is regulated by microtubule-attachment and Aurora B kinase activity. *Journal Cell Sci.* 117:4033-4042.

Brennan, D.J., E. Rexhepaj, S.L. O'Brien, E.M. McSherry, D.P. O'Connor, A. Fagan, A.C. Culhane, D.G. Higgins, K. Jirstrom, R.C. Millikan, G. Landberg, M.J. Duffy, S.M. Hewitt, and W.M. Gallagher. 2008. Altered cytoplasmic-to-nuclear ratio of survivin is a prognostic indicator in breast cancer. . *Clinical Cancer Research* 14:2681-2689.

Capalbo, G., K. Dittman, C. Weiss, S. Reichert, E. Hausmann, C. Rodel, and F. Rodel. 2010. Radiation-induced survivin nuclear accumulation is linked to DNA damage repair. *Int. J. Radiat. Onc. Biol. Phys.* . 77:226-234.

Chakravarti, A., G.G. Zhai, M. Zhang, R. Malhotra, D.E. Lathman, M.A. Delaney, P. Robe, U. Nestler, Q. Song, and J. Loeffler. 2004. Survivin enhances radiation resistance in primary human glioblastoma cells via caspase-independent mechanisms. *Oncogene.* 23:7494-7506.

Chan, K.-S., C.-H. Wong, Y.-F. Huang, and H.-L. Li. 2010. Survivin withdrawal by nuclear export failure as a physiological switch to commit cells to apoptosis. *Cell Death and Disease.* epub.

Colnaghi, R., C.M. Connell, R.M.A. Barrett, and S.P. Wheatley. 2006. Separating the anti-apoptotic and mitotic roles of survivin. *J. Biological Chemistry.* 281:33450-33456.

Connell, C.M., R. Colnaghi, and S.P. Wheatley. 2008a. Nuclear survivin has reduced stability and is not cytoprotective. *J. Biological Chemistry.* 238:3289-96.

Connell, C.M., S.P. Wheatley, and I.A. McNeish. 2008b. Nuclear survivin abrogates multiple cell cycle checkpoints and enhances virus oncolysis. *Cancer Research.* 68:7923-7931.

Dohi, T., F. Xia, and D.C. Altieri. 2007. Compartmentalized phosphorylation of IAP by protein kinase A regulates cytoprotection. *Molecular Cell.* 27:17-28.

Engelsma, D., J.A. Rodriguez, A. Fish, G. Giaccone, and M. Fornerod. 2007. Homodimerization antagonizes nuclear export of survivin. *Traffic.* 11:1495-1502.

Fortugno, P., N.R. Wall, A. Giodini, D.S. O'Connor, J. Plescia, K.M. Padgett, S. Tognin, P.C. Marchisio, and D.C. Altieri. 2002. Survivin exists in immunochemically distinct subcellular pools and is involved in spindle microtubule function. *J.Cell Sci.* 115:575-585.

Fukuda, M., and L.M. Pelus. 2006. Survivin, a cancer target with an emerging role in normal adult tissues. *Mol. Cancer Therapy.* 5:1087-1098.

Kelly, A.E., C. Ghenoiu, J.Z. Xue, C. Zierhut, H. Kimura, and H. Funabiki. 2010. Survivin Reads Phosphorylated Histone H3 Threonine 3 to Activate the Mitotic Kinase Aurora B. *Science.* 330:235-239.

Klein, U.R., E.A. Nigg, and U. Gruneberg. 2006. Centromere targeting of the chromosomal passenger complex requires a ternary subcomplex of borealin, survivin, and the N-terminal domain of INCENP. *Mol. Biol. Cell.* 17:2547-2558.

Knauer, S.K., O.H. Kramer, T. Knosel, K. Engels, F. Rodel, K. A.F., W. Dietmaier, K.-H. L., N. Habtemichael, A. Schweitzer, J. Brieger, C. Rodel, W. Mann, I. Petersen, T. Heinzel, and R.H. Stauber. 2007. Nuclear export is essential for the tumour-promoting activity of survivin. *FASEB J.* 21:207-216.

Li, F., J. Yang, N. Ramnath, M.M. Javle, and D. Tan. 2005. Nuclear or cytoplasmic expression of survivin: What is the significance? *Int. J. Cancer.* 114:509-512.

Li, J., M. Xing, M. Zhu, X.C. Wang, M. Wang, S. Zhou, N. Li, R. Wu, and M. Zhou. 2008. Glycogen synthase kinase 3 beta induces apoptosis in cancer cells through increase in survivin nuclear localization. . *Cancer Letters.* 272:91-101.

Mahotka, C., J. Liebmann, M. Wenzel, C.V. Suschek, M. Schmitt, H.E. Gabbert, and C.D. Gerharz. 2002. Differential subcellular localization of functionally divergent survivin splice variants. *Cell Death Differ.* 9:1334-1342.

Mahotka, C., M. Wenzel, E. Springer, H.E. Gabbert, and C.D. Gerharz. 1999. Survivin-{{Delta}}Ex3 and Survivin-2B: two novel splice variants of the apoptosis inhibitor survivin with different antiapoptotic properties. *Cancer Res.* 59:6097-6102.

Noton, E.A., R. Colnaghi, S. Tate, C. Starck, A. Carvalho, P.K. Ferrigno, and S.P. Wheatley. 2006. Molecular analysis of survivin isoforms: evidence that alternatively spliced variants do not play a role in mitosis. *J. Biological Chemistry.* 281:1286-1295.

Otto, K., M.H. Andersen, A. Eggert, P. Keikavoussi, L.O. Pedersen, J.C. Rath, M. Bock, E.-B. Brocker, P. Strathen, E. Kampgen, and J.C. Becker. 2005. Lack of taxocity of therapy-induced T cell responses against the universal tumour antigen survivin. *Vaccine.* 23:884-889.

Pettersen, E.F., T.D. Goddard, C.C. Huang, G.S. Couch, D.M. Greenblatt, E.C. Meng, and T.E. Ferrin. 2004. A visualization system for exploratory research and analysis. *J. Comput.Chem.* 25:1605-1612.

Rexhepaj, E., K. Jirstrom, D.P. O'Connor, S.L. O'Brien, G. Landberg, M.J. Duffy, D.J. Brennan, and W.M. Gallagher. 2010. Validation of cytoplasmic-to-nuclear ratio of survivin as an indicator of improved prognosis in breast cancer. *BMC Cancer.* 10:639-651.

Rodriguez, J.A., S.M.A. Lens, S.W. Span, G. Vader, R.H. Medema, F.A.E. Kruyt, and G. Giaccone. 2006. Subcellular localization and nucleocytoplasmic transport of the chromosomal passenger proteins before nuclear envelope breakdown. *Oncogene.* 25:4867-4879.

Rodriguez, J.A., S.W. Span, C.G.M. Ferreira, F.A.E. Kruyt, and G. Giaccone. 2002. CRM1-mediated nuclear export determines the cytoplasmic localisation of the antiapoptotic protein survivin. *Experimental Cell Research.* 275:44-53.

Ruchaud, S., M. Carmena, and W.C. Earnshaw. 2007. Chromosomal passengers: conducting cell division. *Nature Reviews in Molecular Cell Biology.* 8:798-812.

Stauber, R.H., W. Mann, and S.K. Knauer. 2007. Nuclear and cytoplasmic survivin: molecular mechanism, prognostic, and therapeutic potential. *Cancer Research.* 67:5999-6002.

Suzuki, A., M. Hayashida, T. Ito, H. Kawano, T. Nakano, M. Miura, K. Akahane, and K. Shiraki. 2000. Survivin initiates cell cycle entry by the competitive interaction with Cdk4/p16$^{INK4a}$ and Cdk2/Cyclin E complex activation. *Oncogene.* 19:3225-3234.

Takeno, S., S.-i. Yamashita, Y. Takahashi, K. Ono, M. Kamei, T. Moroga, and K. Kawahara. 2010. Survivin expression in oesophageal squamous cell carcinoma: its prognostic impact and splice variant expression. *European Journal of Cardiac-Thoracic Surgery.* 37:440-445.

Temme, A., P. Diestelkoetter-Bachert, M. Schmitz, A. Morgenroth, B. Weigle, M.A. Rieger, A. Kiessling, and E.P. Rieber. 2005. Increased p21ras activity in human fibroblasts transduced with survivin enhances cell proliferation. *Biochem. Biophys. Res. Comm.* 327:765-773.

Velculescu, V.E., S.L. Madden, L. Zhang, A.E. Lash, J. Yu, C. Rago, A. Lal, C.J. Wang, G.A. Beaudry, K.M. Ciriello, B.P. Cook, M.R. Dufault, A.T. Ferguson, Y. Gao, T.-C. He, H. Hermeking, S.K. Hiraldo, P.M. Hwang, M.A. Lopez, H.F. Luderer, B. Mathews, J.M. Petroziello, K. Polyak, L. Zawel, W. Zhang, X. Zhang, W. Zhou, F.G. Haluska, J. Jen, S. Sukumar, G.M. Landes, G.J. Riggins, B. Vogelstein, and K.W. Kinzler. 1999. Analysis of human transcriptomes. *Nature Genetics.* 23:387-388.

Verdecia, M.A., H. Huang, E. Dutil, D.A. Kaiser, T. Hunter, and J.P. Noel. 2000. Structure of the human anti-apoptotic protein survivin reveals a dimeric arrangement. *Nat Struct Biol.* 7:602-8.

Wang, H.J., M.P. Holloway, L. Ma, Z.A. Cooper, M. Riolo, A. Samkari, K.S.J. Elenitoba-Johnson, Y.E. Chin, and R.A. Altura. 2010. Acetylation directs survivin nuclear localization to repress STAT3 oncogenic activity. *J. Biol. Chem.* 285:36129-36137.

Xie, D., Y.X. Zeng, H.J. Wang, J.M. Wen, Y. Tao, J.S.T. Sham, and X.Y. Guan. 2006. Expression of cytoplasmic and nuclear survivin in primary and secondary human glioblastoma. *British J. of Cancer*. 94:108-114.

Yamagishi, Y., T. Honda, Y. Tanno, and Y. Watanabe. 2010. Two histone marks establish the inner centromere and chromosome bi-orientation. *Science*. 330:239-243.

# Part 3

## Promising Anticancer Plants

# 16

# Anticancer Properties of Curcumin

Varisa Pongrakhananon[1,2] and Yon Rojanasakul[2]
[1]*Chulalongkorn University, Department of Pharmacology and Physiology*
*Faculty of Pharmaceutical Sciences, Bangkok,*
[2]*West Virginia University*
*Department of Basic Pharmaceutical Sciences, Morgantown, West Virginia*
[1]*Thailand*
[2]*USA*

## 1. Introduction

Curcumin is a major biological active compound from turmeric or *Curcuma longa*. This non-toxic natural compound has been reported to possess several biological activities that are therapeutically beneficial to cancer treatment. It has been reported to increase the efficacy of other chemotherapeutic agents and to reduce their toxic side effects which are the major drawback of most chemotherapeutic agents. Curcumin is also well known for its anti-inflammatory activity (Amanda and Robert, 2008). Since cancer often develops under chronic inflammatory conditions, curcumin has the potential to be a preventive treatment agent against cancer. Furthermore, unlike most chemotherapeutic agents which act on a specific process of cancer development, i.e., cell growth or apoptosis, curcumin exerts its effect on various stages of cancer development, i.e., oncogene activation (Singh and Singh, 2009), cancer cell proliferation (Simon et al., 1998), apoptosis evasion (Han et al., 1999), anoikis resistance (Pongrakhananon et al., 2010), and metastasis (Chen et al., 2008) (Figure 1). Therefore, curcumin has the potential to overcome chemoresistance which is a major problem in cancer chemotherapy. This chapter will provide an overview of the anticancer activities of curcumin and present pre-clinical and clinical evidence supporting the use of curcumin as an anticancer agent.

Cancer is known to be associated with genetic instability in which *c-myc* serves as a major modifier of many targeted genes (Mai and Mushinski, 2003). Likewise, the mutation of proto-oncogene *ras* has been identified in many types of tumor (Rajalingam et al., 2007). The dysregulation of these oncogenes is well recognized as an initial step in the development of tumorigenesis. Interestingly, curcumin has been reported to have a suppressive effect on the oncogenes and inhibit their downstream effectors such as cell cycle promoting and proapoptotic proteins (Singh and Singh, 2009). Curcumin also exhibits anticancer properties through its ability to inhibit cell proliferation and induce apoptosis. The anti-proliferative effect of curcumin is dependent on its concentration, duration of treatment, and specific cell type. At low doses, curcumin causes cell cycle arrest, while at higher doses it induces apoptosis. Cell proliferation is controlled by several cell cycle regulating proteins, notably the family of cyclin and cyclin-dependent kinases (Kastan and Bartek, 2004) whose expression is tightly associated with tumorigenesis (Diehl, 2002). Curcumin inhibits cell cycle progression by downregulating cyclin D1 and the transition from G1 to S phase in human head and neck squamous carcinoma cells (Aggarwal et al., 2004). It also inhibits bladder cancer cell proliferation through the downregulation of cyclin A and upregulation of p21 (Park et al., 2006).

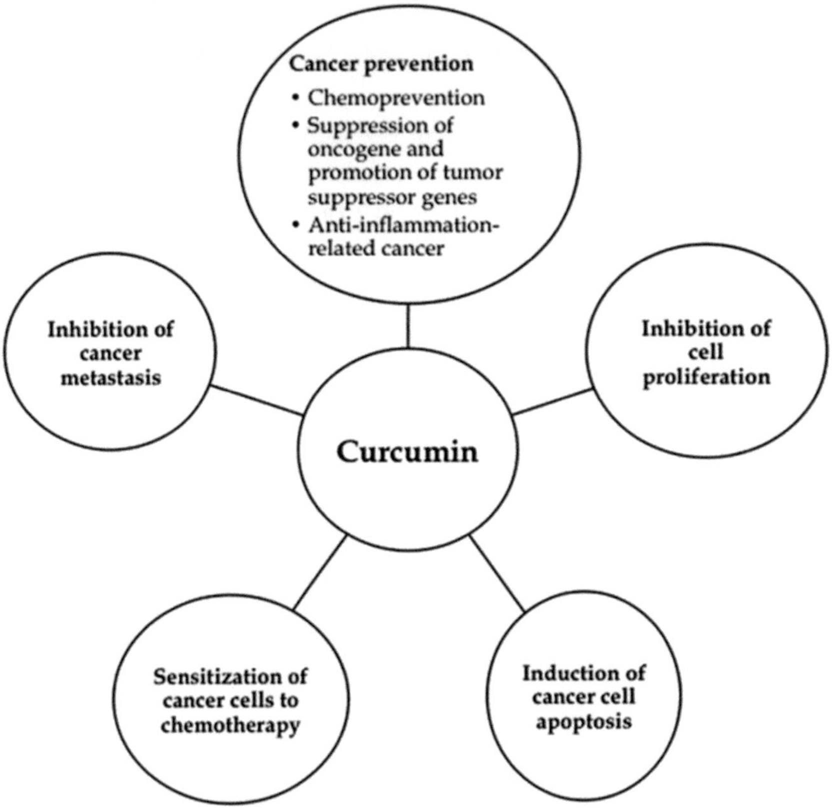


Fig. 1. Anticancer properties of curcumin

Curcumin possesses apoptosis-inducing activity causing cancer cell death primarily through the mitochondrial death pathway. It induces an upregulation of the proapoptotic protein Bax and downregulation of the antiapoptotic protein Bcl-2 in breast cancer cells (Chiu and Su, 2009), resulting in the loss of mitochondrial function, release of cytochrome c, and activation of caspase-9 and -3 (Chen et al., 2010). Curcumin also potentiates the cytotoxic effect of chemotherapeutic agents such as cisplatin (Chanvorachote et al., 2009), doxorubicin (Notarbartolo et al., 2005), tamoxifen (Chuang et al., 2002), and placitaxel (Genta and Amiji, 2009). The use of curcumin as a chemo-sensitizing agent in combination therapy has the potential to overcome chemoresistance which is common in advance staged cancers and is a major cause of cancer-related death.

An increasing number of reports have described the inhibitory effect of curcumin on cancer metastasis. Metastasis is a multi-step process involving tumor vascularization, cancer cell detachment, avoidance of anoikis, and increased cell invasion. The vascularization induced by tumor is an essential step providing nutrients, oxygen, and removing waste products for tumor growth and metastasis. A key mechanism that cancer cells utilize during metastasis is the acquisition of anoikis resistance. Anoikis or detachment-induced apoptosis is recognized as an important mechanism preventing cancer cell dissemination and invasion to form

secondary tumors. A recent study by our group has shown that curcumin is able to sensitize lung cancer cells to undergo anoikis through a mechanism that involves post-translational modification of Bcl-2 via the ubiquitin-proteasome pathway (Pongrakhananon et al., 2010). Curcumin also acts as a negative regulator of cancer cell migration and invasion through diverse signaling pathways including MMP-9, MMP-2 and COX-2 (Philip et al., 2004, Lee et al., 2005; Hong et al., 2006; Lin et al., 2009).
Animal and clinical studies of curcumin have been well investigated. In mice, curcumin markedly inhibits DMBA and TPA-induced skin tumor formation (Azuine et al., 1992). In a xenograft model, curcumin administration significantly decreases the incidence of breast cancer metastasis to the lung (Aggarwal et al., 2005). In phase 1 clinical studies, oral administration of curcumin was shown to be well tolerated with no dose-limiting toxicity (Sharma et al., 2004; Lao et al., 2006). In patients with intestinal metaplasia, curcumin treatment showed a significant improvement in the precancerous lesion (Cheng et al., 2001), supporting the clinical use of curcumin as a preventive treatment agent against cancer. Although curcumin has demonstrated promising pharmacological effects and safety both *in vitro* and *in vivo*, poor bioavailability and tissue accumulation have been observed with the compound. Further studies on proper drug delivery, dose optimization, and biodistribution are needed.

## 2. Chemistry of curcumin

For thousands of years, plants and some parts of animal have been used as dietary agents which have been identified to be biologically active. These natural compounds have gained considerable interest for their potential as treatment and preventive agents for human diseases. Curcumin (diferuloylmethane) is a major biologically active compound extracted from the dried rhizome of turmeric or *Curcuma longa*. It has been widely used for centuries as medicinal plant and food additive due to its yellow color. Its medicinal properties are attributed to curcuminoids, which include curcumin (curcumin I), demethoxycurcumin (curcumin II), and bisdemethoxycurcumin (curcumin III) (Figure 2). Curcumin I (77%) is a

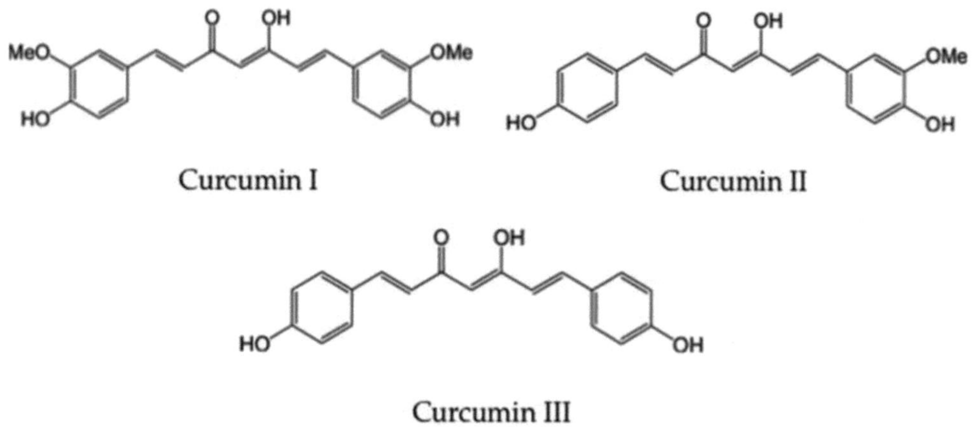


Fig. 2. Chemical structure of curcuminoids

major component found in commercial curcumin, while curcumin II and III constitute approximately 17% and 3% respectively. Cucumin is a water-insoluble compound, but dissolves well in ethanol, dimethylsulfoxide, and other organic solvents. The molecular weight of curcumin is 368.37 and melting point is 183 °C. It shows a spectrophotometric maximum absorption (λmax) at 450 nm in methanol (Prasad and Sarasija, 1997). Fluorescence of curcumin occurs at 524 nm in acetonitrile and 549 nm in ethanol (Chignell et al., 1994). Curcumin undergoes rapid degradation in phosphate buffer and serum-free media, i.e., 90% within 30 minutes (Wang et al., 1997). In serum-containing (10%) media and human blood, curcumin is more stable with less than 20% degradation in 1 hour, and about 50% after 8 hours. Its degradation products are *trans*-6-(4'-hydroxy-3'-methoxyphenyl)-2,4-dioxo-5-hexenal (major) and vanillin, ferulic acid, and feruloyl methane (minor) (Wang et al., 1997).

## 3. Anticancer properties of curcumin

Curcumin has long been used as a dietary ingredient with known health benefits. Extensive research over the last decade has shown that curcumin possesses anticancer activities and could be used as a preventive or treatment agent against cancers, either as a single or combination therapy with chemotherapeutic agents. Curcumin exhibits biological activities in various stages of carcinogenesis including inhibition of oncogene activation, prevention of cancer-related inflammation, inhibition of cancer cell proliferation, induction of apoptosis and anoikis, prevention of metastasis, and sensitization of cancer cells to chemotherapy.

### 3.1 Cancer prevention

#### 3.1.1 Chemopreventive properties

Carcinogenesis is a multistep process driven by genetic instability. Continuous exposure to environmental and endogenous genotoxic agents can cause substantial DNA damage. The damaged molecules can be transmitted during cell division producing mutated clones that can give rise to the expansion of premalignant cell population possessing uncontrolled proliferative and invasive properties. Curcumin has been established as a chemopreventive agent that has the ability to suppress or retard the carcinogenic process induced by various chemical carcinogens (Table 1). In animal models of gastric and colon cancer, curcumin inhibits the development of cancerous and precancerous lesions induced by N-methyl-N'-nitro-N-nitrosoguanosine (MNNG), a known mutagenic agent causing DNA methylation (Ikesaka et al., 2001). In the study, MNNG was given in drinking water at the concentration of 100 ppm for 8 weeks, and then 0.2% or 0.5% of curcumin was fed to the rats for 55 weeks. The results showed that the number of atypical hyperplasia in curcumin-treated rats was significantly less than that in the control group. Similarly, the curcumin analog bis-1,7-(2-hydroxyphenyl)-hepta-1,6-diene-3,5-dione was shown to inhibit the tumorigenic effect of 1,2-dimethylhydrazine in rats (Devasena et al., 2003). Furthermore, natural and synthetic curcuminoids exhibit an inhibitory effect on mutagenesis induced by 2-acetamidofluorene (2-AAF) (Anto et al., 1996). In the study, up to 87% of 2-AAF-induced papilloma was inhibited by bis-(p-hydroxycinnamoyl)methane (curcuminoid III), while 70% and 68% of the papilloma were inhibited by feruloyl-p-hydroxycinnamoylmethane (curcuminiod II) and diferuloylmethane (curcuminoid I), respectively. The most potent curcuminoid was salicylcurcuminoid which completely inhibited the papilloma formation.

#### 3.1.2 Suppression of oncogenes and upregulation of tumor suppressor genes

As mentioned earlier, genetic instability is linked to the initiation of carcinogenesis. This irreversible process involves several molecular events that either promote the activity of oncogenes such as myc and ras or impede the function of tumor suppressor genes such as p53 (Vogelstein and Kinzler, 2004). Curcumin has been shown to suppress oncogenes and activate tumor suppressor genes in various cancer cell types (Table 1). In an *in vivo* study, curcumin suppresses c-fos and c-Ha-ras activation induced by environmental mutagenic agents (Limtrakul et al., 2001). Dietary administration of curcumin (0.1-0.2%) prevents 2-dimethylbenz(α)anthracene (DMBA) and 12-O-tetradecanoylphorbol-13-acetate (TPA)-induced skin tumor in mice. There is an increase in the oncogene (c-fos and ras) expression in this tumor model, which is suppressed by the dietary curcumin. Similarly, c-myc is also a target oncogene attenuated by curcumin in the TPA-induced tumor model (Kakar and Roy, 1994).

| Chemopreventive properties | | | |
|---|---|---|---|
| Cancer | Carcinogen | Animal | References |
| Stomach cancer | MNNG | Rat | Ikesaki et al., 2001 |
| Colon cancer | DMH | Rat | Devasena et al., 2003 |
| Papilloma | 2-AAF | - | Anto et al., 1996 |
| Mammary tumor | DMBA | Rat | Pereira et al., 1996 |
| Skin tumor | TPA | Mouse | Lu et al., 1993 |
| Liver cancer | Diethylnitrosamine | Mouse | Chuang et al., 2000 |
| **Oncogene suppression and tumor suppressor gene activation** | | | |
| Cancer | Mechanism | | References |
| Skin tumor | Suppress c-fos and c-Ha-ras-activation by DMBA | | Limtrakul et al., 2001 |
| B cell lymphoma | Suppress c-myc | | Han et al., 1999 |
| Mouse skin cancer | Suppress c-myc activated by TPA | | Kakar & Roy, 1994 |
| Human colon adenocarcinoma | Enhance p53 activity | | Song et al., 2005 |
| Human breast cancer | Enhance p53 activity | | Choudhuri et al., 2002 |
| Human glioma | Enhance p53 activity | | Liu et al., 2007 |
| **Anti-inflammation -related cancer** | | | |
| Cancer | Mechanism | | References |
| - | Inhibit NO synthase in macrophages | | Brouet & Ohshima, 1995 |
| Human mantle cell lymphoma | Inhibit constitutive NF-κB activation | | Shishodia et al., 2005 |
| Mouse melanoma | Inhibit constitutive NF-κB activation | | Marin et al., 2007 |
| Human oral cancer | Inhibit constitutive NF-κB activation | | Sharma et al., 2006 |
| Non-small cell lung carcinoma | Inhibit constitutive NF-κB activation and COX expression | | Shishodia et al., 2003 |

Table 1. Cancer preventive properties of curcumin

### 3.1.3 Anti-inflammatory activity

Epidemiological studies have supported the concept that cancers frequently originate at the site of chronic inflammation. This event has increasingly been accepted as the seventh hallmark of cancer (Colotta et al., 2009). Inflammation is a vital physiological process in response to injury, which leads to the mediation of inflammatory cells in the presence of enzymes and cytokines for repairing tissue damage. The linkage between cancer and inflammation is generally characterized as being intrinsic or extrinsic (Mantovani et al., 2008). The extrinsic pathway is induced by inflammation that facilitates cancer development, while the intrinsic pathway is driven by genetic instability causing inflammatory environment-related cancer. Both processes mediate the transcription factors involved in cell proliferative function and persistent activation of this event can lead to cancer. A considerable number of reports have described the linkage between cancer preventive properties and anti-inflammatory action of curcumin (Table 1). Mechanistically, curcumin inhibits the induction of nitric oxide synthase (NOS) by activated macrophages (Brouet and Ohshima, 1995). Nitric oxide (NO) and its derivatives such as peroxynitrite play a critical role in the inflammation process causing fibroblast proliferation and fibrosis (Romanska et al., 2002). Treatment of macrophages with lipopolysaccharide (LPS) and IFN-$\gamma$ induces an inflammatory response that leads to the release of NO, which is inhibited by curcumin. Curcumin also suppresses the transcription of inducible NOS which is activated by LPS and IFN-$\gamma$. Since NO is implicated in tumor promotion, the attenuation of NO by curcumin hence suppresses tumor development.

Numerous studies have suggested that NF-κB plays a key role in promoting cancer development during chronic inflammation. NF-κB regulates the expression of several genes involved in the immune and inflammatory responses as well as in cell proliferation and apoptosis (Karin et al., 2002). It is required for the expression of a wide range of inflammatory cytokines and adhesion molecules, and is important in the cellular proliferative function by activating growth factor genes, proto-oncogenes and cell cycle regulators that contribute to carcinogenesis. In a study using human mantle cell lymphoma (MCL), curcumin inhibits constitutive NF-κB activation leading to the suppression of NF-κB regulated genes (Shishodia et al., 2005). MCL expresses a high level of cyclin D1, a cell cycle promoting factor and target transcription of NF-κB, which is a key survival factor of this cancer type. Curcumin treatment causes downregulation of constitutive NF-κB activation, inhibits IκBα kinase (IKK) and phosphorylated IκBα and p65, leading to cell cycle arrest and apoptosis. NF-κB is overexpressed in various tumors and cancer cell lines including melanoma cells. Electrophoretic mobility shift and gene reporter assays have demonstrated that curcumin suppresses constitutive NF-κB activation in melanoma cells and increases the number of cells in the sub G1 phase of cell cycle (Marin et al., 2007). Interestingly, curcumin shows selectivity in inducing apoptosis of melanoma cells but not melanocytes.

Other mechanisms of the anti-inflammatory-related cancer effect of curcumin have been proposed including suppression of cyclooxygenase 2 (COX-2). A wide range of stimuli mediates COX-2 expression and overexpression of this molecule is found in various cancer types in association with accelerated cell growth, antiapoptotic activity, angiogenesis, and metastasis (Prescott and Fitzpatrick, 2000). In a cigarette-smoking (CS) study using non-small cell lung cancer model, CS exposure activates NF-κB and subsequently induces COX-2 expression, which is inhibited by pre-treatment with curcumin (Shishodia et al., 2003). This chemopreventive property of curcumin is also observed in smokeless-tobacco mediated activation of NF-κB and its downstream target COX-2 (Sharma et al., 2006). Since inflammation contributes to tumor initiation, and curcumin possesses anti-inflammatory activity, curcumin could be beneficial in cancer prevention.

### 3.2 Inhibition of tumor growth and cell proliferation

Excessive proliferation is a hallmark of cancer (Hanahan and Weinberg, 2000). Aberrational cell division is an important basis of cancer development allowing formation and expansion of tumor growth. In normal cells, cell proliferation requires the growth signal that is generated by cell-cell interaction, neighbour cells and extracellular matrix. Cancer cells can further generate their own growth signals, upregulate growth receptors, and be desensitized to antigrowth factors. Upon transmitting the growth signals to their receptors, downstream mediators are activated which drive the quiescent cells to proliferative cycle (Evan and Vousden, 2001). Curcumin has been shown to modulate the expression and activity of growth factors, including epidermal growth factor (EGF) and insulin-like growth factor (IGF) (Table 2). Overexpression of EGF and its receptor, EGFR, was found in human prostate cancer cells undergoing rapid growth expansion (Cai et al., 2008). It has been demonstrated that curcumin blocks the EGF pathway through downregulation of EGFR, suppression of intrinsic EGFR tyrosine kinase activity, and inhibition of ligand-induced EGFR activity in both androgen-dependent and androgen-independent prostate cancer cells (Dorai et al., 2000).

| Inhibition of cancer proliferation and tumor growth | | |
|---|---|---|
| Cancer | Mechanism | References |
| Prostate cancer cells | Downregulation of EGFR, suppression of intrinsic EGFR tyrosine kinase activity, and inhibition ligand-induced EGFR activity | Dorai et al., 2000 |
| Prostate and breast cancer cells | Downregulation of cyclin D1 | Mukhopadhyay et al., 2002 |
| Breast cancer cells | Suppression IGF system | Xia et al., 2007 |
| Breast cancer cells | Induction of cell cycle arrest at S, G2/M phase by upregulation of p21 | Chiu & Su, 2009 |
| Human epidermoid carcinoma cells | Inhibit EGFR activity | Korutla & Kumar, 1994 |
| Colon carcinoma cells | Induction of cell cycle arrest at S, G2/M phase | Chen et al., 1999 |
| Human head and neck squamous carcinoma cells | Downregulation of cyclin D1 | Aggarwal et al., 2004 |
| Human biliary cancer cells | Downregulation of cyclin D1 | Prakobwong et al., 2011 |
| Human hepatocarcinoma cells | Induction of cell cycle arrest at S, G2/M phase | Cheng et al., 2010 |

Table 2. Inhibition of cancer proliferation and tumor growth

Likewise, insulin-like growth factor has been implicated in the regulation of normal cell growth, in which its atypical expression is found in human cancer cells (Samani et al., 2007). Curcumin abrogates IGF-1 system in MCF-7 human breast carcinoma cells (Xia et al., 2007). It decreases IGF-1 secretion in concomitant with the increasing IGF binding protein IGFBP-3 in a dose-dependent fashion. Furthermore, it abolishes IGF-1-stimulated MCF-7 growth through the suppression of IGF-1 mediated receptor activity and downregulation of IGF receptor mRNA expression.

Deregulation of cell cycle causes limitless replicative potential of cancer. Curcumin exhibits antiproliferative activity via the regulation of cell cycle (Table 2). It disrupts the progression of cell cycle by increasing the number of cancer cells at S, G2/M phase, hence preventing cell entering next cycle (Chen et al., 1999). Additional mechanistic studies indicate that curcumin downregulates cyclin D1 expression through inhibition of its promoter activity and enhanced degradation (Mukhopadhyay et al., 2002). Cyclin D1 is a subunit of cyclin-dependent kinase (Cdk)-4 and Cdk-6 which plays a key role in determining the cell cycle progression from G1 to S phase (Baldin et al., 1993) and overexpression of this gene is a common event in several forms of cancer (Knudsen et al., 2006). Similarly, in the presence of curcumin, cyclin D1 is suppressed as a result of NF-κB inhibition as observed in human head carcinoma, neck squamous carcinoma, and biliary cancer cells (Aggarwal et al., 2004; Prakobwong et al., 2011).

### 3.3 Induction of cancer cell apoptosis

Apoptosis plays an essential role in various physiological and pathological processes (Hengartner, 2000). Tissue homeostasis maintains the balance of cell proliferation and cell death as part of normal tissue development. Dysregulation of this process can lead to several diseases including cancer. Avoidance of apoptotic cell death is a major characteristic of malignant cells in response to stress conditions, which is achieved by activating the antiapoptotic signals or inhibiting proapoptotic signals (Hanahan and Weinberg, 2000). Several strategies have been developed to overcome this defective mechanism in cancers and curcumin has shown promising activities that modulate this mechanism in favor of cancer cell apoptosis.

Apoptosis generally occurs through two main pathways, intrinsic and extrinsic (Lavrik et al., 2005). The intrinsic pathway is initiated by several cellular stresses such as DNA damage which activates proapoptotic proteins, notably the Bcl-2 family proteins, causing mitochondrial membrane permeabilization and subsequent activation of the caspase cascade. In the extrinsic pathway, the interaction between death ligands and death receptors results in the assembly of death-inducing signaling complex (DISC) and the activation of initiator caspases. Curcumin is known to overcome the apoptosis resistance of cancer cells through both pathways (Table 3). In human acute myelogenous leukemia HL-60 cells, curcumin induces apoptosis by suppressing the expression of antiapoptotic Bcl-2 and Bcl-xL, causing cytochrome c release, caspase-3 activation, and PARP cleavage (Anto et al., 2002). Curcumin also stimulates the death receptor pathway through caspase-8 activation but overexpression of the DISC protein FADD cannot protect the cells from apoptosis in response to curcumin. In A549 lung adenocarcinoma cells, curcumin treatment up-regulates the mitochondrial Bax protein expression, suggesting the intrinsic pathway as a major pathway of curcumin-induced apoptosis in this cell type (Chen et al., 2010).

| Molecular mechanisms of curcumin-induced apoptosis | | |
|---|---|---|
| Cancer | Mechanism | References |
| Human acute myelogenous leukemia cells | Downregulation of Bcl-2 and Bcl-xL | Anto et al., 2002 |
| Lung adenocarcinoma cells | Upregulation of Bax and Downregulation of Bcl-2 | Chen et al., 2010 |
| Rat histocytoma cells | Induction of ROS production | Bhaumik et al., 1999 |
| Human gingival fibroblasts and human submandibular gland carcinoma cells | Induction of ROS production | Atsumi et al., 2006 |
| Human breast cancer cells | Downregulation of anti-apoptotic and upregulation of proapoptotic proteins in a p53-dependent manner | Choudhuri et al., 2002 |
| Human breast cancer cells | Inhibition of PI3K/Akt pathway | Squires et al., 2003 |
| Human breast and hepatic cancers cells | Glutathione depletion and ROS production | Syng-Ai et al., 2004 |
| Human ovarian cancer cells | Upregulation of caspase-3 and downregulation of NF-κB expression | Zheng et al., 2002 |
| Human colon cancer cells | Induction of ROS production and deactivation of JNK pathway | Moussavi et al., 2006 |
| Human colon adenocarcinoma cells | Downregulation of anti-apoptotic and upregulation of proapoptotic proteins in a p53-dependent manner | Song et al., 2005 |
| Human melanoma cells | Activation of caspase-3, and -8, Fas receptor aggregation, suppression of NF-κB activation, and downregulation of XIAP expression | Bush et al., 2001 |
| T cell leukemia cells | Inhibition of PI3K/Akt pathway | Hussain et al., 2006 |
| Prostate cancer cells | Inhibition of PI3K/Akt pathway | Shankar & Srivastava, 2007 |
| Human glioblastoma cells | Increasing Bax:Bcl-2 ratio, activation of caspase-8, -9, and -3, downregulation of NF-κB | Karmakar et al., 2006 |
| Breast cancer cells | Inhibition of MAPK and PI3K/Akt pathway | Squires et al., 2003 |

Table 3. Molecular mechanisms of curcumin-induced apoptosis

In human melanoma cells, curcumin induces apoptosis through the extrinsic pathway by activating caspase-8 (Bush et al, 2001). Inhibition of caspase-8 by specific caspase-8 inhibitor or pan-caspase inhibitor prevents cancer cell apoptosis, whereas specific caspase-9 inhibitor lacks this ability. The underlying apoptosis mechanism involves the induction of Fas receptor oligomerization independent of Fas ligand, supporting the role of death receptor modification in curcumin-induced apoptosis. In some cancers such as human glioblastoma T98G cells, curcumin induces apoptosis through both pathways (Karmakar et al., 2006).

The activation of apoptotic pathwas by curcumin is regulated by reactive oxygen species (ROS). In various cancer cell types including H460 non-small cell lung cancer cells (Chanvorachote et al., 2009), AK5 rat histocytoma cells (Bhaumik et al., 1999), human gingival fibroblasts (HGF), and human submandibular gland carcinoma (HSG) cells (Atsumi et al., 2006), the induction of apoptosis by curcumin requires ROS generation. Likewise, in MCF-7, MDAMB, and HepG2 cells, apoptosis is mediated through oxidative stress induced by curcumin as a result of glutathione depletion (Syng-Ai et al., 2004). In colon cancer cells, curcumin-induced cell death is associated with ROS generation that converges on JNK activation (Moussavi et al., 2006).

Other mechanisms of curcumin-induced apoptosis have been reported. In human HT-29 colon adenocarcinoma (Song et al., 2005) and breast cancer cells (Choudhuri et al., 2002), curcumin upregulates proapoptotic proteins and downregulates antiapoptotic proteins in the Bcl-2 family through p53-dependent mechanism. In T cell leukemia (Hussain et al., 2006) and breast cancer cells (Squires et al., 2003), apoptosis induced by curcumin involves PI3K/Akt signaling pathway. Curcumin inhibits Akt phosphorylation and upregulates p53 expression which induces the proapoptotic Bcl-2 family proteins facilitating cell apoptosis (Shankar and Srivastava, 2007).

### 3.4 Sensitization of cancer cells to chemotherapy

In addition to its direct apoptosis-inducing effect, curcumin has been reported to sensitize cancer cells to chemotherapy-induced cell death. The main problem of cancer chemotherapy is the acquisition of apoptosis resistance of cancer cells and the cytotoxicity to normal cells. Combination therapy is an alternative approach that can overcome this problem by potentiating the effects of combination drugs and reducing their cytotoxicity by using optimal dosage regimens. Curcumin is one such agent that has been investigated for its effect in combination therapy (Table 4). In non-small cell lung cancer cells, we have recently shown that cotreatment of the cells with cisplatin and curcumin results in a substantial increase in cancer cell death as compared to cisplatin treatment alone (Chanvorachote et al., 2009). Since cisplatin-based therapy is the first line drug for treatment of lung cancer and the efficacy of this drug is frequently attenuated by the development of drug resistance especially in advanced stage cancer (Chang, 2011), curcumin has the potential to overcome this resistance problem. Curcumin promotes the apoptotic effect of cisplatin by inducing superoxide anion and downregulating the anti-apoptotic Bcl-2 protein which facilitates the cancer cell killing by cisplatin.

In pancreatic cancer cells, the acquisition of apoptosis resistance to the combination therapy of gemcitabine and capecitabine (a prodrug of 5-fluorouracil, 5-FU) is frequently observed. It is thought that overexpression of the multidrug resistance-associated protein 5 (MRP5), which promotes cellular efflux of the drugs (Szakacs et al., 2006), contributes to the resistance. Curcumin was shown in a recent study to inhibit MRP5 activity and increase the sensitivity of pancreatic cancer cells to 5-FU-induced toxicity in a dose-dependent manner (Li et al., 2010).

| Cancer cells | Chemotherapeutic drugs | References |
|---|---|---|
| Non-small cell lung cancer cells | Cisplatin | Chanvorachote et al., 2009 |
| Pancreatic cancer cells | 5-Fluorouracil | Li et al., 2010 |
| Hela cells | Taxol | Bava et al., 2005 |
| Human hepatic cancer cells | Doxorubicin | Notarbartolo et al., 2005 |
| Hepatocellular carcinoima cells | Doxorubicin | Chuang et al., 2002 |
| Human ovarian adenocarcinoma cells | Paclitaxel | Ganta & Amiji, 2009 |
| Human melanoma cells | Tamoxifen | Chatterjee & Pandey, 2011 |
| Human colorectal cancer cells | Oxaliplatin | Howells et al., 2010 |
| Bladder cancer cells | Gemcitabine | Tharakan et al., 2010 |

Table 4. Curcumin potentiates chemotherapeutic agent-induced cancer cell death

Curcumin also augments the therapeutic effect of taxol in Hela cells (Bava et al., 2005). The synergistic mechanism involves the inhibition of NF-κB activation and Akt phosphorylation which results in increased apoptosis and decreased DNA synthesis of cancer cells independent of tubulin polymerization. The increased susceptibility of cancer cells to chemotherapeutic agents by curcumin might overcome the drug resistance problem, thus improving the clinical outcomes.

### 3.5 Inhibition of cancer metastasis

Cancer metastasis is the spread of cancer cells from the initiation site to other parts of the body, and particularly presented in several advanced stage cancers which are difficult to treat (Gubta and Massagué, 2006). Cancer metastasis is a multistep process involving complex interactions between the disseminating cancer cells and their microenvironment. When transformed cells are initiated and continue to grow at the primary site, angiogenic factors are synthesized for vascularization which increases the likelihood of tumor cells to enter in the blood stream or lymphatic system and colonize at distant sites. Once at the new sites, the extravasation of cancer cells allows the formation and growth of secondary tumors which complete the metastatic process (Fidler, 2003). Agents that inhibit metastasis provide a major advantage in treating cancers. Several studies have shown that curcumin inhibits cancer angiogenesis, migration and invasion by interacting with key regulatory molecules as summarized in Table 5.

It is well established that vascular endothelial growth factor (VEGF) and matrix metallo-proteinase family proteins (MMP) are essential factors in the angiogenesis and invasion of cancer cells (Carmeliet, 2005; Helmestin et al., 1994). In non-small cell lung cancer cells, VEGF, MMP-9 and MMP-2 are inhibited by curcumin through MEKK and ERK-dependent pathways, resulting in inhibition of cell migration and invasion (Lin et al., 2009). Similarly, in a human glioblastoma xenograft mouse model, curcumin inhibits tumor growth, suppresses angiogenesis, and increases animal survival through the inhibition of MMP-9 and neovascularization (Perry et al., 2010). Curcumin also acts as a potent inhibitor of breast cancer cell motility and invasion through the attenuation of MMP-3 which acts as an invasive factor in this cancer cell type (Boonrao et al., 2010).

| Cancer | Effects | Mechanism | References |
|---|---|---|---|
| Human non-small cell lung cancer | Inhibition of cell invasion and migration | Inhibition of VEGF, MMP-9, and MMP-2 through MEKK and ERK pathway | Lin et al., 2009 |
| Human glioblastoma | Suppression of angiogenesis | Inhibition of MMP-9 | Perry et al., 2010 |
| Human breast cancer | Inhibition of cancer motlity and invasion | Attenuation of MMP-3 activity | Boonrao et al., 2010 |
| Human non-small cell lung cancer | Sensitization of cancer cell anoikis | Downregulation of Bcl-2 through proteasomal degradation | Pongrakhananon et al., 2010 |
| Human lung cancer | Inhibition invasion and metastasis | Activation of tumor suppressor HLJ1 through JNK/JunD pathway | Chen et al., 2008 |
| Human colon cancer | Inhibition of migration | Inhibition of neurotensin-mediated activator protein-1 and NF-κB activation, and suppression of neurotensin-stimulated IL-8 gene induction | Wang et al., 2006 |
| Prostate cancer | Inhibition of invasion | Downregulation of MMP-2 and MMP-9 | Hong et al., 2006 |
| Human fribosarcoma | Inhibition of migration and invasion | Downregulation of MMP-2, MMP-9, uPA, MT1-MMP, and TIMP-2 | Yodkeeree et al., 2008 |

Table 5. Antimetastatic properties of curcumin

Several studies have investigated the molecular mechanisms of cancer cell survival during metastasis. Survival of primary cancer cells in the circulation is a key factor determining its metastatic ability. In general, most adherent cells undergo apoptosis when detached due to improper environmental conditions. This detachment-induced apoptosis or anoikis which is often impaired in metastatic cancers (Mehlen and Puisieux, 2006) has increasingly been recognized as an important mechanism for controlling cancer cell dissemination and invasion to secondary sites. A recent study by our group has shown that curcumin can sensitize non-small cell lung cancer cells to anoikis (Pongrakhananon et al., 2010) through a mechanism that involves Bcl-2 downregulation through ubiquitin-proteasomal degradation. This process is dependent on ROS generation, partcularly superoxide anion which mediates the Bcl-2 degradation process, consistent with the previous findings on the pro-oxidant properties of curcumin (Bhaumik et al., 1999; Khar et al., 2001; Wang et al., 2008).

### 3.6 Animal studies

Several animal studies have been reported on the anticancer and chemopreventive effects of curcumin in various cancer types. Since the *in vivo* chemopreventive effect of curcumin has earlier been described under 3.1.1 and summarized in Table 1, we will focus on the direct *in vivo* anticancer properties of curcumin.

The anticancer property of curcumin in prostate cancer was investigated by using prostate cancer cells implanted into nude mice (Dorai et al., 2001). Dietary curcumin at the concentration of 2% was given to the mice, and after 6 weeks of treatment the animals were examined for tumor growth, apoptosis, and vascularity. The results showed that curcumin was able to decrease tumor volume, increase cancer cell apoptosis, and inhibit vascular angiogenesis as indicated by the reduction in microvessel density. A similar study using a murine xenograft model of human lung carcinoma cells was reported (Su et al., 2010). In this study, NCI-H460 cells were implanted subcutaneously into nude mice, and curcumin (30 and 45 mg/kg of bodyweight) was intraperitoneally injected into the mice every 4 days after the tumor reached 100 $mm^3$ in size. Curcumin was shown to significantly decrease the tumor size as compared to non-treated control.

The antitumor property of curcumin-encapsulated nanoparticles was investigated in the xenograft mouse model of human pancreatic cancer (Bisht et al., 2010). The nanoparticle formulation was injected twice daily for 3 weeks into the xenografted mice. Plasma concentration of curcumin was sustained in the treated mice at Tmax of 2.75 ± 1.50 h and Cmax of 17,176 ± 5,176 ng/ml. Tumor volume was substantially decreased in curcumin treated group. A greater antitumor effect was observed when curcumin was combined with gemcitabine. Curcumin also exhibited antimetastatic activity which was greatly enhanced by the combination treatment. The underlying mechanism of curcumin action involves NF-κB activation and downregualtion of cyclin D1 and MMP-9.

Curcumin also improves the therapeutic activity of paclitaxel in breast cancer (Aggarwal et al., 2005). Since most metastatic breast cancers acquire apoptosis resistance to paclitaxel, which is the first line therapy for breast cancer, a combination therapy with apoptosis-sensitizing agents such as curcumin could be beneficial. In a mouse model of breast cancer metastasis, curcumin was shown to decrease the incidence of breast cancer metastasis to the lung as compared to paclitaxel treatment alone. Tissue sections from treated animals showed that NF-κB, MMP-9, and COX-2 expression were increased in the paclitaxel-treated group but suppressed in the curcumin co-treatment group, supporting the ability of curcumin to abrogate paclitaxel resistance in this metastatic breast cancer model.

### 3.7 Clinical studies

Several clinical studies are ongoing to investigate the efficacy and safety of curcumin as a preventive treatment agent for a variety of cancers. In prospective phase I clinical trials, curcumin was shown to be safe even at high doses (Cheng et al., 2001). In this study, patients with premalignant lesions caused by oral leukoplakia, intestinal metaplasia, uterine cervical intraepithelial neoplasia, skin Bowen's disease, and bladder cancer were given a curcumin tablet which was taken orally for the period of three months at the daily dose of 500, 1000, 2000, 4000, and 8000 mg. No toxicity was observed in these patients even the highest dose (8000 mg/day). However, this dose was unacceptable by the patients due to its bulky volume. Peak serum concentration of curcumin after the 4000 mg administration was 0.51±0.11 μM, and 0.63±0.06 μM and 1.77±1.87 μM respectively after the 6000 mg and 8000 mg dosing. A similar study showed that a single dose of curcumin up to 12,000 mg had no

dose-limiting toxic effect in healthy volunteers, not even minor adverse effects such as diarrhea (Lao et al., 2006).
Expanding from the above findings, another phase I clinical study was conducted in patients with colon adenocarcinoma to investigate the phamacodynamic of curcumin (Sharma et al., 2004). Curcuminoid, formulated as 500 mg in soft gelatin capsule containing 450 mg of curcumin, 40 mg of desmethoxycurcumin, and 10 mg of bisdesmethoxycurcumin, was taken orally at the dose of 450, 900, 1800, and 3600 mg/day of curcumin for 4 months. Since curcumin is known to induce glutathione S-transferase (GST), suppress prostaglandin E2 (PGE2) production, and inhibit oxidative DNA adduct (M1G) formation, these biomarkers are frequently used to indicate curcumin efficacy. Curcumin and its metabolites were collected from plasma, urine, and feces, and analyzed to assess the pharmacokinetic parameters. The results showed that curcumin was well tolerated by the patients without a dose-limiting toxicity, except in a few cases where patients reported a minor gastrointestinal upset. The result also showed that curcumin at the dose of 3600 mg/day was suitable for phase II evaluation. Curcumin was shown to inhibit PGE2 without affecting GST and M1G, suggesting that GST and M1G may not be useful as indicators for curcumin efficacy. Furthermore, curcumin and its glucuronide and sulfate metabolites were found in the plasma and urine. The presence of these metabolites at all time points indicates that curcumin has poor systemic availability when given orally.
Consistent with the above finding, numerous other studies have demonstrated low systemic bioavailability of curcumin resulting from poor absorption, rapid metabolism, and rapid systemic elimination (Hsu et al., 2007; Ireson et al., 2001; Maiti et al., 2007; Garcea et al., 2004). Glucuronide and sulfate metabolites of curcumin are rapidly detected in the peripheral and portal circulation after curcumin administration (Garcea et al., 2004). In this study, patients with liver metastasis from colorectal adenocarcinoma were administered orally with curcumin at the daily dose of 450, 1800, and 3600 mg for a week. No curcumin or its metabolites was detected in the bile or hepatic tissue, indicating that curcumin is not suitable for treating patients with tumors distant from the absorption site.
In a phase II clinical study conducted in patients with advanced pancreatic cancer, curcumin was administered orally at the dose of 8 g/day for 8 weeks (Dhillon et al., 2008). The treatment was well tolerated by the patients with no systemic side effects, while effectively reducing the tumor size and the activation of NF-κB and COX-2. Mechanistically, curcumin induces cancer cell apoptosis through an upregulation of p53 in the tumor tissues (He et al., 2011).

## 4. Conclusion

Curcumin has a great potential in cancer therapy and is gaining wide acceptance as a preventive treatment agent due to its safety. It affects multiple steps in the carcinogenic process, which is important in avoiding chemoresistance. Clinical studies have indicated its efficacy as a single agent or in combination therapy; however, more rigorous testing are needed. Furthermore, problems associated with the low bioavailability of curcumin, including poor absorption, rapid metabolism, and limited tissue distribution, must be addressed. Current strategies that have been investigated to overcome these problems include alternative administration routes, chemical modifications, and various drug delivery and formulation strategies. These strategies will likely benefit the development of curcumin as an anticancer agent.

## 5. Acknowledgment

This work was supported by NIH grants R01-HL076340, R01-HL076340-04S1, and R01-HL095579.

## 6. References

Aggarwal, S., Takada, Y., Singh, S., Myers, J.N., & Aggarwal, B.B. (2004) Inhibition of growth and survival of human head and neck squamous cell carcinoma cells by curcumin via modulation of nuclear factor-kappaB signaling. *International Journal of Cancer*, Vol. 111, No. 5, (September 2004), pp. 679-692, ISSN 1097-2015

Aggarwal, B.B., Shishodia, S., Takada, Y., Banerjee, S., Newman, R.A., Bueso-Ramos, C.E., & Price, J.E. (2005) Curcumin suppresses the paclitaxel-induced nuclear factor-kappaB pathway in breast cancer cells and inhibits lung metastasis of human breast cancer in nude mice. *Clinical Cancer Research*, Vol. 11, No. 20, (October 2005), pp. 7490-7498, ISSN 1078-0432

Amanda, M.G., & Robert, A.O. (2008) Curcumin and resveratrol inhibit nuclear factor-kappaB-mediated cytokine expression in adipocytes. *Nutrition and Metabolism*, Vol. 12, No. 5, (June 2008), pp. 1-13, ISSN 1743-7075

Anto, R.J., George, J., Babu, K.V., Rajasekharan, K.N., & Kuttan, R. (1996) Antimutagenic and anticarcinogenic activity of natural and synthetic curcuminoids. *Mutation Research*, Vol. 370, No. 2, (September 1996), pp. 127-131, ISSN 1383-5742

Anto, R.J., Mukhopadhyay, A., Denning, K., & Aggarwal, B.B. (2002). Curcumin (diferuloylmethane) induces apoptosis through activation of caspase-8, BID cleavage and cytochrome c release: Its suppression by ectopic expression of bcl-2 and bcl-xl. *Carcinogenesis*, Vol. 23, No. 1, (January 2002), pp. 143-150, ISSN 0143-3334

Atsumi, T., Tonosaki, K., & Fujisawa, S. (2006). Induction of early apoptosis and ROS-generation activity in human gingival fibroblasts (HGF) and human submandibular gland carcinoma (HSG) cells treated with curcumin. *Archives of Oral Biology*, Vol. 51, No. 10, (October 2006), pp. 913-921, ISSN0003-9969

Azuine, M.A., Kayal, J.J., & Bhide, S.V. (1992) Protective role of aqueous turmeric extract against mutagenicity of direct-acting carcinogens as well as benzopyrene-induced genotoxicity and carcinogenicity. *Journal of Cancer Research and Clinical Oncology*, Vol. 118, No. 6, pp. 447-452, ISSN 1432-1335

Baldin, V., Lukas, J., Marcote, M.J., Pagano, M. & Draetta, G. (1993) Cyclin D1 is a nuclear protein required for cell cycle progression in G1. *Genes & Development*, Vol. 7, No. 5, (May 1993), pp. 812-21, ISSN1549-5477

Bava, S.V., Puliappadamba, V.T., Deepti, A., Nair, A., Karunagaran, D., & Anto, R.J. (2005). Sensitization of taxol-induced apoptosis by curcumin involves down-regulation of nuclear factor-kappaB and the serine/threonine kinase akt and is independent of tubulin polymerization. *The Journal of Biological Chemistry*, Vol. 280, No. 8, (February 2005), pp. 6301-6308, ISSN 1083-351X

Bhaumik, S., Anjum, R., Rangaraj, N., Pardhasaradhi, B.V.V., & Khar, A. (1999) Curcumin mediated apoptosis in AK-5 tumor cells involves the production of reactive oxygen intermediates. *FEBS Letters*, Vol. 456, No. 2, (August 1999), pp.311-314, ISSN 0014-5793

Bisht, S., Mizuma, M., Feldmann, G., Ottenhof, N.A., Hong, S.M., Pramanik, D., Chenna, V., Karikari, C., Sharma, R., Goggins, M.G., Rudek, M.A., &Maitra, A. (2010). Systemic administration of polymeric nanoparticle-encapsulated curcumin (NanoCurc) blocks tumor growth and metastases in preclinical models of pancreatic cancer. *Molecular Cancer Therapeutics*, Vol. 9, No. 8, (August 2010), pp. 2255-2264, ISSN 1535-7163

Boonrao, M., Yodkeeree, S., Ampasavate, C., Anuchapreeda, S., & Limtrakul, P. (2010). The inhibitory effect of turmeric curcuminoids on matrix metalloproteinase-3 secretion in human invasive breast carcinoma cells. *Archives of Pharmacal Research*, Vol. 33, No. 7, (July 2010), pp. 989-998, ISSN 1976-3786

Brouet, I., & Ohshima, H. (1995)Curcumin, an anti-tumor promoter and anti-inflammatory agent, inhibits induction of nitric oxide synthase in activated macrophages.*Biochemical and Biophysical Research Communications*, Vol. 206, No. 2, (January 1995), pp. 533-540, ISSN 1090-2104

Bush, J.A., Cheung, K.J.,Jr, & Li, G. (2001). Curcumin induces apoptosis in human melanoma cells through a fas receptor/caspase-8 pathway independent of p53. *Experimental Cell Research*, Vol. 271, No. 2, (December 2001), pp. 305-314, ISSN 0014-4827

Cai, C.Q., Peng, Y., Buckley, M.T., Wei, J., Chen, F., Liebes, L., Gerald, W.L., Pincus, M.R., Osman, I. & Lee, P. (2008). Epidermal growth factor receptor activation in prostate cancer by three novel missense mutations. *Oncogene*, Vol. 27, No. 22, (January 2008), pp. 3201-3210, ISSN 0950-9232

Carmeliet, P. (2005). VEGF as a key mediator of angiogenesis in cancer. *Oncology*, Vol. 69, No. Suppl 3, (November 2005), pp. 4-10, ISSN 1423-0232

Chang, A. (2011). Chemotherapy, chemoresistance and the changing treatment landscape for NSCLC. *Lung Cancer (Amsterdam, Netherlands)*, Vol. 71, No. 1, (January 2011), pp. 3-10, ISSN 0169-5002

Chanvorachote, P., Pongrakhananon, V., Wannachaiyasit, S., Luanpitpong, S., Rojanasakul, Y., & Nimmanit U (2009) Curcumin sensitizes lung cancer cells to cisplatin-induced apoptosis through superoxide anion-mediated Bcl-2 degradation. *Cancer Investigation*, Vol. 26, No. 6, (July 2009), pp. 624-635, ISSN 1532-4192

Chatterjee, S.J., & Pandey, S. (2011). Chemo-resistant melanoma sensitized by tamoxifen to low dose curcumin treatment through induction of apoptosis and autophagy. *Cancer Biology & Therapy*, vol. 11, No. 2, (January 2011), pp. 216-228, ISSN 1555-8576

Chen, H., Zhang, Z.S., Zhang, Y.L., & Zhou, D.Y. (1999). Curcumin inhibits cell proliferation by interfering with the cell cycle and inducing apoptosis in colon carcinoma cells. *Anticancer Research*, Vol. 19, No.5A, (Septober-October 1999), pp. 3675-3680, ISSN 1791-7530

Chen, H.W., Lee, J.Y., Huang, J.Y., Wang, C.C., Chen, W.J., Su, S.F., Huang, C.W., Ho, C.C., Chen, J.J., Tsai, M.F., Yu, S.L., & Yang, P.C. (2008) Curcumin inhibits lung cancer cell invasion and metastasis through the tumor suppressor HLJ1. *Cancer Research*, Vol. 68, No. 18, (September 2008), pp. 7428-7438, ISSN 1538-7445

Chen, Q.Y., Lu, G.H., Wu, Y.Q., Zheng, Y., Xu, K., Wu, L.J., Jiang, Z.Y., Feng, R., & Zhou, J.Y. (2010) Curcumin induces mitochondria pathway mediated cell apoptosis in A549 lung adenocarcinoma cells. *Oncology Report*, Vol. 23, No. 5, (May 2010), pp. 1285-1292, ISSN 1792- 2431

Cheng, A.L., Hsu, C.H., Lin, J.K., Hsu, M.M., Ho, Y.F., Shen, T.S., Ko, J.Y., Lin, J.T., Lin, B.R., Ming-Shiang, W., Yu, H.S., Jee, S.H., Chen, G.S., Chen, T.M., Chen, C.A., Lai, M.K., Pu, Y.S., Pan, M.H., Wang, Y.J., Tsai, C.C., & Hsieh, C.Y. (2001) Phase I clinical trial of curcumin, a chemopreventive agent, in patients with high-risk or pre-malignant lesions. *Anticancer Research*, Vol. 21, No. 4B, (July-August 2001), pp. 2895-2900, ISSN 1791-7530

Cheng, C.Y., Lin, Y.H., & Su, C.C. (2010). Curcumin inhibits the proliferation of human hepatocellular carcinoma J5 cells by inducing endoplasmic reticulum stress and mitochondrial dysfunction. *International Journal of Molecular Medicine*, Vol. 26, No. 5, (November 2010), pp. 673-678, ISSN 1791-244X

Chignell, C.F., Bilski, P., Reszka, K.J., Motten, A.G., Sik, R.H., & Dahl, T.A. (1994). Spectral and photochemical properties of curcumin. *Photochemistry and Photobiology*, Vol. 59, No. 3, (March 1994), pp. 295-302, ISSN 1751-1097

Chiu, T.L., & Su, C.C. (2009) Curcumin inhibits proliferation and migration by increasing the Bax to Bcl-2 ratio and decreasing NF-kappaBp65 expression in breast cancer MDA-MB-231 cells. *International Journal of Molecular Medicine*, Vol. 23, No. 4, (April 2009), pp. 469-475, ISSN 1791- 244X

Choudhuri, T., Pal, S., Agwarwal, M.L., Das, T., & Sa, G. (2002). Curcumin induces apoptosis in human breast cancer cells through p53-dependent bax induction. *FEBS Letters*, Vol. 512, No.1-3, (February 2002), pp. 334-340, ISSN 0014-5793

Chuang, S.E., Cheng, A.L., Lin, J.K., & Kuo, M.L. (2000). Inhibition by curcumin of diethylnitrosamine-induced hepatic hyperplasia, inflammation, cellular gene products and cell-cycle-related proteins in rats.*Food and Chemical Toxicology : An International Journal Published for the British Industrial Biological Research Association*, Vol. 38, No. 11, (November 2000), pp. 991-995, ISSN 1873-6351

Chuang, S.E., Yeh, P.Y., Lu, Y.S., Lai, G.M., Liao, C.M., Gao, M., & Cheng, A.L. (2002) Basal levels and patterns of anticancer drug-induced activation of nuclear factor-kappaB (NF-kappaB), and its attenuation by tamoxifen, dexamethasone, and curcumin in carcinoma cells. *Biochemical Pharmacology*, Vol. 63, No. 9, (May 2002), pp. 1709-1716, ISSN 1873-2968

Colotta, F., Allavena, P., Sica, A., Garlanda, C., &Mantovani, A. (2009)Cancer-related inflammation, the seventh hallmark of cancer: links to genetic instability. *Carcinogenesis*, Vol. 7, No. 30, (May 2009), pp. 1073-1081, ISSN 1460-2180

Devasena, T., Rajasekaran, K.N., Gunasekaran, G., Viswanathan, P., & Menon, V.P. (2003)Anticarcinogenic effect of bis-1,7-(2-hydroxyphenyl)-hepta-1,6-diene-3,5-dione a curcumin analog on DMH-induced colon cancer model. *Pharmacological Research*, Vol. 47, No. 2, (Febrauary 2003), pp. 133-140, ISSN 1096-1186

Dhillon, N., Aggarwal, B.B., Newman, R.A., Wolff, R.A., Kunnumakkara, A.B., Abbruzzese, J.L., Ng, C.H., Badmaev, E., & Kurzrock, R. (2008). Phase II trial of curcumin in patients with advanced pancreatic cancer. *Clinical Cancer Research : An Official*

*Journal of the American Association for Cancer Research*, Vol. 14, No. 14, (July 2008), pp. 4491-4499, ISSN 1557-3265

Diehl, J.A. (2002) Cycling to cancer with cyclin D1. *Cancer Biology & Therapy*, Vol. 1, No. 3, (May- June 2002), pp. 226-231, ISSN 1555-8576

Dorai, T., Gehani, N., & Katz, A. (2000). Therapeutic potential of curcumin in human prostate cancer. II. curcumin inhibits tyrosine kinase activity of epidermal growth factor receptor and depletes the protein. *Molecular Urology*, Vol. 4, No. 1, pp. 1-6, ISSN 1091-5362

Dorai, T., Cao, Y.C., Dorai ,B., Buttyan, R., &Katz, A.E. (2001) Therapeutic potential of curcumin in human prostate cancer. III. Curcumin inhibits proliferation, induces apoptosis, and inhibits angiogenesis of LNCaP prostate cancer cells in vivo. *The prostate*, Vol. 47, No. 4, (June 2001), pp. 293-303, ISSN 1097-0045

Evan, G.I., & Vousden, K.H. (2001) Proliferation, cell cycle and apoptosis in cancer. *Nature*, Vol. 6835, No. 411, (May 2001), pp. 342-348, ISSN 1476-4687

Fidler, I.J. (2003) The pathogenesis of cancer metastasis: the seed and soil hypothesis revisited. *Nature Reviews Cancer*, Vol. 3, No.6, (June 2003), pp. 453-458, ISSN 1474-1768

Ganta, S., &Amiji, M. (2009) Coadministration of paclitaxel and curcumin in nanoemulsion formulations to overcome multidrug resistance in tumor cells. *Molecular Pharmacology*, Vol. 6, No. 3, (May-June 2009), pp. 928-939, ISSN 1543-8392

Garcea, G., Jones, D.J., Singh, R., Dennison, A.R., Farmer, P.B., Sharma, R.A., Steward, W.P., Gescher, A.J., & Berry, D.P. (2004). Detection of curcumin and its metabolites in hepatic tissue and portal blood of patients following oral administration. *British Journal of Cancer*, Vol. 90, No. 5, (March 2004), pp. 1011-1015, ISSN 0007-0920

Gupta, G.P., & Massague, J. (2006). Cancer metastasis: Building a framework. *Cell*, Vol. 127, No. 4, (November 2006), pp. 679-695, ISSN 0092-8674

Han, S.S., Chung, S.T., Robertson, D.A., Ranjan, D., & Bondada, S. (1999) Curcumin causes the growth arrest and apoptosis of B cell lymphoma by downregulation of egr-1, c-myc, bcl-XL, NF- kappa B, and p53. *Clinical Immunology*, Vol. 93, No. 2, (November 1999), pp. 152-161, ISSN 1521-7035

Hanahan, D.,& Weinberg, R.A. (2000) The Hallmarks of cancer. *Cell*, Vol. 1, No. 100, (January 2000), pp. 57-70, ISSN0092-8674

He, Z.Y., Shi, C.B., Wen, H., Li, F. L., Wang, B.L., & Wang, J. (2011). Upregulation of p53 expression in patients with colorectal cancer by administration of curcumin. *Cancer Investigation*, Vol. 29, No. 3, (March 2011), pp. 208-213, ISSN 0735-7907

Hengartner, M.O. (2000) The biochemistry of apoptosis. *Nature*, Vol. 407, No. 6805, (October 2000), pp. 770–776, ISSN 0028-0836

Himelstein, B.P., Canete-Soler, R., Bernhard, E.J., Dilks, D.W., & Muschel, R.J. (1994). Metalloproteinases in tumor progression: The contribution of MMP-9. *Invasion & Metastasis*, Vol. 14, No. 1-6, pp. 246-258, ISSN 0251-1789

Hong, J.H., Ahn, K.S., Bae, E., Jeon, S.S., & Choi, H.Y. (2006) The effects of curcumin on the invasiveness of prostate cancer in vitro and in vivo. *Prostate Cancer and Prostatic Diseases*, Vol. 9, No. 2, (January 2006), pp. 147-52, ISSN 1476-5608

Howells, L.M., Sale, S., Sriramareddy, S.N., Irving, G.R., Jones, D.J., Ottley, C.J., Pearson, D.G., Mann, C.D., Manson, M.M., Berry, D.P., Gescher, A., Steward, W.P., &Brown,

K. (2010). Curcumin ameliorates oxaliplatin-induced chemoresistance in HCT116 colorectal cancer cells in vitro and in vivo. *International Journal of Cancer.Journal International Du Cancer*, (Septemper 2010), ISSN 1097-0215

Hsu, C.H., & Cheng, A.L. (2007) Clinical studies with curcumin. *Advances* in *Experimental Medicine and Biology*, Vol. *595*, pp. 471-480, ISSN 0065-2598

Hussain, A.R., Al-Rasheed, M., Manogaran, P.S., Al-Hussein, K.A., Platanias, L.C., Al Kuraya, K., & Uddin, S. (2006). Curcumin induces apoptosis via inhibition of PI3'-kinase/AKT pathway in acute T cell leukemias. *Apoptosis : An International Journal on Programmed Cell Death*, Vol. 11, No. 2, (February 2006), pp. 245-254, ISSN 1573-675X

Ikezaki, S., Nishikawa, A., Furukawa, F., Kudo, K., Nakamura, H., Tamura, K., & Mori, H. (2001)Chemopreventive effects of curcumin on glandular stomach carcinogenesis induced by N-methyl-N'-nitro-N-nitrosoguanidine and sodium chloride in rats. *Anticancer Research*,Vol. 21, No. 5, (September-October 2001), pp. 3407-3411, ISSN 1791-7530

Ireson, C., Orr, S., Jones, D.J., Verschoyle, R., Lim, C.K., Luo, J.L,Howells, L., Plummer, S., Jukes, R., Williams, M., Steward, W.P., &Gescher, A. (2001). Characterization of metabolites of the chemopreventive agent curcumin in human and rat hepatocytes and in the rat in vivo, and evaluation of their ability to inhibit phorbol ester-induced prostaglandin E2 production. *Cancer Research*, Vol. 61, No. 3, (February 2001), pp. 1058-1064, ISSN 1538-7445

Jagetia, G.C., & Rajanikant, G.K. (2005) Curcumin treatment enhances the repair and regeneration of wounds in mice exposed to hemibody gamma irradiation. *Plastic and Reconstructive Surgery*, Vol. 115, No. 2, (February 2005), pp. 515-528, ISSN 1529-4242

Kakar, S. S., & Roy, D. (1994). Curcumin inhibits TPA induced expression of c-fos, c-jun and c-myc proto-oncogenes messenger RNAs in mouse skin. *Cancer Letters*, Vol. 87, No. 1, (November 1994), pp. 85-89, ISSN 0304-3835

Karin, M., Cao, Y., Greten, F.R., & Li, Z.W. (2002)NF-kB in cancer: from innocent bystander to major culprit. *Nature Reviews Cancer*, Vol. 4, No. 2, (April 2002), pp. 301-310, ISSN 1474-1768

Karmakar, S., Banik, N.L., Patel, S.J., & Ray, S.K. (2006). Curcumin activated both receptor-mediated and mitochondria-mediated proteolytic pathways for apoptosis in human glioblastoma T98G cells.*Neuroscience Letters*, Vol. 407, No. 1, (October 2006), pp. 53-58, ISSN 0304-3940

Kastan, M.B., & Bartek, J. (2004) Cell-cycle checkpoints and cancer. *Nature*, Vol. 432, No. 7015, (November 2004), pp. 316-23, ISSN 1476-4687

Khar, A., Ali, A.M., Pardhasaradhi, B.V.V., Varalakshmi, C., Anjum, R., & Kumari, A.L. (2001) Induction of stress response renders human tumor cell lines resistant to curcumin-mediated apoptosis: role of reactive oxygen intermediates. *Cell Stress Chaperones*, Vol. 6, No. 4, (October 2006), pp. 368-376, ISSN1466-1268

Knudsen, K.E., Diehl, J.A., Haiman, C.A., & Knudsen, E.S. (2006). Cyclin D1: Polymorphism, aberrant splicing and cancer risk. *Oncogene*, Vol. 25, No. 11, (March 2006), pp. 1620-1628, ISSN1476-5594

Korutla, L., & Kumar, R. (1994). Inhibitory effect of curcumin on epidermal growth factor receptor kinase activity in A431 cells. *Biochimica Et Biophysica Acta*, Vol. 1224, No. 3, (December 1994), pp. 597-600. ISSN 0006-3002

Lao, C.D., Ruffin, M.T. 4th, Normolle, D., Heath, D.D., Murray, S.I., Bailey, J.M., Boggs, M.E., Crowell, J., Rock, C.L., & Brenner, D.E. (2006) Dose escalation of a curcuminoid formulation.*BMC Complementary and Alternative Medicine*, Vol. 12, No. 6, (March 2006), pp. 10, ISSN 1472-6882

Lavrik, I.N., Golks, A., & Krammer, P.H. (2005) Caspases: pharmacological manipulation of cell death. *The Journal of Clinical Investigation*, Vol. 115, No. 10, (October 2005), pp. 2665-2672, ISSN 1558-8238

Lee, K.W., Kim, J.H., Lee, H.J., & Surh, Y.J. (2005) Curcumin inhibits phorbol ester-induced upregulation of cyclooxygenase-2 and matrix metalloproteinase-9 by blocking ERK1/2 phosphorylation and NF-kappaB transcriptional activity in MCF10A human breast epithelial cells. *Antioxidant and Redox Signaling*, Vol. 7, No. 11-12, (November-December 2005), pp. 1612-1620, ISSN 1523-0864

Li, Y., Revalde, J.L., Reid, G., & Paxton, J.W. (2010). Modulatory effects of curcumin on multi-drug resistance-associated protein 5 in pancreatic cancer cells. *Cancer Chemotherapy and Pharmacology*,(November 2010), ISSN 1432-0843

Limtrakul, P., Anuchapreeda, S., Lipigorngoson, S., & Dunn, F.W. (2001). Inhibition of carcinogen induced c-ha-ras and c-fos proto-oncogenes expression by dietary curcumin. *BMC Cancer*, Vol. 1, No. 1, (Junuary 2011), ISSN 1471-2407

Lin, S.S., Lai, K.C., Hsu, S.C., Yang, J.S., Kuo, C.L., Lin, J.P., Ma, Y.S., Wu, C.C., & Chung, J.G. (2009) Curcumin inhibits the migration and invasion of human A549 lung cancer cells through the inhibition of matrix metalloproteinase-2 and -9 and vascular endothelial growth factor (VEGF). *Cancer Letters*, Vol. 285, No. 2, (May 2009), pp. 127-133, ISSN 1872-7980

Liu, E., Wu, J., Cao, W., Zhang, J., Liu, W., Jiang, X., & Zhang, X. (2007). Curcumin induces G2/M cell cycle arrest in a p53-dependent manner and upregulates ING4 expression in human glioma. *Journal of Neuro-Oncology*, Vol. 85, No. 3, (December 2007), pp. 263-270, ISSN 1573-7373

Lu, Y.P., Chang, R.L., Huang, M.T., & Conney, A.H. (1993). Inhibitory effect of curcumin on 12-O-tetradecanoylphorbol-13-acetate-induced increase in ornithine decarboxylase mRNA in mouse epidermis.*Carcinogenesis*, Vol. 14, No. 2, (February 1993), pp. 293-297, ISSN 1460-2180

Mai, S.,& Mushinski, J.F. (2003) c-Myc-induced genomic instability. *Journal of Environmental Pathology, Toxicology and Oncology*, Vol. 22, No. 3, pp. 179-199, ISSN 0731-8898

Maiti, K., Mukherjee, K., Gantait, A., Saha, B.P., & Mukherjee, P.K. (2007). Curcumin-phospholipid complex: Preparation, therapeutic evaluation and pharmacokinetic study in rats. *International Journal of Pharmaceutics*, Vol. 330, No. 1-2, (February 2007), pp. 155-163, ISSN 0378-5173

Mantovani, A., Allavena, P., Sica, A., & Balkwill, F. (2008) Cancer-related inflammation. *Nature*, Vol. 7203, No. 454, (July 2008), pp. 436-444, ISSN 1476-4687

Marin, Y.E., Wall, B.A., Wang, S., Namkoong, J., Martino, J.J., Suh, J., Lee, H.J., Rabson, A.B., Yang, C.H., Chen, S., & Ryu, J.H. (2007). Curcumin downregulates the constitutive activity of NF-kappaB and induces apoptosis in novel mouse melanoma cells. *Melanoma Research*, Vol. 17, No. 5, (October 2007), pp. 274-283, ISSN 1473-5636

Mehlen, P., & Puisieux, A. (2006) Metastasis: a question of life or death. *Nature Reviews Cancer*, Vol. 6, No. 6, (June 2006), pp. 449-458, ISSN 1474-1768

Moussavi, M., Assi, K., G6mez-Muñoz, A., & Salh, B. (2006) Curcumin mediates ceramide generation via the de novo pathway in colon cancer cells. *Carcinogenesis*, Vol. 27, No. 8, (August 2006), pp. 1636-1644, ISSN 1460-2180

Mukhopadhyay, A., Banerjee, S., Stafford, L.J., Xia, C., Liu, M., & Aggarwal, B.B. (2002). Curcumin-induced suppression of cell proliferation correlates with down-regulation of cyclin D1 expression and CDK4-mediated retinoblastoma protein phosphorylation. *Oncogene*, Vol. 21, No. 57, (December 2002), pp. 8852-8861, ISSN 1476-5594

Notarbartolo, M., Poma, P., Perri, D., Dusonchet, L., Cervello, M., & D'Alessandro, N. (2005) Antitumor effects of curcumin, alone or in combination with cisplatin or doxorubicin, on human hepatic cancer cells. analysis of their possible relationship to changes in NF-kB activation levels and in IAP gene expression. *Cancer Letters*, Vol. 224, No. 1, (June 2005), pp. 53-65, ISSN 1872- 7980

Park, C., Kim, G.Y., Kim, G.D., Choi, B.T., Park, Y.M., & Choi, Y.H. (2006) Induction of G2/M arrest and inhibition of cyclooxygenase-2 activity by curcumin in human bladder cancer T24 cells. *Oncology Reports*, Vol. 15, No. 5, (May 2006), pp. 1225-1231, ISSN 1791-2431

Pereira, M.A., Grubbs, C.J., Barnes, L.H., Li, H., Olson, G.R., Eto, I., Juliana, M., Whitaker, L.M., Kelloff, G.J., Steele, V.E., & Lubet, R.A. (1996). Effects of the phytochemicals, curcumin and quercetin, upon azoxymethane-induced colon cancer and 7,12-dimethylbenz[a]anthracene-induced mammary cancer in rats. *Carcinogenesis*, Vol. 17, No. 6, (June 1996), pp. 1305-1311, ISSN 1460-2180

Perry, M.C., Demeule, M., Regina, A., Moumdjian, R., & Beliveau, R. (2010). Curcumin inhibits tumor growth and angiogenesis in glioblastoma xenografts. *Molecular Nutrition & Food Research*, Vol. 54, No. 8, (August 2010), pp. 1192-1201, ISSN 1613-4133

Philip, S., Bulbule, A., & Kundu, G.C. (2004) Matrix metalloproteinase-2: mechanism and regulation of NF-kappaB-mediated activation and its role in cell motility and ECM-invasion. *Glycoconjugate Journal*, Vol. 21, No. 8-9, (November 2004), pp. 429-441, ISSN 1573-4986

Pongrakhananon, V., Nimmannit, U., Luanpitpong, S., Rojanasakul, Y., & Chanvorachote, P. (2010) Curcumin sensitizes non-small cell lung cancer cell anoikis through reactive oxygen species- mediated Bcl-2 downregulation. *Apoptosis*, Vol. 15, No. 5, (May 2010), pp. 574-585, ISSN 1360- 8185

Prakobwong, S., Gupta, S.C., Kim, J.H., Sung, B., Pinlaor, P., Hiraku, Y., Wongkham, S., Sripa, B., Pinlaor, S., & Aggarwal, B.B. (2011). Curcumin suppresses proliferation and induces apoptosis in human biliary cancer cells through modulation of multiple cell signaling pathways. *Carcinogenesis*, (February 2011), ISSN1460-2180

Prasad, N.S., & Sarasija, S. (1997) Spectrophotometric estimationof curcumin. *Indian Drugs*, vol. 34, pp. 227-228, ISSN 0019-462X

Prescott, S.M., & Fitzpatrick, F.A. (2000) Cyclooxygenase-2 and carcinogenesis. *Biochimica et biophysica acta*, Vol. 1470, No. 2, (March 2000), pp. M69-78, ISSN 0006-3002

Rajalingam, K., Schreck, R., Rapp, U.R., & Albert, S. (2007) Ras oncogenes and their downstream targets. *Biochimica et Biophysica Acta*, Vol. 1773, No. 8, (January 2007), pp. 1177-1195, ISSN 0006-3002

Romanska, H.M., Polak, J.M., Coleman, R.A., James, R.S., Harmer, D.W., Allen, J.C., & Bishop, A.E. (2002)iNOS gene upregulation is associated with the early proliferative response of human lung fibroblasts to cytokine stimulation. *The Journal of Pathology*, Vol. 3, No. 197, (July 2002),pp. 372–379, ISSN 1096-9896

Samani, A.A., Yakar, S., LeRoith, D., & Brodt, P. (2007) The role of the IGF system in cancer growth and metastasis: overview and recent insights. *Endocrine Reviews*, Vol. 28, No. 1, (Febrauary 2007), pp. 20-47, ISSN 1945-7189

Shankar, S., & Srivastava, R.K. (2007). Involvement of bcl-2 family members, phosphatidylinositol 3'-kinase/AKT and mitochondrial p53 in curcumin (diferulolylmethane)-induced apoptosis in prostate cancer.*International Journal of Oncology*, Vol. 30, No.4, (April 2007), pp. 905-918, ISSN 1019-6439

Sharma, C., Kaur, J., Shishodia, S., Aggarwal, B.B., & Ralhan, R. (2006). Curcumin down regulates smokeless tobacco-induced NF-kappaB activation and COX-2 expression in human oral premalignant and cancer cells. *Toxicology*, Vol. 228, No. 1, (November 2006), pp. 1-15, ISSN 0300-483X

Sharma, R.A., Euden, S.A., Platton, S.L., Cooke, D.N., Shafayat, A., Hewitt, H.R., Marczylo, T.H., Morgan, B., Hemingway, D., Plummer, S.M., Pirmohamed, M., Gescher, A.J., & Steward, W.P. (2004) Phase I clinical trial of oral curcumin: biomarkers of systemic activity and compliance. *Clinical Cancer Research*, Vol. 15, No. 20, (October 2004), pp. 6847-6854, ISSN 1078-0432

Shishodia, S., Potdar, P., Gairola, C.G., & and Aggarwal, B.B. (2003)Curcumin (diferuloylmethane) down-regulates cigarette smoke-induced NF-kBactivation through inhibition of IkBa kinase in human lung epithelial cells:correlation with suppression of COX-2, MMP-9 and cyclin D1. *Carcinogenesis*, Vol.24, No.7, pp.1269-1279, ISSN 1460-2180

Shishodia, S., Amin, H.M., Lai, R., & Aggarwal, B.B. (2005). Curcumin (diferuloylmethane) inhibits constitutive NF-kappaB activation, induces G1/S arrest, suppresses proliferation, and induces apoptosis in mantle cell lymphoma. *Biochemical Pharmacology, Vol. 70, No.* 5, (September 2005), pp. 700-713, ISSN 1873-2968

Simon, A., Allais, D.P., Duroux, J.L., Basly, J.P., Durand-Fontanier, S., & Delage, C. (1998) Inhibitory effect of curcuminoids on MCF-7 cell proliferation and structure-activity relationships. *Cancer Letters*, Vol. 129, No. 1, (July 1998), pp. 111-116, ISSN 1872-7980

Singh, M., & Singh, N. (2009) Molecular mechanism of curcumin induced cytotoxicity in human cervical carcinoma cells *Molecular and Cellular Biochemistry*, Vol. 325, No. 1-2, (February 2009), pp. 107-119, ISSN 1573-4919

Song, G., Mao, Y.B., Cai, Q.F., Yao, L.M., Ouyang, G.L., & Bao, S.D. (2005). Curcumin induces human HT-29 colon adenocarcinoma cell apoptosis by activating p53 and regulating apoptosis-related protein expression. *Brazilian Journal of Medical and Biological Research*, Vol. 38,No. 12, (December 2005), pp. 1791-1798, ISSN 1414-431X

Squires, M.S., Hudson, E.A., Howells, L., Sale, S., Houghton, C.E., Jones, J.L., Fox, L.H., Dickens, M., Prigent, S.A. & Manson, M.M. (2003). Relevance of mitogen activated protein kinase (MAPK) and phosphotidylinositol-3-kinase/protein kinase B (PI3K/PKB) pathways to induction of apoptosis by curcumin in breast cells. *Biochemical Pharmacology*, Vol. 65, No. 3, (February 2003), pp. 361-376, ISSN1873-2968

Su, C.C., Yang, J.S., Lu, C.C., Chiang, J.H., Wu, C.L., Lin, J.J., Lai, K.C., Hsia, T.C., Lu, H.F., Fan, M.J., & Chung, G.J. (2010). Curcumin inhibits human lung large cell carcinoma cancer tumour growth in a murine xenograft model. *Phytotherapy Research : PTR*, Vol. 24, No. 2, (February 2010), pp. 189-192, ISSN 1099-1573

Syng-Ai, C., Kumari, A.L., & Khar, A. (2004). Effect of curcumin on normal and tumor cells: Role of glutathione and bcl-2. *Molecular Cancer Therapeutics*, Vol. 3, No. 9, (September 2004), pp. 1101-1108, ISSN 1538-8514

Szakacs, G., Paterson, J.K., Ludwig, J.A., Booth-Genthe, C. & Gottesman, M.M. (2006) Targeting multidrug resistance in cancer. *Nature Reviews. Drug Discovery*, Vol. 5, No. 3, (March 2006), pp. 219-234, ISSN 1474-1784

Tharakan, S.T., Inamoto, T., Sung, B., Aggarwal, B.B., & Kamat, A.M. (2010). Curcumin potentiates the antitumor effects of gemcitabine in an orthotopic model of human bladder cancer through suppression of proliferative and angiogenic biomarkers. *Biochemical Pharmacology*, Vol. 79, No. 2, (January 2010), pp. 218-228, ISSN 0006-2952

Ventura, A., Kirsch, D.G., McLaughlin, M.E., Tuveson, D.A., Grimm, J., Lintault, L., Newman, J., Reczek, E.E., Weissleder, R., & Jacks, T. (2007) Restoration of p53 function leads to tumour regression in vivo. *Nature*, Vol. 445, No.7128, (February 2007), pp. 661-665, ISSN 0028-0836

Vogelstein, B., & Kinzler, K.W. (2004) Cancer genes and the pathways they control. *Nature Medicine*, Vol. 8, No. 10, (August 2004), pp. 789-799, ISSN 1546-170X

Wang, L., Chanvorachote, P., Toledo, D., Stehlik, C., Mercer, R.R., Castranova, V., & Rojanasakul, Y. (2008) Peroxide is a key mediator of Bcl-2 down-regulation and apoptosis induction by cisplatin in human lung cancer cells. *Molcular Pharmacology*, Vol. 73, No. 1, (October 2007), pp. 119-127, ISSN 1521-0111

Wang, X., Wang, Q., Ives, K.L., & Evers, B.M. (2006). Curcumin inhibits neurotensin-mediated interleukin-8 production and migration of HCT116 human colon cancer cells. *Clinical Cancer Research : An Official Journal of the American Association for Cancer Research*, Vol. 12, No. 18, (September 2006), pp. 5346-5355, ISSN 1557-3265

Wang, Y.J., Pan, M.H., Cheng, A.L., Lin, L.I., Ho, Y.S., Hsieh, C.Y., & Lin, J.K. (1997). Stability of curcumin in buffer solutions and characterization of its degradation products. *Journal of Pharmaceutical and Biomedical Analysis*, Vol. 15, No. 12, (August 1997), pp. 1867-1876, ISSN 1873-264X

Xia, Y., Jin, L., Zhang, B., Xue, H., Li, Q., & Xu, Y. (2007). The potentiation of curcumin on insulin-like growth factor-1 action in MCF-7 human breast carcinoma cells. *Life Sciences*, Vol. 80, No. 23, (May 2007), pp. 2161-2169, ISSN 0024-3205

Yang, F., Lim, G.P., Begum, A.N., Ubeda, O.J., Simmons, M.R., Ambegaokar, S.S., Chen, P.P., Kayed, R., Glabe, C.G., Frautschy, S.A., & Cole, G.M. (2005) Curcumin inhibits formation of amyloid beta oligomers and fibrils, binds plaques, and reduces amyloid in vivo. *Journal of Biological Chemistry*, Vol. 280, No. 7, (December 2004), pp. 5892-5901, ISSN 1083-351X

Yodkeeree, S., Garbisa, S., & Limtrakul, P. (2008). Tetrahydrocurcumin inhibits HT1080 cell migration and invasion via downregulation of MMPs and uPA. *Acta Pharmacologica Sinica*, Vol. 29, No.7, (July 2008), pp. 853-860, ISSN 1745-7254

Zheng, L.D., Tong, Q.S., & Wu, C.H. (2002). Inhibitory effects of curcumin on apoptosis of human ovary cancer cell line A2780 and its molecular mechanism. *Ai Zheng Chinese Journal of Cancer*, Vol. 21, No. 12, (December 2002), pp. 1296-1300, ISSN 1000-467X

17

# Salograviolide A: A Plant-Derived Sesquiterpene Lactone with Promising Anti-Inflammatory and Anticancer Effects

Isabelle Fakhoury and Hala Gali-Muhtasib
*American University of Beirut*
*Lebanon*

## 1. Introduction

Natural products are chemical substances produced by living organisms of the Biota superdomain, namely plants, animals, fungi and bacteria (G. & C. Merriam Co., 1913). Up to 80% of all drugs discovered prior to 1981 and 50% of all approved drugs between the years 1994 and 2007 are of natural product origin (Harvey, 2008). The contribution of natural products derived from plants, particularly to the well-being of mankind, extends very far back in history. Some of the most famous findings supportive of this fact come from the Middle East region and include documented medical papyri of ancient Egyptians dating back to ca. 1,850 B.C., as well as recent studies revealing their use of medicinal herbs dispensed in grape wine ca. 3,150 B.C. (McGovern et al., 2009). Incidentally, the oldest evidence for the use of herbal medicine to be so far discovered dates back to the prehistoric Neanderthal man who lived also in the Middle East region around 60,000 years ago (Solecki, 1971).

Several world heritages of medicinal plants have also inspired and greatly contributed to the development of modern medicine (Azaizeh et al., 2008). Indeed some of the early drugs were derived from plants. Morphine, for instance, was the first pharmacologically active pure compound to be extracted from a plant over 200 years ago (Jesse et al., 2009). Clinical, pharmacological, and chemical studies have since then led to the identification of a lengthy list of drugs derived from plants covering a wide range of diseases from diabetes, malaria, microbial infections, osteoporosis to inflammation and cancer.

The story of the discovery of plants exhibiting anticancer properties in particular, began almost fifty years ago. With the increase in cancer incidences, there has been an increase of interest in screening for anti-tumor agents from diverse sources including plants. For that purpose, in 1960 the National Cancer Institute (NCI) launched a large-scale screening of 35,000 sample plants. The program resulted among others, in the discovery in 1967 of the best-selling anticancer drug today; Taxol (Cragg, 1998). This breakthrough boosted cancer researchers all over the world and especially those in regions with high diversity to explore the indigenous plants' active ingredients efficacy against cancer. Considering that more than 60% of anticancer drugs available for clinical use today are derived from natural products including plants (Balunas et al., 2005; Newman and Cragg, 2007), one cannot deny that there has been a successful contribution of plants to the fight against cancer (reviewed in Gali-Muhtasib and Bakkar, 2002; Darwiche et al., 2007).

Lebanon falls within the Levantine Uplands center of diversity. Compared to other Mediterranean countries, it stands second after Turkey in its floristic diversity with 2600 plant species distributed around its humble 10452 $km^2$ (Nehmeh, 1977). About 311 plants corresponding to 12% of the total plant species are endemic to Lebanon and have been used in part by Lebanese folk medicine practitioners and Lebanese people for preventive and therapeutic purposes (Nehmeh, 1977). As members of the Nature Conservation Center for Sustainable Futures (IBSAR), we have been leading research over the past 10 years for the understanding and evaluation of Lebanese indigenous plant properties against various conditions, especially cancer. The following chapter aims at retracing our adventure with "Salograviolide A" (Sal A), and bringing to light this peculiar molecule that exhibits both anti-inflammatory and anticancer effects.

## 2. Sesquiterpene lactones in traditional and conventional medicine

Sesquiterpene lactones (SLs) are generally colourless bitter phytochemicals of lipophylic nature. Thousands of molecules are classified in the SLs subfamily of the terpenoids group of plant secondary metabolites. They are predominantly isolated from leaves or flowering heads of plants of the sunflower family Asteraceae and to a limited extent from Umbelliferae and Magnoliaciae (Heywood et al., 1977). The percentage of SLs per plant dry weight often exceeds 1% (Heywood et al., 1977).

The benefits of many plants enriched with SLs have been described in depth in Mediterranean folk literature with emphasis on their laxative values as well as their potential for the treatment of sores, wounds, sprains, fever, pain, headaches, malaria, anaemia, microbial infections, arthritis, cough, bronchitis, diabetes, hypertension and inflammation (Awadallah, 1984; Moukarzel, 1997).

Similarly, scientific literature supports most of the SLs activities attributed to their plants of origin in traditional medicine such as the hypoglycemic (Genta et al., 2010), antibacterial (Bach et al., 2011), antifungal (Vajs et al., 1999), antiplasmodial (Medjroubi et al., 2005), antinociceptive, antipyretic (Akkol et al., 2009) and anti-inflammatory (Al-Saghir et al., 2009) effects.

There are to date around 1500 publications that have reported the anticancer and anti-inflammatory properties of SLs. Three major SLs and/or many of their synthetic derivatives have reached phase I-II cancer clinical trials, namely thapsigargin from *Thapsia garganica* (Apiaceae), artemisinin and artesunate from *Artemisia annua,* and parthenolide from *Tanacetum parthenium* (Fig. 1) (reviewed in Ghantous et al., 2010). These SLs have properties that enable them to target tumor cells and cancer stem cells while sparing normal cells. They also affect different cancers or inflammation conditions. For example, thapsigargin demonstrated promising results against advanced solid tumors (breast, kidney and intestine) while parthenolide had an effect on blood and lymph nodes tumors (reviewed in Ghantous et al., 2010). Artemisinin showed efficacy against lupus nephritis, metastatic breast and colorectal cancer while clinical evidence indicated that artesunate is effective against nonsmall cell lung cancer, metastatic uveal melanoma and laryngeal squamous cell carcinoma (Berger et al., 2005; Christensen et al., 2009; Efferth, 2006; Guzman et al., 2007, as cited in Ghantous et al., 2010). The chemical basis for the observed biological activities of SLs has been reviewed by our group recently (Ghantous et al., 2010).

*Centaurea* is one of the largest genera of the Asteracae family with almost 250 species (Font et al., 2008). Plants belonging to the *Centaurea* genus are native to Eurasia. They were introduced to North America around the late 1800's and can now be found all around the world. *Centaurea* extracts have also been used in traditional medicine for their effects as stimulants, diuretics, analgesics, anti-rheumatics, anti-microbial, anti-diabetics and anti-inflammatory (refer to www.ibsar.org). Anecdotally; the genus' name is a dedication to the centaur Chiron who, according to Greek mythology, had discovered the curative properties of these medicinal plants (Nehmeh, 1977). Scientists eventually investigated the medicinal properties traditionally attributed to the *Centaurea* genus and isolated a multitude of SLs in addition to other various types of compounds such as alkaloids, lignans, acetylenes and flavonoids. When entering on PubMed the search terms "Centaurea and sesquiterpene lactones", and adding to them the hits from the search "Centaurea and cancer", 46 results get displayed. We investigated the number, nature and biological activity of SLs in the different species and summarized some of them in Table 1.

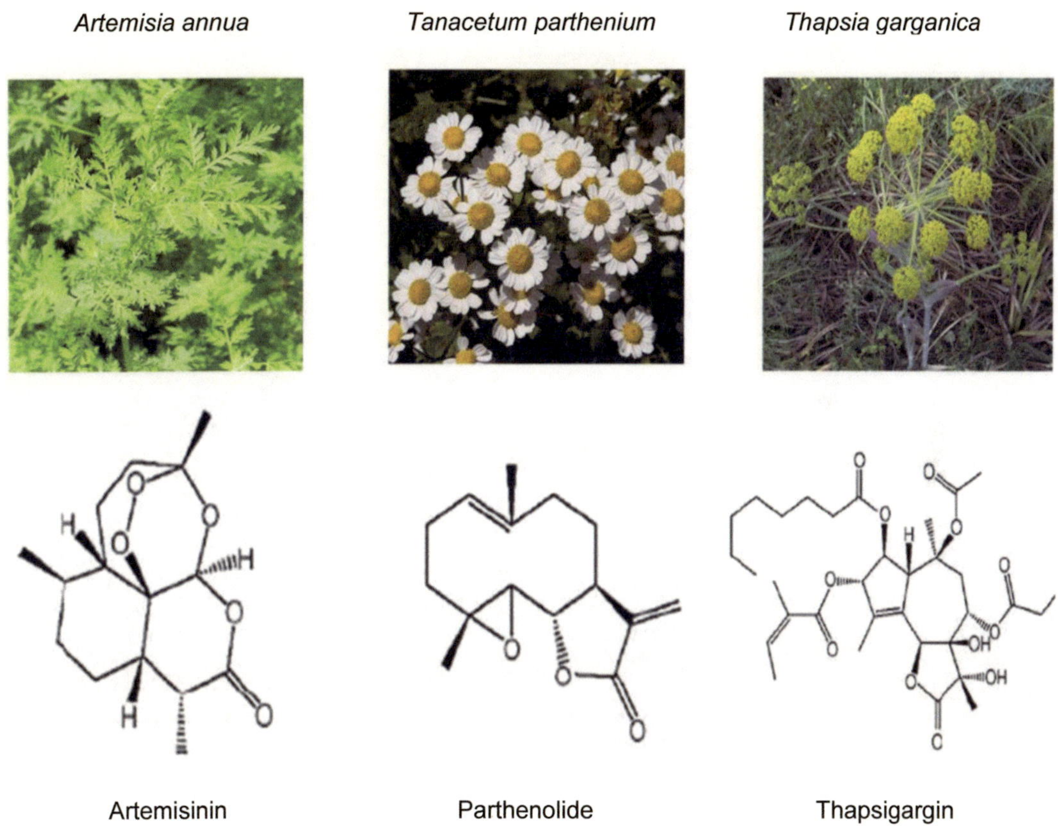


Fig. 1. Illustration of the sesquiterpene lactones that have reached clinical trials, namely thapsigargin extracted from *Thapsia garganica*, artemisinin from *Artemisia annua* L., and parthenolide from *Tanacetum parthenium*. The plants pictures are courtesy of Mr. Luigi Rignanese, Mr. Peter Griffee and Mr. Paul Drobot, respectively.

Table 1 indicates that there are at least 89 SLs in 10 *Centaurea* species. As expected, the amount of the SLs as well as their nature is species-specific. Also, the activities of the represented SLs cover most of those attributed to the plants in traditional medicine. Aside from Sal A, several articles have reported anticancer properties of SLs extracted from *Centaurea* species (Bruno et al., 2005; Chicca et al., 2011; Csupor-Löffler et al., 2009; El-Najjar et al., 2007; Ghantous et al., 2007; González et al., 1980; Koukoulista et al., 2002; Saroglou et al., 2005).

| Plant | Number of SLs | Example of SLs | Activity | Reference |
|---|---|---|---|---|
| *C. bella* | 26 | Repin | Anti-tumor | 1, 2 |
| *C. musimomum* | 11 | Cynaropicrin | Antiplasmodial<br>Cytotoxic | 3, 4 |
| *C. napifolia* | 4 | Cnicin | Antibacterial<br>Cytotoxic | 1, 5 |
| *C. nicolai* | 5 | Kandavanolide | Antifungal | 6 |
| *C. pullata* | 10 | Melitensin | Antibacterial<br>Antifungal | 7 |
| *C. scoparia* | 9 | Chlorohyssopifolin | Anti-tumor<br>Antiviral<br>Antimicrobial | 8, 9, 10 |
| *C. solstitialis* | 7 | Solstitialin A | Hypoglycemic<br>Antiviral<br>Antimicrobial | 11, 12, 13, 14 |
| *C. spinosa* | 10 | Malacitanolide | Antibacterial<br>Cytotoxic | 15 |
| *C. sulphurea* | 3 | Sulphurein | - | 16 |
| *C. tweediei* | 4 | Onopordopicrin | Antibacterial<br>Antifungal<br>Cytotoxic | 5, 17, 18 |

1: Bruno et al., 2005 - 2: Nowak et al., 1993- 3: Cho et al., 2004 - 4: Medjroubi et al., 2005- 5: Bach et al., 2011 - 6: Vajs et al., 1999 - 7: Djeddi et al., 2007, 2008 - 8: González et al., 1980 - 9: Ozçelik et al., 2009 - 10: Youssef et al., 1994, 1998 - 11: Akkol et al., 2011 - 12: Cheng et al., 1992 - 13: Gürbüz et al., 2007 - 14: Ozçelik et al., 2009 - 15: Saroglou et al., 2005 - 16: Lakhal et al., 2010 - 17: Fortuna et al., 2001 - 18: Lonergan et al., 1992.

Table 1. Sesquiterpene lactones of different *Centaurea* species and their biological activities.

## 3. Salograviolide A: Isolation and chemical characterization

In 1992, Daniewski et al. isolated an unusually hydroxylated SL from the aerial parts of the plant *Centaurea salonitana* Vis. of Bulgarian origin collected in the Greek region Gravia (Fig. 2a). The compound was baptised "Salograviolide A" with the prefix "salo" referring to the

species *salonitana* from which it was isolated, "gravi" in allusion for the region Gravia and finally the suffix "olide" indicating the presence of a lactone group.
The first procedure used for the isolation and characterization of Sal A (Fig. 2b) included drying the plant and grinding it to a powder. This was followed by dividing the dry material (600 g) into three parts that were each soaked in 1 l of methanol (MeOH) for 24 h. The extracts were afterwards combined, evaporated (7.5 g) and dissolved in a mixture of equal amounts of water and chloroform ($H_2O$-$CHCl_3$ (1:1)). The aqueous layer was extracted three times with chloroform alone and the final step consisted of evaporating the extract and subjecting it to two separate chromatography techniques for optimal purification, thin layer chromatography (TLC) and column chromatography (CC). Infra Red (IR), high resolution Mass Spectrum (MS) and $^1H$ and $^{13}C$ Nuclear Magnetic Resonance (NMR) spectroscopy techniques enabled the identification of the structure of Sal A that was later confirmed by Rychlewska et al. (1992) using crystal X-ray diffraction techniques.
Sal A is a 3β-acetoxy-8α, 9β-dihydroxy-lαH, 5αH, 6βH, 7αH-guaian-4(15), 10(14), 11(13)-trien-6, 12-olide with the molecular formula $C_{17}H_{20}O_6$. It is classified according to its carbocyclic skeleton in the guaianolides group, one of the major groups of SLs. Comprised of 15 carbons (15-C) as indicated by the prefix "sesqui", Sal A has 3 isoprene (5-C) units and a lactone group (cyclic ester) (Fig. 2c). The presence of this α-methylene-γ-lactone is thought to be responsible for the biological activity of Sal A because of its ability to react with nucleophiles by a Michael-type addition (Ghantous et al., 2010).
Sal A was subsequently isolated from other *Centaurea* species, namely from *C. nicolai* Bald (Vajs et al., 1999) and from *C. ainetensis* Bois by bioguided fractionation following an extraction scheme adopted from Harborne (1998) (Saliba et al., 2009).

## 4. IBSAR efforts for bringing Sal A to the forefront

Ibsar, AUB's nature conservation center for sustainable futures, is an interdisciplinary and interfaculty center founded in the year 2002 by AUB faculty. Ibsar's mission is "to promote the conservation and sustainable utilization of biodiversity in arid and Mediterranean regions by providing an open academic platform for innovative research and development", and its vision is "for societies to become guardians and primary beneficiaries of biodiversity in the region" (www.ibsar.org).
Very early in its establishment, Ibsar recognized that the Lebanese floristic richness also represents an untapped resource for the potential discovery of new therapeutic agents and/or useful dietary supplements. As a result, one of the key program areas in Ibsar has been to integrate traditional knowledge and biotechnology. The objective of this program is to discover useful therapeutic agents that may be hidden in wild Lebanese plants and to develop products attractive to biotechnology industries. Towards this end, plants from the region are collected, extracted and tested for their potential effects on major diseases such as cancer, inflammation, microbial infections, skin diseases and diabetes as well as their value in nutrition and use for general health purposes.
*C. ainetensis* (Arabic name; Qanturyun Aynata or Shawk al-dardar) whose specimen is deposited at the herbarium of the American University of Beirut (Lebanon), is an endemic plant to Lebanon. It flowers from May to June, has purplish tube of anthers and can only be found growing wild in stony, sterile or bushy places in particular areas in Lebanon, mainly Dayr-ul-Ahmar to Aynata region at elevations of 1200–1800 m above sea level respectively, and in Anti-Lebanon Mountain range above Ayn-Burday at 1250–1300 m (Dinsmore, 1932 as cited in Talhouk et al., 2008).

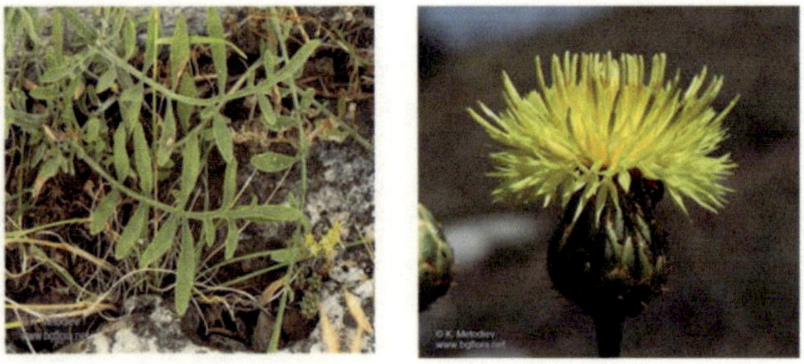

(a) Left: Photo of the plant *Centaurea salonitana* of Portuguese origin. Right: The aerial part of the plant

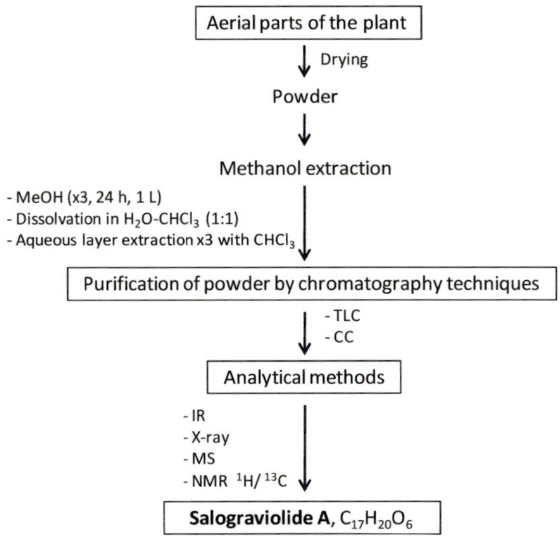


(b) Procedure for extraction of Sal A, $C_{17}H_{20}O_6$

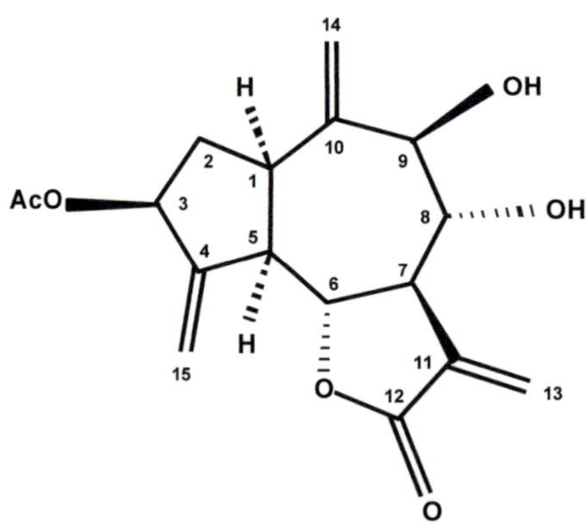


(c) Chemical structure of Sal A.

Fig. 2. Illustration of *Centaurea salonitana*, the procedure of Sal A extraction and its chemical structure.

The plant was collected during its flowering season and water extract was obtained from it by decoction. Briefly, the plant was air dried and soaked either entirely or only its ground flower head in hot boiling water for 20-30 min with a ratio of plant material weight to water volume of 1/8 (1 g of plant for every 8 ml of water). The solution was filtered either through 3 mm Whatman filter or through Sterile Gauze sponges 30x30 cm which yielded a residue and a filtrate named the "crude water extract". The resulting aqueous layer was sterilized using 0.2 µm non-pyrogenic sterile-R filter before storing it at -20°C until use.

*C. ainetensis* water extract is claimed in Lebanese folk literature to have anti-inflammatory effects. However, no research paper prior to 2004 investigating this plant's biological activity had ever been published. A screening of 29 plants reported by traditional medicine practitioners to have anti-inflammatory effects led to the validation of this activity for *C. ainetensis* water extract (Talhouk et al., 2008). Moreover, a screening of 109 wild Lebanese plant extracts, including 41 crude water, 34 methanol and 34 chloroform extracts, has resulted in the identification of selective and anti-proliferative bioactivity against several cancer cell lines in four wild Lebanese plant species namely, *Achillea damascene* also known as *Achillea falcata, Centaurea ainetensis, Onopordum cynarocephalum* and *Ranunculus myosuroudes* (Table 2). Although, *in vitro,* the three other plant extracts showed higher activities than *C. ainetensis,* the latter extract demonstrated the highest tumor growth inhibition ranging from 73 to 79% when tested *in vivo* in a mouse model of colorectal cancer (El-Najjar et al, 2007).

It was also shown later, that *C. ainestensis* water extract was mildly toxic but largely inhibited metastasis of leukemic cells (El-Sabban, unpublished findings).

Finally the extract was tested against the Infectious Bursal Disease (Gumboro) Virus (IBDV) in broilers and showed a mild reduction of IBDV viral antigens in the Bursa of Fabricius as well as a mild reduction in bursal lesions (Barbour, unpublished findings).

In an attempt to unravel the underlying causes for *C. ainetensis* water extract activity, we isolated the bioactive compound Sal A. The plant was subjected to bio-assay guided fractionation which consisted of testing the anti-tumor, anti-inflammatory and cytotoxicity effects of each fraction of the plant extract. Fractions of the crude water extract were inactive; however, Sal A was obtained from a fractionation of the methanol crude extract. Sal A manifested the same biological activities as the crude water extract with greater efficacy at lower concentrations. A parallel study was conducted to assess the effect of both the water crude extract and methanol crude extract of *C. ainetensis* along with 26 other indigenous Lebanese plants against nine microbial species. The results showed that the crude water extract was inactive against all microbial species whereas the methanol extract was effective against 88.8% of the tested microorganisms (Barbour et al., 2004).

Fig. 3 summarizes the acid-base extraction procedure used to fractionate the methanol crude extract and isolate Sal A. First the methanol crude extract was obtained by soaking the dried plant flowers in methanol with w/v of 1/10 for 16 h.

The mixture was then incubated on a shaker for 2 h at 20°C. The extract was filtered and yielded a residue and a filtrate named the "methanol crude extract". For further fractionation, the residue issued from the methanol extraction was soaked in EtOAc mixture in a ratio of 10/1 w/v. It was then separated by filtration into a residue and a filtrate consisting of fat and waxes and numbered I.1. To the crude methanol extract, concentrated $H_2SO_4$ solution was then added drop-wise till the pH reached 2. Following, a mixture of $CHCl_3$-$H_2O$ (2:1 ratio) was added. The $CHCl_3$ phase enriched with terpenoids and phenols was collected and labeled as I.2. The aqueous layer, on the other hand, was basified to pH 10

| Plant | Name in Arabic | Concentration (%)* | Growth Inhibition (%) | Cell line |
|---|---|---|---|---|
| *Achillea damascene* | Akhilia zat al-alf waraqah | | | Breast: |
| | | 0.5 | 65 | Scp2 |
| | | | | Colon/intestine: |
| | | 3 | 85 | HCT-116 |
| | | 3 | 80 | HT-29 |
| | | 3 | 70 | Mode K |
| *Centaurea ainetensis* | Quanturyun Aynata/ Shawk al-dardar | | | Breast: |
| | | 3 | 60 | Scp2 |
| | | | | Colon/intestine: |
| | | 3 | 60 | HCT-116 |
| | | 3 | 80 | HT-29 |
| | | 5 | 50 | Mode K |
| | | | | Skin: |
| | | 3 | 40 | PMK |
| | | 3 | 87 | SP1 |
| | | 3 | 65 | 308 |
| | | 3 | 67 | PAM212 |
| | | 3 | 40 | 17 |
| *Onopordum cynarocephalum* | Aqsun harshafi al ra's | 0.1 | | Breast: |
| | | | 50 | Scp2 |
| | | 0.5 | | Colon/intestine: |
| | | 0.5 | 70 | HCT-116 |
| | | 1.5 | 50 | HT-29 |
| | | | 50 | Mode K |
| *Ranunculus myosuroudes* | Hawdhan | | | Skin: |
| | | 2 | 36 | PMK |
| | | 2 | 98 | SP1 |
| | | 2 | 64 | 308 |
| | | 2 | 61 | PAM212 |
| | | 2 | 20 | 17 |

Table 2. Representation of the four Lebanese plant extracts with anticancer potentials. The following results were obtained for the water extracts of *A. damascene*, *C. ainetensis* and *O. cynarocephalum* and the methanol extract of *R. myosuroudes*. Cell proliferation and cytotoxicity were determined using the CellTiter 96 Non-Radioactive Cell Proliferation Assay and the CytoTox 96 Non-Radioactive Cytotoxicity Assay (both kits from Promega, Madison, WI) according to the manufacturer's suggestions.
* % = Volume extract/ Volume media

by adding concentrated $NH_4OH$ drop-wise and then resuspended in a $CHCl_3$-MeOH mixture (3:1 ratio) to be later separated into two organic and aqueous layers labeled I.3 containing alkaloids and I.4, respectively. I.1, I.2, I.3 and I.4 were evaporated to dryness under reduced pressure and weighed. A known amount of each subfraction was dissolved in a known volume of suitable solvent for further chromatographic and or/bioassays analysis.

Fraction "I.2" was the only of three other fractions to exhibit activity against cancer cells and in models of inflammation. Therefore TLC, thick layer chromatography and CC were used to further subdivide the I.2 bioactive fraction and yielded six subfractions I.2.1-I.2.6. Additional testing showed that only subfraction I.2.2 exhibited the anti proliferative, anti-inflammatory activity observed with the fraction I.2. This subfraction also maintained its bioactivity after it was purified using Solid Phase Extraction.

Finally, UV, IR, NMR and MS enabled the identification of the bioactive compound Sal A.

In conclusion, three research papers on *C. ainetensis* water extracts and three on Sal A anti-inflammatory and anti-tumor activities have been so far published by Ibsar while a fourth one is in progress (Al-Saghir et al., 2009; Barbour et al., 2004; El-Najjar et al., 2007; Ghantous et al., 2007; Saliba et al., 2009; Talhouk et al., 2008). Prior to our work, there was only one published article on Sal A's biological activity since its isolation (Vajs et al., 1999). Therefore, Ibsar has had a major contribution in identifying Sal A's biological activity and determining its mechanisms of action.

## 5. Salograviolide A: Overview of biological activities

To date, *C. ainetensis* water extract was shown to have antifungal, antibacterial, anti-viral, anticancer and anti-inflammatory activities. Sal A on the other hand, was only shown to have antifungal, anticancer and anti-inflammatory properties. The group of Vajs et al. discovered in 1999 the antifungal activity of Sal A while Ibsar faculty revealed the two others. It is unfortunate that no study has so far assessed whether Sal A is responsible for the antimicrobial and antiviral potentials exhibited by *C. ainetensis* water extract.

Following its isolation from *C. nicolai,* Sal A was tested against seven fungal species: *Aspergillus niger, A. ochraceus, Penicillium ochrochloron, Cladosporium cladosporoides, Fusarium tricinctum, Phomopsis helianthi* and *Trichoderma viride* (Vajs et al., 1999). Each strain was inoculated in the center of a plate with or without Sal A addition to the nutritional agar media. After incubation at 20°C for three weeks, the percentage of fungi inhibition was determined by comparing the diameter of each fungal strain colony inoculated in the presence of Sal A to that of the control inoculated without Sal A. The results showed that Sal A inhibited all the fungi strains except *Trichoderma viride*. Subsequently the use of different concentrations of Sal A enabled the determination of the Minimum Inhibitory Concentration (MICs) to inhibit the mycelial growth of the respective fungal species.

To test for the inflammation potential of *C. ainetensis* water extract, the pro-inflammatory cytokine interleukin-6 (IL-6) was chemically induced in mammary epithelial cells (CID-9 and Scp2) by treatment with endotoxin (ET)). The ability of the extract to reverse or prevent IL-6 production was then assessed and the results demonstrated that *C. ainetensis* water extract inhibited IL-6 in a dose-dependent manner (Talhouk et al., 2008). It was also shown that the extract reversed chemically induced paw edema signs in ET-pretreated Sprague-Dawley rats as well as thermal hyperalgesia in rats subjected to the hot plate test. Sal A was isolated from the water extracts and shown to be responsible for its observed bioactivity. In

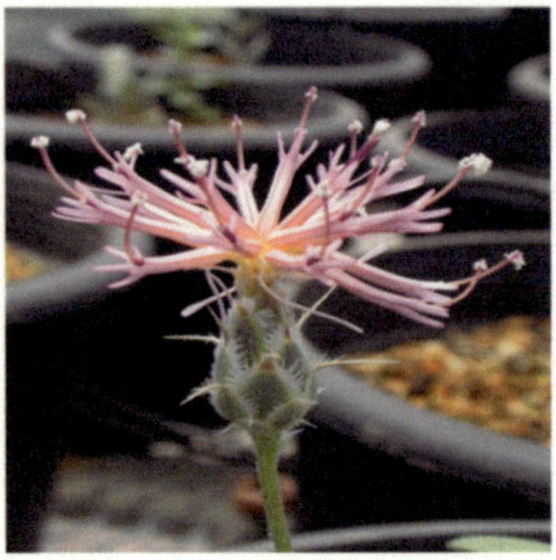

| Kigndom | Plantae |
|---|---|
| Subkingdom | Tracheobionta |
| Division | Magnioliophyta |
| Class | Magnoliopside |
| Subclass | Asteridae |
| Order | Asterales |
| Family | Asteraceae |
| Genus | *Centaurea* L. |
| Species | *ainetensis* |

(a) *Centaurea ainetensis* and its taxonomy

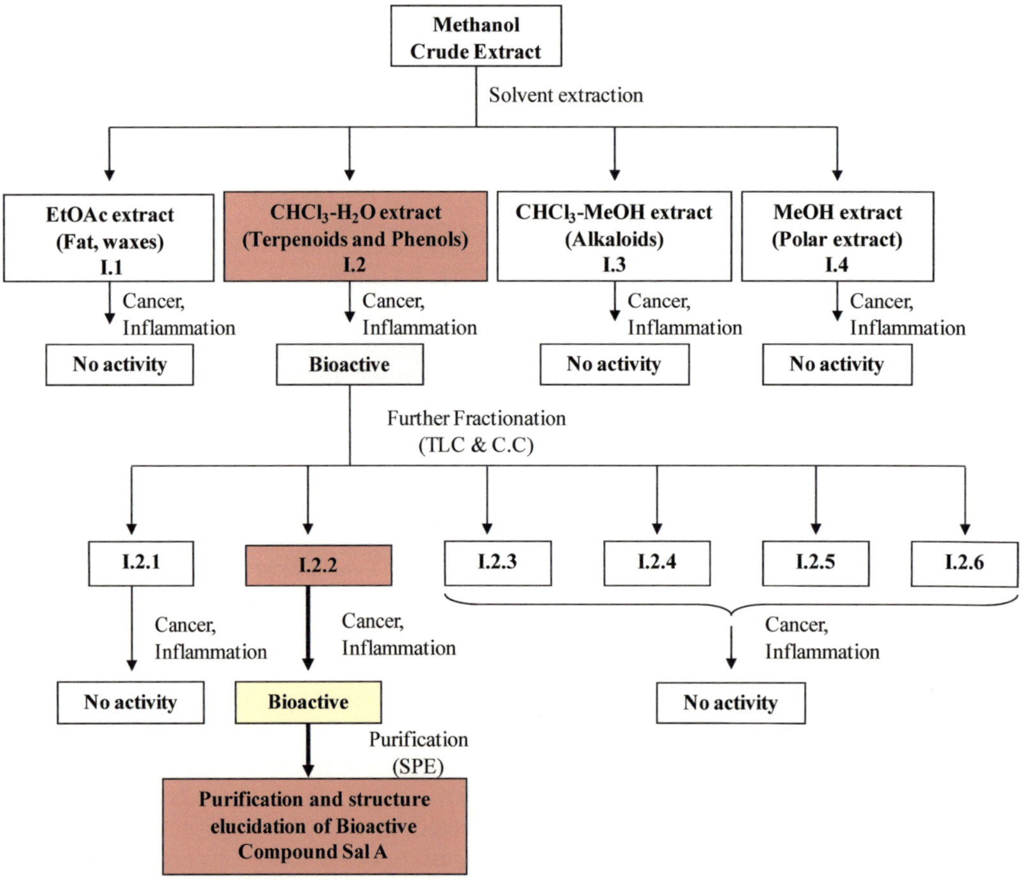


(b) The bioguided fractionation procedure

Fig. 3. Illustration of the indigenous Lebanese plant *Centaurea ainetensis* and the bioguided fractionation procedure that enabled the isolation of Salograviolide A. The plant picture is courtesy of Mr. Khaled Sleem.

parallel, the anti-inflammatory property of Sal A was demonstrated in a murine intestinal epithelial cell model (Mode K cells) treated with IL-1 and in *vivo* in a rat model of colonic inflammation induced by rectal injection of iodoacetoamide (Al-Saghir et al., 2009). The results showed that, similarly to *C. ainetensis* water extract, Sal A significantly reduced inflammatory cytokines and acted as a preventive agent to reduce inflammation.

*C. ainetensis* water extract and Sal A were also tested against different types of cancers (El-Najjar et al., 2007; Ghantous et al., 2007). *In vitro,* they were both non cytotoxic to normal primary murine keratinocytes while they preferentially inhibited neoplastic benign tumors and squamous cell carcinoma growth in a dose-dependent manner. The selective antiproliferative effects were confirmed in leukemic cells at the metastatically invasive stages as well as in human colon carcinomas. Sal A was also tested in combination with another sesquiterpene lactone, the Iso-seco-tanapartholide (TNP) extracted from *Achillea damascene,* against human colon cancer cell lines (Gali-Muhtasib, unpublished findings). The study demonstrated a synergistic apoptotic effect of both sesquiterpene lactones that failed to induce apoptosis when tested alone at the same low concentrations. Finally *in vivo,* the intraperitoneal water extract injection in Balb/c mice before chemically inducing colon cancer reduced drastically the mean size of aberrant crypt foci which is indicative of the extract's cancer preventive activity.

## 6. Salograviolide A and inflammation: Mechanisms and targets

Natural products derivatives have contributed over the last 25 years to approximately one fourth of the anti-inflammatory drugs used in the clinic (Newman & Cragg, 2007). In 2008, 18 additional natural product derived drugs were being tested at different clinical stages (Harvey, 2008). Terpenoids including sesquiterpene lactones have also reached clinical trials as potential anti-inflammatory agents. For instance, andrographolide; a labdane diterpenoid derived from the plant *Andrographis paniculata* of the Acanthacaea family, reached phase II clinical trials for rheumatoid arthritis. The sesquiterpene lactone parthenolide that made it to phase I cancer clinical trials, has also reached phase II and III clinical trials for the treatment of allergic contact dermatitis (refer to http://www.clinicaltrials.gov/).

Drugs with anti-inflammatory activities have common targets and modes of action that lead to the downregulation of the signs of inflammation as well as the chemical mediators controlling the mechanisms of inflammation. Elements of the complement system, angiogenic factors, prostaglandins, cytokines such as interleukins and matrix metalloproteinases (MMPs) are some of the most common inflammatory mediators.

Prostaglandins play a role in the modulation of blood flow. They are derived from the arachidonic acid due to the action of two prostaglandins H synthases isoforms known as the cyclooxygenases 1 and 2 (COX-1 and COX-2). COX-1 is constitutively expressed in different tissues while COX-2 is induced by inflammatory stimuli and is therefore thought to be the only isoform involved in propagating the inflammatory response (Larsen & Henson, 1983).

IL-6 secreted by the macrophages releases proteinases and elastases which bind to IL-6 receptor and generate signals implicated in humoral inflammation (Heinrich et al., 2003). IL-1, on the other hand, induces the mobilization of the arachidonic acid and its metabolism into prostaglandins thus contributing to cellular inflammation. It was also shown that IL-1 induces the synthesis of COX-2 through the activation of the nuclear factor Kappa B (NF-κB) transcription factor (Larsen & Henson, 1983). NF-κB is a key modulator of inflammation and is implicated in inflammation-induced tumor formation as well (Karin & Greten, 2005). It is

known to promote the expression of target genes of the inflammation response such as interleukins, COX-2, and inducible nitric-oxide synthase (iNOS) (Mazor et al., 2000).
Finally, components of the MMP family have been reported to act in wound healing and embryogenesis (Mainardi et al., 1991). Gelatinase A or MMP-2 (72 KDa) and gelatinase B or MMP-9 (92 KDa) have been identified as pro-inflammatory agents. They enable the digestion of components of the basement membrane; a function that is referred to as gelatinolysis (Birkedal-Hansen et al., 1993).
Sal A and *C. ainetensis* water extract were shown to modulate some of these major players of the inflammatory response. They both inhibit IL-6 expression (Talhouk et al., 2008) and IL-1-induced COX-2 expression by interfering with their synthesis (Al-Saghir et al., 2009). Only the effect of the water extract on the expression levels of the gelatinases A and B was assessed. The results indicate that the water extract decreased the expression of both proteins with preferential inhibition of gelatinase B 9 h post treatment with endotoxin (Talhouk et al., 2008). Similarly, only the effect of Sal A on the NF-κB signaling was investigated. NF-κB is composed of the two subunits p50 and p65 and is only active after translocation of the subunits into the nucleus and their dimerization. In normal conditions, NF-κB is inactive due to its retention in the cytoplasm by the inhibitor of NF-κB (IκB). Pro-inflammatory stimuli such as IL-1 cause the phosphorylation of the IκB by the inhibitor of NFκB- β (IKK). The phosphorylation in return leads to IκB degradation enabling thus the translocation to the cytoplasm and the dimerization of the NF-κB subunits, their binding to target DNA sequences, initiation of transcription and activation of the NF-κB transduction pathway (Baeuerele & Baltimore, 1996).
It was demonstrated that Sal A inhibits the NF-κB activation by two mechanisms. The first involved the stabilization of IκB, since combination treatment of Sal A with IL-1 decreased the degradation of IκB observed in response to treatment with IL-1 alone. The second involved inhibiting NF-κB translocation and binding to DNA, since the incubation of cells with Sal A after IL-1 addition (hence after IκB degradation) still caused a reduction in the activity of NF-κB (Fig. 4) (Al-Saghir et al., 2009).

## 7. Salograviolide A and cancer: Mechanisms and targets

The mechanism behind the anticancer activity of sesquiterpene lactones has been extensively investigated. For example, parthenolide was shown to induce cell cycle arrest, promote cell differentiation and trigger apoptosis (Pajak et al., 2008). The molecular basis for parthenolide activity in cancer cells include among others, inhibiting NF-κB and stimulating apoptosis by accumulation of reactive oxygen species (ROS) as well as by regulating the levels of anti-apoptotic and pro-apoptotic proteins (Pajak et al., 2008). Interestingly, parthenolide showed a synergistic effect when used in combination with paclitaxel and increased apoptosis in breast cancer cells (Patel et al., 2000).
As mentioned earlier, *C. ainetensis* crude extract and Sal A were tested against skin, colon and blood cancer cell lines and showed selective antineoplastic effects with no cytotoxicity to normal cells. At the cellular level, *C. ainetensis* crude extract induced $G_0/G_1$ cell cycle arrest in neoplastic epidermal cells while Sal A increased the population in Pre-$G_1$. In accordance with this finding, the levels of cyclin D1 whose activity is required for the $G_1/S$ transition were reduced (Li et al., 2011). On the other hand, the levels of the tumor suppressors p16 and p21 which are associated with greater susceptibility to chemotherapy

and with calcium induced differentiation in keratinocytes, respectively were increased (Hochhauser, 1997; Di Cunto et al., 1998, as cited in Ghantous et al., 2007). Moreover, p21 proteins were differentially regulated: they were upregulated in the presence of the crude extract which was consistent with the observed $G_0/G_1$ cell cycle arrest, whereas their upregulation in the presence of Sal A was found to be transient. This transient upregulation of p21 has been reported as critical for its role in differentiation (Di Cunto et al., 1998).

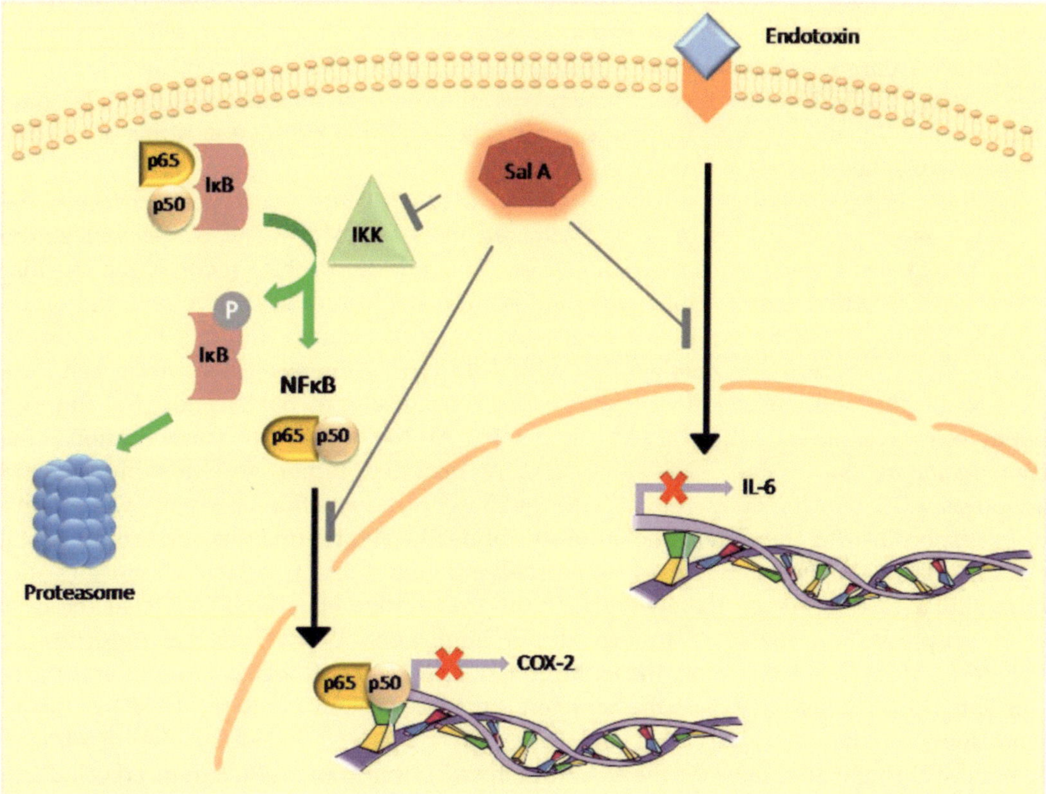


Fig. 4. Anti-inflammatory cascade triggered by Sal A. Details of the mechanism are explained in section 6 above.

In addition to cell cycle modulation, characteristic signs of apoptosis such as the partial and complete condensation of the chromatin were noted in the presence of Sal A. Furthermore, the ratio of the pro-apoptotic protein Bax to the anti-apoptotic protein Bcl-2 was found to be elevated. Bax and Bcl-2 have counteracting roles regarding the mitochondrial membrane permeabilization and thus the high ratio of Bax to Bcl-2 reflects the permeabilization of the mitochondrial membrane to release factors such as cytochrome c and the apoptosis inducing factor that will induce cell death. In conjunction, a considerable amount of ROS accumulated in the cells in the presence of Sal A. In fact, the accumulation of ROS was even shown to precede the growth inhibition and indicated an oxidant role of Sal A in these cells. Finally, the crude extract and Sal A had a contradictory regulatory effect on NF-κB. The crude plant extract decreased in a dose-dependent manner the binding of NF-κB to the DNA without affecting the expression level of IκB, whereas Sal A increased it. It is worth noting that in cancer, the role of NF-κB activation or inhibition is in itself conflicting. NF-κB can be best described as a double edged sword for its activation can promote tumorigenesis (by inducing inflammatory mediators) or promote differentiation and thus inhibit tumorigenesis (Seitz et al., 1998, as cited in Ghantous et al., 2007).

In addition, the crude extract was assessed in human colon cancers and showed both an increase in p21 protein level of expression and in the ratio of Bax to Bcl-2 proteins. In colon cancer, cyclin B1 levels were decreased by the extract, while they were found to be unaffected by neither Sal A nor the extract in skin cancer. Cyclin B1 decrease is important for the exit from mitosis and for the cytokinesis (Takizawa & Morgan, 2000, as cited in El-Najjar et al., 2007). Another protein which was differentially modulated in skin *vs* colon cancer is p53. In colon cancer, the crude extract increased the expression levels of the p53 protein, while the levels were unaffected in skin cancer.

In leukemic cells, similarly to what was shown with the other two types of cancers, the extract induced pre-$G_1$ cell cycle arrest, increased the levels of p53 and p21 as well as the ratio of Bax to Bcl-2, and decreased cyclin D1 levels. In addition, the secretion of the vascular endothelial growth factor (VEGF) was significantly decreased by Sal A and the crude extract, adding VEGF to the list of targets of Sal A (El-Sabban, unpublished findings). Finally, Sal A was tested in combination with TNP against human colon cancer cell lines (Gali-Muhtasib, unpublished findings). At low concentrations, Sal A and TNP induced $G_2/M$ cell cycle arrest when tested separately. At the same low concentrations, the combination of Sal A and TNP synergistically inhibited tumor growth and triggered apoptosis. ROS, which increased by a factor of 25 upon combination treatment, were found to be responsible for the synergistic-induced cell death. The pretreatment of the colorectal cancer cells with the antioxidant N-acetyl-L-cysteine (NAC), which diminishes the intracellular ROS, reversed the synergistic anti-proliferative effect and protected the cells from apoptosis and therefore confirmed the implication of ROS in the induction of apoptosis. Moreover, p38 kinase, the extracellular signal regulated kinase (ERK) and the c-Jun N-terminal kinase (JNK) of the mitogen-activated protein kinases (MAPK) pathway were found to be phosphorylated and thus induced after the combination treatment. Literature strongly advocates for the MAPK pathway implication in ROS induced cell death (Zhang et al., 2003). Using specific inhibitors of both ERK (usually involved in mitogenic signals and cellular proliferation), and of p38 (associated with stress along with JNK and commonly known as the stress activated protein kinases (Lewis et al., 1998)) abolished the apoptotic synergistic effect of the combination treatment and emphasized the pathway's association to cell death. Further studies with Sal A and TNP suggested a cross-talk between ROS, JNK and Bcl-2 family in the induction of apoptosis. ROS accumulation was found to induce Bax relocalization to the mitochondrial membrane on the one hand and to decrease the ani-apoptotic Bcl-2 expression levels on the other (Gali-Muhtasib, unpublished findings). Bcl-2 decrease was also associated with a maximal JNK activation which suggested that JNK might play a role in further inactivation of Bcl-2. In accordance with our findings several studies have reported the involvement of JNK but not ERK nor p38 in the phosphorylation and inactivation of Bcl-2 (Srivasta et al., 1999).

Taken together these results indicate a promising chemotherapeutic effect for using Sal A alone or in combination against various cancer types.

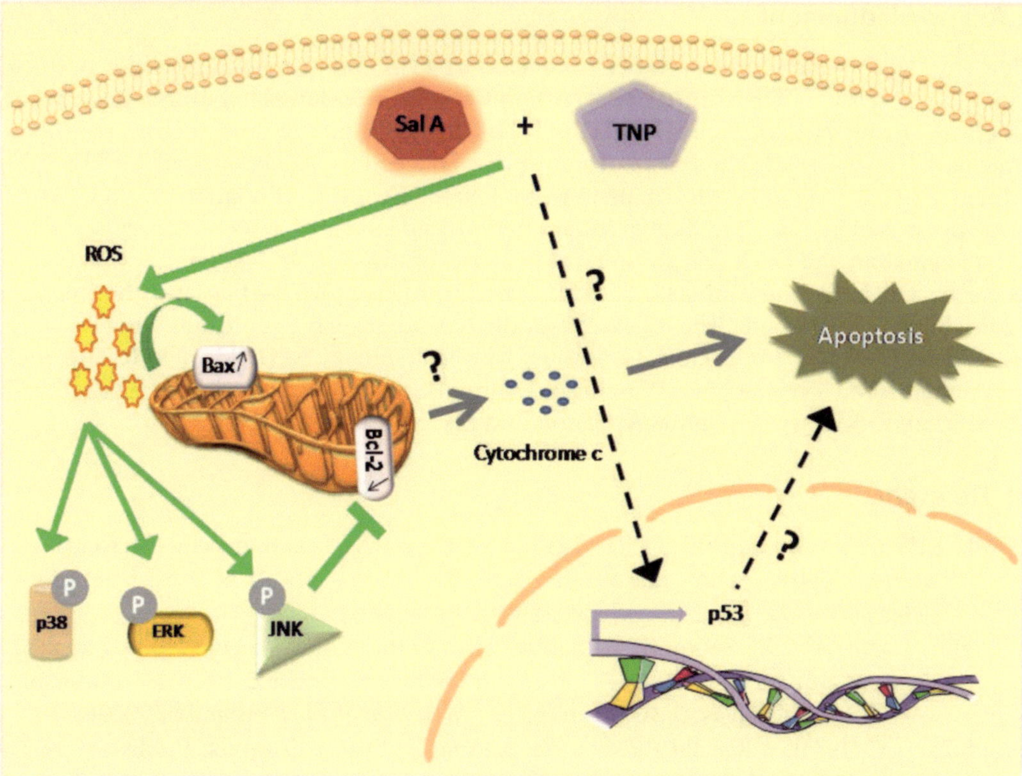


Fig. 5. Anticancer cascade triggered by the combination of Sal A and TNP in colon cancer cells. The combination caused increase in ROS and activation of MAPK molecules, ERK, JNK and p38 leading to apoptosis. It is still unclear whether apoptosis is associated with the modulation of p21, p53, and cyclin B1 proteins or the release of cytochrome c from mitochondria.

## 8. Conclusion and future direction

Cancer progression is characterized by seven hallmarks: sustaining proliferative signaling, insensitivity to growth suppressors, evading apoptosis, acquisition of replicative immortality, induction of angiogenesis, activation of invasion and metastasis and finally chronic inflammation (Colotta F. Et al., 2009).

In a nutshell, the evidence that has been collected so far by multiple investigators suggests that Sal A is a promising compound for cancer drug discovery for it acts at least on three cancer hallmarks: it upregulates tumor suppressors, triggers apoptosis and downregulates the mediators of inflammation. Its selectivity toward tumor cells and ability to target multiple pathways involved in inflammation and cancer imply that this compound is unlikely to have a single target that is responsible for its biological activities. Although a large body of information supports the role of Sal A against cancer and inflammation, there are yet no studies assessing its toxicology profiles or its absorption, distribution and metabolism in animals and humans. Such studies are warranted to better determine its potential for future applications in the clinical setting whether alone or in combination with standard clinical drugs.

## 9. Acknowledgement

This work was supported by grants from UNISANTIS and the research was conducted under the direction of the Nature Conservation Center for Sustainable Futures (Ibsar) at the American University of Beirut, Lebanon. Dr. Salma Talhouk and many researchers contributed to the establishment of Ibsar. Plant collection was supervised by Dr. Salma Talhouk and carried out by Mr. Khaled Sleem. Extraction and fractionation of plant extracts were supervised by Dr. Najat Saliba. Inflammation studies on Sal A were supervised by Dr. Fadia Homeidan and Dr. Rabih Talhouk, skin cancer studies by Dr. Nadine Darwiche, colon cancer by Dr. Hala Gali-Muhtasib, leukemia by Dr. Marwan El-Sabban and the microbial studies by Dr. Elie Barbour. The following graduate students have contributed to this work: Ms. Nahed El-Najjar, Mr. Akram Ghantous, Mr. Mohammad Salla, Ms. Saada Dakdouki, Mr. Ahmad Abou Tayyoun, Mr. Wassim El-Jouni, Ms. Melody Saikaly, Mr. Houssam Shaib, Ms. Myriam El-Khoury, Ms. Jamal Al-Saghir and Ms. Noura Abdallah.

## 10. References

Akkol, EK.; Arif, R.; Ergun, F. & Yesilada, E. (2009). Sesquiterpene lactones with antinociceptive and antipyretic activity from two Centaurea species. *J Ethnopharmacol.* 122, 2 (March 2009), pp. 210-5.

Al-Saghir, J.; Al-Ashi, R.; Salloum, R.; Saliba, NA.; Talhouk, RS. & Homaidan FR. (2009). Anti-inflammatory properties of Salograviolide A purified from Lebanese plant Centaurea ainetensis. *BMC Complement Altern Med.* 9, 36, (September 2009).

Awadallah, A. (1984). *Al'Ilaj Bil Aa'shab Wal Nabatat Al Shafiya* (Arabic). Published by Dar Ikraa, Beirut, Lebanon.

Azaizeh, H., Saad, B., Cooper, E. & Said, O. (2008). Traditional Arabic and Islamic Medicine, a Re-emerging Health Aid. *Evid Based Complement Alternat Med.* 7, 4, (Jun 2008), pp. 419-424.

Bach, SM.; Fortuna, MA.; Attarian, R.; de Trimarco, JT.; Catalán, CA.; Av-Gay, Y. & Bach, H. (2011). Antibacterial and cytotoxic activities of the sesquiterpene lactones cnicin and onopordopicrin. *Nat Prod Commun.* 6, 2, (February 2011), pp. 163-6.

Baeuerle, PA. & Baltimore, D. (1996). NF-kappa B: ten years after. *Cell.* 87, 1, (October 1996), pp. 13-20.

Balunas, MJ. & Kinghorn, AD. (2005). Drug discovery from medicinal plants. *Life Sci.* 78, 5, (December 2005), pp. 431-41. Review.

Barbour, EK.; Al Sharif, M.; Sagherian, VK.; Habre, AN.; Talhouk, RS. & Talhouk, SN. (2004). Screening of selected indigenous plants of Lebanon for antimicrobial activity. *J Ethnopharmacol.* 93, 1, (July 2004), pp. 1-7.

Birkedal-Hansen, H.; Moore, WGI.; Windsor, LJ.; Birkedal-Hansen, B.; DeCarlo, A. & Engler, JA. (1993). Matrix metalloproteinases: A Review. *Crit Rev Oral Biol And Med.* 4, 2, pp. 197-250

Bruno, M.; Rosselli, S.; Maggio, A.; Raccuglia, RA.; Bastow KF., Wu CC & Lee, KH. (2005). Cytotoxic activity of some natural and synthetic sesquiterpene lactones. *Planta Med.*71, 12, (December 2005), pp. 1176-8.

Cheng, CH.; Costall, B.; Hamburger, M.; Hostettmann, K.; Naylor, RJ.; Wang, Y. & Jenner, P. (1992). Toxic effects of solstitialin A 13-acetate and cynaropicrin from Centaurea solstitialis L. (Asteraceae) in cell cultures of foetal rat brain. *Neuropharmacology*.31, 3, (March 1992), pp. 271-7.

Chicca, A.; Tebano, M.; Adinolfi, B.; Ertugrul, K.; Flamini, G. & Nieri, P. (2011). Anti-proliferative activity of aguerin B and a new rare nor-guaianolide lactone isolated from the aerial parts of Centaurea deflexa. *Eur J Med Chem.* (March 2011).

Cho, JY.; Kim, AR.; Jung, JH.; Chun, T.; Rhee, MH. & Yoo, ES. (2004). Cytotoxic and pro-apoptotic activities of cynaropicrin, a sesquiterpene lactone, on the viability of leukocyte cancer cell lines. *Eur J Pharmacol.* 492, 2-3, (May 2004), pp. 85-94.

Clinical trials (2010): http://www.clinicaltrials.gov/ct2/search/browse?brwse=intr_cat_Infl

Colotta, F.; Allavena, P.; Sica, A.; Garlanda, C. & Mantovani, A. (2009). Cancer-related inflammation, the seventh hallmark of cancer: links to genetic instability. *Carcinogenesis*. 30, 7, (July 2009), pp. 1073-81. Review.

Cragg, G.M. (1998). Paclitaxel (Taxol): a success story with valuable lessons for natural product drug discovery and development. *Med Res Rev.*18, 5 (September 1998), pp. 315-31.

Csupor-Löffler, B.; Hajdú, Z.; Réthy, B.; Zupkó, I.; Máthé, I.; Rédei, T.; Falkay, G. & Hohmann, J. (2009). Antiproliferative activity of Hungarian Asteraceae species against human cancer cell lines. Part II. *Phytother Res.* 23, 8, (August 2009), pp. 1109-15.

Daniewski, W.M.; Nowak, G.; Routsi, E.; Rychlewska, U.; Szczepanska, B. & Skibicki, P. (1992). Salogravilide A, A Sesquiterpene From Centaurea Salonitana. *Phytochemistry*. 31, 8, pp. 2891-2893.

Darwiche, N.; El-Banna, S. & Gali-Muhtasib, H. (2007). Cell cycle modulatory and apoptotic effects of plant-derived anticancer drugs in clinical use or development. *Expert Opinion on Drug Discovery*. 2, 3, (March 2007), pp. 361-379.

Djeddi, S.; Karioti, A.; Sokovic, M.; Koukoulitsa, C. & Skaltsa, H. (2008). A novel sesquiterpene lactone from Centaurea pullata: structure elucidation, antimicrobial activity, and prediction of pharmacokinetic properties. *Bioorg Med Chem.* 16, 7, (April, 2008), pp. 3725-31.

Djeddi, S.; Karioti, A.; Sokovic, M.; Stojkovic, D.; Seridi, R. & Skaltsa, H. (2007). Minor sesquiterpene lactones from Centaurea pullata and their antimicrobial activity. *J Nat Prod.* 70, 11, (November 2007), pp. 1796-9.

El-Najjar, N.; Dakdouki, S.; Darwiche, N.; El-Sabban, M.; Saliba, NA. & Gali-Muhtasib, H. (2008). Anti-colon cancer effects of Salograviolide A isolated from Centaurea ainetensis. *Oncol Rep.* 19, 4, (April 2008), pp. 897-904.

Font, M.; Garcia-Jacas, N.; Vilatersana, R.; Roquet, C. & Susanna, A. (2009). Evolution and biogeography of Centaurea section Acrocentron inferred from nuclear and plastid DNA sequence analyses. *Ann Bot.* 103, 6, (April 2009), pp. 985-97.

Fortuna, AM.; de Riscala, EC.; Catalan, CA.; Gedris, TE. & Herz, W. Sesquiterpene lactones from Centaurea tweediei. *Biochem Syst Ecol.* 29, 9, (October 2001), pp. 967-971.

Gali-Muhtasib, H. & Bakkar, N. (2002). Modulating Cell Cycle: Current Applications and Prospects for Future Drug Development. *Current Cancer Drug Targets.* 2, 4, (December 2002), pp. 309-336.

Genta, SB.; Cabrera, WM.; Mercado, MI.; Grau, A.; Catalán, CA. & Sánchez, SS. (2010). Hypoglycemic activity of leaf organic extracts from Smallanthus sonchifolius: Constituents of the most active fractions. *Chem Biol Interact.* 185, 2, (April 2010), pp. 143-52.

Ghantous, A.; Tayyoun, AA;, Lteif, GA.; Saliba, NA.; Gali-Muhtasib, H.; El-Sabban, M. & Darwiche, N. (2008). Purified Salograviolide A Isolated From Centaurea ainetensis Causes Growth Inhibition and Apoptosis in Neoplastic Epidermal Cells. *Int J Oncol.* 32, 4, (April 2008), pp. 841-9.

Ghantous, A.; Gali-Muhtasib, H.; Vuorela, H.; Saliba, NA. & Darwiche, N. (2010). What made sesquiterpene lactones reach cancer clinical trials? *Drug Discov Today.* 15, 15-16, (August 2010), pp. 668-78.

González, AG.; Darias, V.; Alonso, G. & Estévez, E. (1980). The cytostatic activity of the chlorohyssopifolins, chlorinated sesquiterpene lactones from Centaurea. *Planta Med.* 40, 2, (October 1980), pp. 179-84.

Gürbüz, I. & Yesilada, E. Evaluation of the anti-ulcerogenic effect of sesquiterpene lactones from Centaurea solstitialis L. ssp. solstitialis by using various in vivo and biochemical techniques. *J Ethnopharmacol.* 112, 2, (Jun 2007), pp. 284-91.

Harvey, AL. Natural products in drug discovery. (2008). *Drug Discov Today.* 13, 19-20, (October 2008), pp. 894-901. Review.

Heinrich, PC.; Behrmann, I.; Haan, S.; Hermanns, HM.; Müller-Newen, G. & Schaper, F. (2003). Principles of interleukin (IL)-6-type cytokine signaling and its regulation. *Biochem J.* 15, 374(Pt 1), (August 2003), pp. 1-20. Review.

Heywood, V.H.; Harborne, J.B. & Turner, B.L. (1997). The biology and chemistry of the compositae, vols I and II, *Academic press: New York.*

Ibsar: Traditional Knowledge and Biotechnology > plants > Centaurea ainetensis (2010) http://www.ibsar.org/research/Traditional%20Knowledge%20and%20Biotechnology/plants/Centaurea%20ainetensis.htm.

Karin, M. & Greten, FR. (2002). NF-kappaB: linking inflammation and immunity to cancer development and progression. *Nat Rev Immunol.* 5, 10, (October 2005), pp. 749-59. Review.

Koukoulitsa, E.; Skaltsa, H.; Karioti, A.; Demetzos, C. & Dimas, K. (2002). Bioactive sesquiterpene lactones from Centaurea species and their cytotoxic/cytostatic activity against human cell lines in vitro. *Planta Med.* 68, 7, (July 2002), pp. 649-52.

Lakhal, H.; Boudiar, T.; Kabouche, A.; Kabouche, Z.; Touzani R.; & Bruneau, C. (2010). New sesquiterpene lactone and other constituents from Centaurea sulphurea (Asteraceae). *Nat Prod Commun.* 5, 6, (Jun 2010), pp. 849-50.

Larsen, GL. & Henson, PM. (1983). Mediators of inflammation. *Annu Rev Immunol.* 1983, 1, pp. 335-59. Review.

Lewis, T S.; Shapiro, P S. & Ahn, N G. (1998). Signal transduction through MAP kinase cascades. *Advances in Cancer Research.* 1998, 74, pp. 49-139.

Li, J.; Huang, X.; Xie, X.; Wang, J. & Duan, M. (2011). Human telomerase reverse transcriptase regulates cyclin D1 and G1/S phase transition in laryngeal squamous carcinoma. *Acta Otolaryngol.* 131, 5, (May 2011), pp. 546-51.

Lonergan, G.; Routsi, E.; Georgiadis, T.; Agelis, G.; Hondrelis, J.; Matsoukas, J.; Larsen, LK. & Caplan, FR. (1992). Isolation, NMR studies, and biological activities of onopordopicrin from Centaurea sonchifolia. *J Nat Prod.* 55, 2, (February, 1992), pp. 225-8.

Mainardi, CL.; Pourmotabbed, TF. & Hasty, KA. (1991). Inflammation phagocytes and connective tissue degrading metalloproteinases. *Am J Med Sci.* 302, 3, (September 1991), pp. 171-175.

Mazor, R L.; Menendez, I Y.; Ryan, M A.; Fiedler, M A. & Wong, H R. (2000). Sesquiterpene lactones are potent inhibitors of interleukin 8 gene expression in cultured human respiratory epithelium. *Cytokine.* 12, 3, (March 2000), p. 239-45.

McGovern, PE.; Mirzoian, A. & Hall, GR. (2009). Ancient Egyptian herbal wines. *Proc Natl Acad Sci USA.* 106, 18, (May 2009), pp. 7361-6.

Medjroubi, K.; Benayache, F. & Bermejo, J. Sesquiterpene lactones from Centaurea musimomum. (2005). Antiplasmodial and cytotoxic activities. *Fitoterapia.* 76,7-8, (December 2005), pp. 744-6.

Moukarzel K., 1997 Al Tadawi Bil Nabatat Al Tabi'iya, Kitab Tob Cha'bi Mouzawad Bil Souwar Wal Fahares (Arabic) published by Dar Al Hadara, Beirut, Lebanon.

Nehmeh M., 1977. Wild Flowers of Lebanon, National Council for Scientific Research, Beirut, Lebanon.

Newman, DJ. & Cragg, GM. (2007). Natural products as sources of new drugs over the last 25 years. *J Nat Prod.* 70, 3, (March 2007), pp. 461-77. Review.

Nowak, G. (1993). Chromatography of Twentysix Sesquiterpene Lactones from Centaurea bella. *Chromatographia.* 35, 5/6, (March 1993)

Ozçelik, B.; Gürbüz, I.; Karaoglu, T. & Yeşilada, E. (2007). Antiviral and antimicrobial activities of three sesquiterpene lactones from Centaurea solstitialis L. ssp. solstitialis. *Microbiol Res.* 164, 5, (July 2007), p. 545-52.

Pajak, B.; Gajkowska, B. & Orzechowski, A. (2008). Molecular basis of parthenolide-dependent proapoptotic activity in cancer cells. *Folia Histochem Cytobiol.* 46, 2, pp. 129-35. Review.

Patel, N M.; Nozaki, S.; Shortle, N H.; Bhat-Nakshatri, P.; Newton, T R.; Rice, S.; Gelfanov, V.; Boswell, S H.; Goulet, R J.; Sledge, G W. & Nakshatri H. (2000). Paclitaxel sensitivity of breast cancer cells with constitutively active NF-kappaB is enhanced by IkappaBalpha super-repressor and parthenolide Oncogen. 19, 36, (August, 2000), pp. 4159-69.

Rychlewska, U.; Szczepafiska, B.; Daniewski, W.M. & Nowak G. (1992). Crystal structure of salograviolide A, a guaiane-type sesquiterpene lactone. *Journal of Crystallographic and Spectroscopic Research.* 22, 6, (February 1992), pp. 659-663.

Saliba, NA.; Dakdouki, S.; Homeidan, FR.; Kogan, J.; Bouhadir, K.; Talhouk, SN. & Talhouk, RS. (2009). Bio-guided identification of an anti-inflammatory guaianolide from Centaurea ainetensis. *Pharmaceutical Biology.* 47, 8, (August 2009), pp. 701-707.

Saroglou, V.; Karioti, A.; Demetzos, C.; Dimas, K. & Skaltsa, H. (2005). Sesquiterpene lactones from Centaurea spinosa and their antibacterial and cytotoxic activities. *J Nat Prod.* 68, 9, (September 2005), pp. 1404-7.

Solecki, R.S. (1975). Shanidar IV, a Neanderthal flower burial in northern Iraq. *Science*. 190, 4217, ( 1975), pp. 880–881.

Talhouk RS, El-Jouni W, Baalbaki R, Gali-Muhtasib H, Kogan J & Talhouk SN. Anti-inflammatory bio-activities in water extract of Centaurea ainetensis Journal of *Medicinal Plants Research*. 2, 2, (February 2008), pp. 024-033.

Vajs, V.; Todorović, N.; Ristić, M.; Tesević, V.; Todorović, B.; Janaćković, P.; Marin, P. & Milosavljević, S. (1999). Guaianolides from Centaurea nicolai: antifungal activity. *Phytochemistry*. 52, 3, (October 1999), pp. 383-6.

Webster's Revised Unabridged Dictionary. Published in 1913 by C. & G. Merriam Co. Edited by Noah Porter. United States of America.

Zhang, X.; Shan, P.; Sasidhar, M.; Chupp, G L.; Flavell, R A.; Choi, A M. & Lee, P J. (2003). Reactive oxygen species and extracellular signal-regulated kinase 1/2 mitogen-activated protein kinase mediate hyperoxia-induced cell death in lung epithelium. *American journal of respiratory cell and molecular biology*. 28, 3, (March 2003), pp. 305-315.

# Part 4

## Inflammation, Immune System and Cancer

# 18

# The Role of Inflammation in Cancer

O'Leary D.P., Neary P.M. and Redmond H.P.
*Department of Academic Surgery, Cork University Hospital*
*Ireland*

## 1. Introduction

Cancer is a pro-inflammatory disease. The link between inflammation and cancer was first noticed over 150 years ago. In 1863, Virchow observed that tumours tend to occur at sites of chronic inflammation (Balkwill, 2001).

Epidemiological studies have recently emerged which support the association between cancer and inflammation. Viruses and bacteria cause chronic inflammation and are significant risk factors in the development of malignancy. Human papilloma viruses, hepatitis B, hepatitis C and helicobacter pylori are well studied examples of this phenomenon which result in cervical cancer, hepatocellular cancer, lympho-proliferative disorders and gastric cancer respectively. Furthermore, increased risk of malignancy is associated with chronic inflammation caused by chemical and physical agents (Gulumian, 1999). In addition to epidemiological data, gene-cluster polymorphisms that lead to increased levels of pro-inflammatory cytokine release are associated with a poorer prognosis and disease severity in cancer patients (Warzocha, 1998; El-Omar, 2000). Moreover, the fact that chronic use of NSAIDs, such as aspirin are shown to reduce the incidence of numerous cancer types including colon, lung and stomach, gives additional supporting evidence for the link between inflammation and cancer (Wang, 2003).

## 2. NF-κB – A key player

Recent studies have implicated an inflammation-induced protein called nuclear factor kappa B (NF-κB) as a central figure in the link between cancer and inflammation. In 1986, Baltimore et al., originally discovered NF- κB as a factor in the nucleus of B cells that binds to the enhancer of the kappa light chain of immunoglobulin (Sen, 1986). NF- κB activity is considered a hallmark of inflammation. It is shown that NF-κB manipulation can convert inflammation-driven tumour growth into inflammation-induced tumour regression (Luo, 2004). Furthermore, many oncogenes and carcinogens can cause activation of NF-κB, whereas chemicals with chemo-protective properties can interfere with NF-κB activation (Bharti, 2002).

In unstimulated cells, the majority of NF-κB complexes are kept predominantly cytoplasmic and in an inactive form by binding a family of inhibitors known as Inhibitor-κB (IκB). The NF-κB pathway can be activated by numerous stimuli including bacteria, viruses and pro-inflammatory cytokines especially tumour necrosis factor (TNF). Phosphorylation of NF-κB bound I-kappa-B kinases (IκK) on two conserved serine residues within the N-terminal domain of the IκB proteins, which allows for proteasomal degradation and resultant NF-κB liberation. Activation of the NF-κB signalling cascade results in complete degradation of IκB allowing translocation of NF-κB to the nucleus where it induces transcription. The NF-κB family of transcription factors is composed of homodimers and heterodimers derived from 5 subunits - including REL-A(p65), c-REL, REL-B, p50(NF-κB1) and p52 (NF-κB2). When these subunits enter the nucleus, they can mediate transcription of target genes (Hayden, 2004). All family members share a highly conserved Rel homology domain responsible for DNA binding, dimerization domain and interaction with IκBs, the intracellular inhibitor of NF-κB. Cellular stresses including ionising radiation and chemotherapeutic agents can also activate NF-kB. The subsequent release of pro-inflammatory mediators (CSF-1, COX-2, IL-6, IL-1, VEGF, TNF) (Luo, 2004; Marx, 2004) and known anti-apoptotic regulators (BCL-2 and GADD45β) are thought to potentiate tumour growth. In 2004, Karin et al discovered the mechanism that NF-κB contributes to tumourigenesis (Luo, 2004). Prior to this study evidence implicating NF-κB and cancer was mostly circumstantial. Using a murine model of colitis-associated cancer, researchers were able to use genetically altered mice which had the NF-κB activator enzyme IκK knocked out of intestinal epithelial cells and macrophages. In the absence of the IκK gene, neither cell could activate NF-κB. Interestingly, loss of NF-κB activity in both macrophages and epithelial cells individually reduced tumour incidence. They also found that this occurred through two different mechanisms. Tumour incidence decreased by approximately 50% with the loss of NF-κB activity in macrophages through a reduction in growth factors produced by inflammatory cells normally induced by NF-κB activation. Secondly, the loss of NF-κB activity in intestinal epithelial cells resulted in an 80% drop in tumour incidence. The mechanism seen here was different to that seen with the macrophages. Inflammation was not reduced as with the macrophages, instead, apoptosis was no longer inhibited in intestinal cells (Karin, 2004). Pikarsky et al had similar findings in a murine model of inflammation-associated liver cancer where they inhibited NF-κB by adding a gene encoding for IκB, a natural NF-κB inhibitor (Pikarsky, 2004).

The NF-κB family of transcription factors plays a key role in regulation of immune and inflammatory responses including apoptosis and oncogenesis (Baldwin, 2001). NF-κB regulated gene products including those encoding ICAM-1, the extracellular matrix protein tenascin C, vascular endothelial growth factor (VEGF), the chemokine IL-8, the pro-inflammatory enzyme COX2 and matrix metalloprotease 9 (MMP9) are associated with tumour progression and metastasis (Karin, 2002). However NF-κB may also control the expression of apoptosis promoting cytokines such as TNF alpha and FAS ligand (Kasibhatla, 1998).

NF-κB activation is required for endotoxin induced tumour growth. Lou et al showed both tumour nodule numbers and lung weights in the Lipopolysaccharide (LPS) challenged CT26 and CT26 vector groups were significantly higher than the controls (<0.05) (Luo, 2004). This demonstrates that inhibition of NF-κB activity in cancer cells converts the LPS-induced proliferative response to an apoptotic response. LPS was shown to induce NF-κB dependent genes in tumour cells. TNF alpha was shown to mediate LPS induced tumour growth and NF-κB activation. TRAIL mediates LPS induced regression of NF-κB deficient tumours. Overall, NF-κB in CT26 cells is responsible for induction of several anti-apoptotic proteins including Bcl-2 and Bcl-X. Most importantly the inhibition of NF-κB converted the growth promoting effect of LPS mediated by TNF alpha into a cytocidal effect. Trail is a weak inducer of inflammation which is an important characteristic, most likely related to its poor

NF-κB activating ability. In addition to preventing the expression of anti-apoptotic proteins, inhibition of NF-κB also led to increased expression of the Trail receptor DR5. Type I and II interferons (IFN) are efficient inducers of Trail. The authors postulate that IFN based therapy with anti-TNF alpha medications may reduce inflammation associated toxicities, block inflammation induced tumour growth and potentiate Trail dependent tumour killing.
The bcl-2 family of proto-oncogenes are a critical regulator of apoptosis and are frequently deregulated in a wide variety of cancers. They have recently been identified as having an NF-κB binding site in the bcl-2 p2 promoter (Catz, 2001). Thus chemotherapeutic drugs that activate NF-κB can also activate bcl-2 family proteins in various cancer cell lines. Activated NF-κB binds to specific DNA sequences in target genes, designated as kB elements and regulates transcription of over 400 genes involved in immunoregulation, growth, inflammation, carcinogenesis and apoptosis.
Several chemotherapeutic agents including 5-fluorouracil (5-FU) have been reported to induce NF-κB activation in various cell lines (Cusack, 1999). Cytotoxic drugs induce NF-κB with delayed kinetics. This delay is due to the time required to induce nuclear DNA damage and relay the damage signal to the cytoplasmic IκK complex. Treatment with 5-FU can also induce activation of NF-κB in colorectal cancer cells (Wang, 2003). Using RKO human colorectal cell line and two NF-κB signalling deficient RKO mutants, Fukuyama et al demonstrated that 5-FU stimulates NF-κB and RKO cell survival through induction of IκK activity (Fukuyama, 2007). Several studies have shown that inhibition of NF-κB activation results in reversal of chemoresistance (Jones, 2000; Arlt, 2001; Cusack, 2001). It was shown that the inhibition of inducible NF-κB by a NF-κB decoy could induce apoptosis and reduce chemoresistance against 5-FU (Uetsuka, 2003). Inhibition of NF-κB activity reduces chemoresistance to 5-fluorouracil (5-FU) in human stomach cancer. Ionising radiation (IR) has been reported to activate NF-κB in both in vitro and in vivo studies (Rithidech, 2005; Ahmed, 2006). Laszlo et al recently reported that IkB-alpha depletion in the late phase of IR is a result of a combined regulation at both transcription and translation levels (Laszlo, 2008).

## 3. Toll-like receptors

### 3.1 Overview

Inflammation is initiated through many cellular transmembrane receptors of which the best characterised are the TLR family. Toll like receptors (TLRs) have been the subject of extensive investigation since their discovery in 1996. The first Toll receptor was discovered in Drosophila and it was revealed that the innate immune system may be activated once the receptor was bound by an extracellular ligand (Belvin, 1996). Subsequent research has revealed a total of 13 mammalian TLRs, 11 of which are expressed in humans. They are involved in the recognition by immune and non-immune cells of stimuli such as lipopolysaccharides (LPS) and dsRNA. They signal through the use of adapter proteins such as TRIF-related adaptor molecule (TRAF) and myeloid differentiation factor 88 (Myd88) (Killeen, 2009). Recognition of pathogen–associated molecular patterns (PAMPS) through TLRs, either alone or in heterodimerization with other TLRs or non-TLRs, triggers signals responsible for activation of the innate and adaptive immune responses. Most TLRs are found in innate immune cells such as polymorphonuclear neutrophils, monocytes/macrophages and dendritic cells where they trigger an immediate response. More recently TLRs have been shown to be expressed in a number of different cancer cells (Cheadle, 2002; Huang, 2008). Recent experimental evidence shows that TLRs display both tumouricidal and tumourigenesis properties (Salaun, 2006; Killeen, 2008). Each TLR recognises a different ligand. All TLRs (except for TLR3) signal through the adapter protein MyD88. MyD88 has been found to play a key role in inflammation induced tumour growth, principally through the innate immune system (Rakoff-Nahoum S, 2007). MyD88 mediates NF-κB activation through the canonical pathway (O'Neill, 2008; Akira, 2006). MyD88 is capable of NF-κB signalling selectively via TLR2 (Fitzgerald, 2003; Horng, 2001). Hence, both TLR2 and TLR4 both of which are expressed on the plasma membrane of cells appear to be involved in NF-κB inflammation-associated tumourigenesis. TLR2 is stimulated by numerous pro-inflammatory stimuli and helps activate the innate immune system.

Several TLRs are responsible for NF-κB activation. TLR4 induces tumour growth through NF-κB activation mediated by TNF-α (Luo, 2004). Interestingly, endotoxin or LPS, which binds specifically to TLR4 in cells is shown to be capable of inducing tumour growth (Pigeon, 1999). Endotoxin is a molecule found in the outer membrane of Gram-negative bacteria and elicits a strong inflammatory response in animals. Hence, it appears that the pro-tumorigenic effects of endotoxin occur through TLR4 mediated NF-κB activation. The focus of recent cancer immunology and medical oncology research has been aimed at activating the immune system in order to inhibit cancer cell growth and induce cancer cell apoptosis. Thus, TLRs offer a unique target for cancer therapy.

### 3.2 Toll-like receptor-3

TLR3 is a type 1 trans-membrane receptor protein located intracellularly on the endosome of eukaryotic cells. TLR3 has been shown to be an important "danger" signalling receptor that has a dual role in controlling the delicate balance between tolerance and inflammation on one hand and inflammation and disease on the other hand (Vercammen, 2008). TLR3 is composed of an ectodomain (ECD) containing multiple leucine rich repeats (LRRs), a transmembrane region and a cytoplasmic tail containing the Toll interleukin-1 receptor (TIR) domain (Vercammen, 2008). The LRRs form a horse shoe shaped solenoid structure which is capped at one end by a LRR N-terminal (LRR-NT) and at the other end by a LRR C-terminal (LRR-CT) (Bell, 2005). The TLR3 ectodomain (ECD) binds dsRNA. This can only occur in an acidic environment (pH<6.5) reflecting the endosomal location of the receptor. DsRNA binding initiates a signalling pathway that recruits the TIR domain containing adaptor protein (TRIF) to its cytoplasmic domain. TLR3 is the sole TLR to interact directly with TRIF. The TIr domain of TLR3 then binds to TRIF. This indirectly activates several transcription factors including NFκB and IRF3. TRIF knockout mice have shown impaired Interferon-B production in response to a TLR3 ligand which proves that TRIF is essential to the signalling pathway (Takeuchi, 2003). TRIF is an adaptor molecule which is essential for TLR-3 signalling pathways (Yamamoto, 2003). The activity of TRIF allows indirect activation of several transcription factors such as NF-κB and IRF-3.

TLR3 is the critical sensor of the dsRNA. In response to dsRNA stimulation, specific signalling pathways are activated leading to activation of transcription factors such as nuclear factor- κB (NF-κB) and interferon regulatory factor 3 (IRF-3). This response acts as a defence mechanism against a viral insult to the body. The dsRNA itself is produced during viral replication (Jacobs, 1996). Strong or sustained TLR-3 signalling is potentially harmful and in some cases fatal to the host cell. It appears that the mammalian cells have adapted to this using a negative feedback mechanism. PIK3 and RIP-1 binding to TRIF has been shown to inhibit the actions of TRIF signalling (Meylan, 2004). Polyribosinic:polyriboctidic acid (poly I:C) is a stable synthetic dsRNA which acts as an agonist on the TLR3 receptor. It has been the subject of anti-cancer immunotherapy trials for decades. However its activity on the TLR3 receptor as well as RIG-1 and MDA-5 has only been recently identified. It activates the human innate system which subsequently regulates adaptive immunity. Poly I:C is recognised by both endosomal receptor TLR3 and cytosolic receptors including RNA helicases such as RIG-1 melanoma differentiation associated gene 5 (MDA5). TLR3 preferentially recognizes synthetic poly(I:C) rather than a virus derived dsRNA (Okahira, 2005). The important role played by TLR3 in poly I:C recognition was shown in one study which used TLR3 deficient mice. These mice demonstrated reduced responses to poly I:C and produced lower levels of inflammatory cytokines (Alexopoulou, 2001). Poly I:C has several side effects such as nephrotoxicity, coagulopathies and hypersensitivity reactions. In order to reduce this toxicity a modified form of poly I:C known as Poly I:$C_{12U}$ has been produced. This substitutes uridine for cytosine at a ratio of 1:12 and results of a clinical trial of patients with HIV have proven Poly I:$C_{12u}$ to be very safe. Studies using differing lengths of poly I:C showed that longer duplexes are better inducers of TLR3 signalling (Boone, 2004; Okahira, 2005). There are various alternatives to Poly I:C available. Poly I:$C_{12}$U is a mismatched dsRNA helix in which uridine has replaced cytosine. It has a rapid half-life compared to Poly I:C which has opened the door for its use as a clinically useful drug. Poly I:$C_{12}$U is more specific in its binding to TLR3 and this may account for its reduced toxicity and safe use in clinical trials (Mitchell, 2006). No evidence exists of dose limiting organ toxicity including haematological, liver or renal toxicity following intravenous administration to HIV positive patients (Thompson, 1996). Poly I:C mediates a potent adjuvant effect in cells expressing TLR3 and this strongly enhances antigen specific CD8+ T-cell responses, promotes antigen cross presentation by dendritic cells (Cui, 2006; Schulz, 2005) and directly acts on effector CD8+ T and natural killer cells to alter the release of IFN-γ (Tabiasco, 2006). It is the most potent type 1 interferon stimulant that is recognised by TLR3 (Yoneyama, 2004; Matsumoto, 2008).

TLR3 stimulation by dsRNA can cause direct apoptosis and inhibit cell proliferation in various types of cancer cells including colon, breast and melanoma (Taura, 2010; Salaun, 2006, 2007). It is now known that expression and function of TLR3 is dependent on p53 activation (Taura, 2008). Salaun et al recently used poly I:C to treat a breast cancer cell line by triggering apoptosis (Salaun, 2006). They showed that poly I:C can directly cause apoptosis without the involvement of the immune system. They also showed that poly I:C induced apoptosis occurred through the Fas-associated protein death domain-caspase 8 signalling pathway. The extrinsic apoptotic pathway was also shown to be involved by the same group in selected cancer cells (Salaun, 2007). Polyadenylic:polyuridylic acid (poly A:U) is another synthetic double stranded RNA. Poly A:U is unique as it only signals through TLR3. Poly A:U has been used with moderate success to treat breast and gastric cancer as a monotherapy (Laplanche, 2000; Jeung, 2010). Interferons (IFN) are a group of cytokines that can cause antiviral, antiproliferative and apoptotic effects through the Jak/STAT pathway signal transducers (Stark, 2007). In particular, IFN-α, a type I IFN has been shown to induce TLR3 expression and thus significantly enhance tumour cell apoptosis when combined with Poly I:C compared to each treatment alone (Taura 2010). The same study combined IFN-α, Poly I:C and 5-FU which resulted in a significant increase in cancer cell death in a colon cancer cell line. They also showed that by inhibiting the JAK/STAT pathway, induction of TLR3 by INF- α caused a reduced response of TLR3 to INF- α stimulation. Several clinical trials have examined the effect of combining a TLR3 agonist and INF-α with or without a chemotherapeutic agent. Wadler et al combined 5-FU with INF-α and achieved a good response in colon cancer cells however this combination was not effective in clinical trials (Wadler, 1990). Early clinical trials involving a TLR3 agonist as a single adjuvant therapy in colorectal cancer showed mixed results. Lacour et al showed that Poly A:U alone as an adjuvant therapy in colorectal cancer patients who had undergone a resection of the primary tumour was unable to improve the overall survival of patients after five years compared to a placebo (Lacour, 1992). However, when used as a combination therapy there have been very positive results in a clinical trial to demonstrate a positive role for Poly A:U in cancer treatment. After a 14 year median follow-up Laplanche et al reported the results of a trial which combined Poly A:U with loco-regional radiotherapy versus chemotherapy with cyclophosphamide, methotrexate and fluorouracil (CMF) in women with operable breast cancer. They reported that the Poly A:U combination group had a significantly improved disease free survival (p=0.03) and significantly reduced the incidence of metastasis when compared to the CMF group. This trial did not however differentiate the role that Poly A:U and radiotherapy had as single therapies (Laplanche, 2000). Several studies have reported that caspase 3 is up-regulated by TLR3 agonist activity which would suggest a role for caspase 3 in cancer cell apoptosis induced by TLR3 agonists (Salaun, 2006; Khvalevsky, 2007). A recent study by Conforti et al demonstrated the synergistic effects between vaccines, chemotherapy and poly A:U (Conforti, 2010). A vaccine (OVA plus CpG) was administered prior to the combination of oxaliplatin and poly A:U and this significantly reduced tumour growth and prolonged survival. Interestingly these results were not demonstrated in nude and TRIF knockout mice.

### 3.3 Toll-like receptor-4

TLR4 was first discovered in 1998. Lipopolysaccharide (LPS) is a cell wall protein in gram negative bacteria and works as a ligand for TLR4. The recognition of LPS by TLR4 requires other proteins including LPS binding protein, CD14 and MD2. In resting cells TLR4 is located in the Golgi apparatus. The translocation of TLR4 from the Golgi apparatus to the plasma membrane and the binding of LPS is dependent on MD2 (Nagai, 2002; Shimazu, 1999). TLR4 signals through two pathways: the MyD88-dependant pathway and the MyD88-independant pathway. In the MyD88-dependant pathway, MyD88 binds to the Toll-IL-1 receptor domain of the TLR4 receptor and activates IL-1 receptor associated kinase (IRAK). IRAK in turn phosphorylates TRAF6, which in turn activates a MAP-3-kinase called TAK1, and TAK1 phosphorylates and activates the IκK complex. IκK then liberates NFκB. Killeen et al showed that bacterial endotoxins directly promote tumour cell adhesion and invasion through up-regulation of urokinase plasminogen activator and urokinase plasminogen activator receptor through TLR4 dependant activation of NFκB (Killeen 2009). TLR4 can also signal through the MyD88-independant pathway to stimulate the production of Interferon-B. Wang et al showed that TLR4/MyD88 over-expression was frequently detected in colo-rectal cancer with liver metastasis and TLR4/MyD88 levels were significantly higher in these patients (Wang, 2010). Although there have been a number of studies investigating the role of TLR4 in colo-rectal cancer, the exact impact of TLR4 signalling in comparison to TLR3 signalling in colon cancer cells has yet to be established.

TLR4 signalling has been shown to promote resistance of cancer cells to apoptosis following introduction of a TLR4 ligand in colon cancer cells (Cianchi, 2010). TLR4 signalling appears to promote the development of colitis associated cancer by mechanisms including enhanced

Cox-2 expression and increased EGFR signalling (Fukata, 2007). Recent experimental studies have shown that TLR4 induced inflammatory factors may cause tumour cell escape from immune surveillance and resistance to chemotherapy and radiotherapy (He, 2007).

One proposed mechanism by which tumour cells resist treatment involves an impairment of the immune response by the inflammatory microenvironment at the tumour site (Coussens, 2002). TLR4 upregulation has been shown to increase the secretion of immunosuppressive cytokines TGF-β, VEGF and pro-angiogenic chemokine IL-8 in human lung cancer cells and induces resistance of human lung cancer cells to TNF-α and TRAIL induced apoptosis (He, 2007). The same study demonstrated secretion of VEGF and IL-8 is p38MAPK dependent and the ERK1/2 and JNK1/2 proteins are not activated. NF-κB activation contributes to apoptosis resistance of human lung cancer cells after LPS stimulation and LPS-induced apoptosis is dependent on NF-κB activation in human lung cancer cells. NF-κB is an anti-apoptotic transcriptional factor induced by cellular components such as LPS, radiation and various chemotherapy drugs.

Contrasting evidence for the role of TLR4 in chemotherapy and radiotherapy resistance was reported by Apetoh et al who demonstrated reduced tumour growth and prolonged survival in immunocompetent wild type mice when treated with chemotherapeutic agents such as oxaliplatin and doxorubicin but this effect was significantly less in TLR4$^{-/-}$ mice and nu/nu mice (Apetoh, 2007). These findings were also demonstrated in TRIF$^{-/-}$ mice which behaved like the wild type mice but Myd88$^{-/-}$ mice behaved like TLR$^{-/-}$ mice. This suggests a certain dependence of tumour treatment resistance on the MyD88 dependent pathway in TLR4 signalling. These results show that when TLR4 itself is knocked out this will lead to a reduction in tumour growth when the tumour is exposed to an appropriate chemotherapeutic agent or radiotherapy. However, when TLR4 is up regulated in the presence of LPS, this results in resistance to chemotherapy and arguably radiotherapy treatment.

Various agents have been suggested as having a role in reversing TLR4 induced tumour apoptotic resistance. Rapamycin is one such agent. Rapamycin is a macrolide antifungal agent and is a potent immunosuppressive medication that is used as an anti-inflammatory and immunosuppressive drug for the treatment of autoimmune diseases such as Systemic lupus erythematosus (SLE) and transplantation rejection (Fernandez, 2006; Hackstein, 2003). In terms of cancer treatment Rapamycin has been shown to display a number of useful anti-cancer cell properties including inhibition of cancer cell proliferation and induction of apoptosis (Hartford, 2007; Zhang, 2007). Rapamycin can also inhibit invasion and metastasis of tumour cells (Abraham, 2007). One study focused on Rapamycins ability to reverse the apoptotic resistance that can occur following TLR4 stimulation with LPS. Sun et al showed that Rapamycin reverses TLR4 ligation induced apoptotic resistance in colon cancer cells (Sun, 2008). Interestingly this same study showed that Rapamycin inhibits anti-apoptotic protein bcl-xL expression and activation of Akt and NF-κB pathways following LPS treatment of cells and this was shown to reverse apoptosis when Akt and NF- κB were inhibited. Paclitaxel has been described as a potential ligand to TLR4 (Asselin, 2001). Kelly et al demonstrated that TLR4 signalling promotes tumour growth and paclitaxel chemo-resistance in ovarian cancer cells (Kelly, 2006). This behaviour was mediated by MyD88 expression.

## 4. Role of chemokines and cytokines

### 4.1 Overview

Both TLR3 and TLR4 signalling produce a pro-inflammatory response including chemokines and it has previously been shown that the pro-inflammatory response may contribute to tumorigenesis (Kelly, 2006). Chemokines and cytokines are markers of inflammation which normally recruit leucocytes and aid in blood vessel remodelling. Pathophysiological roles for chemokines include acting as autocrine growth factors, disruption of basement membranes, increasing motility and tumour invasion (Rollins, 2006; Balkwill 2004).

### 4.2 CXCL-8/IL-8

A recent paper examined the presence of cytokines, chemokines and their receptors in colon cancer using a Taqman Low Density Array with probes for 24 ligands and 17 receptors. This revealed CCL3, CCL4 and CXCL8 levels to be significantly increased in colon cancer samples compared to normal tissue (Erreni, 2009). Further analysis of the levels of CCL3, CCL4 and CXCL8 mRNA expression showed that CCL4 and CCL3 levels were higher in normal and tumour tissue. However, CXCL8 expression was significantly increased in tumour tissue ($p<0.0001$). There was no correlation with tumour stage for all three inflammatory markers. SW620 and HT29 cell lines showed low but detectable levels of CXCL8 which increased with stimulation with TNFα and TGFβ. Interestingly there was high levels of two anti-angiogenic chemokines found in these samples also, CXCL9 and CXCL10 but their receptor was not significantly expressed.

The main function of CXCL8 is the recruitment of neutrophils. These leucocytes have a short life span and have no presence or role in the tumour micro-environment. CXCL8 has however been reported to have a role in the tumour micro-environment by stimulating tumour advancement and invasion by stimulating the process of neoangiogenesis and by activating tumour matrix proteases (Zhu, 2004; Bates, 2004). However, CCL3 and CCL4 are not products of TLR3 and TLR4 signalling, but CXCL8 is produced as a result of signalling by TLR3 and TLR4. Elevated levels of CXCL8 or Interleukin-8 has been associated with increased angiogenesis in normal and transformed tissue adjacent to colon cancer tumours (Fox, 1998; Kuniyasi, 2000). Also, increased CXCL8 protein expression in primary colo-rectal tumours increases the risk of metastasis (Haraguchi, 2002). To date CXCL8 has two known receptors, CXCR1 and CXCR2. These receptors are known broadly as G-protein coupled receptors (GPCR). Recently GPCR antagonists have been developed which can block the biological effects of GPCR signalling. [D-Arg$^{1}$, D-Trp$^{5,7,9}$,Leu$^{11}$]SP or substance P antagonist is a potent GPCR antagonist and has been shown to inhibit small cell lung cancer cell proliferation both in vitro and in vivo (Seckl, 1997) and in pancreatic cancer cell proliferation in vitro and in vivo (Guha, 2005). The GPCR ligand/receptor interaction has been shown to result in neuropeptide-induced $Ca^{2+}$ mobilisation which increases intra-cellular $Ca^{2+}$ and this proves useful as a marker of GPCR function (Ryder, 2001). A GPCR antagonist has previously been shown to prevent GPCR agonist induced increase in $Ca^{2+}$, DNA synthesis and anchorage independent growth in pancreatic cancer cells (Guha, 2005). The role of a GPCR antagonist in colon cancer has yet to be established. IL-8 is produced and has been shown to be produced by tumour cells and the level of its production correlates directly with the metastatic potential of the tumour (Abdollahi, 2003; Bruserud, 2004).

## 5. Immuno-surveillance

The interaction between cancer cells and the innate and adaptive immune system is complex. As described previously, pro-inflammatory cytokines promote tumour growth; however the immune system has a means of restricting cancer development through immuno-surveillance and immuno-editing. The pro-tumorigenic effect of the inflammatory immune response appears generally to be a consequence of the innate immune system, whereas the adaptive immune system exerts anti-tumorigenic effects (Karin, 2005).

Cancer immunosurveillance is a theory formulated in 1957 by Burnet and Thomas, who proposed that lymphocytes act as sentinels in recognising and eliminating continuously arising transformed cells (Dunn, 2002; Burnet, 1957). Cancer immunosurveillance appears to be an important host protection process that inhibits carcinogenesis and maintains regular cellular homeostasis (Kim 2007). It has been shown that when mice are deficient in genes that encode for cells integral to the adaptive immune response such as T cells, B cells and natural killer T (NKT) cells, tumour incidence and tumour growth are increased (Shankaran, 2001). With the aid of additional studies, natural killer cells and T cells now appear to be the dominant cells involved in tumour immuno-surveillance. Interestingly, interferon-γ (IFN-γ) is produced by both NKT and T cells. Furthermore, IFN-γ is the most influential cytokine released by these cells. Recent studies have now shown that mice deficient in IFN-γ are more susceptible to spontaneous carcinogenesis (Shankaran, 2001).

The mechanism involved in the anticancer protective effect of the immune system is complex. Generally, it is theorised that cells of the immune system recognise the presence of a growing tumour which has undergone stromal remodelling, causing local tissue damage. This is followed by the induction of inflammatory signals which recruits natural killer cells, NKT cells and macrophages to the tumour site. During this phase, the infiltrating lymphocytes such as the natural killer cells and NKT cells are stimulated to produce IFN-γ. Newly synthesised IFN-γ then induces tumour death as well as promoting the production of chemokines which play an important role in promoting tumour death by blocking the formation of new blood vessels.

Similarly, IL-4 is released in large quantities by NKT cells upon activation and is a key regulator in the adaptive immunity. Therapeutic attempts to recruit the immune system to curtail cancer growth have now become a keen area of interest. Although, attempts have met with limited success thus far, this is the basis of vaccine guided anti-cancer therapy which is a rapidly progressing area of research (Dranoff, 2004).

It is clear that elements of the immune system can restrict tumour growth. However, as discussed previously pro-inflammatory cytokine release initiated by the immune system can also promote tumour growth. Therefore, the immune system appears to have the effect of a double edged sword on cancer growth. If we had full understanding and control of these pathways, this could potentially lead to successful cures for cancer.

### 5.1 Vaccines

Recently vaccines have been developed to take advantage of the role played by the immune system in cancer. The discovery of tumour associated antigens (TAA) expressed by colorectal carcinoma as well as recent advances in tumour immunology are providing new focus to develop biologically targeted immunotherapeutic strategies. It has been reported that immuno-deficient animals as well as humans, e.g. transplant patients, are at greater risk of developing malignancy (Penn, 2000). It has also been reported that cytotoxic T lymphocytes (CTL) and antibodies specific for TAA have been demonstrated in patients with cancers including colorectal cancer (Nagorsen, 2000). Therefore there is an ideal niche in cancer treatment for an active specific immunotherapy. Previously identified or undefined TAAs can be administered to cancer patients in order to cause a systemic immune response which will lead to malignant cell destruction (Rosenberg, 2001).

Despite the huge amount of evidence and theoretical potential of this treatment strategy, the clinical results are limited to date. There is evidence to support the tumouricidal effects of active specific immunotherapy however it appears cancer cells are able to survive the tumouricidal effects as the disease progresses. This phenomenon has become known as 'tumour immune escape'. Several mechanisms have been proposed as to how this phenomenon occurs. One body of evidence shows evidence that cancer genetic instability leads to TAA/HLA downregulation as well as to disruption of the TAA processing/presenting machinery which then allows malignant cells to evade the surveillance of immune sentinels (Seliger, 2001; Yang, 2003). Another proposed mechanism lies in the ability of cancer cells to produce immunosuppressive cytokines e.g. IL-10, and thus counteract the immune system response (Mocellin, 2001; Walker, 1997). The challenge for tumour immunologists currently is to overcome this 'tumour immune escape' and increase the proportion of patients mounting an immune response and increase the rate of responses from the targeted tumour.

The role of macrophages in the development of colorectal cancer is controversial. One study demonstrated that increased numbers of macrophages in all areas of the tumour correlated with an advanced tumour stage (Bailey, 2007). On the other hand Forssell et al showed that the presence of macrophages positively influenced prognosis in colorectal cancer (Forssell, 2007). Another group demonstrated that macrophages have the ability to inhibit or stimulate tumour growth according to their polarisation and state of activation (Mantovani, 2005). This group showed that M1-polarised macrophages activated by IFNγ and bacterial products like LPS display tumouricidal effects whereas M2 macrophages differentiated in the presence of Th2 cytokines, IL-4, IL-13 or IL-10, have the opposite effect. These macrophages favour tumour cell proliferation and stimulate tumour progression and tumour invasion. These studies are crucial in demonstrating the important role that inflammatory mediators such as chemokines and cytokines play in the establishment of the tumour microenvironment. The tumorgenicity of proinflammatory mediators such as interleukin-6 and tumour necrosis factor-α (TNFα) was shown by Coussens et al (Coussens, 2002).

## 6. Surgery, inflammation and tumourigenesis

At present, the only recognised curative treatment for cancer is surgery. As a result, surgery is the mainstay treatment for tumours. However, surgery is not indicated for all patients with a cancer diagnosis. Surgery is only indicated in these patients if the cancer has not dissipated and spread to distant organs. In fact, surgery in these patients worsens outcome and survival. This begs the question, is surgery tumorigenic? Numerous studies have examined the role of surgery itself on tumour growth. Interestingly, cancer surgery in the presence of micrometastases increases metastatic burden and enhances peri-operative tumour growth (Pigeon, 1999; MS, 1997; Coffey, 2002). The presence of undetected micro-metastases is thought to be largely responsible for these recurrences. Cancer patients often harbour micrometastases which are undetectable at the time of surgery. Surgical intervention in these patients is thought not only to accelerate their progression but also to be responsible for activating dormant micrometastases that may have remained inactive in the absence of surgery. In addition, the extent of the surgery is proportional to the post-operative recurrence rate. This is evidenced by the meta-analyses that show that minimally invasive surgery is more effective than open surgery in improving tumour recurrence, and cancer-related survival (Hensler, 1997), although equally studies exist that do not support this idea (Jayne, 2010). Considering surgery is the only curative treatment of solid tumours, this knowledge has prompted efforts to understand this undesired effect of surgery. It is hoped that this understanding will eventually help develop therapeutic treatments that may attenuate or eliminate this unwelcome consequence of surgery.

### 6.1 Mechanisms of surgery induced tumourigenesis

Considering what is already known concerning the role of inflammation in tumourigenesis, it is not surprising that surgery is tumorigenic. Surgery confers a traumatic insult to the body which like all traumas induce a potent pro-inflammatory response. Surgery is followed by a biologic period of repair to help restore homeostasis. It induces an early hyper-inflammatory response, which is characterised by pro-inflammatory TNF-α, IL-1 and IL-6 cytokine release (Walker, 1999) and neutrophil activation (Hensler, 1997). Several of these cytokines have been shown to potentiate tumour growth (Coussens, 2004). The massive and continuous IL-6 release subsequently accounts for the up-regulation of major anti-inflammatory mediators, such as $PGE_2$, IL-10, and TGF-ß (Walker 1999). The magnitude and duration of this hyper-inflammatory response is proportional to the severity of the trauma which may explain how laparoscopic versus open surgery may result in lower tumour recurrence (Colacchio, 1994; Baigrie, 1992). Following surgery, angiogenesis is also stimulated as the body initiates a period of healing and biological repair. Pro-angiogenic substances such as VEGF become elevated post-operatively. Moreover, anti-angiogenic substances such as endostatin and angiostatin are not detectable in the serum shortly after tumour excision (Li, 2001; Holmgren 1995; O'Reilly, 1994). This incites the formation of capillaries and new blood vessels not only to the areas of tissue insult but also to all parts of the body including areas of residual metastatic disease which promotes tumour growth.

Furthermore, surgery also influences immune system function. Immuno-suppression is a feature of the post-operative stress response and is also associated with anaesthesia, blood transfusion and the release of acute-phase proteins (Lee, 1977). The immune system appears to be an important regulator in identifying and eliminating any abnormal cells with cancerous potential. Hence, any disruption of immune function as a result of surgery can also lead to potentiating tumour growth. Interestingly, this immuno-suppression is greater dependent on the extent of surgery (Da Costa, 1998; Da Costa, 1999). The immunosuppressive effects of surgery can last anywhere from between 4 to 14 days depending on the size of surgical trauma induced but peaks day three post-operatively in most cases. Likewise, this may explain why laparoscopic versus open surgery in colon cancer patients confers a greater survival advantage, although the evidence supporting this is not equivocal.

Endotoxaemia also occurs following surgery involving bowel manipulation. Endotoxin, a potent inflammatory mediator, is a component on the wall of Gram negative bacteria often found in the lumen of the gastrointestinal system. Upon manipulation, endotoxin or LPS translocates across the intestinal lumen and enters the circulation. Endotoxaemia further potentiates the hyper-inflammatory response following surgery such as colorectal cancer resection. One study examined the effect of endotoxin administration on a murine breast cancer model (Pigeon, 1999). Interestingly, they found enhanced metastatic growth in the endotoxin treated group compared to controls. In a later study the same group found that endotoxin-induced metastatic growth was associated with increased angiogenesis, vascular permeability and tumour cell invasion and migration (Harmey, 2002). Therefore, this is another potential mechanism of surgically induced tumour growth especially in regard to colorectal cancer operations. In addition, the actual manipulation of the tumour during surgery results in the dissemination of tumour cells into the circulation. These tumour cells can potentially seed in distant sites throughout the body facilitating metastatic spread. Surgeons will make efforts to minimise tumour manipulation intra-operatively to minimise this potential.

Peri-operative tumour growth appears to significantly impact on tumour recurrence following "curative" surgery. Following a deeper understanding of this mechanism, therapeutic efforts are now being sought. Peri-operative immunomodulators such as IL-2, known to abrogate the immune changes that follow excisional cancer surgery, are being investigated as potential peri-operative treatments showing promising initial results (Den Otter, 1996). Even current chemotherapeutic regimes known to induce cell death in rapidly dividing cells have been given immediately post-operatively resulting in increased long-term survival. However, most of these treatments are limited by their toxicities as tissue and wound healing are essential in the immediate post-operative period.

## 7. Conclusion

Overall, our understanding of the relationship between inflammation and cancer has improved greatly since Virchow first made his observation over 150 years ago. The unravelling of signalling pathways shared by cancer and inflammation will provide the focus for future cancer treatment strategies.

## 8. References

Abdollahi T, Robertson NM, Abdollahi A, Litwack G. 2003. Identification of interleukin 8 as an inhibitor of tumor necrosis factor-related apoptosis-inducing ligand-induced apoptosis in the ovarian carcinoma cell line OVCAR3. Cancer Res. 63, 4521–4526.

Abraham RT, Gibbons JJ. The mammalian target of rapamycin signaling pathway: twists and turns in the road to cancer therapy. Clin Cancer Res 2007;13:3109–14.

Ahmed KM, Dong S, Fan M, Li JJ. Nuclear factor-kappaB p65 inhibits mitogen activated protein kinase signaling pathway in radioresistant breast cancer cells. Mol. Cancer Res. 4 (2006) 945–955

Akira S, Uematsu S, Takeuchi O. Pathogen recognition and innate immunity. Cell 2006;124(4):783-801.

Alexopoulou, L., A. C. Holt, R. Medzhitov, and R. A. Flavell. 2001. Recognition of double-stranded RNA and activation of NF-kB by Toll-like receptor 3. Nature 413:732–738.

Apetoh L, Ghiringhelli F, Tesniere A. Toll-like receptor 4-dependent contribution of the immune system to anticancer chemotherapy and radiotherapy. Nature Medicine. 2007;13(9):1050–1059.

Arlt A, Vorndamm J, Breitenbroich M, Folsch UR, Kalthoff H, Schmidt WE, Schafer H. Inhibition of NF-kappaB sensitizes human pancreatic carcinoma cells to apoptosis induced by etoposide (VP16) or doxorubicin, Oncogene 20 (2001) 859–868.

Asselin E, Mills GB, Tsang BK. XIAP regulates Akt activity and caspase-3-dependent cleavage during cisplatin-induced apoptosis in human ovarian epithelial cancer cells. Cancer Res 2001;61:1862–8.

Baigrie R, Lamont P, Kwiatkowski D, Dallman M, Morris P. Systemic cytokine response after major surgery. British Journal of Surgery 1992;79(8): 757–760.

Bailey C, Negus R, Morris A, Ziprin P, Goldin R et al. Chemokine expression is associated with the accumulation of tumour associated macrophages (TAMs) and progression in human colorectal cancer, Clin. Exp. Metastasis 24 (2007), pp. 121–130

Baldwin, A.S., Jr. (2001). Series introduction: The transcription factor NF-B and human disease. J. Clin. Invest. 107, 3–6.

Balkwill F, Mantovani A. Inflammation and cancer: back to Virchow? The Lancet 2001;357(9255): 539-545.

Balkwill F. Cancer and the Chemokine Network. Nature Reviews, Cancer 2004;4:540–50.

Bates RC, DeLeo MJ, Arthur M. The epithelial–mesenchymal transition of colon carcinoma involves expression of IL-8 and CXCR-1-mediated chemotaxis. Mercurio Experimental Cell Research 299 (2004) 315- 324.

Baud V, Karin M. Is NF-kappaB a good target for cancer therapy? Hopes and pitfalls, Nat. Rev. Drug Discov. 8 (2009) 33–40

Bell JK. Proc. Natl. Acad. Sci. U.S.A. 102, 10976 (2005).

Belvin MP, Anderson KV. A CONSERVED SIGNALING PATHWAY: The Drosophila Toll-Dorsal Pathway. Annual Review Cell Dev. Biol. 1996. 12:393–416

Bharti AC AB. Chemopreventive agents induce suppression of nuclear factor-kappaB leading to chemosensitization. Ann N Y Acad Sci 2002;973(Nov): 392-395.

Böhm B, Schwenk W, Hucke H, Stock W. Does methodic long-term follow-up affect survival after curative resection of colorectal carcinoma? Diseases of the Colon & Rectum 1993;36(3): 280-286.

Boone DL, Turer EE, Lee EG, Ahmad RC, Wheeler MT et al. 2004. The ubiquitin-modifying enzyme A20 is required for termination of Toll-like receptor responses. Nat. Immunol.5:1052–1060.

Braumann C, Winkler G, Rogalla P, Menenakos C, Jacobi C. Prevention of disease progression in a patient with a gastric cancer-re-recurrence. Outcome after intravenous treatment with the novel antineoplastic agent taurolidine. Report of a case. World Journal of Surgical Oncology 2006;4(1): 34.

Bruserud O, Ryningen A, Wergeland L, Glenjen NI, Gjertsen BT. 2004. Osteoblasts increase proliferation and release of pro-angiogenic interleukin 8 by native human acute myelogenous leukemia blasts. Haematologica 89, 391–402.

Burnet F. Cancer-A biological approach. 37. Med J 1957;1: 779-841.

Catz SD, Johnson JL, Transcriptional regulation of bcl-2 by nuclear factor kappa B and its significance in prostate cancer, Oncogene 20 (2001) 7342–7351.

Cheadle EJ, Jackson AM. (2002) Bugs as drugs for cancer. Immunology 107:10–19

Coffey J, Doyle M, O'Mahony L. Probiotics confer protection against perioperative metastatic tumour growth. Ann Surg Oncol 2002;9: 93.

Colacchio T, Yeager M, Hildebrandt L. Perioperative immunomodulation in cancer surgery. American journal of surgery 1994;167(1): 174

Conforti R, Ma Y, Morel Y, Paturel C, Terme M, Viaud S, Ryffel B, Ferrantini M, Uppaluri R, Schreiber R, Combadière C, Chaput N, André F, Kroemer G, Zitvogel L. Opposing effects of toll-like receptor (TLR3) signaling in tumors can be therapeutically uncoupled to optimize the anticancer efficacy of TLR3 ligands. Cancer Res. 2010 Jan 15;70(2):490-500.

Coussens L. Inflammation and cancer. Toxicologic Pathology 2004;32(6): 732-734.

Coussens LM, Werb Z. Inflammation and cancer. Nature 2002; 420: 860–66.

Cui Z, Qiu F. Synthetic double-stranded RNA poly(I:C) as a potent peptide vaccine adjuvant: therapeutic activity against human cervical cancer in a rodent model. Cancer Immunol Immunother 2006;55: 1267–79.

Cusack JC, Liu R, Baldwin AS. NF- kappa B and chemoresistance: potentiation of cancer drugs via inhibition of NF- kappa B, Drug Resist. Updat. 2 (1999) 271–273

Cusack JC, Liu R, Houston M, Abendroth K, Elliott PJ, Adams J, Baldwin AS. Enhanced chemosensitivity to CPT-11 with proteasome inhibitor PS-341: implications for systemic nuclear factor-kappaB inhibition, Cancer Res. 61(2001) 3535–3540.

Da Costa M, Redmond H, Bouchier-Hayes D. The effect of laparotomy and laparoscopy on the establishment of spontaneous tumor metastases. The Journal of Urology 1999;162(2): 633-634.

Da Costa M, Redmond H, Finnegan N, Flynn M, Bouchier-Hayes D. Laparotomy and laparoscopy differentially accelerate experimental flank tumour growth. British Journal of Surgery 1998;85(10).

Den Otter W, De Groot J, Bernsen M, Heintz A, Maas R, Jan Hordijk G, Hill F, Klein W, Ruitenberg E, Rutten V. Optimal regimes for local IL-2 tumour therapy. International Journal of Cancer 1996;66(3).

Dranoff G. Cytokines in cancer pathogenesis and cancer therapy. Nature Reviews Cancer 2004;4(1): 11-22.

Dunn G, Bruce A, Ikeda H, Old L, Schreiber R. Cancer immunoediting: from immunosurveillance to tumor escape. Nature immunology 2002;3(11): 991-998.

Erreni M, Bianchi P, Laghi L, Mirolo M, Fabbri M et al. Expression of Chemokines and Chemokine Receptors in Human Colon Cancer Methods in Enzymology, Volume 460, 2009, Pages 105-121.

Fernandez D, Bonilla E, Mirza N, Niland B, Perl A. Rapamycin reduces disease activity and normalizes T cell activation-induced calcium fluxing in patients with systemic lupus erythematosus. Arthritis Rheum 2006;54:2983–8.

Fitzgerald KA, McWhirter SM, Faia KL, Rowe DC, Latz E, Golenbock DT, Coyle AJ, Liao SM, Maniatis T. IKKε and TBK1 are essential components of the IRF3 signaling pathway. Nature immunology 2003;4(5): 491-496.

Forssell J, Oberg A, Henriksson ML, Stenling R, Jung A, Palmqvist R. High macrophage infiltration along the tumor front correlates with improved survival in colon cancer, Clin. Cancer Res. 13 (2007), pp. 1472–1479

Fox SH, Whalen GF, Sanders MM, Burleson JA, Jennings K, Kurtzman S, Kreutzer D. Angiogenesis in normal tissue adjacent to colon cancer. Journal of Surgical Oncology 1998;69:230–4.

Fukata M, Chen A, Vamadevan AS, Cohen J, Breglio K, Krishnareddy S, Hsu D, Xu R, Harpaz N, Dannenberg AJ, Subbaramaiah K, Cooper HS, Itzkowitz SH, Abreu MT (2007) Toll-like receptor-4 promotes the development of colitis-associated colorectal tumors. Gastroenterology 133: 1869–1881.

Fukuyama R, Ng KP, Cicek M, Kelleher C, Niculaita R, Casey G, Sizemore N. Role of IKK and oscillatory NFkappaB kinetics in MMP-9 gene expression and chemoresistance to 5-fluorouracil in RKO colorectal cancer cells, Mol. Carcinog. 46 (2007) 402–413.

Guha S, Eibl G, Kisfalvi K, Fan R, Burdick M. Broad-Spectrum G Protein–Coupled Receptor Antagonist, [D-Arg1,D-Trp5,7,9,Leu11]SP: A Dual Inhibitor of Growth and Angiogenesis in Pancreatic Cancer. Cancer Res April 1, 2005 65; 2738.

Gulumian M. The role of oxidative stress in diseases caused by mineral dusts and fibres: current status and future of prophylaxis and treatment. Molecular and cellular biochemistry 1999;196(1): 69-77.

Hackstein H, Taner T, Zahorchak AF, Morelli AE, Logar AJ, Gessner A, et al. Rapamycin inhibits IL-4-induced dendritic cell maturation in vitro and dendritic cell mobilization and function in vivo. Blood 2003;101:4457–63.

Haraguchi M, Komuta K, Akashi A, Matsuzzaki S, Furui J, Kanematsu T. Elevated IL-8 levels in the drainage vein of resectable Duke's C colorectal cancer indicate high risk for developing hepatic metastasis. Oncology Reports 2002;9:159–65.

Harmey J, Bucana C, Lu W, Byrne A, McDonnell S, Lynch C, Bouchier-Hayes D, Dong Z. Lipopolysaccharide-induced metastatic growth is associated with increased angiogenesis, vascular permeability and tumor cell invasion. International Journal of Cancer 2002;101(5): 415-422.

Hartford CM, Ratain MJ. Rapamycin: something old, something new, sometimes borrowed and now renewed. Clin Pharmacol Ther 2007;82:381–8.

Hayden MS, Ghosh S. Signaling to NF- B. Genes & development 2004;18(18): 2195-2224.

He W, Liu Q, et al. (2007). TLR4 signaling promotes immune escape of human lung cancer cells by inducing immunosuppressive cytokines and apoptosis resistance. Molecular immunology 44(11): 2850-2859.

Hensler T, Hecker H, Heeg K, Heidecke C, Bartels H, Barthlen W, Wagner H, Siewert J, Holzmann B. Distinct mechanisms of immunosuppression as a consequence of major surgery. Infection and immunity 1997;65(6): 2283.

Holmgren L, O'Reilly M, Folkman J. Dormancy of micrometastases: balanced proliferation and apoptosis in the presence of angiogenesis suppression. Nature Medicine 1995;1(2): 149-153.

Horng T, Barton GM, Medzhitov R. TIRAP: an adapter molecule in the Toll signaling pathway. Nature immunology 2001;2(9): 835-841.

Huang B, Zhao J, Li H, He KL, Chen Y, Chen SH, et al. Toll-like receptors on tumor cells facilitate evasion of immune surveillance. Cancer Res 2005;65:5009–14.

Huang B, Zhao J, Unkeless JC, Feng ZH, Xiong H. (2008) TLR signalling by tumor and immune cells: a double-edged sword. Oncogene 27:218–224.

Jacobi C, Peter F, Wenger F, Ordemann J, Müller J. New therapeutic strategies to avoid intra- and extraperitoneal metastases during laparoscopy: results of a tumor model in the rat. Dig Surg 1999;16: 393-399.

Jacobi C, Sabat R, Ordemann J, Wenger F, Volk H, Müller J. Peritoneal instillation of taurolidine and heparin for preventing intraperitoneal tumor growth and trocar metastases in laparoscopic operations in the rat model. Langenbecks Archiv für Chirurgie 1997;382(4 Suppl 1): S31.

Jacobs BL, Langland JO. When two strands are better than one: the mediators and modulators of the cellular responses to double stranded RNA. Virology 1996 219:339-349.

Jayne D, Thorpe H, Copeland J, Quirke P, Brown J, Guillou P. Five year follow up of the Medical Research Council CLASICC trial of laparoscopically assisted versus open surgery for colorectal cancer. Br J Surg. 2010 Nov;97(11):1638-45.

Jeung HC, Moon YW, Rha SY, et al. Phase III trial of adjuvant 5-fluorouracil and Adriamycin versus 5-fluorouracil, Adriamycin, and Optimizing Poly(A:U) Anticancer Therapy. Cancer Res; 70(2) January 15, 2010 499.

Jones DR, Broad RM, Madrid LV, Baldwin AS, Mayo MW. Inhibition of NFkappaB sensitises non-small cell lung cancer cells to chemotherapy-induced apoptosis, Ann. Thorac. Surg. 70 (2000) 930–936 discussion 936–937.

Karin M, Greten F. NF- B: linking inflammation and immunity to cancer development and progression. Nature Reviews Immunology 2005;5(10): 749-759.

Karin M, Lin A. (2002). NF-B at the crossroads of life and death. Nat. Immunol. 3, 221–27 227.

Kasibhatla, S., Brunner, T., Genestier, L., Echeverri, F., Mahboubi, A., Green, D.R. (1998). DNA damaging agents induce expression of Fas and subsequent apoptosis in T lymphocytes via the activation of NF-kB and AP-1. Mol. Cell 1, 543–551.

Kelly MG, Alvero AB, Chen R, et al. TLR-4 signaling promotes tumor growth and paclitaxel chemoresistance in ovarian cancer. Cancer Res 2006;66:3859–68.

Khvalevsky E, Rivkin L, Rachmilewitz J, Galun E, Giladi H. TLR3 signaling in a hepatoma cell line is skewed towards apoptosis. J Cell Biochem 2007;100: 1301–12.

Killeen SD, Wang JH, Andrews EJ, Redmond HP (2008) Exploitation of the Toll-like receptor system in cancer: a doubled-edged sword? Br J Cancer 95: 247–252.

Killeen SD, Wang JH, Andrews EJ, Redmond HP. Bacterial endotoxin enhances colorectal cancer cell adhesion and invasion through TLR-4 and NF-kB-dependent activation of the urokinase plasminogen activator system. British Journal of Cancer (2009) 100, 1589 - 1602.

Kim R, Emi M, Tanabe K. Cancer immunoediting from immune surveillance to immune escape. Immunology 2007;121(1):1.

Knight B, Skellern G, Smail G, Browne M, Pfirrmann R. NMR studies and GC analysis of the antibacterial agent taurolidine. Journal of Pharmaceutical Sciences 1983;72(6): 705-707.

Kuniyasu H, Yasui W, Shinohara H, Yano S, Ellis LM, Wilson MR, Bucana CD, Rikita T, Tahara, E, Fidler I. Induction of angiogenesis by hyperplastic colonic mucosa adjacent to colon cancer. American Journal of Pathology 2000;157:1523–35.

Lacour J, Laplanche A, Malafosse M, Gallot D, Julien M et al. Polyadenylic-polyuridylic acid as an adjuvant in resectable colorectal carcinoma: a 6 1/2 year follow-up analysis of a multicentric double blind randomized trial. Eur J Surg Oncol. 1992 Dec;18(6):599-604.

Laplanche A, Alzieu L, Delozier T, Berlie J, Veyret C, Fargeot P, Luboinski M, Lacour J. Polyadenylic-polyuridylic acid plus locoregional radiotherapy versus chemotherapy with CMF in operable breast cancer: a 14 year follow-up analysis of a randomized trial of the F´ed´eration Nationale des Centres de Lutte Contre le Cancer (FNCLCC). Breast Cancer Research and Treatment 64: 189-191, 2000.

Laszlo CF, Wu S. Mechanism of UV-induced IkappaBalpha-independent activation of NF-kappaB, Photochem. Photobiol. 84 (2008) 1564–1568

Lee SJ, Lim KT. UDN glycoprotein regulates activities of manganese-superoxide dismutase, activator protein-1, and nuclear factor-kappaB stimulated by reactive oxygen radicals in lipopolysaccharide-stimulated HCT-116 cells. Cancer Lett 2007;254:274–87.

Lee Y. Effect of anesthesia and surgery on immunity. Journal of Surgical Oncology 1977;9(5).

Li T, Kaneda Y, Ueda K, Hamano K, Zempo N, Esato K. The influence of tumour resection on angiostatin levels and tumour growth—an experimental study in tumour-bearing mice. European Journal of Cancer 2001;37(17): 2283-2288.

Little D, Regan M, BOUCHIER-HAYES D. Perioperative immune modulation. Surgery 1993;114(1): 87-91.

Luo JL, Maeda S, Hsu LC, Yagita H, Karin M. Inhibition of NF- B in cancer cells converts inflammation-induced tumor growth mediated by TNF to TRAIL-mediated tumor regression. Cancer Cell 2004;6(3): 297-305.

Mantovani A. Cancer: Inflammation by remote control, Nature 435 (2005), pp. 752–753.

Marx J. Cancer research: Inflammation and cancer: The link grows stronger. In; 2004. p. 966-968.

Matsumoto M, Seya T. TLR3: Interferon induction by double-stranded RNA including poly(I:C). Adv Drug Deliv Rev 2008; 60:805-12.

Meylan, E., K. Burns, K. Hofmann, V. Blancheteau, F. Martinon, M. Kelliher, and J. Tschopp. 2004. RIP1 is an essential mediator of Toll-like receptor 3-induced NF-_B activation. Nat. Immunol. 5:503–507.

Mitchell W. 2006. Review of Ampligen clinical trials in chronic fatigue syndrome. J. Clin. Virol. 37:S113.

Mocellin S, Wang E, Marincola FM. Cytokines and immune response in the tumor microenvironment. J Immunother 2001;24:392–407

MS O, Boehm T, Shing Y, Fukai N, Vasios G, Lane W, Flynn E, Birkhead J, Olsen B, Folkman J. Endostatin: an endogenous inhibitor of angiogenesis and tumor growth. Cell 1997;88(2): 277-285.

Nagai Y, Akashi S, Nagafuku M, Ogata M, Iwakura Y, Akira S, Kitamura T, Kosugi A et al. Essential role of MD-2 in LPS responsiveness and TLR4 distribution. Nat Immunol 3 (2002), pp. 667–672.

Nagorsen D, Keilholz U, Rivoltini L. Schmittel A, Letsch A, Asemissen AM, Berger G, Buhr HJ, Theil E, Scheibenbogen C. Natural T-cell response against MHC class I epitopes of epithelial cell adhesion molecule, her-2/neu, and carcinoembryonic antigen in patients with colorectal cancer. Cancer Res 2000;60:4850–4854.

Okahira S, Nishikawa F, Nishikawa S, Akazawa T, Seya T, Matsumoto M. 2005. Interferon-beta induction through Toll-like receptor 3 depends on double-stranded RNA structure. DNA Cell Biol. 24:614–623.

O'Neill LAJ. The interleukin-1 receptor/Toll-like receptor superfamily: 10 years of progress. Immunological Reviews 2008;226(1):10.

O'Reilly M, Holmgren L, Shing Y, Chen C, Rosenthal R, Moses M, Lane W, Cao Y, Sage E, Folkman J. Angiostatin: a novel angiogenesis inhibitor that mediates the suppression of metastases by a Lewis lung carcinoma. Cell 1994;79(2): 315-328.

Penn I. Post-transplant malignancy: the role of immunosuppression. Drug Saf 2000;23:101–113.

Pidgeon G, Harmey J, Kay E, Da Costa M, Redmond H, Bouchier-Hayes D. The role of endotoxin/lipopolysaccharide in surgically induced tumour growth in a murine model of metastatic disease. British journal of cancer 1999;81(8): 1311-1317.

Pikarsky E, Porat RM, Stein I, Abramovitch R, Amit S, Kasem S, Gutkovich-Pyest E, Urieli-Shoval S, Galun E, Ben-Neriah Y. NF- B functions as a tumour promoter in inflammation-associated cancer. Nature 2004;431(7007): 461-466.

Rakoff-Nahoum S, Medzhitov R. Regulation of spontaneous intestinal tumorigenesis through the adaptor protein MyD88. Science 2007;317(5834):124.

Reith H. Therapy of peritonitis today. Surgical management and adjuvant therapy strategies. Langenbecks Archiv für Chirurgie 1997;382(4 Suppl 1): S14.

Rithidech KN, Tungjai M, Arbab E, Simon SR. Activation of NF-kappaB in bone marrow cells of BALB/cJ mice following exposure in vivo to low doses of (137)Cs gamma-rays, Radiat. Environ. Biophys. 44 (2005) 139–143.

Rollins B. Inflammatory chemokines in cancer growth and progression. European Journal of Cancer. 2006;42:760–7.

Rosenberg SA. Progress in human tumour immunology and immunotherapy. Nature 2001;411:380–384.

Ryder NM, Guha S, Hines OJ, Reber HA, Rozengurt E. G protein-coupled receptor signaling in human ductal pancreatic cancer cells: neurotensin responsiveness and mitogenic stimulation. J Cell Physiol 2001; 186: 53–64.

Salaun B, Coste I, Rissoan MC, Lebecque SJ, Renno T. TLR3 can directly trigger apoptosis in human cancer cells. J Immunol 2006; 176: 4894–901.

Salaun B, Lebecque S, Matikainen S, Rimoldi D, Romero P. Toll-like receptor 3 expressed by melanoma cells as a target for therapy? Clin Cancer Res 2007;13: 4565–74.

Schulz O, Diebold SS, Chen M, et al. Toll-like receptor 3 promotes cross-priming to virus-infected cells. Nature 2005;433:887–92.

Seckl MJ, Higgins T, Widmer F, Rozengurt E. [DArg1,D-Trp5,7,9,Leu11]substance P: a novel potent inhibitor of signal transduction and growth in vitro and in vivo in small cell lung cancer cells. Cancer Res 1997:57;51–4

Seliger B, Wollscheid U, Momburg F, Blankenstein T, Huber C. Characterization of the major histocompatibility complex class I deficiencies in B16 melanoma cells. Cancer Res 2001;61:1095–1099

Sen R, Baltimore D. Inducibility of kappa immunoglobulin enhancer-binding protein Nf-kappa B by a posttranslational mechanism. Cell 1986;47(6): 921-928.

Shankaran V, Ikeda H, Bruce A, White J, Swanson P, Old L, Schreiber R. IFN and lymphocytes prevent primary tumour development and shape tumour immunogenicity. Nature 2001;410(6832): 1107-1111.

Shimazu R, Akashi S, Ogata H, Nagai Y, Fukudome K, Miyake K, Kimoto M. MD-2, a molecule that confers lipopolysaccharide responsiveness on Toll-like receptor 4. J Exp Med 189 (1999), pp. 1777–1782.

Stark GR. How cells respond to interferons revisited: from early history to current complexity. Cytokine Growth Factor Rev 2007; 18: 419–23.

Sun Q, Zheng Y, Liu Q, Cao X. International Immunopharmacology 8 (2008) 1854–1858.

Tabiasco J, Devevre E, Rufer N, et al. Human effector CD8+ T lymphocytes express TLR3 as a functional coreceptor. J Immunol 2006;177:8708–13.

Takeuchi, M. Sugiyama, M. Okabe, K. Takeda, and S. Akira. 2003. Role of adaptor TRIF in the MyD88-independent Toll-like receptor signaling pathway. Science 301:640–643.

Taura M, Eguma A, Suico MA et al. p53 regulates Toll-like receptor 3 expression and function in human epithelial cell lines. Mol Cell Biol 2008; 28: 6557–67.

Taura M, Fukuda R, Suico MA, Eguma A, Koga T et al. TLR3 induction by anticancer drugs potentiates poly I:C-induced tumor cell apoptosis. Cancer Sci | July 2010 | vol. 101 | no. 7 | 1615

Thompson KA, Strayer DR, Salvato, PD, Thompson CE, Klimas N, Molavi A et al. Results of a double blinded placebo controlled study of the double stranded RNA drug poly1:polyC12U in the treatment of HIV infection. Eur J Clin Microbiol Infect Dis 1996;15(7):580-7.

Uetsuka H, Haisa M, Kimura M, Gunduz M, Kaneda Y et al. Inhibition of inducible NF-kappaB activity reduces chemoresistance to 5-fluorouracil in human stomach cancer cell line, Exp. Cell Res. 289 (2003) 27–35.

Vercammen E, Staal J, Beyaert R. Sensing of Viral Infection and Activation of Innate Immunity by Toll-Like Receptor 3. CLINICAL MICROBIOLOGY REVIEWS, Jan. 2008, p. 13–25 Vol. 21, No. 1.

Wadler S, Schwartz EL. Antineoplastic activity of the combination of interferon and cytotoxic agents against experimental and human malignancies: a review. Cancer Res 1990; 50: 3473–86.

Walker C, Bruce D, Heys S, Gough D, Binnie N, Eremin O. Minimal modulation of lymphocyte and natural killer cell subsets following minimal access surgery. American journal of surgery 1999;177(1): 48.

Walker PR, Saas P, Dietrich PY. Role of Fas ligand (CD95L) in immune escape: the tumor cell strikes back. J Immunol 1997;158:4521–4524

Wang EL, Qian ZR, Nakasono M, Tanahashi T, Yoshimoto K, Bando Yet al. High expression of Toll-like receptor 4/myeloid differentiation factor 88 signals correlates with poor prognosis in colorectal cancer. British Journal of Cancer (2010) 102, 908 - 915.

Wang L, Liu Q, Sun Q, Zhang C, Chen T, Cao X. TLR4 signaling in cancer cells promotes chemoattraction of immature dendritic cells via autocrine CCL20. Biochem Biophys Res Commun 2008;366:857–61.

Wang WH, Huang JQ, Zheng GF, Lam SK, Karlberg J, Wong BCY. Non-steroidal anti-inflammatory drug use and the risk of gastric cancer: a systematic review and meta-analysis. jnci 2003;95(23): 1784-1791.

Warzocha K, Ribeiro P, Bienvenu J, Roy P, Charlot C, Rigal D, Coiffier B, Salles G. Genetic polymorphisms in the tumor necrosis factor locus influence non-Hodgkin's lymphoma outcome. Blood 1998;91(10): 3574.

Wiemann B, Starnes CO. Coley's toxins, tumor necrosis factor and cancer research: a historical perspective. Pharmacol Ther. 1994;64(3):529-64.

Yakovlev VA, Barani IJ, Rabender CS, Black SM, Leach JK et al. Tyrosine nitration of IkappaBalpha: a novel mechanism for NF-kappaB activation. Biochemistry 46 (2007) 11671–11683.

Yamamoto M, Sato S, Hemmi H, Hoshino K, Kaisho T, Sanjo H, Takeuchi O, Sugiyama M, Okabe M, Takeda K, Akira S. Role of adaptor TRIF in the MyD88-independent toll-like receptor signaling pathway. Science. 2003 Aug 1;301(5633):640-3.

Yang T, McNally BA, Ferrone S, Liu Y, Zheng P. A single-nucleotide deletion leads to rapid degradation of TAP-1 mRNA in a melanoma cell line. J Biol Chem 2003;278:15291–15296

Yoneyama M, Kikuchi M, Natsukawa T, Shinobu N, Imaizumi T, Miyagishi M, et al. The RNA helicase RIG-I has an essential function in double-stranded RNA-induced innate antiviral responses. Nat Immunol 2004; 5:730-7.

Zhang JF, Liu JJ, Lu MQ, Cai CJ, Yang Y, Li H, et al. Rapamycin inhibits cell growth by induction of apoptosis on hepatocellular carcinoma cells in vitro. Transpl Immunol 2007;17:162–8.

Zhu YM, Webster SJ, Flower D, Woll PJ. Interleukin-8/CXCL8 is a growth factor for human lung cancer cells. British Journal of Cancer (2004) 91, 1970 – 1976.

19

# CD277 an Immune Regulator of T Cell Function and Tumor Cell Recognition

Jose Francisco Zambrano-Zaragoza[1,2] et al.*
[1]*INSERM, UMR 891, CRCM, Institut Paoli-Calmettes, Universite Medierranée, Marseille, France*
[2]*Universidad Autónoma de Nayarit, Ciencias Químico Biológicas y Farmacéuticas, Tepic Nayarit, Mexico*

## 1. Introduction

Molecules involved in tumor cell recognition are potentially important targets in cancer therapeutics. Therefore, research on the identification of tumor cell antigens as well as, immune-regulatory molecules is essential. The study of new co-stimulatory molecules has attracted special interest due to, their role in activation and/or inhibition of effector function of immune cells. In this chapter, we focused on the study of CD277 and its putative counter-receptor, and their possible role in activation or inhibition of immune cells and recognition of cancer cells.

CD277 has been involved in immune cells regulation, because of its role in activating or inhibiting effector, cytokine secretion and cytotoxic functions, depending on the activating conditions of these cells. Moreover, the fact that the stimulation of tumor cell lines with anti-CD277 leave to a better recognition and killing by γδ and αβ T cells lead us to postulate that these molecules is involved also in tumor recognition. We will discuss different aspects of CD277 and its counter-receptor in this chapter.

Classically, the immune response has been divided into innate and adaptive immunity, with distinct properties. The innate immune response uses a small number of receptors that detect a limited set of conserved antigens. Induction of the adaptive immune response involves antigen presenting cells (APC) and T cells (Borghesi & Milcarek, 2007). The interaction between the T cell and the APC is the pivotal step that controls a series of events, including T cell activation, cell division and effector differentiation (Zhu & Chen, 2009). However, recognition of the processed antigenic peptide coupled to Major

---

* Nassima Messal[1], Sonia Pastor[1], Emmanuel Scotet[3], Marc Bonneville[3], Danièle Saverino[4], Marcello Bagnasco[5], Crystelle Harly[3], Yves Guillaume[1], Jacques Nunes[1], Pierre Pontarotti[6], Marc Lopez[1] and Daniel Olive[1]
[1]*INSERM, UMR 891, CRCM, Institut Paoli-Calmettes, Universite Medierranée, Marseille, France*
[2]*Universidad Autónoma de Nayarit, Ciencias Químico Biológicas y Farmacéuticas,Tepic Nayarit, Mexico*
[3]*Centre de Recherche en Cancerologie de Nantes Angers, IRT UN, INSERM UMR 892, Nantes France*
[4]*Department of Experimental Medicine-Section Human Anatomy, University of Genova, Italy*
[5]*Medical and Radio metabolic Therapy Unit, Department of Internal Medicine, University of Genova, Italy*
[6]*Université Aix Marseille 1, UMR 6632 Marseille, France*

Histocompatilibity Complex (MHC) class I or II molecules on APC is not enough to activate T cells, they require an antigen independent second signal involving the B7 family molecules. The lack of this co-stimulatory signal induces anergy (Ledbetter *et al.*, 1990).

CD28 and the related molecule CTLA-4, together with their natural ligands CD80 and CD86 are the classical co-stimulatory molecules (Ward, 1996). CD28 is constitutively expressed on T cells and is involved in their activation through signal transduction. CTLA-4, which delivers a strong inhibitory signal, is expressed on the T cell surface after engagement of TCR. CD80 and CD86 belong to the B7 co-signalling receptors family, they are cell surface glycoproteins that are essential to modulate and tune the T cell receptor (TCR)-mediated activation of T lymphocytes (Moretta & Bottino, 2004). Other members of this family are PD1 and their ligands PDL-1 and PDL-2 with inhibitory properties on T cell activation and ICOS and ICOSL, involved in T cell activation (Moretta & Bottino, 2004; Rietz & Chen, 2004).

Members of the related B7 family belong to the immunoglobulins superfamily (IgSF). They have two Ig extracellular domains and show similarity to the variable (V) and the constant (C) domains of Ig. Previous studies have shown that IgV-like domains of B7.1 and B7.2 share similarity with myelin oligodendrocyte glycoprotein (MOG), chicken blood group system protein (BG) and butyrophillin (BT). Thus, these five proteins depict a subfamily in the IgSF. MOG is expressed only in the central nervous system (CNS) as a component of the myelin sheath and is involved as autoantigen in the pathogenesis of multiple sclerosis; BG proteins are only expressed in chicken and are associated with immunological functions acting as strong adjuvants when used in co-immunization with other proteins and; BT is a glycoprotein that forms a major component of milk fat globule membrane and is expressed in mammary gland at the end of pregnancy and during lactation but its function remains unknown. Whereas MOG and BG have only one extracellular IgV-like domain, BT has a B7-"like" structure with an IgV-like and an IgC-like domain (Henry *et al.*, 1999). Furthermore, BT has an intracellular domain of 166 amino acids named B30.2 and is presumably involved in the regulation of intracellular superoxide concentrations (Henry *et al.*, 1997).

Interestingly, the human *bt* and *mog* genes map to the distal part of the MHC class I region and six additional BT members were identified in this region. The six genes could be divided in two groups called BT2 and BT3 and are named using three different nomenclatures. Within these groups, there are BT2.1 (also called BTF1or BTN2A1], BT2.2 (also called BTF2 or BTN2A2], BT2.3 (also called BTF1 or BTN2A1], BT3.1 (also called BTF5 or BTN3A1], BT3.2 (also called BTF4 or BTN3A2], BT3.3 (also called BTF3 or BTN3A3]. The degree of identity between members of BT2 and BT3 groups is around 50 %, while identity is around 95% within the same sub-family. Among these molecules BT3.1 or CD277 has a wide tissue distribution and its ligands are expressed on T cells suggesting that it could play a role in immune functions (Compte *et al.*, 2004). Other members of this family have also been identified on chromosome 6 (BTNL2) or other chromosomes.

Expasy site annotates 15 butyrophilin-like genes in humans including BT and MOG. Butyrophilin proteins typically have a signal peptide, an IgV-like and IgC-like domain, and a transmembrane and cytoplasmic domain. In addition, they often possess a heptad repeat which is a 7-aa sequence encoded by a single exon. Many butyrophilin molecules also contain a 166 aa B30.2 domain in the cytoplasmic region also found in tripartite motif (TRIM) proteins and stonutoxin. The precise function of the B30.2 domain in butyrophilin remains unclear. The B30.2 domain is also present in the C terminal part of various types of proteins which N-terminal globular domain may either contain Ig fold (butyrophilin), a

RING finger domain or a leucine zipper. It has been recently found that the protein TRIM5 interacts with HIV via its B30.2 domain. Xanthine oxidase interacts with B30.2 and may indirectly regulate nitric oxid production.

In pathological settings, proteins possessing B30.2 domain have been reported in over exuberant inflammatory responses such as Familial Mediterranean Fever (FMF) which is caused by mutation in the B30.2 domain of pyrin/marenostrin. In addition, mutations within this domain in the MID1 protein are also associated to the Opitz syndrome.

Because the IgV-like domains of B7.1 and B7.2 are more similar to the IgV-like domain of butyrophilin than to any other sequence, Linsley et al. proposed that B7 and butyrophilin molecules might have evolved from a common ancestral gene to compose a subfamily within the Ig superfamily. It is unclear whether B7 and butyrophilin molecules share common functions in regulating immune responses (Linsley *et al.*, 1994).

CD277 is thought to be involved in immune response because their expression can be modulated by pro-inflammatory cytokines such as TNF-α and IFN-γ (Compte *et al.*, 2004). Stimulation of BTN3 molecules results in phosphorylation BTN3A3 molecules leading to the attenuation of proliferation and cytokine secretion in CD4+ and CD8+ T cells in a CD4+CD25+ independent manner, demonstrating the agonistic properties of BTN3 to mediate negative-signal transduction (Yamashiro *et al.*, 2010).

In order to expand our knowledge about the CD277 and their role in tumor cell recognition, we analyzed different aspects of stimulation of leukaemia cell lines and some strategies to be used in the identification of the CD277 counter-receptor.

## 2. CD277: Its role in immune regulation and tumor cell recognition

The CD277 molecule is expressed on αβ, γδ T cells, B and NK lymphocytes, monocytes, dendritic cells and hematopoietic precursors as identified by mRNA expression and flow cytometry. Moreover, the CD277 surface expression is constitutive on endothelial cells and it is increased by pro-inflammatory cytokines such as TNF-α and IFN-γ, suggesting that these molecules might be involved in the early events of tissue damage and inflammation (Compte *et al.*, 2004). Even though there are some reports regarding the effects of CD277 on immune cells, little is known about the functions of the CD277 counter-receptor in leukaemia and tumor cells. Here, we report our findings on functional properties of this counter-receptor and propose some strategies to determine the identity of this molecule.

### 2.1 Engagement of CD277 regulates αβ T cells functions

Two different monoclonal antibodies (mAb) recognizing CD277 have been reported, 1) BT3.1, obtained from mice immunized with the extracellular domain of BTN3A1 (Compte *et al.*, 2004) and, 2) 232-5, obtained from mice immunized with the extracellular domain of BTN3A3 (Yamashiro *et al.*, 2010). In both cases, no differences in the recognition of the different isoforms of CD277 have been found. Therefore, these antibodies were used for the study of the immunomodulatory functions of CD277 on T cells. Yamashiro *et al.*, have evaluated the proliferation of CD4+ and CD8+ T cells populations in PBMC stimulated with anti-CD3 and anti-CD277 mAb. Interestingly, they found that the proliferation of both CD4+ and CD8+ T cells were suppressed by 232-5 but not by BT3.1 mAb. Moreover, IFN-γ and IL-4 production in CD4 T cells and IFN-γ in CD8+ T cells were down-regulated by 232-5 but not by BT3.1 mAb. Additionally, they report that this effect requires the cross-link of CD277 in the cell surface because the observed effects with the 232-5 mAb were lost when the Fab fragment was used (Yamashiro *et al.*, 2010).

These result suggest the negative effect of CD277 on T cell activation, but considering that the affinity of the BT3.1 mAb is lower than those observed with the 232-5 mAb and that the BT3.1 mAb did not show any effect on the T cell population analyzed it is possible that different effects could be attributed to CD277 on αβ T cells. Using another mAb (20.1) we found that CD277 engagement enhanced the CD3 or CD3/CD28 co-stimulation at the proliferation and cytokine production levels. The effect of this mAb was associated with an increased intracellular signalling (Messal et al., submitted).

On the other hand, T cells expressing γδ TCRs have emerged as an important component of the immune repertoire and are included as component of the innate immune response (Nedellec *et al.*, 2010; Saenz *et al.*, 2010). In humans, the γδ T cells are also located in peripheral organs and peripheral blood. Circulating γδ T cells express a TCR comprising mainly Vδ2 and Vγ9 and cells with this phenotype represent 2% of mononuclear cells. These Vγ9Vδ2 T cells are activated by TCR stimulation with small non peptidic phosphorylated compounds also referred as phosphoantigens (Tanaka *et al.*, 1995). Unlike the conventional T cells, their activation does not require activating co-signals provided by CD28 - CD80 and CD86 interaction. However, their activation can be regulated by NKR (Das *et al.*, 2001; Halary *et al.*, 1997) and TLR (Deetz *et al.*, 2006; Wesch *et al.*, 2006). Moreover, engagement of NKG2D can activate them, without TCR stimulation (Rincon-Orozco *et al.*, 2005). Thus, considering the role of γδ T cells in the anti-tumoral immune response (Tokuyama *et al.*, 2008) it is important to analyze the effects of CD277 on the functions of γδ T cells as well.

### 2.2 CD277 and dendritic cells

We have reported that CD277 is expressed on the surface of resting and activated monocytes and monocyte-derived dendritic cells (iDC). The effect of CD277 on monocytes and iDC was analyzed in freshly isolated monocytes and monocyte-derived dendritic cells stimulated with anti-CD19 or anti-CD277 (anti-BT3.1). We found that upon stimulation for 24 h, anti-CD277 triggered the activation of monocytes, measured by up-regulation of the expression of CD86 on the cell surface as compared to cells treated with isotype-matched control. No effect was observed when control antibody (anti-CD19) or soluble anti-CD277 were used, indicating that cross-linking is required for the cellular activation observed (Simone *et al.*, 2010). Further, these results demonstrate that receptors for the Fc fragment of immunoglobulins (FcRs) dependent signalling are not responsible for cell activation.

On the other hand, a wide variety of receptors regulate the activity of cells of the myeloid lineage. We have also analyzed the effects of CD277 as co-receptor in proinflammatory responses triggering by pathogenic stimuli by stimulating monocytes and iDC with anti-CD277 in presence of different doses of Toll-like receptors (TLR) ligands (LPS and R-848). We observed that secretion of proinflammatory cytokines (IL8/CXCL8, IL-1β and IL-12/p70) are increased in monocytes cultured with both anti-CD277 and TLR ligands compared with individual stimuli. Parallel experiments performed with iDC shown that cytokine secretion is similar to those observed with monocytes (Simone *et al.*, 2010).

These data suggest a possible role of CD277 as activation receptor on monocytes and dendritic cells. The need of cross-linking to obtain a biological effect on both monocytes and iDC is consistent with their possible agonist nature.

These data suggest a possible role of CD277 molecules as activation receptors on monocytes and dendritic cells. In addition, the need of cross-linking to obtain a biological effect on both monocytes and iDC is consistent with their possible agonist nature.

### 2.3 CD277 and tumor recognition

The effect of CD277 stimulation on αβ T cells and monocytes and iDC described above, suggests the regulatory role of CD277, by activating or inhibiting the effector functions of immune cells. Moreover, the presence of the putative CD277 counter-receptor in the immune environment may play a critical role in defining where and when CD277 is engaged. We have reported that leukaemia cell lines and solid tumor cells lines such as HeLa and MCF-7, Raji, C91, HUT78 and JA16 (Compte *et al.*, 2004) express both CD277 and the CD277 counter-receptor. In addition, we have recently found (Harly et al., in preparation) that Raji cells stimulated with anti-CD277 are better recognized and killed by Vγ9Vδ2 T cells. We postulated that the effect of CD277 stimulation on Raji cells would stand at the level of regulation of the antigen stimulation of Vγ9Vδ2 T cells and/or over-expression of the counter-receptor for CD277, thus, we investigated the effect of CD277 stimulation on the expression of CD277 counter-receptor in Raji cells. We used these cells because they express low levels of CD277 counter-receptor on the cell surface, therefore its regulation can be followed up by flow cytometry using the CD277-Fc fusion protein.

To analyze the expression of CD277 on different cell lines after treatment with anti-CD277, anti-CD80 or the Fab portion of anti-CD277 monoclonal antibodies, Raji, C91, TF1 or HUT78 cells were plated onto 96 round bottom wells ($10^6$ cells/well) and incubated with or without these antibodies at different concentrations (from 10 to 0.078125 μg/mL) for 2 hours. Then cells were extensively washed on PBS-FCS and incubated with or without 15 μg/mL of CD277-Fc fusion protein (Compte *et al.*, 2004) for 30 minutes at 4°C. After incubation, cells were washed twice on PBS-2% FCS and stained with 1/100 goat-anti-human-Fc-PE for 15 min at room temperature. After wash, the cells were fixed with PBS - 1% formaldehyde and acquisition was done in a LSRII (BD bioscience). Data were analyzed with flow-jo software.

We found that the expression of CD277 counter-receptor is weak on non-stimulated Raji cells (Figure 1). However, the stimulation of Raji cells with anti-CD277 antibodies enhances the expression of CD277 counter-receptor compared to non-stimulated or stimulated with anti-CD80 antibodies controls (Figure 1A, B and C). These data suggest that up-regulation in the expression of CD277 counter-receptor is due to the CD277 engagement, because Raji cells stimulated with anti-CD80 express the counter-receptor at similar levels as non-stimulated cells non-stimulated (Figure 1B).

This effect was also observed on different cell lines such as C91, HUT78 and TF1. Although different basal levels of CD277 counter-receptor expression was found in these cells, in all cases stimulation with anti-CD277 antibodies lead to a higher expression of the counter-receptor on the cell surface (Figure 2). Additionally, stimulation with the Fab portion of the anti-CD277 has no effect on the expression of the counter-receptor; therefore it is necessary to cross-link CD277 on the cell surface to have the stimulatory effect observed (Figure 3). Moreover, the effect observed was dose-dependent, as shown in Figure 4.

### 2.4 Stimulation by CD277 and the regulation of the expression of CD277

We know that the expression of CD277 on immune cells is constitutive and that it is increased by proinflammatory cytokines such as IFN-γ and TNF-α (Compte *et al.*, 2004), however, little is known regarding the effect of CD277 stimulation on its own expression.

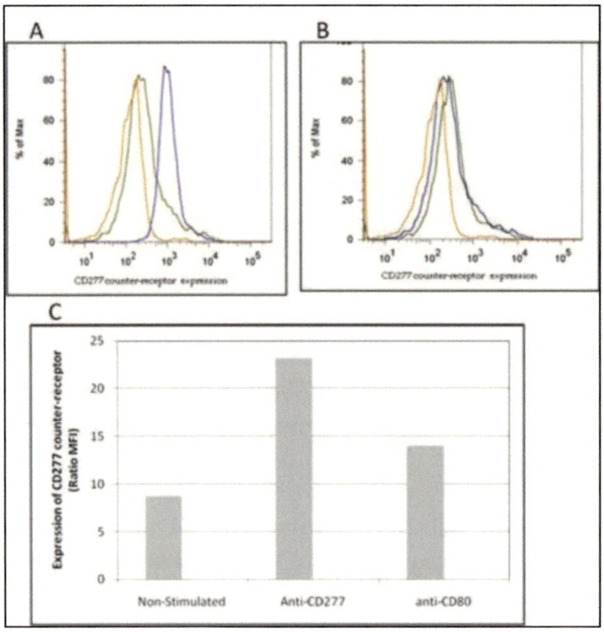


Fig. 1. Effect of CD277 stimulation in the CD277 counter-receptor expression on Raji cells. A) CD277 counter receptor expression in Raji cells after stimulation with anti-CD277 antibodies: Orange, basal fluorescence; green, expression of CD277 counter-receptor in non-stimulated and; blue, expression of CD277 counter-receptor in cells stimulated with anti-CD277 antibodies. B) CD277 counter-receptor expression in Raji cells after stimulation with anti CD80 antibodies(control): Orange, basal fluorescence , green, expression of CD277 counter-receptor in non-stimulated and; Blue, expression of CD277 counter-receptor in cells stimulated with anti-CD80 antibodies. C) MFI ratio was calculated by dividing the fluorescence intensity of cells in different conditions by the fluorescence intensity of the isotype control.

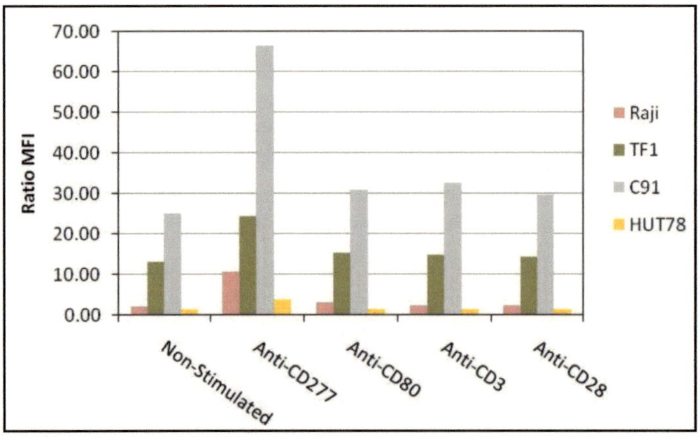


Fig. 2. CD277 counter-receptor expression on Raji, TF1, C91 and HUT78 cell lines stimulated by CD277. Each bar represents the mean fluorescence of triplicates divided by mean fluorescence of the isotype control.

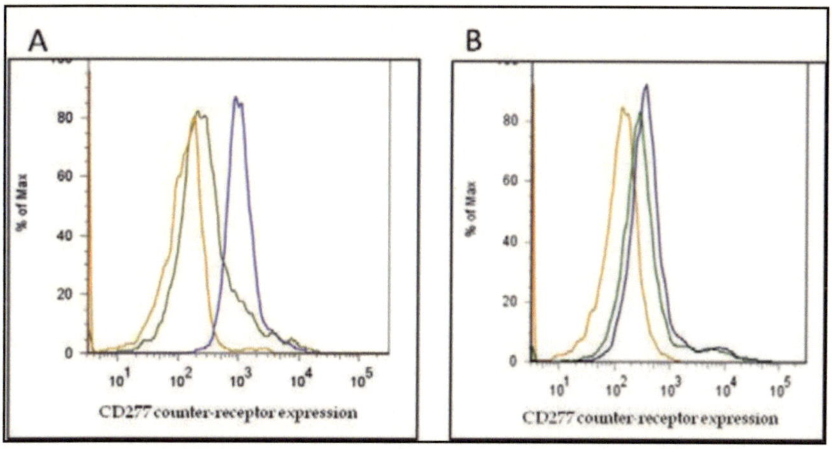


Fig. 3. Effect of CD277 cross-link on the CD277 counter-receptor expression in Raji cells. Orange, basal fluorescence; green, expression of CD277 counter-receptor in non-stimulated and Raji cells and; blue, expression in Raji cells stimulated with (A) anti-CD277 antibodies or (B) Fab of anti-CD277 antibodies.

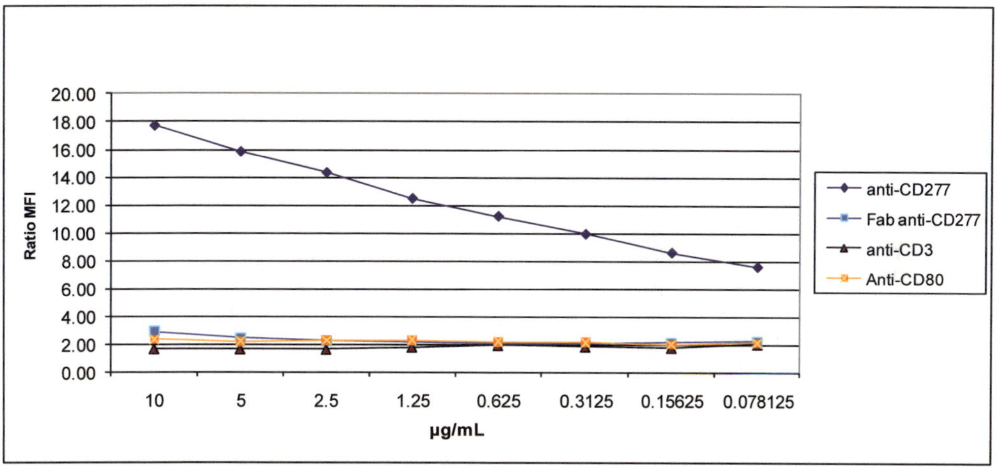


Fig. 4. Over-expression of CD277 counter-receptor in Raji cells is dose-dependent. Raji cells were tested with increasing concentrations of the anti-CD277, the Fab portion of the anti-CD277, anti-CD3 or anti-CD80 monoclonal antibodies and expression of CD277 counter-receptor was followed by flow cytometry.

To test this hypothesis, Raji cells (10 X $10^6$) were cultured in RPMI 1640 + 10% FCS and stimulated with 10 µg/mL of either anti-CD277 or anti-CD80 monoclonal antibodies for 0, 2, 4, 6 or 24 hours at 37°C in a 5% $CO_2$ atmosphere. RNA was extracted with trizol® and RT-PCR using Taqman assays (Applied Biosystems) for CD277 isoforms (BTN3A1, BTN3A2, BTN3A3), and GAPDH, as endogenous housekeeping gene, was done. Expression of the CD277 isoforms was calculated as follows:

$$\Delta CT_{stimulated} = CT_{Probe} - CT_{GAPDH}$$

$$\Delta\Delta CT = \Delta CT_{stimulated} - \Delta CT_{time=0}$$

Where $CT_{Probe}$ is the CT for the CD277 isoforms, obtained from Raji cells stimulated with either anti-CD277 or anti-CD80, and $\Delta CT_{time=0}$ is the $\Delta CT$ value for the CD277 isoforms at time = 0 hours (control).
The relative quantity (RQ) expression by using the formula:

$$RQ = 2^{-\Delta\Delta CT}$$

We found that the expression of BTN3A1 and BTN3A3 molecules but not BTN3A2, at 2, 4 and 6 hours is higher in Raji cells stimulated with anti-CD277 monoclonal antibodies and that this effect is lost after 24 hours (Figure 5). Taken together, our data suggest multiple functions of CD277: Promotion of the expression of CD277 counter-receptor and up-regulation of the expression of the CD277 molecules itself.
Although the CD277 monoclonal antibodies tested cannot differentiate between BTN3A1, BTN3A2 and BTN3A3 isoforms, we know that differences in the intracellular region of BTN3 molecules stand mainly with BTN3A2 which lacks the B30.2 domain. Therefore, since our data point out that signal transduction due to CD277 can be mediated by BTN3A1 and BTN3A3 isoforms, it seems likely that the B30.2 domain is involved this effect.

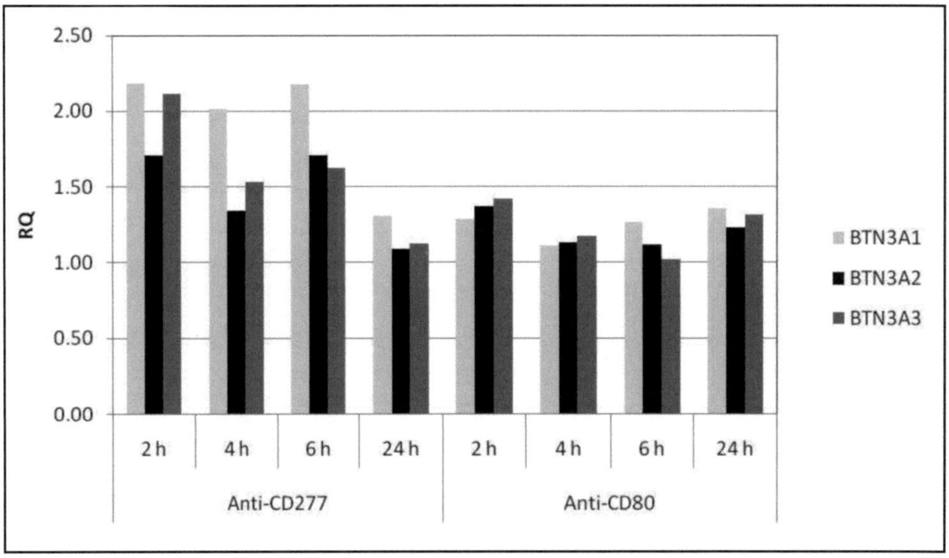


Fig. 5. A representative experiment on the gene expression of BTN3 isoforms on Raji cells stimulated by CD277. BTN3A1, A2 and A3 are the reported isoforms for CD277. The RQ was calculated as described. A RQ value higher than 2.0 was considered as indicative of gene over expression.

### 2.5 Effect of cytokines on the expression of CD277 counter receptor

It has been reported that cells stimulated by CD277 secrete inflammatory cytokines such as IFN-γ and TNF-α (Cubillos-Ruiz *et al.*, 2010; Yamashiro *et al.*, 2010) and that these cytokines may influence the expression of CD277. However, little is known about the modulation of the expression of the CD277 counter-receptor by these proinflammatory cytokines.

To further investigate the regulatory effects of inflammatory signals on the expression of CD277, C91 cells (50,000 cels/well) were treated with IFN-γ (5, 50, 500 and 5000 ng/mL), TNF-α (0.4, 4, 40 and 400 ng/mL), TGF-β (0.02. 0.2 and 2 ng/mL) and IL-22 (1, 10, 100 and 1000 ng/mL) for 24 hours at 37°C in a 5% $CO_2$ atmosphere. Following washes with PBS-FCS, the cells were incubated with or without (control) 15 μg/mL of CD277-Fc fusion protein for 30 minutes at 4°C. After incubation, the cells were washed twice on PBS-2% FCS and stained with 1/100 goat-anti-human-Fc-PE for 15 min at room temperature. After wash, cells were fixed on PBS- 1% formaldehyde and expression of CD277 was assessed by flow cytometry (LSRII, BD bioscience). Analysis was done with flow-jo software. Our results show that stimulation with IFN-γ, TNF-α, TGF-β or IL-22 has no effect on the expression of CD277 counter-receptor in C91 cells (Figure 6).

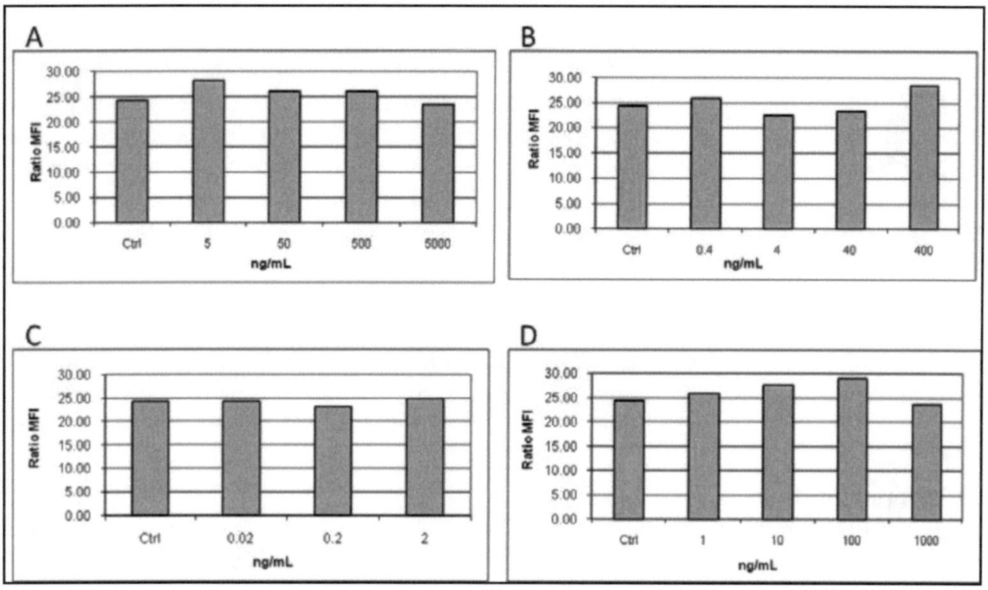


Fig. 6. A representative experiment on the expression of CD277 counter-receptor in C91 cells stimulated with different concentrations of (A) IFN-γ (B) TNF-α (C) TGFβ and (D) IL-22 for 24 hours. Cells were stained with CD277-Fc fusion protein and analyzed by flow cytometry.

### 2.6 Strategies for CD277 counter receptor identification

The identity of CD277 counter-receptor is one of the main challenges in the near future, for a better understanding of the mechanisms involved in immune cell regulation and tumor cell recognition.

#### 2.6.1 Methods to determine the CD277-counter receptor identity

In spite of the weak expression of the counter-receptor in different cell lines (Compte *et al.*, 2004), C91 cells were selected because of the expression profile is higher than in other cell lines such as Raji, TF1, HUT78 or JA16. In order to obtain a cell population with a stable expression of the CD277 counter-receptor, C91 cells were stained with the CD277-Fc fusion protein as described above. The positive population was identified by comparing to unstained control and the 1% most positive population was selected and purified using a

FacsAria (BD Bioscience). These cells were then cultured in RPMI 1640 supplemented with 10% FCS and antibiotics. Expression of CD277 counter-receptor was followed by flow cytometry to corroborate that its surface expression was stable.

The cells obtained, were used in two different approaches to determine the identity of the CD277 counter-receptor. First, the use of cross-linking assays with Bis (sulfosuccinimidyl) suberate (BS3) a homobifunctional, water-soluble, non-cleavable and membrane impermeable crosslinker and; second, a classical co-immunoprecipitation assay from post-nuclear membranes.

In the first approach, C91T3.3 cells were incubated with 30 µg/mL of the CD277-Fc fusion protein and then the interaction was covalently stabilized by using 3 mM of BS3. After crosslink a standard co-immunoprecipitation protocol was carried out using anti-CD277 monoclonal antibodies and protein G. A 4-12% polyacrilamide gel electrophoresis-sodium dodecyl sulfate (PAGE-SDS) and western-blot were then used to detect the CD277-Fc crosslinked, bands were then cut from the PAGE-SDS gel and sent to be identified by MALDI (Matrix-Assisted Laser Desorption/Ionization)-TOF in a mass-spectrometry assay.

The second strategy to determine the identity of CD277 counter-receptor involves a procedure to obtain the postnuclear membranes. This procedure leads us to enrich the membrane proteins and eliminate the nuclear contaminants that can interfere with the interaction between CD277 and its counter-receptor. In this approach, the C91T3.3 cells were treated with 3 mM imidazole for cell membrane lysis but not the nuclear membrane. After centrifugation, membranes were recovered and used in a classical co-immunoprecipitation assay with CD277-Fc and CTLA4-Fc as a control. A 4-12% PAGE-SDS was carried out to cut the putative counter-receptors for CD277-Fc and CTLA4-Fc, compared with a control without recombinant proteins. Bands that are in the assay but not in the controls were selected to be identified by MALDI-TOF.

### 2.6.2 Experimental results

The procedure to enhance the expression of CD277 counter-receptor was done twice and cells obtained were named C91T and C91T2. The expression of CD277 counter-receptor in C91T2 was higher than it was in C91T (Figure 8). A third assay to enrich the cell population expressing CD277 counter-receptor by this method was not possible, because the expression after the procedure was not stable.

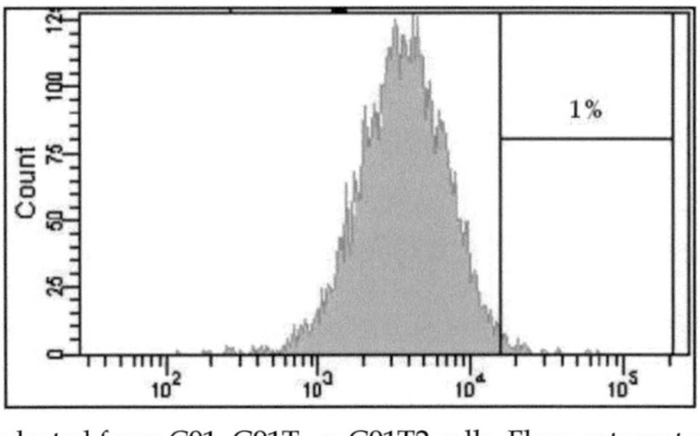


Fig. 7. Population selected from C91, C91T, or C91T2 cells. Flow cytometry was carried out to enhance the stable expression of the CD277 counter-receptor.

From C91T2 cells stained with the CD277-Fc fusion protein we proceeded to clone from the 1% most positive cells (Figure 7). Cloned cells were followed to measure the CD277 counter-receptor expression and the most positive clone obtained was selected and named C91T3.3. As shown in figure 8, increasing expression levels of CD277 counter-receptor were reached with enrichment each step. However, after C91T3.3 no more clones with stable expression of CD277 counter-receptor were obtained. Thus, the highest stable expression of CD277 counter-receptor was that obtained in C91T3.3 cells.

In the first approach to identify the CD277-counter receptor, our preliminary results shown only the homo-polymerization of CD277-Fc by the crosslinking agent BS3 and its detection by mass spectrometry (MALDI-TOF) led us to postulate that this approach is appropriate to determine the identity of CD277 counter-receptor. Nonetheless, the use of additional controls such as CTLA4-Fc is needed to further validate the results. Moreover, as can be seen in our results, it is possible that these homo-polymers mask the potential CD277-Fc - CD277 counter-receptor heterodimerization. Therefore they should be eliminated as collateral products of the reaction in order to select the appropriate band to be analyzed.

Representative 4-12% PAGE-SDS and western-blot analysis are shown in figure 9. The selected bands were analyzed by MALDI-TOF, but only the polymerization of CD277-Fc fusion protein was identified.

The use of the appropriated controls, negative and positive, is essential to validate the results. As a positive control, we used CTLA4-Fc fusion protein in C91 cells (positive by flow cytometry). However, the determination of the identity of CD277 counter-receptor is in process.

In both approaches used (crosslink and co-immunoprecipitation with post-nuclear membranes) the CD80/86 molecules were used to validate these methods. We hypothesized that if detecting CD80/86 was possible, this methodological approach would be useful for the CD277 counter-receptor identification. However, we were not able to detect CD80/86 by any of the strategies tested. Thus, even though this kind of approach has been used in similar circumstances, like the identification of the B7_H6 counter-receptor (Brandt *et al.*, 2009), technical modifications are needed in order to have the validated conditions for the detection of the CD277 counter-receptor.

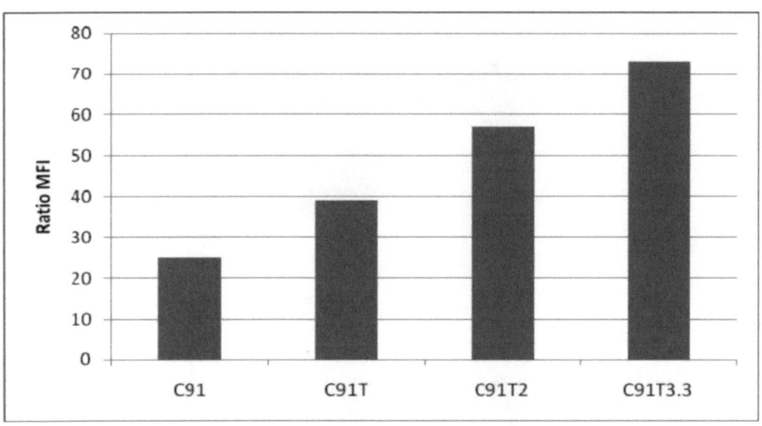


Fig. 8. Enhanced expression of CD277 counter-receptor in C91, C91T, C91T2 and C91T3.3 cells after cell sorting and cloning. Expression was followed-up using CD277-Fc fusion protein by flow cytometry.

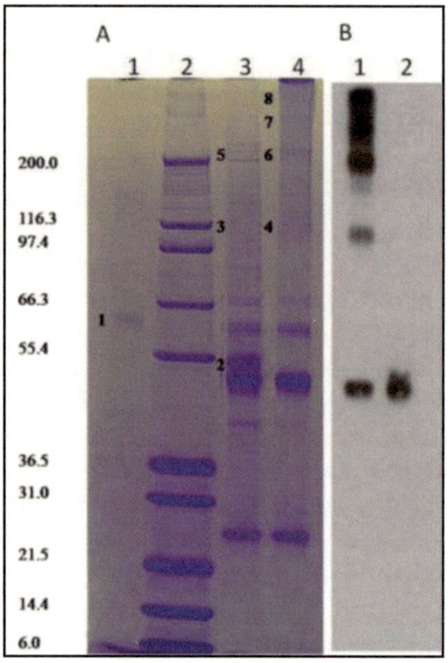


Fig. 9. A typical PAGE-SDS and western-blot analysis for the identification of CD277 counter-receptor. A) 1.- control BSA 2.- molecular weight markers, 3.- assay without BS3 and 4.- with BS3. B) Western-blot line 1 with BS3, line 2 without BS3 and line 3 molecular weight markers. Numbers indicate the selected band to be analyzed by MALDI-TOF.

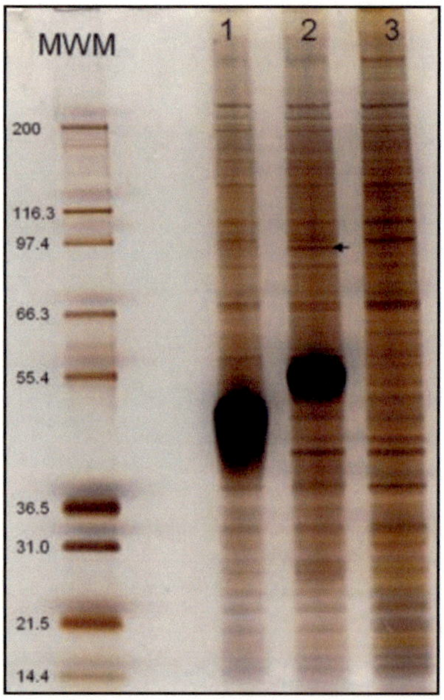


Fig. 10. A typical PAGE-SDS used in co-immunoprecipitation assays using the post-nuclear membranes. 1) Using CTLA4-Fc 2) Using CD277-Fc and 3) control without recombinant proteins. The arrow shows the band to be analyzed.

### 2.6.3 Monoclonal antibodies against the CD277 counter receptor

The production and use of monoclonal antibodies is another attractive strategy to enhance our knowledge of CD277 counter-receptor. However, the identity of the receptor or a recombinant counter-receptor is not available yet. Thus, we decided to obtain monoclonal antibodies to recognize this counter-receptor using cells expressing it as the immunogenic stimulus. With this rationale we immunized rats with C91T3.3 cells, which as described above, enhanced expression of the CD277 counter-receptor. Spleen cells from these immunized rats were used for the production of hybridomas following standard protocols. Important to note is the fact that when using this type of approach, the screening systems are crucial to identify the relevant hybridomas to be clone and antibodies to be purified.

Considering that the rat immune system will produce antibodies against many of the cell surface proteins of C91T3.3, a first screening was done using the CD277 counter-receptor expressing human erythroleukaemic cell line TF1. Hybridomas secreting antibodies against TF1 cells were selected for a second screening. In addition, since Raji cells stimulated with anti-CD277 mAbs show enhanced expression of the CD277 counter-receptor, these cells were used for a second screening of the clones selected in the first one. This second screening was done in parallel with an inhibitory test using C91T3.3 cells and the CD277-Fc.. With this system, hybridomas secreting antibodies against the Raji cells and with inhibitory activity on C91T3.3 were selected for cloning.

In figure 11 a representative figure is shown. The basal fluorescence of Raji cells is shown (11A). The percentage of positive non-stimulated Raji cells is shown in red and it is compared to the amount of positive stimulated Raji cells (blue) (11B). This supernatant was a potentially useful, thus it was tested for inhibitory activity on C91T3.3 cells (Figure 12). We can see that effectively the antibodies in this supernatant have an inhibitory effect on the CD277-Fc binding. Interestingly, we found that some supernatants enhance the CD277-Fc binding on C91T3.3. These clones were selected too, because they could recognize some accessory molecules for the counter-receptor.

We selected a total of 6 clones with inhibitory activity on C91T3.3 cells. We also obtained one clone whose supernatant has the ability to enhance the CD277-Fc binding on C91T3.3 cells. The identification of the proteins recognized by these antibodies is in progress.

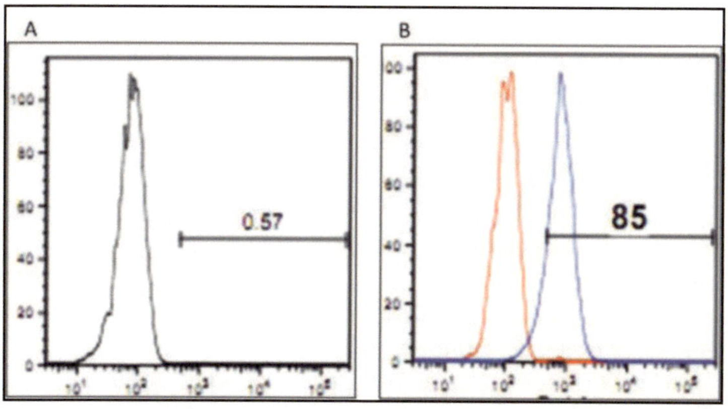


Fig. 11. Representative flow cytometry pattern of a selected clone. A) Basal fluorescence and B) fluorescence of supernatant tested on Raji non stimulated (red) and stimulated with anti-CD277 (blue). The percentage of positive cells is indicated in each pattern.

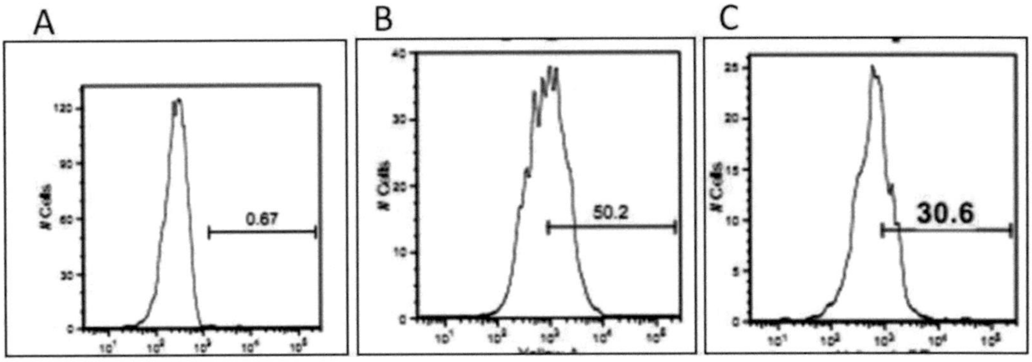


Fig. 12. Representative flow cytometry pattern of a selected clone tested on C91T3.3 cells. A) Basal fluorescence; B) Normal binding of CD277-Fc fusion protein; and C) Inhibitory test showing a reduction in the CD277-Fc binding. The percentage of positive cells is indicated in each pattern.

### 2.7 Perspectives on the potential use of CD277 and its counter-receptor in cancer therapy

The wide variety of function of CD277 described in this chapter shown the future potential of the use of mAbs anti-CD277 to regulate the immune response against tumor cells. The fact that stimulation of different cells by CD277 lead to the secretion of different cytokines, activation of different signalling pathways, enhance the proliferation of T cells, can be useful to modulate the immune response against tumor cells. Moreover, our results showing that Raji cells stimulated by CD277 are better killed by γδ T cells are potentially useful for cancer therapy.

However, it is necessary to elucidate the mechanisms by which these molecules act and to identify the counter-receptor for CD277. The use of mAbs should be a tool to elucidate the mechanisms, but to be used no to mark the tumor cells, but to modulate the response that lead to kill them.

In the near future, regulation of the expression or activity of molecules such as CD277 or its counter-receptor can be useful for enhance the anti-tumoral immune response, however it is necessary the molecular and fully functional characterization of these molecules, and the mechanisms involved in the observed functions, to be used as modulators of immune response in cancer.

## 3. Conclusion

Immune responses can be regulated by CD277 in different ways. CD277 affects different immune cells in various ways including inhibition of proliferation, regulation of cytokine secretion in CD4+ and CD8+ T cells, as well as activating monocytes and iDC. Moreover, CD277 promotes the expression of its counter-receptor and this effect may be important for recognition of leukaemia and solid tumor cells.

Proteomics and production and use of monoclonal antibodies are two different approaches we have tested to determine the identity of the CD277 counter-receptor.. However, although functional analysis of CD277 and its counter-receptor has demonstrated a biological effect, it is necessary to identify the counter-receptor and elucidate the signalling pathways involved in the observed response.

## 4. Acknowledgment

This work was supported by Institut National du Cancer, Institut Paoli Calmettes, Institut National de la Santé et de la Recherche Médicale. J. F Z-Z was a Post-doctoral fellow from Universidad Autónoma de Nayarit.

## 5. References

Borghesi, L. & Milcarek, C. (2007). Innate versus adaptive immunity: a paradigm past its prime? *Cancer Res* 67(9): 3989-3993.

Brandt, C. S., Baratin, M., Yi, E. C., Kennedy, J., Gao, Z., Fox, B., Haldeman, B., Ostrander, C. D., Kaifu, T., Chabannon, C., Moretta, A., West, R., Xu, W., Vivier, E. & Levin, S. D. (2009). The B7 family member B7-H6 is a tumor cell ligand for the activating natural killer cell receptor NKp30 in humans. *J Exp Med* 206(7): 1495-1503.

Compte, E., Pontarotti, P., Collette, Y., Lopez, M. & Olive, D. (2004). Frontline: Characterization of BT3 molecules belonging to the B7 family expressed on immune cells. *Eur J Immunol* 34(8): 2089-2099.

Cubillos-Ruiz, J. R., Martinez, D., Scarlett, U. K., Rutkowski, M. R., Nesbeth, Y. C., Camposeco-Jacobs, A. L. & Conejo-Garcia, J. R. (2010). cd277 is a Negative Co-stimulatory Molecule Universally Expressed by Ovarian Cancer Microenvironmental Cells. *Oncotarget* 1(5): 329-338.

Das, H., Groh, V., Kuijl, C., Sugita, M., Morita, C. T., Spies, T. & Bukowski, J. F. (2001). MICA engagement by human Vgamma2Vdelta2 T cells enhances their antigen-dependent effector function. *Immunity* 15(1): 83-93.

Deetz, C. O., Hebbeler, A. M., Propp, N. A., Cairo, C., Tikhonov, I. & Pauza, C. D. (2006). Gamma interferon secretion by human Vgamma2Vdelta2 T cells after stimulation with antibody against the T-cell receptor plus the Toll-Like receptor 2 agonist Pam3Cys. *Infect Immun* 74(8): 4505-4511.

Halary, F., Peyrat, M. A., Champagne, E., Lopez-Botet, M., Moretta, A., Moretta, L., Vie, H., Fournie, J. J. & Bonneville, M. (1997). Control of self-reactive cytotoxic T lymphocytes expressing gamma delta T cell receptors by natural killer inhibitory receptors. *Eur J Immunol* 27(11): 2812-2821.

Henry, J., Miller, M. M. & Pontarotti, P. (1999). Structure and evolution of the extended B7 family. *Immunol Today* 20(6): 285-288.

Henry, J., Ribouchon, M., Depetris, D., Mattei, M., Offer, C., Tazi-Ahnini, R. & Pontarotti, P. (1997). Cloning, structural analysis, and mapping of the B30 and B7 multigenic families to the major histocompatibility complex (MHC) and other chromosomal regions. *Immunogenetics* 46(5): 383-395.

Ledbetter, J. A., Imboden, J. B., Schieven, G. L., Grosmaire, L. S., Rabinovitch, P. S., Lindsten, T., Thompson, C. B. & June, C. H. (1990). CD28 ligation in T-cell activation: evidence for two signal transduction pathways. *Blood* 75(7): 1531-1539.

Linsley, P. S., Peach, R., Gladstone, P. & Bajorath, J. (1994). Extending the B7 (CD80) gene family. *Protein Sci* 3(8): 1341-1343.

Moretta, A. & Bottino, C. (2004). Commentary: Regulated equilibrium between opposite signals: a general paradigm for T cell function? *Eur J Immunol* 34(8): 2084-2088.

Nedellec, S., Bonneville, M. & Scotet, E. (2010). Human V gamma 9V delta 2 T cells: From signals to functions. *Seminars in Immunology* 22(4): 199-206.

Rietz, C. & Chen, L. (2004). New B7 family members with positive and negative costimulatory function. *Am J Transplant* 4(1): 8-14.

Rincon-Orozco, B., Kunzmann, V., Wrobel, P., Kabelitz, D., Steinle, A. & Herrmann, T. (2005). Activation of V gamma 9V delta 2 T cells by NKG2D. *J Immunol* 175(4): 2144-2151.

Saenz, S. A., Noti, M. & Artis, D. (2010). Innate immune cell populations function as initiators and effectors in Th2 cytokine responses. *Trends Immunol* 31(11): 407-413.

Simone, R., Barbarat, B., Rabellino, A., Icardi, G., Bagnasco, M., Pesce, G., Olive, D. & Saverino, D. (2010). Ligation of the BT3 molecules, members of the B7 family, enhance the proinflammatory responses of human monocytes and monocyte-derived dendritic cells. *Molecular Immunology* 48(1-3): 109-118.

Tanaka, Y., Morita, C. T., Nieves, E., Brenner, M. B. & Bloom, B. R. (1995). Natural and synthetic non-peptide antigens recognized by human gamma delta T cells. *Nature* 375(6527): 155-158.

Tokuyama, H., Hagi, T., Mattarollo, S. R., Morley, J., Wang, Q., Fai-So, H., Moriyasu, F., Nieda, M. & Nicol, A. J. (2008). V gamma 9 V delta 2 T cell cytotoxicity against tumor cells is enhanced by monoclonal antibody drugs--rituximab and trastuzumab. *Int J Cancer* 122(11): 2526-2534.

Ward, S. G. (1996). CD28: a signalling perspective. *Biochem J* 318 ( Pt 2): 361-377.

Wesch, D., Beetz, S., Oberg, H. H., Marget, M., Krengel, K. & Kabelitz, D. (2006). Direct costimulatory effect of TLR3 ligand poly(I:C) on human gamma delta T lymphocytes. *J Immunol* 176(3): 1348-1354.

Yamashiro, H., Yoshizaki, S., Tadaki, T., Egawa, K. & Seo, N. (2010). Stimulation of human butyrophilin 3 molecules results in negative regulation of cellular immunity. *Journal of Leukocyte Biology* 88(4): 757-767.

Zhu, Y. & Chen, L. (2009). Turning the tide of lymphocyte costimulation. *J Immunol* 182(5): 2557-2558.

# 20

# Transcription Regulation and Epigenetic Control of Expression of Natural Killer Cell Receptors and Their Ligands

Zhixia Zhou, Cai Zhang, Jian Zhang and Zhigang Tian
*Institute of Immunopharmacology & Immunotherapy,*
*School of Pharmaceutical Sciences, Shandong University*
*China*

## 1. Introduction

Throughout the life of an individual organism, a successful host defense relies on the coordination of innate and adaptive immunity (McQueen and Parham, 2002). Natural killer (NK) cells are characteristic cytolytic cells that are integral components of innate immunity and play a major role both in the direct destruction of infected or transformed cells and in the production of cytokines and chemokines that mediate inflammatory responses and exert a regulatory effect on the adaptive immune responses (McQueen and Parham, 2002; Moretta et al., 2006). Cells become susceptible to NK cell-mediated killing following downregulation of cell surface MHC class I expression after virus infection, which ultimately leads to escape from the MHC-restricted adaptive immune system; a phenomenon also seen in metastasized tumor cells. MHC class I-specific NK receptors (NKR) have acquired the ability to detect immune escape variants and in rodents and primates can be grouped into two distinct classes of MHC class I-specific receptor families based on protein structure: the C-type lectin superfamily (Cl-SF) and the immunoglobulin superfamily (Ig-SF). Humans possess a large family of killer cell immunoglobulin-like receptors (KIR) that belong to the Ig superfamily, whereas mice express lectin-like Ly49 receptors that are now not present in humans, except for a single nonfunctional gene fragment (Lanier, 1998, 2001; Vilches and Parham, 2002; Takei et al., 2001). A third family of NKR, the lectin-like CD94/NKG2 heterodimers, are structurally and functionally conserved between rodents and primates and interact with their ligands: nonclassical MHC class I molecules and some specific ligands that are differentially expressed in different tissues in response to different stresses (McQueen and Parham, 2002; Moretta et al., 2006; Raulet et al., 2001; Uhrberg et al., 1997; Valiante et al., 1997). The actions of NK cells, therefore, are thought to be mediated by the complex interactions between inhibitory and activating signals sent by cell-surface receptors following ligation (Lanier, 2005; Ravetch and Lanier, 2000).

Malignant cells in tumor growth frequently demonstrate alterations in MHC class I expression that play a major role in their ability to escape immune recognition and killing (Dunn et al., 2002; Campoli et al., 2005). NK cells enhance their cytotoxic function and immune regulation by using their stimulatory and inhibitory receptors to maintain the constant balance in the immune system (Chang and Ferrone, 2006). There are major questions, however, regarding the molecular mechanisms that govern the shape of the NK-cell receptors and MHC class I molecules or other ligands that exhibit an exceptionally high degree of genetic polymorphism in a clonally distributed fashion. Studies, therefore, that focus on the molecular mechanisms that govern the expression of NK-cell receptors and their ligands may provide improved strategies of active-specific immunotherapy for the treatment of cancer, infection and other diseases (Campoli and Ferrone, 2008; Krukowski et al., 2011; Gao et al., 2009). Some stimulators, including viruses, tumor cells and heat shock, could promote the expression of NK-cell receptors and their ligands via activation of certain transcription factors that are capable of regulating activity of NKG2 promoters. Epigenetic mechanisms, including DNA methylation and histone posttranslational modification, are also critical for expression of NK-cell receptors and their ligands, and may control the clonal distribution of some NK-cell receptors. These effects may influence the performance of NK-cell functions. In this review, we will discuss the recent advances in transcriptional regulation and epigenetic control of the expression of NK-cell receptors and their ligands (and of KIR and NKG2 receptor families in particular).

## 2. Regulation of gene expression – An introduction in the transcriptional level

Mechanisms that underlie the control of gene expression, which drives the processes of gene morphogenesis and distribution, are complex. Transcription regulation at every step of the process is subject to dynamic regulation in the cell (Beckett, 2009; Pan et al., 2010). This regulation includes structural changes in the chromatin to make a particular gene accessible for transcription, transcription of DNA into RNA, splicing of RNA into mRNA, editing and other covalent modifications of the mRNA, translation of mRNA into protein, and, finally, posttranslational modification of the protein into its mature functional form. Information on molecular details of each of these regulatory steps is becoming increasingly available (Fry and Peterson, 2002; Mitchell and Tjian, 1989).

### 2.1 Transcriptional factor regulation

Regulation at the transcriptional level is a critical mechanism of controlling gene expression. Transcription is controlled by trans-acting factors that regulate spatiotemporal gene expression by associating with cis-acting elements such as promoters, enhancers, and other regulatory regions. Transcription factors perform this function either alone or with other proteins in a complex and by promoting or blocking the transcription of genetic information from DNA to RNA (Mitchell and Tjian, 1989; Alexander and Beggs, 2010; Brivanlou and Darnell, 2002; Karin, 1990). A defining feature of transcription factors is that they contain one or more DNA-binding domains (DBDs), which attach to specific DNA sequences adjacent to the genes that they regulate. In eukaryotes, an important class of transcription factors, called general transcription factors (GTFs), is necessary for transcription to occur. Many of these GTFs do not actually bind to DNA but are parts of the large transcription preinitiation complex that interact directly with RNA polymerase. The most common GTFs are transcription factor II members (TFIIA/B/D/E/F and TFIIH). There are also some nonclassical transcription factors that play crucial roles in gene regulation, including coactivators, chromatin remodelers, histone acetylases, deacetylases, kinases, and methylases, which lack DNA-binding domains (Brivanlou and Darnell, 2002; Karin, 1990; Dowell, 2010; van Nimwegen, 2003).

### 2.2 Epigenetic control

Transcription is also controlled by epigenetic regulation that is defined as gene-regulation activity that does not involve changes in the underlying DNA code and includes DNA methylation and a variety of histone protein posttranslational modifications (Feng et al., 2010; Furumatsu and Ozaki, 2010). DNA methylation usually occurs in CpG islands, CG-rich regions that are "upstream" of the promoter region. The letter "p" here signifies that C and G are connected by a phosphodiester bond. In humans, DNA methylation is carried out by a group of enzymes called DNA methyltransferases. These enzymes not only determine DNA methylation patterns during early development, but are also responsible for copying these patterns to the strands generated from DNA replication. DNA methylation can alter condensed chromatin structure by influencing histone–DNA and histone–histone contact. Methylation of the promoter and 5′ region of the gene and methylation of histone are associated with transcriptional silencing (Bird, 2002; Bird and Wolffe, 1999; Law and Jacobsen, 2010).

Acetylation and methylation of histones are the most general and important histone modifications associated with transcriptional activation. Histone acetylation is catalysed by histone acetyl transferases (HATs), whereas the reverse reaction is performed by histone deacetylases (HDACs) (Furumatsu and Ozaki, 2010). HATs and HDACs are classified into many families that are often conserved throughout evolution from yeast to humans. Histone H3 is primarily acetylated at several lysine residues, Lys9, 14, 18, 23, 27 and 56, whereas histone H4 is acetylated at Lys5, 8, 12 and 16 (Su et al., 2004). Interestingly, methylation is often modified at lysine and arginine residues in histones H3 and H4. It has been suggested that these modifications constitute a "histone code"; the "code" hypothesis speculates that this modification pattern is read by proteins that recognize distinct modifications specifically and then regulate chromatin dynamics and genome function (Wang et al., 2004; Kisliouk et al., 2010). Whether these modifications form a true code is still under discussion. The processes of histone modification and DNA methylation can both influence each other. Moreover, DNA methylation and suppressive histone modifications may prevent transcription, even when transcription factors are abundant. In turn, transcription factors may cause alterations in DNA methylation and histone modifications (Furumatsu and Ozaki, 2010; Fernandez-Morera et al., 2010; Strahl and Allis, 2000). Molecular details of the transcriptional regulators involved in expression of many NK-cell receptors and their ligands are becoming increasingly available, especially for the NKG2 and KIR receptor families and their ligands.

## 3. Transcription factor regulation and epigenetic control of the expression of NK-cell receptors and their ligands

### 3.1 NKG2 receptor family

In humans, the NKG2 receptor family comprises seven members called NKG2A, NKG2B, NKG2C, NKG2D, NKG2E, NKG2F and NKG2H; NKG2A/B and NKG2E/H pairs are splice variants of the same gene (Brostjan et al., 2000; Glienke et al., 1998). All members of the NKG2 family, except NKG2D, share substantial sequence homology, are closely linked, and of the same transcriptional orientation; they contain conserved sequences at the transcriptional start site and at other transcription factor-binding sites, such as the TCF-1 (testosterone conversion factor-1) and GATA-1 (GATA-binding factor 1) sites. These members of the NKG2 family form disulfide-linked heterodimers with CD94. Each member of the NKG2 family, however, has a unique repeat Alu sequence that functions as a gene promoter. Alu repeats are the putative binding sites for several transcription factors: activator protein-1/3 (AP-1/3), cAMP response element binding/activating transcription factors (CREB/ATF), CCAAT/enhancer binding protein (C/EBP), transcription factor-1 (Sp1), nuclear factor-1/CCAAT transcription factor (NF-1/CTF) and lymphocyte-specific DNA-binding protein-1 (LyF-1), and may contribute to differences in gene regulation among family members (Brostjan et al., 2000; Glienke et al., 1998). The CD94 protein associates with different NKG2 isoforms to form heterodimeric receptors that function either to inhibit or to trigger cytotoxicity of NK cells, depending on the NKG2 isoform. Functionally, therefore, CD94/NKG2 heterodimers are divided into activating (NKG2C, NKG2E/H) or inhibitory (NKG2A/B) isotypes (Glienke et al., 1998). It has also been shown that several cytokines, including interleukin (IL)-12 (Derre et al., 2002), transforming growth factor (TGF)-β (Bertone et al., 1999), IL-15 (Mingari et al., 1998) and IL-10 (Romero et al., 2001), are capable of inducing expression of CD94/NKG2 in human NK or T cells, in which IL-15 and TGF-β can upregulate CD94/NKG2A, but not other CD94/NKG2 receptors (Wilhelm et al., 2003). NKG2D is a special activating receptor that is not covalently associated with CD94. NKG2D is downmodulated by TGF-β, but markedly upregulated by IL-15, interferon (IFN)-α and IL-12 stimulation in primary NK cells (Dasgupta et al., 2005). IFN-α can stimulate the expression of NKG2D, but inhibits the expression of the inhibitory receptor NKG2A, and therefore alters the balance of stimulatory and inhibitory receptors in favor of activation, leading to NK-cell-mediated cytotoxicity. IFN-γ addition exerts the opposite effect (Zhang et al., 2005).

CD94 is a C-type lectin and is required for the dimerization of the CD94/NKG2 family of receptors, which are expressed on NK cells and T-cell subsets. The CD94 and NKG2 genes are located in the center of the NK-gene complex between the NKRP1 and PRB3 loci in the region containing the STS markers D12S77 and D12S1093. All six genes are closely linked and are situated 100 to 200 kb proximal to the D12S77 STS marker (Sobanov et al., 1999). The CD94 gene is placed in the opposite orientation relative to the NKG2 gene family members (which all have the same transcriptional orientation). CD94 gene expression is regulated by distal and proximal promoters that transcribe unique initial exons specific for each promoter. Both promoters contain elements with IFN-γ-activated and E26 transformation-specific (ETS)-binding sites (called GAS and EBS respectively). The two promoters differentially regulate expression of the CD94 gene in response to treatment with IL-2 or IL-15 (Lieto et al., 2003).

### 3.2 Ligands of NKG2D-MIC

The two types of NKG2D ligands are MHC class I chain-related proteins (MICA and MICB) and UL16-binding proteins (ULBP) (Sutherland et al., 2001; Bauer et al., 1999). MICA and MICB are located in the MHC complex within the 6q21.3 chromosomal region. The ULBP family contains 10 genes, of which five are expressed (ULBP1–5). ULBPs are located outside the MHC gene complex, in the 6q24.2–25.3 region (Samarakoon et al., 2009). These molecules exhibit highly restricted expression in healthy tissues but are widely expressed on epithelial tumors. In hematological malignancies they are upregulated in nontumor and tumor cells by genotoxic stress (Kim et al., 2006; Venkataraman et al., 2007). Aligned cosmid-derived regions 1.5 kb upstream of the translation start codon (ATG) in MICA and MICB share approximately 90% sequence identity. The 5′-end flanking regions of MICA and

MICB contain putative heat shock elements (HSE) that are prototypic transcription inducer sites in heat shock protein-70 (HSP70) genes and that bind activated trimeric heat shock factor protein-1 (HSF1). Cytomegalovirus (CMV) infection results in up to a 10-fold increase in cell surface MIC expression and is associated with induced HSP70 expression. TATA-like elements and Sp1 consensus sites, as with HSE, are located unusually far "upstream" from MIC gene, but can also moderately or profoundly affect stress-induced and proliferation-associated induction. The common integrating conjugative element (ICE), however, appears to be a negative regulator of MICB, but not of MICA. It is an important to note, although the sequences of MICA and MICB promoters are very similar, the baseline transcriptional activity of MICA is higher than that of MICB and they have different regulatory mechanisms for expression. Most MICA transcripts start downstream of the conserved AP-1 TATA-like motif, a region that lacks a recognizable RNA start site. In contrast, most MICB transcripts initiate further upstream, proximal to the HSE–Sp1–ICE elements (Venkataraman et al., 2007). Nuclear factor kappa-light-chain-enhancer of activated B cells (NF-κB) regulates MICA expression on activated T lymphocytes and on HeLa tumor cells by binding to a specific sequence in the long intron 1 region of the MICA gene (Molinero et al., 2004). Histone deacetylase inhibitor (HDAC-I) and sodium valproate (VPA) induced transcription of MICA and MICB in hepatocellular carcinoma cells, leading to increased cell surface, soluble and total MIC protein expression (Armeanu et al., 2005). Similar results have been obtained using histone deacetylase inhibitors FR901228 and SAHA (Skov et al., 2005). In our laboratory, we found that VPA can increase the expression of HSP70 and Sp1 and increase the binding of transcription factors Sp1 and HSF1 to the MICA/B promoter. This activation leads to the upregulation of MICA/B in HeLa and HepG2 tumor cells (Zhang et al., 2009).

### 3.3 Ligands of NKG2D-ULBPs

All expressed ULBPs (ULBP1–5) have good conservation of the coding sequence, but the 5′-end flanking regions of these genes have little homology. This situation suggests that ULBPs are regulated specifically in response to different stimuli or pathogens (Lopez-Soto et al., 2006). Mechanisms that regulate the expression of ULBP1 have been described previously. In the core region of the ULBP1 promoter, there are many binding sites for transcription factors, including a canonical TATA box, three GC boxes, one overlapping sequence GC(4)/AP-2, two cytokinin response element (CRE)-like sequences (CRE1 and CRE2) (Zeng et al., 1997; Wajapeyee and Somasundaram, 2003), and one NF-κB site. Transcription of ULBP1 depends strictly on binding of Sp1 and Sp3 to a CRE1 site located in the ULBP1 minimal promoter. The mutation or deletion of this Sp1/Sp3 binding site abolished ULBP1 transcription; Sp3 is the main transcription factor that regulates ULBP1 through the CRE1 site. AP-2α, however, repressed the expression of ULBP1 by binding to the GC(4)/AP-2α site and interfering with the binding of Sp3 and Sp1 to the ULBP1 promoter (Lopez-Soto et al., 2006). It has been shown that heat shock and ionizing radiation treatment can induce the expression of ULBP1/2/3 in human cancer cell lines; HSP 70 is induced by heat shock but not by ionizing radiation (Kim et al., 2006). Human cytomegalovirus (HCMV) can also induce the expression of ULBP1/2/3 proteins that are predominantly localized in the endoplasmic reticulum of infected fibroblasts together with UL16 (Rolle et al., 2003). There is interplay, however, between virus and host cells depending on the viral dose. At low viral dose, ULBP1 or ULBP2 surface expression is completely inhibited compared with ULBP3, while at a higher viral doses cell surface expression of ULBP1 and ULBP2 is delayed (Rolle et al., 2003). Whether this phenomenon is mediated through the ULBP promoter or through transcription factors needs to be investigated further.

Epigenetic modulations are also likely to play a large part in the observed alteration in ULBP expression. Current observations imply that loss of DNA methylation (deficient in DNA methyltransferase cells) is correlated with increased ULBP2 mRNA levels. It has been shown that both demethylation of the ULPB2 promoter, necessary for increased protein levels, and the RAS/MEK signaling pathway, shown to control DNA methylation (Lund et al., 2006), are necessary for maximal protein expression (Sers et al., 2009). In addition, the HDAC inhibitor trichostatin A (TSA) is reported to upregulate ULBP1–3 expression in tumor cells; Sp3 was found to be crucial for activation of the ULBP1 promoter by TSA. One report showed that HDAC3 is recruited to the ULBP1 promoter and acts as a repressor of ULBP expression in epithelial cancer cells. TSA treatment interfered with this interaction and caused the complete release of HDAC3 from the ULBP1–3 promoters (Lopez-Soto et al., 2009).

### 3.4 KIR receptor family and their ligands

The KIR family is of particular interest because individual members bind to specific subgroups of HLA allele products, such as HLA-A, HLA-B, HLA-C, and HLA-G, although most KIRs show 90–95% amino acid identity. The high level of homology can facilitate exchange of exons between different KIR loci, by some form of crossing over or gene conversion (Wilson et al., 2000). One study found that due to the polymorphism of KIR genes, two KIR haplotypes segregated at roughly equal frequency in a largely Caucasian population. Group A haplotypes contained seven KIR genes and had KIR2DS4 as the only activating receptor. Group B haplotypes had a greater diversity of KIR genes, had more activating receptors, and were characterized by the KIR2DL2, KIR2DS1, KIR2DS2, KIR2DS3, and KIR2DS5 genes (Uhrberg et al., 1997). KIR can also be further subdivided into inhibitory receptors that carry an inhibitory signal motif within their cytoplasmic domain (KIR2DL and KIR3DL) and into stimulatory receptors (KIR2DS and KIR3DS) that lack this motif. Most of the inhibitory KIRs are specific for the products of HLA class I genes like such as HLA-A/-B and HLA-C (Bellon et al., 1999; Colonna et al., 1993; Dohring et al., 1996). The ligand specificities of many stimulatory KIR are uncertain and might include non-HLA class I ligands. KIR2DL4, however, combines structural and functional features of both stimulatory and inhibitory KIR and is reported to bind to the nonclassical class I protein HLA-G (Chan et al., 2003; Martin et al., 2000; Trompeter et al., 2005; Santourlidis et al., 2002). The expression of KIR appears to be largely independent of each other and the impact of the requirement for inhibition by self class I molecules on the shape of the KIR repertoire is rather subtle.

#### 3.4.1 Transcriptional factors regulation of KIR

Different groups of 2–9 KIR genes are expressed in NK clones, but the sequences of the KIR promoters are homogeneous in their 5'-untranslated regions (5' UTR), except for that of KIR2DL4 (Valiante et al., 1997; Wilson et al., 2000). The sequences of KIR genes comprise a continuous loop that extends seamlessly from gene to gene. The repeat of the loop is broken only by a region 14 kb upstream of the KIR2DL4 locus, which displays some unique features and is characterized by L1 repeats. The sequence upstream of KIR2DL4 may be significant because this gene is unique in this group in being expressed in 100% of NK clones (Valiante et al., 1997; Wilson et al., 2000; Martin et al., 2000). Moreover, KIR2DL4 is the only KIR gene that lacks the repeat region in intron 1. All KIR genes lack typical promoter features such as TATA and CAAT boxes, so many transcription factor binding sites have been predicted to be present in the upstream regions of KIR, including sites for transcription factors CREB, SP1, ETS, AP-1 and AP-4 (Chan et al., 2003; Santourlidis et al., 2002). None of these elements alone, however, is required for or significantly increases promoter activity, except for a CREB site located outside the core promoter region. To date, the basic KIR promoter appears to either require undefined transcription factors or alternatively only interacts with the basic transcription machinery of RNA polymerase II (Trompeter et al., 2005). It has been suggested previously that a binding site for the transcription factor AML/Runx (Runt Homology Domain Transcription Factors) at -100 bp can be essential for KIR expression (Vilches et al., 2000). However, a further study suggested that AML has a general inhibitory influence on KIR expression in mature NK cells and that AML exerts its repressor function by binding directly to the promoter of the different KIR genes (Trompeter et al., 2005). Recently, it was reported that the transcription factor c-Myc upregulated KIR gene transcription through direct binding to an upstream distal promoter element in peripheral blood NK cells, and that IL-15 promoted this effect (Cichocki et al., 2009). It was suggested that the role of the traditional transcription factors in KIR gene expression is different from that in other genes.

### 3.4.2 Histone modifications of KIR

It was found that histone H3 and H4 proteins are substantially acetylated at the Lys9 and Lys14 positions and H4 acetylation at the 5th, 8th, 12th, and 16th positions in both KIR3DL1+ and KIR3DL1- NK cells (Chan et al., 2005). The level of KIR3DL1-associated histone acetylation and methylation was higher in KIR3DL1+ NK cells than in KIR3DL1- NK cells; however, histone H3 methylation at Lys4 (H3K4) is only 2.6-fold higher in KIR3DL1+ NK cells than that in KIR3DL1- NK cells, although the histone H3K4 methylation levels correlated well with the KIR3DL1 promoter to lead to upregulation of KIR3DL1 gene expression, named KIR3DL1-associated histone H3K4 methylation. These findings indicate that histone acetylation and trimethylated modifications, but not histone H3 methylation, are preferentially associated with the transcribed allele in NK cells with monoallelic KIR expression (Santourlidis et al., 2002; Chan et al., 2005).

KIR expression is increased on T cells with increasing age, and can contribute to age-related diseases (van Bergen et al., 2004). In these cells, the KIR2DL4 promoter is partially demethylated, and dimethylated H3L4 is increased; all other histone modifications are characteristic of an inactive promoter. In comparison, NK cells have a fully demethylated KIR2DL4 promoter and have the full spectrum of histone modifications indicative of active transcription with H3 and H4 acetylation. These findings suggest that an increased T-cell ability to express KIR2DL4 with age is conferred by a selective increase in H3L4 dimethylation and limited DNA demethylation (van Bergen et al., 2004; Li et al., 2008).

### 3.4.3 DNA demethylation of KIR

Methylation status of CpG islands in NK cells correlates with transcriptional activity of KIR genes. The overall structure of the CpG islands is similar in all expressed KIR, with complete conservation of four CpG dinucleotides upstream of the transcriptional start site, with the exception of KIR2DL4, which shows a highly divergent profile with lower CpG density. In addition, CpG islands with <70% of methylated CpGs are exclusively found in the expressed KIR2DL3, whereas CpG islands of nonexpressed KIR2DL3 and KIR3DL2 are consistently methylated at 70–100% of CpG dinucleotides (Santourlidis et al., 2002). Analysis of the methylation status at individual CpG sites demonstrated that differential methylation of expressed versus nonexpressed KIR is not restricted to specific CpGs, but is consistently found throughout the CpG islands. That is to say, the methylated CpG islands are associated with transcriptionally silent KIR and unmethylated CpG islands with expressed KIR genes (Chan et al., 2003; Santourlidis et al., 2002).

In addition, exposure to a DNA methyltransferase inhibitor, 5-aza-2'-deoxycytidine (5azaC), effectively induced the whole range of KIR expression in NK cells (Gao et al., 2009; Chan et al., 2003; Santourlidis et al., 2002; Chan et al., 2005), but not in other cells of lymphoid or nonlymphoid origin. A weak induction of KIR3DL2 following treatment with 5aza-dC was observed in a T-cell line (Li et al., 2008; Santourlidis et al., 2008). These results suggested that repression of KIR gene transcription is dependent on DNA methylation only in NK cells and T cells, and that allele-specific KIR3DL1 gene expression is not only correlated with promoter but also with 5'-gene DNA hypomethylation. Further studies showed that methylation influenced KIR expression both in immature NK cells and in mature NK cells, because KIR promoter-associated CpG islands are indeed DNA-methylated at an early developmental stage (Li et al., 2008; Liu et al., 2009).

### 3.4.4 A two-step model of epigenetic regulation of KIR

Recent studies suggested that CpG methylation is functionally linked to histone deacetylation, which, in turn, leads to the formation of condensed, transcriptionally repressive chromatin (Bird, 2002; Bird and Wolffe, 1999). Altering the state of histone acetylation using the deacetylase inhibitor TSA did not change transcriptional activity of either expressed or silent KIR genes. Additionally, combined treatment of 5aza-dC and TSA did not lead to a synergistic effect compared with 5aza-dC alone. In particularly, the expression of KIR2DL4, which is expressed by all human NK clones, was not affected by either demethylating or histone-acetylating treatment. This finding indicated that KIR genes in NK cells might have already acquired a state of transcriptionally competent chromatin. Methylation of KIR CpG islands appears to be the priority epigenetic modification required for silencing of specific KIR genes (Santourlidis et al., 2002). In a further study, this point was addressed. Hematopoietic progenitor cell KIR genes exhibited the major hallmarks of epigenetic repression: dense DNA methylation; inaccessibility of chromatin; and a repressive histone signature, characterized by strong H3K9 dimethylation and reduced H4K8 acetylation. In contrast, KIR genes in NK cells showed active histone signatures characterized by absence of H3K9 dimethylation and presence of H4K8 acetylation. In KIR-competent lineages, active histone signatures were also observed in silenced KIR genes and, in this study, were found in combination with dense DNA methylation of the promoter and nearby regions. The study suggested a two-step model of epigenetic regulation in which lineage-specific acquisition of euchromatic histone is a prerequisite for subsequent gene-specific DNA demethylation and expression of KIR genes (Santourlidis et al., 2008).

### 3.4.5 HLA-ligand of KIR

Recently, epigenetic alterations were shown to play a role in HLA changes associated with malignant transformation of cells (Campoli and Ferrone, 2008). HLA-G, initially discovered on the fetal–maternal interface, plays a key role in the maintenance of immune tolerance by inhibition of NK cells via the receptor KIR2DL4 (Hofmeister and Weiss, 2003); it is expressed in some surgically removed melanoma lesions, but there is little expression in established cell lines. Treatment of a HLA-G-negative melanoma cell line with 5azaC restored HLA-G expression; similarly 5azaC activated HLA-G expression in human leukemia cell lines, even in malignant hematopoietic cells isolated from patients with acute myeloid leukemia (AML) and chronic lymphocytic leukemia (B-CLL) (Polakova et al., 2009a; Polakova et al., 2009b). Further research found that HLA-G was silenced as a result of CpG hypermethylation within a 5′ regulatory region upstream of the start codon (Moreau et al., 2003; Yan et al., 2005). These results determined that regulation of HLA-G expression also involved epigenetic mechanisms, such as DNA methylation. There was no significant difference in HLA-G expression, however, detected in tumor and normal ovarian surface epithelial cells (OSE) samples, although HLA-G expression was significantly increased after treatment with 5azaC. There was no correlation between methylation and HLA-G gene expression in ovarian tumor samples and OSE, which suggested that changes in methylation may be necessary, but not sufficient, for HLA-G expression in ovarian cancer (Menendez et al., 2008).

In addition, the expression of HLA-A, HLA-B and HLA-C, specific ligands for inhibitory KIR (KIR3DL2, KIR3DL1, and KIR2DL1/3) was lost or downregulated in human gastric cancer, where the percentage of promoter methylation was higher than in adjacent nontumor tissues (Ye et al., 2010). In esophageal squamous cell carcinoma lesions, it was also shown that hypermethylation in the gene promoter regions of the HLA-A, HLA-B and HLA-C, and altered chromatin structure of the HLA class I heavy chain gene promoters have both been implicated as a major mechanism for transcriptional inactivation of HLA genes (Nie et al., 2001). Furthermore, the MAPK (mitogen-activated protein kinases) and DNA methyltransferases were shown to downregulate HLA-A expression (Sers et al., 2009). These findings suggest an association between promoter hypermethylation and the downregulated expression of HLA class I molecules.

## 4. Regulation expression of NK cell receptors and their ligands as potential therapeutics for cancer

The mechanisms of regulation the gene expression, which requires signalling cascades for transducing and integrating regulatory cues to determine which genes are expressed, are obligatory for tumorigenesis, tumor progression and metastasis (Bhalla, 2005; Samarakoon et al., 2009; Stein et al., 2010). Transcriptional gene regulations, particularly in transcriptional factors and epigenetic level, affect several aspects of tumor cell biology, including cell growth, proliferation, phenotype, differentiation, DNA repair, and cell death. NK cells are the major effector lymphocytes of innate immune system that defend against many forms of viral infections and tumor growth without prior sensitizations, by the interaction of inhibitory and activating receptors with corresponding ligands on the target cells. This raises the strong possibility that regulation expression of NK cell receptors on NK cells and their ligands on tumor cells may be an effective treatment strategy for malignant tumors. This treatment strategy, as mentioned above, including activation and suppression of the transcription factors and promoter activity, modification the DNA methylation in the underlying DNA code, and rearrangement the acetylation and methylation of protein in histone posttranslational level, leads to the induced or suppressed expression of NK cells receptors and their ligands (Fig. 1), so that the NK cell-mediated immunotherapy can be carried out fully to cure malignancies. So the regulation expression of NK cell receptors and their ligands provides a strategy for targeting gene expression in tumor cells, and may be with minimal offtarget consequences (Villar-Garea and Esteller, 2004; Bhalla, 2005; Szyf, 2005, Stein et al., 2010).

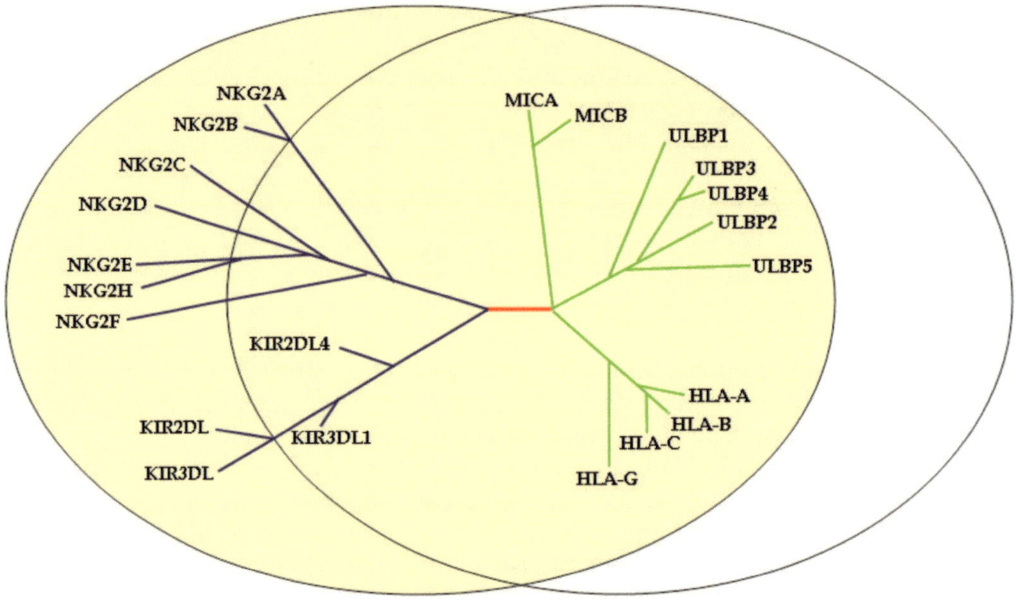


Fig. 1. Transcription regulation and epigenetic control of KIR and NKG2 receptors and their ligands. A dendrogram representing the relatedness of different KIR and NKG2 receptors (blue) and their ligands (green) to each other, and the extent of the sequence relatedness between two genes is shown by the distance of the lines (Raulet, 2003). The left oval shows the gene regulation in transcription factor level, while the right oval shows the gene regulation in epigenetic level, and the overlapping part shows the co-regulation.

## 5. Concluding remarks

NK cells not only are important players of innate effecter responses, but also participate in the initiation and development of antigen-specific responses through secretion of immunoregulatory cytokines (such as IFN-γ, tumor necrosis factor-α (TNF-α) and granulocyte–macrophage colony-stimulating factor (GM–CSF)) and through cell-to-cell contact (Biron et al., 1999). Regulation of the expression of NK-cell receptors and their ligands refers to the control of the amount, the timing of appearance, and the functional products of these genes, leading to the flexibility of NK cells or other immune cells to adapt to a variable environment, external signals, and damages to target cells (Wu et al., 2005). In particular, the modification of NK-cell receptors and their ligands is a potential therapeutic implication for cancer treatment. Although the regulation mechanism of expression of NK-cell receptors and related ligands has acquired important progress at the transcription level, the regulatory mechanisms of a number of crucial receptors and ligands, for example signaling lymphocytic activating molecule (SLAM)-related receptors (CD150, 2B4, Ly-9,

CD84, and NTB-A) (Sidorenko and Clark, 2003; Engel et al., 2003; Morra et al., 2001), are not well understood. More research is needed into other regulated stages of gene expression, such as posttranscriptional modification, RNA transport, translation, and mRNA degradation. Investigation of the regulatory mechanisms of NK-cell receptors and their ligands might aid in the design of therapy against cancer, infection, inflammation, or autoimmune diseases.

## 6. Acknowledgment

This work was supported by grants from the Natural Science Foundation of China (No. 90713033), the National 973 Basic Science Program of China (No. 2007CB815800) and the Important National Science & Technology Specific Projects of China (No. 2008ZX10002-008).

## 7. References

Armeanu, S., Bitzer, M., Lauer, U. M., Venturelli, S., Pathil, A., Krusch, M., Kaiser, S., Jobst, J., Smirnow, I., Wagner, A., Steinle, A. & Salih, H. R. (2005). Natural killer cell-mediated lysis of hepatoma cells via specific induction of NKG2D ligands by the histone deacetylase inhibitor sodium valproate. *Cancer Res*, Vol.65, No.14, pp. 6321-6329, ISSN 1538-7445

Alexander, R. & Beggs, J. D. (2010). Cross-talk in transcription, splicing and chromatin: who makes the first call? *Biochem Soc Trans*, Vol.38, No.5, pp. 1251-1256, ISSN 0300-5127

Bauer, S., Groh, V., Wu, J., Steinle, A., Phillips, J. H., Lanier, L. L. & Spies, T. (1999). Activation of NK cells and T cells by NKG2D, a receptor for stress-inducible MICA. *Science*, Vol. 285, No.5428, pp. 727-729, ISSN 1095-9203

Bellon, T., Heredia, A. B., Llano, M., Minguela, A., Rodriguez, A., Lopez-Botet, M. & Aparicio, P. (1999). Triggering of effector functions on a CD8+ T cell clone upon the aggregation of an activatory CD94/kp39 heterodimer. *J Immunol*, Vol.162, No.7, pp. 3996-4002, ISSN 0732-0582

Bertone, S., Schiavetti, F., Bellomo, R., Vitale, C., Ponte, M., Moretta, L. & Mingari, M. C. (1999). Transforming growth factor-beta-induced expression of CD94/NKG2A inhibitory receptors in human T lymphocytes. *Eur J Immunol*, Vol.29, No.1, pp. 23-29, ISSN 0014-2980

Bird, A. P. & Wolffe, A. P. (1999). Methylation-induced repression--belts, braces, and chromatin. *Cell* , Vol.99, No.5, pp. 451-454, ISSN 0092-8674

Biron, C. A., Nguyen, K. B., Pien, G. C., Cousens, L. P. & Salazar-Mather, T. P. (1999). Natural killer cells in antiviral defense: function and regulation by innate cytokines. *Annu Rev Immunol*, Vol.17, pp. 189-220, ISSN 0732-0582

Brostjan, C., Sobanov, Y., Glienke, J., Hayer, S., Lehrach, H., Francis, F. & Hofer, E. (2000). The NKG2 natural killer cell receptor family: comparative analysis of promoter sequences. *Genes Immun*, Vol.6, No.8, pp. 504-508, ISSN 1466-4879

Brivanlou, A. H. & Darnell, J. E., Jr. (2002). Signal transduction and the control of gene expression. *Science*, Vol.295, No.5556, pp. 813-818, ISSN 0036-8075

Bird, A. (2002). DNA methylation patterns and epigenetic memory. *Genes Dev*, Vol.16, No.1, pp. 6-21, ISSN 1549-5477

Bhalla, K. N. (2005). Epigenetic and chromatin modifiers as targeted therapy of hematologic malignancies. *J Clin Oncol*, Vol.23, No.17, pp. 3971-3993, ISSN 0732-183X

Beckett, D. (2009). Regulating transcription regulators via allostery and flexibility. Proc Natl Acad Sci U S A , Vol.106, No.52, pp. 22035-22036, ISSN 0027-8424 Campoli, M., Ferrone, S., Zea, A. H., Rodriguez, P. C. & Ochoa, A. C. (2005). Mechanisms of tumor evasion. *Cancer Treat Res*, Vol.123, pp. 61-88, ISSN 0927-3042

Colonna, M., Borsellino, G., Falco, M., Ferrara, G. B. & Strominger, J. L. (1993). HLA-C is the inhibitory ligand that determines dominant resistance to lysis by NK1- and NK2-specific natural killer cells. *Proc Natl Acad Sci U S A* , Vol.90, No.24, pp. 12000-12004, ISSN 0027-8424

Chan, H. W., Kurago, Z. B., Stewart, C. A., Wilson, M. J., Martin, M. P., Mace, B. E., Carrington, M., Trowsdale, J. & Lutz, C. T. (2003). DNA methylation maintains allele-specific KIR gene expression in human natural killer cells. *J Exp Med*, Vol.197, No.2, pp. 245-255, ISSN 0022-1007

Chan, H. W., Miller, J. S., Moore, M. B. & Lutz, C. T. (2005). Epigenetic control of highly homologous killer Ig-like receptor gene alleles. *J Immunol*, Vol.175, No.9, pp. 5966-5974, ISSN 0022-1767

Chang, C. C. & Ferrone, S. (2006). NK cell activating ligands on human malignant cells: molecular and functional defects and potential clinical relevance. *Semin Cancer Biol*, Vol.16, No.3, pp. 359-393, ISSN 1044-579X

Campoli, M. & Ferrone, S. (2008). HLA antigen changes in malignant cells: epigenetic mechanisms and biologic significance. *Oncogene*, Vol.27, No.45, pp. 5869-5885, ISSN 0950-9232

Cichocki, F., Hanson, R. J., Lenvik, T., Pitt, M., McCullar, V., Li, H., Anderson, S. K. & Miller, J. S. (2009). The transcription factor c-Myc enhances KIR gene transcription through direct binding to an upstream distal promoter element. *Blood*, Vol.113, No.14, pp. 3245-3253, ISSN 0006-4971

Dohring, C., Scheidegger, D., Samaridis, J., Cella, M. & Colonna, M. (1996). A human killer inhibitory receptor specific for HLA-A1,2. *J Immunol*, Vol.156, No.9, pp. 3098-3101, ISSN 0022-1767

Derre, L., Corvaisier, M., Pandolfino, M. C., Diez, E., Jotereau, F. & Gervois, N. (2002). Expression of CD94/NKG2-A on human T lymphocytes is induced by IL-12: implications for adoptive immunotherapy. *J Immunol*, Vol.168, No.10, pp. 4864-4870, ISSN 0022-1767

Dunn, G. P., Bruce, A. T., Ikeda, H., Old, L. J. & Schreiber, R. D. (2002). Cancer immunoediting: from immunosurveillance to tumor escape. *Nat Immunol*, Vol.3, No.11, pp. 991-998, ISSN 1529-2908

Dasgupta, S., Bhattacharya-Chatterjee, M., O'Malley, B. W., Jr. & Chatterjee, S. K. (2005). Inhibition of NK cell activity through TGF-beta 1 by down-regulation of NKG2D in a murine model of head and neck cancer. *J Immunol*, Vol.175, No.8, pp. 5541-5550, ISSN 0022-1767

Dowell, R. D. (2010). Transcription factor binding variation in the evolution of gene regulation. *Trends Genet*, Vol.26, No.11, pp. 468-475, ISSN 0168-9525

Engel, P., Eck, M. J. & Terhorst, C. (2003). The SAP and SLAM families in immune responses and X-linked lymphoproliferative disease. *Nat Rev Immunol,* Vol.3, No.10, pp. 813-821, ISSN 0732-0582

Fry, C. J. & Peterson, C. L. (2002). Transcription. Unlocking the gates to gene expression. *Science*, Vol.295, No.5561, pp. 1847-1848, ISSN 0036-8075

Feng, S., Jacobsen, S. E. & Reik, W. (2010). Epigenetic reprogramming in plant and animal development.*Science*, Vol. 330, No. 6004, pp. 622-627, ISSN 0036-8075

Fernandez-Morera, J. L., Calvanese, V., Rodriguez-Rodero, S., Menendez-Torre, E. & Fraga, M. F. (2010). Epigenetic regulation of the immune system in health and disease. *Tissue Antigens*, Vol.76, No.6, pp. 431-439, ISSN 0001-2815

Furumatsu, T. & Ozaki, T. (2010). Epigenetic regulation in chondrogenesis. *Acta Med Okayama,* Vol. 64, No.3, pp. 155-161, ISSN 0386-300X

Glienke, J., Sobanov, Y., Brostjan, C., Steffens, C., Nguyen, C., Lehrach, H., Hofer, E. & Francis, F. (1998). The genomic organization of NKG2C, E, F, and D receptor genes in the human natural killer gene complex. *Immunogenetics*, Vol.48, No.3, pp. 163-173, ISSN 0093-7711

Gao, X. N., Lin, J., Wang, L. L. & Yu, L. (2009). Demethylating treatment suppresses natural killer cell cytolytic activity. *Mol Immuno*l, Vol.46, No.10, pp. 2064-2070, ISSN 1672-7681

Hofmeister, V. & Weiss, E. H. (2003). HLA-G modulates immune responses by diverse receptor interactions. Semin Cancer Biol , Vol.13, No.5, pp. 317-323, ISSN 1044-579X

Karin, M. (1990). Too many transcription factors: positive and negative interactions. *New Biol*, Vol.2, No.2, pp. 126-131, ISSN 0090-0028

Kim, J. Y., Son, Y. O., Park, S. W., Bae, J. H., Chung, J. S., Kim, H. H., Chung, B. S., Kim, S. H. & Kang, C. D. (2006). Increase of NKG2D ligands and sensitivity to NK cell-mediated cytotoxicity of tumor cells by heat shock and ionizing radiation. *Exp Mol Med,* Vol.38, No.5, pp. 474-484, ISSN 1226-3613

Kisliouk, T., Ziv, M. & Meiri, N. (2010). Epigenetic control of translation regulation: alterations in histone H3 lysine 9 post-translation modifications are correlated with the expression of the translation initiation factor 2B (Eif2b5) during thermal control establishment. *Dev Neurobiol*, Vol.70, No.2, pp. 100-113, ISSN 1064-0517

Krukowski, K., Eddy, J., Kosik, K. L., Konley, T., Janusek, L. W. & Mathews, H. L. (2011). Glucocorticoid dysregulation of natural killer cell function through epigenetic modification. *Brain Behav Immun*, Vol.25, No.2, pp. 239-249, ISSN 0889-1591

Lanier, L. L. (1998). NK cell receptors. Annu Rev Immunol, Vol.16, No.3, pp. 359-393, ISSN 0732-0582

Lanier, L. L. (2001). On guard--activating NK cell receptors. *Nat Immunol*, Vol.2, No.1, pp. 23-27, ISSN 1529-2908

Lieto, L. D., Borrego, F., You, C. H. & Coligan, J. E. (2003). Human CD94 gene expression: dual promoters differing in responsiveness to IL-2 or IL-15. *J Immunol*, Vol.171, No.3, pp. 5277-5286, ISSN 0022-1767

Lanier, L. L. (2005). "NK cell recognition. *Annu Rev Immunol*, Vol.23, pp. 225-274, ISSN 0732-0582

Lopez-Soto, A., Quinones-Lombrana, A., Lopez-Arbesu, R., Lopez-Larrea, C. & Gonzalez, S. (2006). Transcriptional regulation of ULBP1, a human ligand of the NKG2D receptor.*J Biol Chem*, Vol.281, No.41, pp. 30419-30430, ISSN 0021-9258

Lund, P., Weisshaupt, K., Mikeska, T., Jammas, D., Chen, X., Kuban, R. J., Ungethum, U., Krapfenbauer, U., Herzel, H. P., Schafer, R., Walter, J. & Sers, C. (2006). Oncogenic HRAS suppresses clusterin expression through promoter hypermethylation. *Oncogene*, Vol.25, No.35, pp.4890-4903, ISSN 0950-9232

Li, G., Weyand, C. M. & Goronzy, J. J. (2008). Epigenetic mechanisms of age-dependent KIR2DL4 expression in T cells. *J Leukoc Biol*, Vol.84, No.3, pp. 824-834, ISSN 0741-5400

Liu, Y., Kuick, R., Hanash, S. & Richardson, B. (2009). DNA methylation inhibition increases T cell KIR expression through effects on both promoter methylation and transcription factors. *Clin Immunol*, Vol.130, No.2, pp. 213-224, ISSN 1521-6616

Lopez-Soto, A., Folgueras, A. R., Seto, E. & Gonzalez, S. (2009). HDAC3 represses the expression of NKG2D ligands ULBPs in epithelial tumour cells: potential implications for the immunosurveillance of cancer. *Oncogene*, Vol. 28, No.25, pp. 2370-2382, ISSN 0950-9232

Law, J. A. & Jacobsen, S. E. (2010). Establishing, maintaining and modifying DNA methylation patterns in plants and animals. *Nat Rev Genet*, Vol.11, No.3, pp. 204-220, ISSN 1471-0056

Mitchell, P. J. & Tjian, R. (1989). Transcriptional regulation in mammalian cells by sequence-specific DNA binding proteins.*Science*, Vol.245, No.4916, pp. 371-378, ISSN 0036-8075

Mingari, M. C., Ponte, M., Bertone, S., Schiavetti, F., Vitale, C., Bellomo, R., Moretta, A. & Moretta, L. (1998). HLA class I-specific inhibitory receptors in human T lymphocytes: interleukin 15-induced expression of CD94/NKG2A in superantigen- or alloantigen-activated CD8+ T cells. *Proc Natl Acad Sci U S A*, Vol.95, No.3, pp. 1172-1177, ISSN 0027-8424

Martin, A. M., Freitas, E. M., Witt, C. S. & Christiansen, F. T. (2000). The genomic organization and evolution of the natural killer immunoglobulin-like receptor (KIR) gene cluster. *Immunogenetics*, Vol.51, No. 4-5, pp. 268-280, ISSN 0093-7711

Morra, M., Howie, D., Grande, M. S., Sayos, J., Wang, N., Wu, C., Engel, P. & Terhorst, C. (2001). X-linked lymphoproliferative disease: a progressive immunodeficiency. *Annu Rev Immunol*, Vol.119, pp. 657-682, ISSN 0732-0582

McQueen, K. L. & Parham, P. (2002). Variable receptors controlling activation and inhibition of NK cells. *Curr Opin Immunol*, Vol.14, No.5, pp. 615-621, ISSN 0952-7915

Moreau, P., Mouillot, G., Rousseau, P., Marcou, C., Dausset, J. & Carosella, E. D. (2003). HLA-G gene repression is reversed by demethylation. *Proc Natl Acad Sci U S A*, Vol.100, No.3, pp. 1191-1196, ISSN 0027-8424

Molinero, L. L., Fuertes, M. B., Girart, M. V., Fainboim, L., Rabinovich, G. A., Costas, M. A. & Zwirner, N. W. (2004). NF-kappa B regulates expression of the MHC class I-related chain A gene in activated T lymphocytes. *J Immunol,* Vol.173, No.9, pp. 5583-5590, ISSN0022-1767

Moretta, L., Bottino, C., Pende, D., Castriconi, R., Mingari, M. C. & Moretta, A. (2006). Surface NK receptors and their ligands on tumor cells. *Semin Immunol,* Vol.18, No.3, pp. 151-158, ISSN 1044-5323

Menendez, L., Walker, L. D., Matyunina, L. V., Totten, K. A., Benigno, B. B. & McDonald, J. F. (2008). Epigenetic changes within the promoter region of the HLA-G gene in ovarian tumors. *Mol Cancer,* Vol.7, pp. 43, ISSN 1476-4598

Nie, Y., Yang, G., Song, Y., Zhao, X., So, C., Liao, J., Wang, L. D. & Yang, C. S. (2001). DNA hypermethylation is a mechanism for loss of expression of the HLA class I genes in human esophageal squamous cell carcinomas. *Carcinogenesis,* Vol.22, No.10, pp. 1615-1623, ISSN 0143-3334

Polakova, K., Bandzuchova, E., Sabty, F. A., Mistrik, M., Demitrovicova, L. & Russ, G. (2009a). Activation of HLA-G expression by 5-aza-2 - deoxycytidine in malignant hematopoetic cells isolated from leukemia patients. *Neoplasma,* Vol.56, No.6, pp. 514-520, ISSN 0028- 2685

Polakova, K., Bandzuchova, E., Kuba, D. & Russ, G. (2009b). Demethylating agent 5-aza-2'-deoxycytidine activates HLA-G expression in human leukemia cell lines. *Leuk Res,* Vol.33, No.4, pp. 518-524, ISSN 0145-2126

Pan, Y., Tsai, C. J., Ma, B. & Nussinov, R. (2010). Mechanisms of transcription factor selectivity.*Trends Genet,* Vol.26, No.2, pp. 75-83, ISSN 0168-9525

Raulet, D. H., Vance, R. E. & McMahon, C. W. (2001). Regulation of the natural killer cell receptor repertoire. *Annu Rev Immunol,* Vol.19, pp.291-330, ISSN 0732-0582

Romero, P., Ortega, C., Palma, A., Molina, I. J., Pena, J. & Santamaria, M. (2001). Expression of CD94 and NKG2 molecules on human CD4(+) T cells in response to CD3-mediated stimulation. *J Leukoc Biol,* Vol.70, No.2, pp. 219-224, ISSN 0741-5400

Ravetch, J. V. & Lanier, L. L. (2000). Immune inhibitory receptors. *Science,* Vol.290, No.5489, pp. 84-89, ISSN 0036-8075

Raulet, D. H. (2003). Roles of the NKG2D immunoreceptor and its ligands. *Annu Rev Immunol,* Vol.3, No.10, pp.781-790, ISSN 0732-0582

Rolle, A., Mousavi-Jazi, M., Eriksson, M., Odeberg, J., Soderberg-Naucler, C., Cosman, D., Karre, K. & Cerboni, C. (2003). Effects of human cytomegalovirus infection on ligands for the activating NKG2D receptor of NK cells: up-regulation of UL16-binding protein (ULBP)1 and ULBP2 is counteracted by the viral UL16 protein. *J Immunol,* Vol.171, No.2, pp. 902-908, ISSN 0022-1767

Sobanov, Y., Glienke, J., Brostjan, C., Lehrach, H., Francis, F. & Hofer, E. (1999). Linkage of the NKG2 and CD94 receptor genes to D12S77 in the human natural killer gene complex. *Immunogenetics,* Vol.49, No.2, pp. 99-105, ISSN 1744-313X

Strahl, B. D. & Allis, C. D. (2000). The language of covalent histone modifications. *Nature,* Vol. 403, No. 6765, pp. 41-45, ISSN 0028-0836

Sutherland, C. L., Chalupny, N. J. & Cosman, D. (2001). The UL16-binding proteins, a novel family of MHC class I-related ligands for NKG2D, activate natural killer cell functions. *Immunol Rev,* Vol.181, No.3, pp. 185-192, ISSN 0105-2896

Santourlidis, S., Trompeter, H. I., Weinhold, S., Eisermann, B., Meyer, K. L., Wernet, P. & Uhrberg, M. (2002). Crucial role of DNA methylation in determination of clonally distributed killer cell Ig-like receptor expression patterns in NK cells. *J Immunol*, Vol.169, No.8, pp. 4253-4261, ISSN 0022-1767

Sidorenko, S. P. & Clark, E. A. (2003). The dual-function CD150 receptor subfamily: the viral attraction. *Nat Immunol*, Vol.4, No.1, pp. 19-24, ISSN 1529-2908

Su, R. C., Brown, K. E., Saaber, S., Fisher, A. G., Merkenschlager, M. & Smale, S. T. (2004). Dynamic assembly of silent chromatin during thymocyte maturation." *Nat Genet*, Vol.36, No.5, pp. 502-506, ISSN 1061-4036

Skov, S., Pedersen, M. T., Andresen, L., Straten, P. T., Woetmann, A. & Odum, N. (2005). Cancer cells become susceptible to natural killer cell killing after exposure to histone deacetylase inhibitors due to glycogen synthase kinase-3-dependent expression of MHC class I-related chain A and B. *Cancer Res*, Vol.65, No.23, pp. 11136-11145, ISSN 1538-7445

Szyf, M. (2005). DNA methylation and demethylation as targets for anticancer therapy. *Biochemistry (Mosc)* , Vol.70, No.5, pp. 533-549, ISSN 0006-2979

Santourlidis, S., Graffmann, N., Christ, J. & Uhrberg, M. (2008). Lineage-specific transition of histone signatures in the killer cell Ig-like receptor locus from hematopoietic progenitor to NK cells. *J Immunol*, Vol.180, No.1, pp. 418-425, ISSN0022-1767

Samarakoon, A., Chu, H. & Malarkannan, S. (2009). Murine NKG2D ligands: "double, double toil and trouble". *Mol Immunol*, Vol.46, No.6, pp. 1011-1019, ISSN 1672-7681

Sers, C., Kuner, R., Falk, C. S., Lund, P., Sueltmann, H., Braun, M., Buness, A., Ruschhaupt, M., Conrad, J., Mang-Fatehi, S., Stelniec, I., Krapfenbauer, U., Poustka, A. & Schafer, R. (2009). Down-regulation of HLA Class I and NKG2D ligands through a concerted action of MAPK and DNA methyltransferases in colorectal cancer cells." *Int J Cancer*, Vol.125, No.7, pp. 1626-1639, ISSN 1097-0215

Stein, G. S., Stein, J. L., Van Wijnen, A. J., Lian, J. B., Montecino, M., Croce, C. M., Choi, J. Y., Ali, S. A., Pande, S., Hassan, M. Q., Zaidi, S. K. and Young, D. W. (2010). Transcription factor-mediated epigenetic regulation of cell growth and phenotype for biological control and cancer. *Adv Enzyme Regul*, Vol.50, No.1, pp. 160-167, ISSN 0065-2571

Takei, F., McQueen, K. L., Maeda, M., Wilhelm, B. T., Lohwasser, S., Lian, R. H. & Mager, D. L. (2001). Ly49 and CD94/NKG2: developmentally regulated expression and evolution. *Immunol Rev*, Vol.181, , pp. 90-103, ISSN 0105-2896

Trompeter, H. I., Gomez-Lozano, N., Santourlidis, S., Eisermann, B., Wernet, P., Vilches, C. & Uhrberg, M. (2005). Three structurally and functionally divergent kinds of promoters regulate expression of clonally distributed killer cell Ig-like receptors (KIR), of KIR2DL4, and of KIR3DL3. *J Immunol*, Vol.174, No.7, pp. 4135-4143, ISSN 0022-1767

Uhrberg, M., Valiante, N. M., Shum, B. P., Shilling, H. G., Lienert-Weidenbach, K., Corliss, B., Tyan, D., Lanier, L. L. & Parham, P. (1997). Human diversity in killer cell inhibitory receptor genes. *Immunity*, Vol.7, No.6, pp. 753-763, ISSN1074-7613

Valiante, N. M., Lienert, K., Shilling, H. G., Smits, B. J. & Parham, P. (1997). Killer cell receptors: keeping pace with MHC class I evolution. *Immunol Rev*, Vol.155, pp. 155-164, ISSN 0105-2896

Vilches, C., Gardiner, C. M. & Parham, P. (2000). Gene structure and promoter variation of expressed and nonexpressed variants of the KIR2DL5 gene. *J Immunol*, Vol.165, No.11, pp. 6416-6421, ISSN 0022-1767

Vilches, C. & Parham, P. (2002). KIR: diverse, rapidly evolving receptors of innate and adaptive immunity. *Annu Rev Immunol*, Vol.20, pp. 217-251, ISSN 0732-0582

van Nimwegen, E. (2003). Scaling laws in the functional content of genomes. *Trends Genet* , Vol.19, No.9, pp. 479-484, ISSN 0168-9525

van Bergen, J., Thompson, A., van der Slik, A., Ottenhoff, T. H., Gussekloo, J. & Koning, F. (2004). Phenotypic and functional characterization of CD4 T cells expressing killer Ig-like receptors. *J Immunol*, Vol.173, No.11, pp. 6719-6726, ISSN 0022-1767

Villar-Garea, A. & Esteller, M. (2004). Histone deacetylase inhibitors: understanding a new wave of anticancer agents. *Int J Cancer*, Vol.112, No.2, pp. 171-178, ISSN 1097-0215

Venkataraman, G. M., Suciu, D., Groh, V., Boss, J. M. & Spies, T. (2007). Promoter region architecture and transcriptional regulation of the genes for the MHC class I-related chain A and B ligands of NKG2D. *J Immunol*, Vol.178, No.2, pp. 961-969, ISSN 0022-1767

Wilson, M. J., Torkar, M., Haude, A., Milne, S., Jones, T., Sheer, D., Beck, S. & Trowsdale, J. (2000). Plasticity in the organization and sequences of human KIR/ILT gene families. *Proc Natl Acad Sci U S A*, Vol.97, No.9, pp. 4778-4783, ISSN 0027-8424

Wajapeyee, N. & Somasundaram, K. (2003). Cell cycle arrest and apoptosis induction by activator protein 2alpha (AP-2alpha) and the role of p53 and p21WAF1/CIP1 in AP-2alpha-mediated growth inhibition. *J Biol Chem*, Vol.278, No.52, pp. 52093-52101, ISSN 0021-9258

Wilhelm, B. T., Landry, J. R., Takei, F. & Mager, D. L. (2003). Transcriptional control of murine CD94 gene: differential usage of dual promoters by lymphoid cell types. *J Immunol,* Vol.171, No.8, pp. 4219-4226, ISSN 0022-1767

Wang, Y., Fischle, W., Cheung, W., Jacobs, S., Khorasanizadeh, S. & Allis, C. D. (2004). Beyond the double helix: writing and reading the histone code. *Novartis Found Symp,* Vol.259, pp. 3-17, ISSN 1528-2511

Wu, P., Wei, H., Zhang, C., Zhang, J. & Tian, Z. (2005). Regulation of NK cell activation by stimulatory and inhibitory receptors in tumor escape from innate immunity. *Front Biosci,* Vol.10, pp. 3132-3142, ISSN 1093-9946

Yan, W. H., Lin, A. F., Chang, C. C. & Ferrone, S. (2005). Induction of HLA-G expression in a melanoma cell line OCM-1A following the treatment with 5-aza-2'-deoxycytidine. *Cell Res*, Vol.15, No.7, pp. 523-531, ISSN 1001-0602

Ye, Q., Shen, Y., Wang, X., Yang, J., Miao, F., Shen, C. & Zhang, J. (2010). Hypermethylation of HLA class I gene is associated with HLA class I down-regulation in human gastric cancer. *Tissue Antigens*, Vol.75, No.1, pp. 30-39, ISSN 0001-2815

Zeng, Y. X., Somasundaram, K. & el-Deiry, W. S. (1997). AP2 inhibits cancer cell growth and activates p21WAF1/CIP1 expression. *Nat Genet*, Vol.15, No.1, pp. 78-82, ISSN 1061-4036

Zhang, C., Zhang, J., Sun, R., Feng, J., Wei, H. & Tian, Z. (2005). Opposing effect of IFNgamma and IFNalpha on expression of NKG2 receptors: negative regulation of IFNgamma on NK cells. *Int Immunopharmacol*, Vol.5, No.6, pp. 1057-1067, ISSN 1567- 5769

Zhang, C., Wang, Y., Zhou, Z., Zhang, J. & Tian, Z. (2009). Sodium butyrate upregulates expression of NKG2D ligand MICA/B in HeLa and HepG2 cell lines and increases their susceptibility to NK lysis. *Cancer Immunol Immunother*, Vol.58, No.8, pp. 1275-1285, ISSN 0340-7004

# Part 5

# Cancer Diagnostic Technologies

21

# Non-Invasive Devices for Early Detection of Breast Tissue Oncological Abnormalities Using Microwave Radio Thermometry

Tahir H. Shah, Elias Siores and Chronis Daskalakis
*Institute of Materials Research and Innovation (IMRI),*
*University of Bolton*
*United Kingdom*

## 1. Introduction

Breast cancer is the most common cancer in women worldwide, comprising 16% of all female cancers and is the leading cause of cancer-related deaths in women ages 40-55. Each year in the U.S.A. over 180,000 women are diagnosed with breast cancer and 46,000 women die of this disease. One in twelve women in the United Kingdom develops breast cancer and the annual death toll stands at around 14,000. Over 33,000 new cases are being monitored year on year basis in the UK. In all, 10%-11% of all women can expect to be affected by breast cancer at some time during their lives. The causes of most breast cancers are not yet fully understood. Sixty years ago, MacDonald proposed that the biological behaviour of a neoplasm is established during its preclinical growth phase (MacDonald, 1951). This view is supported by some data on the behaviour of metastatic lesions such as poor cytological differentiation, lymphatic permeation, blood vessel invasion and the invasion of the surrounding soft tissue by the tumour (Nealon et al, 1979). Screening and early diagnosis are currently the most effective ways to reduce mortality from this disease. Early diagnosis and treatment are the keys to surviving breast cancer. Breast cancer survival rates vary greatly worldwide, ranging from over 80% in North America, Sweden and Japan to around 60% in middle-income countries and below 40% in low-income countries. It is believed that the low survival rates in less developed countries are mainly due to the lack of early detection programmes, resulting in a high proportion of women presenting with late-stage disease, as well as by the lack of adequate diagnosis and treatment facilities. Studies from the American National Cancer Institute show that 96 percent of women whose breast cancer is detected early live five or more years after treatment. Early diagnosis remains an important detection strategy, particularly in low- and middle-income countries where the disease is diagnosed in late stages and resources are very limited. There is some evidence that this strategy can produce "down staging" of the disease to stages that are more amenable to less aggressive treatment. Therefore, thousands of lives and considerable healthcare costs could be saved each year with treatment if early symptoms of breast cancer are detected. Taking full advantage of early diagnosis and treatment means that screening technology should have the characteristics that have high detection success rate, speed of procedure, comfort to the subject and very low health risk.

The principal aim of early breast cancer detection is to identify the disease at a more curable stage and thus improve the prognosis and other vital clinical outcomes. Currently breast cancer detection is a three part procedure. The first part is identification of the abnormality in the breast tissue either by physical examination or by an imaging technique. Secondly, the abnormality is diagnosed as a benign or a malignant condition by using additional diagnostic methods or by biopsy and microscopic examination of the tissue morphology. The third part is concerned with biochemical characterisation of the malignant tissue in order to stage the cancer according to the size of the tumour and extent of invasion and metastasis. Of particular importance is the ability to clearly distinguish between malignant and benign tumours and early detection. This then determines the prognosis and appropriate course of treatment. A review of the published literature shows that all current breast cancer detection techniques have limited capability and surgery is often required to establish the true nature of the tumour.

Currently, the frontline strategies for breast cancer detection still depend essentially on clinical and self-examination and mammograms. The limitations of mammography, with its reported sensitivity rate often below 70% are recognized (Sickles, 1984) and the proposed value of self-breast examination is being queried (Thomas et al, 1997). Mammography is accepted as the most reliable and cost-effective imaging technique, however, its contribution continues to be challenged with persistent false-negative results - ranging up to 30% (Moskowitz, 1983 & Elmore et al, 1884). However, most of the research and development activity related to cancer detection and diagnosis is focussed on the analysis of the existing condition and is costly, time-consuming and requires trained personnel to use the equipment. Furthermore, the incidence of the earliest form of breast cancer, Ductal Carcinoma in Situ (DCIS), has increased significantly over the last few years in the United States and this seems to be directly related to successful screening programmes. This clearly shows that there is a need and scope for developing early breast cancer detection techniques that are simple, quick and can be used by women by themselves.

In this chapter a review of some of the most promising techniques that are being developed for breast cancer detection is presented. A comparison of the various breast cancer detection techniques that are in the developmental stages with the established procedures has been carried out and a state-of-the-art in all the areas is briefly described and the concept of a wearable breast cancer detection device - the 'smart bra'- is also discussed. Particular emphasis has been placed on the non-invasive thermometry based methodologies for early detection of the oncological condition. When infrared thermography was first introduced in medicine, the instrumentation was not sensitive enough to detect the subtle changes in temperature that are involved in diseases such as breast cancer. However, more recently the sensitivity of infrared instrumentation has greatly improved and the IR thermography imaging is being developed and used to monitor the health of the breast and detection of cancerous tumours. Recent literature shows that the technique has the ability to detect tumours that are 3cm in size and are located deeper than 7 cm from the skin surface and tumours smaller than 0.5 cm can be detected if they are close to the surface of the skin. Non-invasive techniques based on profiling of the breast tissue using microwave radiometry are also being developed and investigated as early warning systems for breast cancer. These techniques involve the measurement of the passive electromagnetic thermal radiation emitted from human body using suitable combination of microwave antenna internal temperature sensor and infrared surface temperature sensor, with an appropriate configuration to determine the temperature profile of the concerned area of the body.

Microwave radiometry principles can be employed to obtain sensor information from subcutaneous tissues up to a few centimetres in depth. The device based on these principles can provide an early breast cancer detection/warning technique that is simple, quick and may also be used for diagnosis of other types of cancers such as prostate cancer in men.
The evidence indicates that screening mammography, when correctly performed at recommended intervals and combined with appropriate interventions, can reduce, but not eliminate, breast cancer mortality. This conclusion is based on evidence of efficacy in clinical trials and evidence of effectiveness in the general population. The "ideal" breast cancer screening tool has not yet been developed. All of the tests available for the screening and diagnosis of breast cancer have different strengths and limitations. The ideal test would combine the following characteristics:

- The test should present a low risk of harm from screening
- The test should have high degrees of specificity and sensitivity (low rates of false-positive and false-negative results).
- The test results should have uniform high quality and repeatability.
- Interpretation of test results should be straightforward (objective).
- The test should be simple to perform.
- The test should be non-invasive.
- The test should be able to detect breast cancer at a stage that is curable with available treatments.
- The test should have the ability to distinguish life-threatening lesions from those that are not likely to progress.
- The test should be cost-effective (usually considered <$50,000 per quality-adjusted life year saved).
- The test should be widely available.
- The test should be acceptable to women.

Each modality has different strengths and limitations therefore it seems to be feasible to adopt a multi modality approach in order to achieve the optimum methodology for the detection and diagnosis of the breast tissue oncological abnormalities.

### 1.1 Anatomy and physiology of female breast

It is important to consider the physiology of the breast, as the changes seen in the breast during a woman's life will have an effect on the properties of the tissues. The female breast is a complex and sensitive organ, which is composed of a mass of glandular, fatty, and fibrous tissues positioned over the pectoral muscles of the chest wall and attached to the chest wall by fibrous strands called Cooper's ligaments (Figure 1). A layer of fatty tissue surrounds the breast glands and extends throughout the breast. The fatty tissue gives the breast a soft consistency. The glandular tissues of the breast house the lobules and the ducts. The female breast has a network of arteries and capillaries that carry oxygen- and nutrient-rich blood to the breasts. The axillary artery extends from the armpit and supplies blood to the outer half of the breast. The internal mammary artery, which extends down from the neck, supplies blood to the inner part of the breast. The breast also contains lymph vessels. The lymphatic system is part of the immune system and is composed of blood vessels, lymph ducts and lymph nodes. Clusters of lymph nodes are located under the arm, above the collarbone, behind the breastbone and in various other parts of the body.

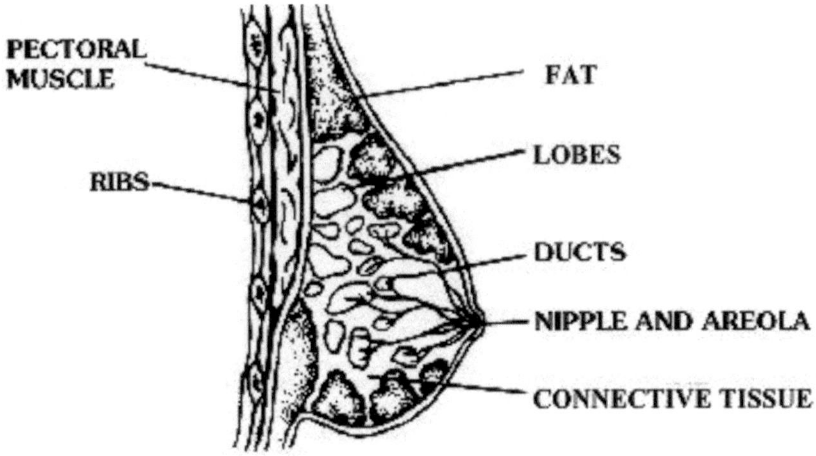


Fig. 1. The anatomical structure of the female breast

The shape and appearance of female breast undergo a number of changes as a woman ages. In young women, the breast skin stretches and expands as the breasts grow, creating a rounded appearance. Young women tend to have denser breasts, due to the presence of more glandular tissue, than older women. The denser breasts lead to poorer contrast between healthy and diseased tissue in x-ray mammography. However the occurrence of breast cancer in younger women is low, with 80 % of breast cancers occurring in women over the age of 50. The growth of breast tissue is mainly influenced by the relative concentrations of progesterone and oestrogen in the body. During each menstrual cycle, breast tissue tends to swell due to variation in the oestrogen and progesterone levels. The milk glands and ducts enlarge resulting in retention of water by the breast. During menstruation, breasts may temporarily appear swollen and this can give rise to breast pain, tenderness, or they may feel lumpy. At menopause, a woman's body stops producing oestrogen and progesterone, which causes a variety of symptoms in many women including hot flushes, night sweats, mood changes and vaginal dryness. During this period breasts also undergo many changes, such as mentioned earlier for the menstrual cycle, and sometimes appearance of cysts may be observed. The glandular tissue tends to shrink after menopause and is replaced with fatty tissue. The breasts also tend to increase in size and droop because the fibrous tissue loses its strength. The breasts become less dense after menopause, which makes the detection of breast cancer often easier in older women. A woman's risk of breast cancer increases with age thus all women are recommended for breast cancer screening at regular interval beyond the age of 40.

### 1.2 Main types of breast cancer

Treatment of cancer depends on the type and stage of the cancer along with other issues such as the individual circumstances of the patient. Mostly breast cancer develops in the glandular tissue and is classified as adenocarcinoma, which is a cancer of the epithelium that originates in the glandular tissue. The common types of breast cancers are:

*Carcinoma in situ:* This term is used for early stage cancer, when it is confined to the place where it started. In breast cancer, it means that the cancer is confined to the ducts or the lobules, depending on where it started. It has not gone into the fatty tissues in the breast nor spread to other organs in the body.

*Ductal carcinoma in situ (DCIS):* This is the most common type of non-invasive breast cancer. DCIS means that the cancer is confined to the ducts. It has not spread through the walls of the ducts into the fatty tissue of the breast. Over 70% of breast cancers are ductal carcinomas, which are associated with the milk ducts. Nearly all women with cancer at this stage can be cured.

*Infiltrating (invasive) ductal carcinoma (IDC):* This type of cancer starts in a duct and breaks through the wall of the duct, and invades the fatty tissue of the breast (Figure 2), then spreading to other parts of the body. IDC is the most common type of breast cancer. It accounts for about 80% of invasive breast cancers.

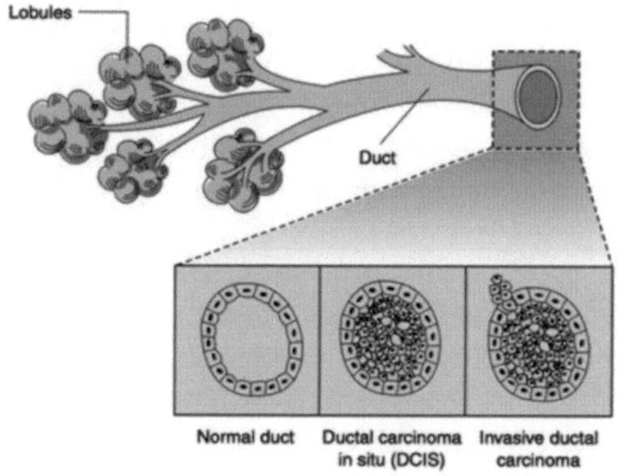


Fig. 2. Growth of ductal carcinoma

Lobular carcinoma in situ (LCIS): This condition begins in the milk-making glands but does not go through the wall of the lobules. Although not a true cancer, having LCIS increases a woman's risk of getting cancer later. For this reason, it is important that women with LCIS follow the screening guidelines for breast cancer. 10% - 15% are lobular carcinomas associated with the lobes, and the rest are relatively rare forms of cancer such as of the connective tissue.

*Infiltrating (invasive) lobular carcinoma (ILC):* This type of cancer starts in the lobules and can spread to other parts of the body (Figure 3). About 10% of invasive breast cancers are of this type.

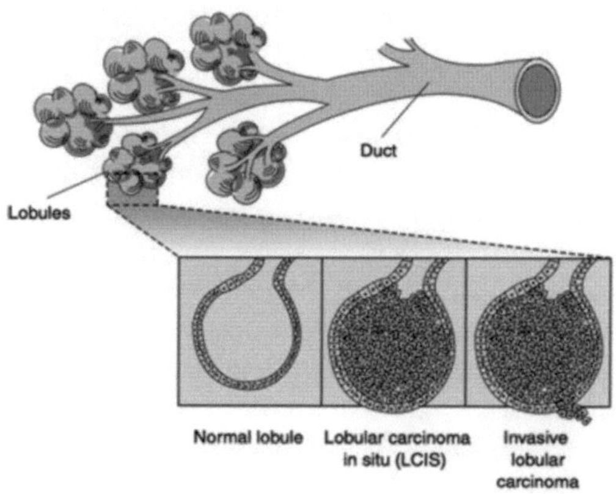


Fig. 3. Growth of lobular carcinoma

*Benign conditions:* There are many lesions and conditions that are non-cancerous but still affect the health of the breast and could be mistaken for cancer. These include fibroadenomas, cysts, mastalgia, breast calcifications, duct ectasia and periductal mastitis, fat necrosis, hyperplasia, intraductal papilloma, phyllodes tumour and sclerosing adenosis.

## 2. Current breast cancer detection modalities and their limitations

Breast is susceptible to a range of pathologic conditions. The most serious of these is breast cancer, which is widely recognised as the most common cancer in women. Other breast conditions include mastalgia, which is referred to a variety of conditions that cause breast pain, and benign lesions such as fibroadenomas and cysts. These conditions are not fatal but they are a source of undesirable symptoms and considerable anxiety for the patients. Improved methods for early detection and diagnosis of breast disease are essential to decrease mortality rates due to cancer. In addition a greater understanding of the physiology of the breast is needed to aid in the diagnosis of disease and in improving treatments.

The breast cancer detection is a three part procedure. The first part is the identification of the abnormality in the breast tissue either by physical examination or by an imaging technique. Secondly the abnormality is diagnosed as a benign or malignant condition by using additional diagnostic methods or by biopsy and microscopic examination of the tissue morphology. The third part is concerned with biochemical characterisation of the malignant tissue in order to stage the cancer according to the size of the tumour and extent of invasion and metastasis. This then determines the prognosis and appropriate course of treatment. The most commonly used imaging modalities are described in the following sections.

The main strategy of breast cancer detection is based on clinical examination and mammography. Mammography is considered to be the 'gold standard' test for breast cancer detection and diagnosis and is accepted as the most cost-effective imaging modality. The performance of a screening test is evaluated by three related measurements: sensitivity, specificity, and a positive predictive value. The sensitivity of a screening test is the proportion of people with the disease who test positive. Specificity is the proportion of people without the disease who test negative. The positive predictive value is the proportion of individuals with a positive screening test result who actually have the disease. In the development of optimum detection modality, there is often a trade-off between sensitivity and specificity, with an increase in one leading to a decrease in the other. The contribution of mammography continues to be challenged with persistent false-negative rates ranging up to 30%.The clinical examination has been challenged with reported sensitivity rates often below 65%. There is also variability in radiologists' interpretation of mammograms with decreasing sensitivity in younger patients and those on oestrogen replacement therapy. In addition, recent data suggests that denser and less informative mammography images are precisely those associated with an increased cancer risk (Boyd et al, 1995). It has also been suggested that mammography procedure cannot be performed by an inexperienced technician or radiologist. With the current emphasis on earlier detection, there is now renewed interest in the development of complimentary imaging techniques that can also exploit the metabolic, immunological, and vascular changes associated with early tumour growth. While promising, techniques such as Doppler ultrasound and MRI are associated with a number of disadvantages, which include the following:

- Duration of the test,

- Limited accessibility,
- Need of intravenous access,
- Patient discomfort,
- Restricted imaging area,
- Difficult interpretation
- Limited availability of the technology

These modalities are in fact more suited as the second-line options to pursue the already abnormal screening evaluations. This stepwise approach currently results in the non-recognition, and thus delayed utilization of any second-line technology in approximately 10% of established breast cancers (Moskowitz, 1995). This view is supported by another study of infrared screening of breast cancer [Keyserlignk & Ahlgren, 1998). A list of the established breast cancer detection modalities approved by FDA is given in Table 1.

| Modality | Description |
|---|---|
| Full-field digital mammography | Detector responds to X-ray exposure, sends electronic signal to computer to be digitized and processed. Separates detector and image display. |
| Computer-assisted detection | Computer programs to aid in identification of suspicious mammograms and classification as benign or malignant. |
| Ultrasound : Compound imaging and Three-dimensional ultrasound imaging | Uses high-frequency sound waves to generate an image. |
| Magnetic resonance imaging (MRI) | Makes use of the property of nuclear magnetic resonance (NMR) to image nuclei of atoms inside the body. Image generated by signals from excitation of nuclear particles in a magnetic field. Breast tumours show increased uptake of contrast agent. |
| Scintimammography | Image created with radioactive tracers, which concentrate more in cancer tissues than in normal tissues. |
| Positron emission tomography (PET) | Uses tracers such as labelled glucose to identify regions in the body with altered metabolic activity. |
| Infrared Thermography | Measures heat emitted by the body. Tumours can raise skin surface temperature, which is detected by infrared cameras. Dynamic area telethermometry detects changes in blood flow. |
| Electrical impedance imaging | Measures voltage at skin surface while passing small current through breast. Changes in cancerous tissue decrease impedance of tissue. |

Table 1. FDA approved modalities for breast cancer detection

## 2.1 X-ray mammography

X-ray mammography is the most common method of imaging the breast at present. The technique involves the breast being compressed between two plates with an x-ray film placed underneath and low energy x-rays are then passed through the breast and the images are recorded. The best contrast between soft tissues is achieved at low energies and hence these are used in x-ray mammography. The x-rays are produced by an electron beam irradiating either a tungsten or molybdenum target depending on the size of the breast to be imaged. At low energies, the transmission is low causing a high dose to the patient. Thus a compromise between contrast and dose is necessary. This problem is reduced by compression of the breast. The breast is compressed to between 2 and 8 cm enabling a high contrast whilst keeping the dose within an acceptable level. Contrast is dependent on the thickness of the breast and the difference in linear attenuation coefficient ($\mu$) between the tissue types. The value of $\mu$ is dependent on the atomic number of the material. Thus tissues with higher atomic numbers will produce a higher attenuation than others (e.g. microcalcifications).

The established sensitivity of mammography is higher than 91% (Brem et al 2003), which is greater than any other imaging modality for breast cancer detection. This is the main reason for the use of mammography in screening programmes. The reported specificity of the technique is quite variable and is considered to be in the region of 72% (Bone et al 1997). This means that nearly a quarter of the benign lesions are diagnosed as suspicious, which leads to unnecessary invasive procedures, biopsies, in order to establish the true nature of the lesion. Furthermore, the sensitivity of mammography for younger women is lower than that for older women. Younger women have denser breasts and less adipose tissue. Adipose tissue provides a greater contrast to calcifications than denser fibrous tissue and so mammography is more successful in older women.

Nearly one quarter of all invasive breast cancers are not detected by x-ray mammography in women aged between 40-49 years. However, the statistics for women above the age of 50 years are significantly better (1 in 10). Treatment of women with undetected invasive cancers, because of false-negative results, may be delayed. Many mammographic abnormalities may not be cancer, but will prompt additional testing and anxiety. Approximately 10 percent of all screening mammograms are read as abnormal. This will result in additional diagnostic tests such as diagnostic mammography, ultrasound, needle aspiration, core biopsy, or surgical biopsy. Given the lower incidence of breast cancer in 40- to 49-year-old women compared with that in older women, false-positive examinations are more common in younger women and the proportion of true-positive examinations increases with increasing age. There is concern that women having abnormal mammograms, both true-positive and false-positive, experience psychosocial stresses, including anxiety, fear, and inconvenience. There is the concern that experiencing a false-positive mammogram may affect subsequent willingness of the patient to undergo future screening mammography at ages when it is of greatest benefit.

The main advantages of x-ray mammography are that the technique has good resolution and microcalcifications can easily be observed. Furthermore, the relatively fast imaging time allows many women to be scanned in one screening session. The major drawbacks of the modality are the use of ionising radiation, which is potentially harmful for the patient and the operator, and interpreting mammograms can be difficult due to differences in the appearance of the normal breast for each woman. The sensitivity is high (91.4% (Brem et al, 2003) but is not 100% and also the specificity is relatively low for some types of tumours.

Particularly, the sensitivity is lower for women with dense breast tissue (e.g. younger women) and breast implants can affect the accuracy of mammography, as silicone implants are not transparent to X-rays. The disadvantages of compressing the breast are that it is, at best, uncomfortable and for many women with sensitive breasts it can be very painful. This limits the maximum time feasible for the imaging process. Also the spatial accuracy of the image can be distorted so that it is difficult to exactly locate an identified lesion.
The risk of radiation-induced breast cancer has long been a concern and has driven the efforts to reduce the radiation dose per examination. Radiation has been shown to cause breast cancer in women, and the risk is proportional to the dose. Especially the younger women are at a greater risk for breast cancer due to the exposure to radiation. Radiation related breast cancers occur at least 10 years after exposure. However, breast cancer as a result of the radiation dose associated with mammography has not been established. Radiation from yearly mammograms during ages 40-49 has been estimated as possibly causing one additional breast cancer death per 10,000 women.

### 2.2 Magnetic resonance imaging (MRI)

The principal imaging modality used for the detection of breast tissue abnormalities is x-ray mammography, which has a high sensitivity, but suffers from a relatively poor specificity for some tumours and breast types, leading to unnecessary biopsies. Thus there is a need for an imaging technique that can non-invasively distinguish between malignant and benign lesions. At the present, magnetic resonance imaging (MRI) and ultrasound (US) can provide additional diagnostic information for this purpose.
The theory of MRI is based on the fact that the nuclei of some atoms have a property known as spin. Such nuclei act like tiny current loops and consequently generate a magnetic field (or magnetic moment), along the spin axis. Under normal circumstances these moments have no fixed orientation so there is no overall magnetic field. When an external magnetic field is applied, the moments will align in certain directions. In the case of hydrogen nuclei, which are the most abundant nuclei in the human body, two discrete energy levels are created. An MRI detection system consists of a magnet, magnetic gradient coils, a radio frequency transmitter and receiver, and a computer that controls the acquisition of signals and computes the MR images obtained. When an atomic nucleus is exposed to a static magnetic field, it resonates when a varying electromagnetic field is applied at an appropriate frequency and an image is computed from the resonance signals.
The signal in MRI arises from the rotating magnetisation, but it decays due to two different relaxation processes. The first process is the spin-lattice relaxation. The second relaxation process is the spin-spin relaxation. During spin-spin relaxation, the detected signal decays over a period of time. However, the spins are also subject to inhomogeneities in the magnetic field causing the signal to decay faster than the natural time period. Part of the signal can be obtained due to the spin-echo effect. This involves the application of a further RF pulse which causes the spins to be flipped by 180°. This means that the phase-position of each spin has been inverted and so nuclei that were precessing faster are now behind spins that were precessing at a slower rate. At the echo time *TE*, the spins will catch each other up and a peak in the signal will be detected. An MRI exam of the breast typically takes between 30 and 60 minutes. Diffusion and perfusion MRI are relatively new procedures. Diffusion MRI measures the mobility of water protons whereas perfusion MRI measures the rate at which blood is delivered to tissue. Both of these factors vary in malignant tissues as compared with benign tissue and therefore can be used as indicators for cancer.

The injection of a contrast agent can enhance the ability of MRI to detect specific features or in the case of dynamic contrast-enhancement MRI the functionality of the tissue can be investigated. The contrast agents used are paramagnetic agents with gadolinium (Gd-DTPA) being the most common. The increased vascularity of tumours produces a preferential uptake of contrast agent and the technique can be used to improve their contrast from surrounding normal tissue. In dynamic contrast-enhancement MRI, scans are repeatedly acquired following the contrast injection and the dynamic nature of contrast uptake can be examined, which may improve the differentiation of benign and malignant disease.

The main advantages of MRI are that the modality is suitable for women with denser breasts and the technique is non-ionising. It is possible to take images in any orientation and determine multi-focal cancers. The technique can also show breast implants and ruptures. The disadvantages of MRI are that a contrast agent is required to provide adequate specificity and that it is immobile, expensive, and unsuitable for some women. The modality cannot image calcifications and can induce feelings of claustrophobia, and require long scan times in comparison to x-ray mammography.

### 2.3 Ultrasound

Ultrasound is defined as a frequency of sound above the threshold of human hearing (i.e. $>$ 20 kHz). The frequency range used in medical ultrasound imaging is 1 - 15 MHz. This allows wavelengths less than 1 mm to be measured and thus produces good spatial resolution. Ultrasound waves interact with tissue in a variety of ways but it is the reflection and transmission at interfaces between tissues of different acoustic impedance that is utilised in medical imaging. If there is a large acoustic mismatch between two tissues then a large fraction of the ultrasound intensity will be reflected. If there is a small difference in the acoustic impedance then most of the intensity will be transmitted. The time between pulse generation and the detection of an echo provides the depth of the reflecting interface, and thus images can be generated. Measuring the magnitude and time difference between different reflected signals can be used to determine the type, depth and size of different tissues.

Ultrasound pulses are generated and detected by a hand-held transducer, based on an array of small piezoelectric crystals. The very low acoustic impedance of air means that any boundary between air and tissue results in a near 100% reflection, so to ensure that the ultrasound waves are coupled into the body an impedance matching gel is used between the breast and the transducer. As there is a large difference between the acoustic impedance of a liquid filled cyst and normal breast tissue, around 23% of the ultrasound wave is reflected at such a boundary, making this technique particularly useful for the diagnosis of such a lesion. The small differences in acoustic impedance between adipose tissue and glandular tissue mean that this technique is of particular use for younger women with denser breasts, where x-ray mammography is often unsuitable. Doppler ultrasound utilises Doppler shifts from Rayleigh backscattered ultrasound waves to determine the velocity at which red blood cells are moving. Doppler ultrasound can be used to monitor blood flow and as a result can be used as an indicator of vascularisation of a malignant tumour in the breast.

Ultrasound is relatively inexpensive and a versatile technique. It can provide excellent contrast resolution, which means suspicious areas are easy to differentiate from normal tissue. X-ray mammograms are frequently followed up with ultrasound imaging to determine whether a lesion that appeared on a mammogram is a cyst or a solid mass. Since a fluid-filled cyst has a different sound signature than a solid mass, radiologists can reliably use ultrasound to identify cysts, which are commonly found in breasts. The technique can be used for younger women and women with breast implants and is entirely safe, and can be used repeatedly. The main disadvantages of the modality are the lack of fine detail, difficulty in detection of microcalcifications, poor ability to see deep lesions and inability to differentiate between certain types of solid breast masses.

### 2.4 Scintimammography

Scintimammography or nuclear medicine imaging is sometimes used alongside x-ray mammography in the diagnosis of breast disease since this technique is able to determine if a located lesion is malignant. The technique involves injection of a radioactive tracer into the patient. The tracer emits radiation, which is detected using a gamma camera. Appropriate image reconstruction algorithms enable the distribution of the tracer within the body to be mapped. Since the tracer accumulates differently in malignant and benign tissues it can be used to distinguish between the two conditions. Several radioactive compounds have been investigated, although only one, technetium-99m sestamibi (MIBI), is approved by FDA for use in breast imaging. A nuclear medicine investigation of the breast usually takes between 45 and 60 minutes. In a typical examination, the radioactive tracer (Tc-99m sestamibi) is injected into the patient's arm. The patient lies face down on a special table with her breast suspended through a hole. The images of the breast are taken from several angles using a gamma camera.

The advantages of scintimammography are that it can be used on patients with dense breasts and it can image large palpable lesions that do not appear with other imaging modalities. The modality involves the use of ionising substance that is injected into a patient (invasive) and is time consuming. Whilst it is 90% accurate for abnormalities over 1cm it is only 40- 60% accurate for smaller size abnormalities. The technique can be used to test tissue remaining from a mastectomy and can also be used to check for metastases in the auxiliary lymph nodes.

## 3. Techniques under development for breast cancer detection

There are several modalities that are at early stages of development but have a considerable potential as breast cancer detection devices. Majority of the imaging technologies for the breast are based on physical, mechanical, electrical, chemical and biological characteristics of the breast tissue. These detection techniques are based on their response to various tissue properties as listed in Table 2.

In an article about controversy over breast cancer screening, Reidy argued that death from malignancy rather than detection of malignancy should be a point of reference in evaluating any screening modality, since fast growing tumours, although detected while small, may have already metastasised. As a result, the number of malignancy related deaths have not altered regardless of their detection stage (Reidy, 1988). This has led to the view that the development of any new breast cancer detection modality must recognise the existence of three biologically distinct breast cancer patient subgroups. Firstly, there is a group of patients, which have slow-growing population of malignant cells that show ability to metastasise until very late. The second group comprises of patients with rapidly growing tumours that can lead to the development of micrometastases long before the tumour is detectable using the current modalities. Finally, there is the group of patients that have moderately fast growing tumours that may or may not be metastatic at the time of detection. The current breast cancer detection modalities are more valuable for the last group of patients. Some of the more likely modalities that can be developed as breast cancer diagnostic tools, which appear to be based on the recognition of the above points, are described in Table 3 and briefly discussed in the following sections.

| Mode of Imaging | Tissue Property |
|---|---|
| Physical | Photon attenuation<br>Temperature |
| Electrical | Conductivity<br>Dielectric coefficient<br>Impedance |
| Mechanical | Architecture<br>Elasticity |
| Biological | Protein (expression/function)<br>Perfusion |

Table 2. Properties of breast tissue exploited by different modes of imaging

| Modality | Description |
|---|---|
| Magnetic resonance spectroscopy | Use of magnetic resonance spectra and "functional" molecular markers to measure biochemical components of cells and tissues. |
| Optical imaging | Use of fibre-optic probes to obtain spectral measurements of elastically scattered light from tissue. Generates spectral signatures that reflect architectural changes at cellular and sub-cellular levels. |
| Optical tomography | Use of light to image the breast |
| Electrical potential measurements | Measurement of electrical potential at the skin surface. Proliferation of epithelial tissue disrupts normal polarization |
| Electronic palpation | Quantitative palpation of breast using pressure sensors. |
| Thermo acoustic computed tomography | Breast is irradiated with radio waves, causing different thermal expansion of tissue and generating sound waves, from which a three-dimensional image is constructed. |
| Microwave imaging | Transmits low-power microwaves into tissue and collects backscattered energy to create three-dimensional image. Higher water content in malignant tissues causes more scatter |
| Hall effect imaging | Induces vibrations by passing electric pulse through tissue while exposed to a magnetic field. |
| Magneto mammography | Tags cancerous tissue with magnetic agents that are imaged with SQUID magnetometers. |

Table 3. Modalities under development for breast cancer detection

### 3.1 Optical imaging

Near infrared imaging is a simple method to determine the optical properties of tissues. It involves placing a light source onto the surface of the tissue and detecting the diffusely reflected light via a fibre/ detector placed some distance from the source. Measurements made in this manner can be used to determine the concentration of different chromophores such as oxy (HbO2) and de-oxy (Hb) haemoglobin within tissue. Optical imaging provides a potential alternative modality to the current breast cancer detection techniques. Diffuse optical tomography (DOT) and spectroscopy (DOS) are non-invasive techniques used to measure the optical properties of tissues. In the near-infrared (NIR) spectral window of 600 - 1000 nm, photon propagation in tissues is dominated by scattering rather than absorption. Photons experience multiple scattering events as they propagate deeply into tissue (up to 10 cm). The technique is based on the study of functional processes and provides several unique measurable parameters with potential to enhance breast tumour sensitivity and specificity. Optical tomography provides a distinction between different tissues based on their optical properties obtained from measurements of transmitted light. The presence of various substances in biological tissues contributes to the absorption of light. Tissue optical absorption coefficients provide access to blood dynamics, total haemoglobin concentration, blood oxygen saturation, water concentration and lipid content. These tissue properties are often substantially different in rapidly growing tumours; for example, high concentrations of haemoglobin with low oxygen saturation are suggestive of rapidly growing tumours due to their high metabolic demand. (Vaupel et al, 1991, 1998 & Weidner, et al 1992). The main substances of interest in optical imaging of breast tissue are water, lipids, haemoglobin and melanin. Of particular interest is the facility to exploit the differences between the absorption spectra of oxy-haemoglobin and deoxy-haemoglobin at near infrared wavelengths to produce images of blood volume and oxygen saturation (Cheng et al, 2003 & Jiang et al, 2003).

Optical tomography involves transillumination of the breast using near infrared (NIR) light. Characteristic absorption by oxy- and deoxy- haemoglobin at NIR wavelengths can be exploited to yield oxygen saturation and blood volume information. This information can provide a distinction between the high vascularisation often associated with malignant lesions and benign or normal breast tissue. Cutler demonstrated the first use of light for breast imaging in 1929 (Cutler, 1929), but it was not until the mid 1980s that interest in the subject became widespread due to the emergence of new source and detector technologies (Hebden et al, 1997). The research activity in this field was further enhanced by the developments in computing technology, which allowed the use of algorithms to reconstruct images representing the optical properties contained within a three-dimensional volume. The constant improvement in processing speeds and detectors has made optical tomography a potential safe alternative imaging technique that, in combination with conventional imaging techniques, can provide greater specificity for breast cancer diagnosis. In a recent study, a 32 channel time-correlated single photon counting system has been utilised to perform the test (Yates, 2005). Specific data extracted from a histogram of the times of flight of photons across the breast is used to reconstruct images of the optical properties. The reconstruction is performed using a non-linear, finite element based algorithm. One system is based on two rings of different diameters to which source and detector bundles are attached. Images displaying heterogeneous features that are unique to specific healthy tissues and reproducible are presented. Pre-diagnosed benign lesions can be identified but they are not always the most dominant feature. A single tumour is identified as a dominant increase in absorption. The second system based on a hemisphere filled with a coupling fluid can also be used. Preliminary findings suggest second method provides superior information to the ring system due to its three dimensional capability and its ability to provide consistent coupling.

### 3.2 Electrical impedance based modalities

Trans-scan (T-scan) and electrical impedance tomography (EIT) modalities are based on the principle that tissues have different conductivities depending on their cell structure and pathology. Cancerous tissue causes alterations in the intracellular and extracellular fluid compartments, cell membrane surface area, ionic permeability, and membrane associated water layers. These histological biochemical changes within the cancerous tissue give rise to measurable changes in tissue electrical impedance. When a small alternating current is placed across the breast, the increase in electrical conductance and capacitance of the cancer tissue distorts the electric field within the breast and the resulting impedance map can be used to highlight a malignant area.

#### 3.2.1 Trans-scan (T-scan)

T-scan is an imaging technique that utilises the inherent differences in electrical impedance between neoplastic and normal tissue and maps noninvasively the distribution of the breast tissue electrical impedance and capacitance. It is a simple device that utilises measurements of electric impedance to distinguish between benign and malignant lesions. The methodology measures low-level bioelectric currents to produce real-time images of the electric impedance properties of the breast. It is considered that a T-scan used in addition to x-ray mammography can increase the specificity of breast cancer diagnosis. During a T-scan 1.0 to 2.5 mA of AC electrical current are generated by the system and conducted through the body via a metallic wand held by the patient. The scanning probe is then moved over the breast, and the current at the surface is measured. This information is then used to construct an image, which is immediately displayed on a computer screen. A gel is used between the skin and the scanning probe to improve the conductivity.
The technique employs relatively small and inexpensive devices and can detect small cancers down to 1 mm. The limitations of the method are that depth information is not available and microcalcifications cannot be detected. Furthermore T-scan cannot be used on patients with pacemakers and is less sensitive to larger tumours. The sensitivity and specificity of the T-scan have not yet been fully investigated, although values of 78% and 53 % respectively have been reported (Tetlow & Hubbard, 2000). T-scan has also been evaluated for symptomatic patients and women with screen-detected abnormalities. Patients undergoing both mammographic and T-scan examinations, which subsequently underwent excision or core biopsy, were retrospectively analysed. The results suggested that the T-scan is a useful addition to the assessment of patients, increasing diagnostic accuracy in terms of both sensitivity and specificity (Barter & Hicks, 2000).

#### 3.2.2 Electrical impedance tomography (EIT)

EIT uses the same principles as a T-scan but utilises a number of measurements obtained by applying different current distributions to reconstruct an image of the electric impedance of the whole breast. The quantities measured by EIT are related to the electric impedance at low frequencies via the Laplace equation. The solution of the Laplace equation is very

sensitive to noise in the measurements and so normalisation techniques are used. Most in-vivo images use linear approximating techniques which attempt to find a solution for a small change in resistivity from a known starting value. Until recently, this change in resistivity was measured over time, and so EIT images displayed physiological function. More recently anatomical images have been produced using the same reconstruction technique, but by imaging changes with frequency (Osterman, et al, 2000).
The advantages of using electric impedance devices are that they are much smaller and cheaper than other imaging modalities and use non-ionising radiation. Also in principle it is possible for EIT to produce thousands of images per second. Its main limitations are low resolution and large variation of images between subjects. The EIT technique still requires further research and development before it is approved for the detection of breast cancer.

### 3.3 Modalities based on histological examination and biomarkers

#### 3.3.1 Fine needle biopsy

If a breast lesion appears to be suspicious or is undefined following examination using the imaging methods described then the patient will undergo a biopsy. There are two degrees of biopsy: fine needle aspiration cytology and core biopsy. In the first biopsy technique a fine needle and syringe are used to obtain a small sample of cells from the suspicious area. If this sample is insufficient or the diagnosis remains inconclusive a core biopsy may be needed which requires a larger needle to remove a larger sample of cells. In both cases the procedure is painful and involves the extraction of potentially diseased tissue through healthy tissue. This is one of the main reasons for a considerable research activity for the development of non-invasive imaging techniques with greater specificity that can reduce the need for biopsy.

#### 3.3.2 Ductal lavage

Ductal lavage is a relatively newer technique used to detect pre-cancerous and cancerous breast cell changes in women who are at high risk for developing breast cancer. It is estimated that over 95% of breast cancers begin in the cells lining the breast ducts. Ductal lavage involves analysing cells that have effectively been washed out from the breast ducts using a breast pump or aspirator. The cells are studied under a microscope to determine whether they have malignant characteristics before they develop into breast cancer. This technique is still in its early stages of development and is a similar idea to the Pap smear used to test for cervical cancer.

#### 3.3.3 Tumour markers

These are substances produced by cancer cells and sometimes normal cells. They can be found in large amounts in the blood or urine of some patients with cancer. Less often, they can also be found in large amounts in the blood or urine of people who do not have cancer. There are many different kinds of tumour markers. Some are produced only by a single type of cancer. Others can be produced by several types of cancer. Most tumour markers used today are proteins or parts of proteins. They are detected by combining the patient's blood or urine with antibodies made to react with that specific protein. The results of any tumour marker test are considered with other laboratory test results and a thorough medical history and physical examination. The American Society of Clinical Oncology first published evidence-based clinical practice guidelines for the use of tumour markers in breast cancer in

1996, which are updated at regular intervals. Thirteen categories of breast tumour markers have been considered that showed evidence of clinical utility and were recommended for use in practice. These include: CA 15-3, CA 27.29, carcinoembryonic antigen, oestrogen receptor, progesterone receptor, human epidermal growth factor receptor 2, urokinase plasminogen activator, plasminogen activator inhibitor 1, and certain multiparameter gene expression assays. Not all applications for these markers were supported, however. The following categories demonstrated insufficient evidence to support routine use in clinical practice: DNA/ploidy by flow cytometry, p53, cathepsin D, cyclin E, proteomics, certain multiparameter assays, detection of bone marrow micrometastases, and circulating tumour cells (Harris et.al, 2007). However, as yet, there are no tumour markers that are useful for diagnosis of early stage breast cancer.

### 3.4 Thermal imaging techniques (TITs) for breast cancer detection

Thermography is based on the principle that metabolism and blood vessel proliferation in both pre-cancerous tissue and the area surrounding a developing breast cancer is almost always higher than in normal breast tissue. Developing tumours increase circulation to their cells by enlarging existing blood vessels and creating new ones in a process called neovascularisation or angiogenesis. This uncontrolled proliferation is considered to be of critical importance in the development of neoplastic condition. The tumour mass is unable to grow to a detectable size (2 $mm^3$) without the establishment of a new blood supply, since passive diffusion of nutrients and waste products is not sufficient for the growing tumour's metabolic requirements. Angiogenesis is induced as a result of the release of a variety of angiogenic peptides that may be produced by the neoplastic cells. These newly developed blood vessels are quite porous and provide easy access to the circulating immediately adjacent tumour cells. For this reason the propensity to metastasise has been related to the number of micro vessels found in a growing mass of tumour. (Nathanson et al, 2000; Wade & Kozolowski, 2007). This process frequently results in an increase in regional temperature of the breast and forms the basis of the thermal modalities for the detection of breast cancer.
The first recorded use of thermo-biological diagnostics can be found in the writings of Hippocrates around 480 B.C. Mud slurry was spread over the patient and allowed to dry. The body areas that dried first were thought to indicate underlying organ pathology. Since then continued research and clinical observations proved that certain temperatures related to the human body were indeed indicative of normal and abnormal physiological processes. There are two thermal based modalities that could have a very significant impact on the detection and diagnosis of breast cancer. These are named as infrared thermography and microwave radiometry. Both techniques detect the changes in the physiology of the tissue rather than evaluating the changes in the tissue anatomical and dielectric features. Figure 4 illustrates that the physiological changes (preclinical phase) in the tissue begin nearly eight years earlier before they become apparent in the form of mass of malignant tumour (Lundgren, 1981).
Although thermography is an appealing method of screening for breast cancer, research over the past 20 years has failed to produce a system that is reliable for such a purpose and therefore thermography is not a widely used modality. However, it is expected that advances such as computerised thermal imaging will provide significant improvement in the cancer detection rate but this remains to be seen. Furthermore, attenuation of infrared radiation in tissue is high. For this reason thermography will only ever be able to provide information on the surface temperature variations and so no depth information is available. This is a severe limitation of infrared thermography in detecting breast cancer.

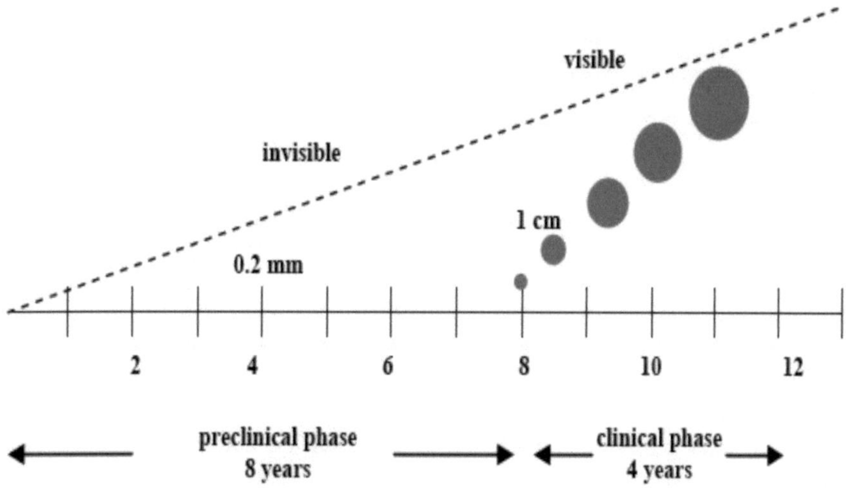


Fig. 4. Kinetics of tumour growth ((Lundgren, 1981)

### 3.4.1 Infrared thermography

Infrared thermal imaging has been used for several decades to monitor the temperature distribution over human skin. Abnormalities such as malignancies, inflammation, and infection cause localized increases in temperature that appear as hot spots or asymmetrical patterns in an infrared thermogram. Thermography, alternatively termed thermometry has been pursued for many years as a technique for breast cancer detection. Studies of thermography have focused on a range of potential uses, including diagnosis, prognosis, and risk indication and as an adjunct to existing technologies; however, the results have been inconsistent and scientific consensus has been difficult to achieve. The research activity in infrared thermography as cancer detection technique was diminished in the 1970s, but the recent technological advances have renewed the interest in the modality. Digital infrared cameras have much-improved spatial and thermal resolutions, and libraries of image processing routines are available to analyze images captured both statically and dynamically.

As an addition to the breast health screening process, infrared imaging has a significant role to play. Due to the technique's unique ability to image the metabolic aspects of the breast, very early warning signals have been observed in long-term studies. A breast tumour can raise the temperature of the skin surface by as much as 3 $^{0}$C compared with the temperature of the skin surface of a woman with normal tissue probably due to the elevated rates of tumour metabolism and elevated levels of vascularity and perfusion. It is for this reason that an abnormal infrared image may be the single most important marker of high risk for the existence of or future development of breast cancer. Furthermore, the proven sensitivity, specificity, and prognostic value of the modality, makes infrared imaging one of the frontline methods for breast cancer screening. The diagnosis of cancer is based on the difference in temperature relative to that for the contralateral breast, which serves as a built-in control. The procedure is non-invasive and does not require compression of the breast or radiation exposure.

### 3.4.2 Microwave radio thermometry (MRT)

The National Cancer Institute (NCI) in the United States of America has funded numerous research projects to improve conventional and develop new technologies to detect, diagnose, and characterize breast cancer. According to the U.S. Institute of Medicine, an ideal breast screening tool is a low risk device that is sensitive to tumours, detects breast cancer at a curable stage, non-invasive, simple to use, cost effective and widely available. The device should also involve minimal discomfort to the user and provides easy to interpret, objective and consistent results. Of particular importance is the ability to clearly distinguish between malignant and benign tumours and early detection. A brief review of the published literature shows that all techniques have limited capability in these respects and surgery is required to establish the nature of the tumour. The research in this area is time consuming since the ultimate test of a technique beyond the proof of concept stage must be clinical trials.

Microwave radio thermometry (MRT) is a modality that uses non ionising electromagnetic radiation for cancer detection in humans. The technique has attracted a great deal of research in the last three decades. An electromagnetic imaging method can be active or passive. In an active system, one or more antennas radiate onto the body, where the electromagnetic field is scattered by tissue dielectric inhomogeneities and then received by the same or other antennas. In multi-frequency active imaging, data is collected at various frequencies and for various locations of the antennas outside the body [Liu et al, 2002; Meaney et al, 2000]. Field data are known terms in the inverse scattering problem, whose solution attempts a retrieval of the contrast of an eventual dielectric anomaly with respect to the background permittivity of healthy tissues. On the other hand time-domain systems exploit higher frequencies and wide-band antennas showing some similarity to ground penetrating radar [Fear & Stuchly, 2000; Li et al, 2004].

Thermal imaging methods include both infrared and microwave radiometry modalities. Both methods detect physiological tissue response, rather than evaluating anatomic dielectric features. Heat is released from the body on the whole electromagnetic spectrum with a maximum at infrared frequencies. There are several physiological features that are related to malignant tissue, which may contribute to the infrared signal. These include increased blood flow in the area surrounding a malignancy, angiogenesis, and the release of vasoactive mediators. The infrared imaging system uses a camera that is highly sensitive to infrared radiation in the appropriate spectrum. Microwave radiometry is based on the measurement of the electromagnetic field spontaneously emitted by a body in the microwave frequency range [Bardati & Solimini, 1983; Edrich, 1979; Leroy et al, 1998; Meyer et al, 1979]. Charged particles in motion are primary sources of incoherent thermal radiation propagating inside the body, where it is partially absorbed and partially radiated externally. Antennas located in the vicinity of the body collect and changes the radiation to an electrical current that fluctuates in the receiver's input unit. Assuming that the body is in a thermodynamic equilibrium, the spectral content of the radiometric signal can be related to the local temperature distribution in the body, allowing its retrieval to be attempted from radiometric data collected at different frequencies and for various antenna positions. A thermal anomaly may be a significant indicator of a malignancy.

The fundamental basis for developing a microwave imaging technique for detecting breast cancer is the significant contrast in the dielectric properties, at microwave frequencies, of normal and malignant breast tissue, as evidenced by experimentally measured data [Li et al, 2005; Bardati et al 2002]. The estimated malignant-to-normal breast tissue contrast is between 2:1 and 10:1, depending on the density and water content of the different tissues. Therefore, microwave modality does not offer the potential for the high spatial resolution provided by X-rays, but it does permit exceptionally high contrast with respect to physical or physiological factors of clinical interest, such as water content, vascularisation or angiogenesis, blood-flow rate, and temperature. Microwave imaging techniques result in a three-dimensional (3-D) volumetric mapping of the relevant tissue properties, and thus offer in situ 3-D positioning of the tissue abnormalities. Furthermore, microwave attenuation in normal breast tissue is low enough to make signal propagation through even large breast volumes quite feasible (~ 4 cm). For these reasons, microwave breast imaging has the potential to overcome some of the limitations of conventional breast cancer screening modalities.

Microwave systems in use or under development may be categorised into three types: passive, active or hybrid. However, the passive technique has been investigated for many years, with clinical trials undertaken with the availability of commercial units that are currently used mainly in conjunction with mammography. The passive method detects regions of increased temperature due to the tumour from the very small "natural" microwave signal from the breast (black body radiation as given by Planck's law). The signals detected are very low and require sensitive electronic systems. Temperature differentials between adjacent areas on the breast are taken as an indication of an abnormality, using a similar area on the other breast as a reference - the approach is somewhat empirical. The increased tumour temperature is thought to arise from "vascularisation" (angiogenesis). There is a great deal of ongoing research, which is related to the development of thermal models of the breast to relate the measured temperature differentials with temperature rises located in the tissue. There is also a considerable focus for the last few years in the USA on the development of detecting antennas. There is evidence that the passive MRT technique can detect malignant tissue abnormality at an early stage, but as yet this cannot be taken as an established fact.

Current understandings of the underlying pathological mechanisms for increased temperature in breast cancer are that breast cancer cells produce nitric oxide, which interferes with the normal neuronal (nervous system) control of breast tissue blood vessel flow by causing regional vasodilation in the early stages of cancerous cell growth, and enhancing angiogenesis in the later stages. The subsequent increased blood flow in the area causes a temperature increase relative to the normal breast temperature, and even deep breast lesions may also contribute to the detectable increase in the heat evolved. These changes relate to physiological breast processes. It is believed that in healthy individuals, temperature is generally symmetrical across the midline of the body. Subjective interpretation of many diagnostic imaging modalities, including microwave thermometry and infrared thermography, rely on the normal contralateral images are relatively symmetrical, and the likelihood that small asymmetries may indicate a tissue abnormalities. Therefore, in breast cancer, thermography/thermometry detects disease by identifying areas of asymmetric temperature distribution on the breast surface.

Microwave radiometry is used for diagnosis of diseases by measuring small changes of internal tissue temperature. The detection and diagnosis is conducted by measuring the intensity of natural electromagnetic radiation of patient's internal tissues at microwave frequencies. The intensity of radiation is proportional to the temperature of the tissues. Cancerous tumours have a significantly different index of refraction and the internal tissue temperature often changes due to inflammation changes in the blood supply or with increased metabolism of cells during oncological transformation of tissues. Microwave radiometry measures the emission of natural radiation from the body in the microwave, or centrimetric, region of the electromagnetic spectrum. All materials above absolute zero emit natural, thermally generated electromagnetic radiation. At body temperature of 37°C the maximum intensity of radiation occurs in the infrared part of the spectrum at wavelengths close to 10 μmeters (Fraseri et al, 1987).

Microwave thermometry may be envisioned as the microwave analogue of infrared thermography (Barrett, et al, 1980). Whereas infrared thermography uses wavelengths of 10 mm (typical), microwave thermometry makes use of much longer wavelengths, typically 1 - 20 cm; this leads to important and fundamental differences between the two techniques as described in the literature(Barrett & Myers, 1975a, 1975b; Barrett et al, 1977, 1980). Microwave radiation is capable of penetrating human tissue and therefore the emission provides information related to subcutaneous conditions within the body. The intensity of microwave emission is linearly proportional to the temperature of the emitter. Therefore, microwave thermometry provides information related to internal body temperatures. The depth of penetration, and hence the depth from which microwave radiation may escape from the body, depends on the wavelength, the dielectric properties of the tissue and the water content of the tissue. Furthermore, the frequency used for microwave breast imaging needs to be low enough to provide adequate depth of penetration, but high enough to allow the use of small antenna array elements. The final resolution of the image depends on both the number of antenna array elements and the frequency. In general, resolution increases with frequency and the number of antenna array elements. In order to obtain useful images, there must be significant contrast between normal and malignant tissue and the greatest contrast in breast tissue occurs in the frequency range 600 MHz-1 GHz.

The distinctive feature of microwave radiometry is an extremely low signal strength entering input of the antenna from the biological tissues. This signal strength is approximately $10^{-13}$ Watt. While conducting the measurement it is necessary to distinguish temperatures differing on a tenth part of degree, which corresponds to signal strength to be $10^{-16}$ Watt. Therefore the special circuits are required for receipt, amplification and treatment of signals. So far, the application of microwave radiometry has been directed at the early detection and diagnosis of breast cancer. Present breast cancer detection techniques, other than radiometry, require that the tumour must have significant mass and contrast with respect to the surrounding tissue (i.e., palpation physical examination, mammography and ultrasound). This results in approximately 85 percent of all determinations of breast disease undergoing extensive surgical procedures. Early detection could lead to a more conservative treatment and a positive attitude toward detection. The diagnosis of breast cancer at a smaller size or earlier stage will allow a woman more choice in selecting among various treatment options.

The passive MRT method is a non-invasive, non-ionizing procedure that determines the thermal activity of the tissue rather than mass and therefore when used in conjunction with one or more other detection modalities, could provide early indication of breast with good accuracy. The determination of thermal activity is a measurement of tumour activity, or growth rate, providing data beyond the physical parameters (i.e., size and depth determined by mammography). Suspicious results found by screening using microwave radiometry could then be referred for further investigation by mammography and other appropriate techniques. Medical microwave radiometry has a number of positive characteristics as follows:

- Early diagnosis of diseases;
- Possibility of non-invasive detection of disease in internal organs before the appearance of structural changes that can be detected by X rays or ultrasound;
- Completely harmless for the patients of all age and with any diseases as well as for medical staff;
- Possibility to conduct the investigation repeatedly (control of treatment):
- Depth of anomaly detection is from 3 to 10 cm;
- Accuracy of measuring the internal averaged temperature ± 0,2 $^{o}$C
- Simplicity of the device handling, the procedure may be conducted by the secondary medical staff.
- Time measuring of one point: 5 - 15 sec.

### 3.5 The concept of the smart bra as an early warning system for breast cancer

The concept of wearable early warning system for breast cancer is under investigation at the Institute of Materials Research and Innovation (IMRI), University of Bolton. The researchers are working on the development of a wearable system that integrates the passive microwave antennae with textile structures. The basic concept of this approach is to present the microwave antennas to the breast in the form of a 'Smart Bra'. Work on developing antenna systems and microelectronics is being carried out. Miniaturisation of the radiometer, antennae and electronics and there integration with appropriate textile structures are the main thrusts of the research and development programmes in progress. It remains to be established how much of the electronics would be mounted on the bra and how critical accurate positioning of the sensors would be. The incorporation of the electronics is the critical part of the research and development programme. Work is also in progress on the development of wearable breast cancer device at De Montfort University, Leicester, UK. This is a low frequency active electrical impedance tomography (EIT) based system, which utilises the differences in electrical properties between healthy and malignant breast tissues and the researchers have introduced the concept of a "Smart Bra" which allows the impedance tomography to be carried out conveniently and rapidly. However, the microwave radio thermometry modality being adopted by the Bolton team is non-contact and passive whereas the EIT is an active modality albeit at low power levels. In the following sections the concept of MRT based wearable early warning system for breast cancer is described.

The microwave radiometer is a device which measures the intensity of electromagnetic radiation from human body in microwave wave length. The noise power at the input of the microwave receiver is proportional to the internal temperature of human body. An array of receivers can resolve the local temperature inside the breast in 3-D and hence provide a signature of local temperature differences inside the breast. The geometrical resolution is determined by the element number and the bandwidth and frequency of operation. Tumour detection relies on temperature difference resolution, which is a function of the noise figure of the receiver, its stability and the bandwidth as well as the test integration time (Skou, 2006).

Traditional microwave radiometers for breast cancer detection known from literature and available on the market are rather large and heavy in weight. Today, only one relatively compact model of microwave radiometer (RTM-01-RES) is available in the market. The radiometer receives energy-emissions from the human body using an infrared sensor and a microwave sensor. The weight of internal temperature sensor is rather high and consequently it is not possible to incorporate such a device in a self-powered wearable system. It is therefore necessary to design miniature balance zero Microwave Radiometer and the Microwave Multi-Channel Electron Switch (MMCES). Miniaturization is essential for both technical reasons, achieving direct coupling to antenna and good stability, as well as for integration into textiles for maximum comfort. In traditional microwave systems antennae are fabricated on rigid substrates, as wires or as hollow structures. Antennae on textiles have been demonstrated earlier but only with limited design variations, mainly as microstrip patch or slot antennae (Klemm et al, 2004, 2005; Locher, 2006; Klemm & Troester, 2005, 2006; Behdad, 2004; & Alomainy et al, 2005). There is a need to explore different structures especially in view of multi-frequency or wideband operation.

The relevant accuracy of measuring the noise power at the input of the receiver is ~ $10^{-3}$. The dielectric constant of a person may change dramatically from 5.5 for fat breast to 50 for muscle. Therefore, the reflection coefficient between antenna and human body tissue may change significantly and as a result about 10% of energy may be reflected from the antenna. However, the accuracy of noise power measurement should remain unchanged. In order to solve this problem it is necessary to use zero balance radiometer with compensation of reflections between antenna and human body tissue. This principle is used in most modern microwave radiometers (Leroy et al, 1998, Hand et al, 2001 & Lee et al, 2002). An overview of microwave radiometry is given in a recent publication (Hand et al, 2001). The balance multi-frequency microwave radiometer has also been described (Leroy et al, 1998). These researchers used 5 frequencies in calculating the temperature profile in the brain. It is very important to use multi-frequency radiometer in order to visualize the temperature inside body. But the increase in the number of frequencies increases the sizes and the weight of the radiometer and decreases the noise imperviousness of the device. The radiation from human body is very small therefore the noise immunity is one of the critical parameters of the microwave radiometer.

It is expected that the multi frequency radiometer will have better accuracy for breast cancer detection in comparison with a single channel radiometer, but it is not evident that the sensitivity will increase greatly. Thousands of measurements during 10 years with the microwave radiometer (RTM-01-RES) have shown that there are about 10 % of breast cancer patients who have no skin temperature increase or brightness temperature increase (Burdina et al, 2005). Thus the probability that these patients will have temperature increase at another frequency is not very high. Due to the weight and sizes limitations for a wearable system, there is no reason to use more than two frequencies. Furthermore, skin temperature information is very important for breast cancer detection.

The fluctuation error of radiometer is dependent on time of integration, the bandwidth and losses of the microwave part of the receiver. Usually for the receiver's bandwidth of 500-600 MHz the measurement time is 5 seconds and fluctuation error is 0.1°C. The increase of bandwidth may decrease the fluctuation error. Another possibility to decrease the fluctuation error is to increase the integration time. Monolithic microwave integrated circuit (MMIC) provides the opportunity to increase the bandwidth of microwave device greatly. Furthermore, for wearable, self-examination devices the time of measurement is not a very important factor, therefore, the fluctuation error may be minimized by choosing the proper value of integration time.

It may be possible to combine a single channel microwave radiometer and a MMCES. In this case, the results of brightness temperature measurement will highly depend on the environment temperature, due to the losses in the MMCES. To overcome this problem, it is necessary to use balance zero radiometer and balance the losses of MMCES and losses of reference noise source. In this situation the losses of MMCES do not decrease the performance of radiometer. Furthermore, it is possible to minimise the losses in MMCES by the utilization of integrated radiometer front-ends. The integration requires the design and fabrication of microwave monolithic integrated circuits with ultra low-noise performance. This can be achieved using state-of-the-art MMIC fabrication processes. Such components are very compact (few square millimetres) and therefore minimize losses and temperature variations. The employed fabrication processes can achieve amplifiers with noise figure below NF<0.5 dB with high gain resulting in excellent radiometer performance (Dabrowski et al, 2004). However, these devices are either large and operate at cryogenic temperatures or are relatively narrowband. There is a need to especially focus on the development of wideband for multi-frequency receiver in order to improve the overall system performance. Yet, another possibility is the introduction of multi-receiver system alleviating the need for an MMCES. This however requires identical channel operation, which can only be fabricated using identical components. In the development of MMIC for the radiometer front-end such a technique becomes feasible.

Introduction of microelectronic microwave components close to the antenna requires appropriate textile integration technologies. This aspect has been dealt within various publications both with woven and nonwoven materials (Catrysse et al, 2004; Coosemans et al, 2005; Hermans et al, 2005; Van Langenhove et al, 2003a, 2003b; Scilingo et al, 2005 & Paradiso et al, 2005). However, only little data is available on the microwave properties of different woven and nonwoven materials (Locher, 2006). Interconnection to the microwave monolithic integrated circuit is an important area of research and development. One possible approach is the implementation of ribbon type interconnects, which can efficiently be used for power supply and low frequency output signals. The active components need to be developed with MMIC operating over a wide range. Low-noise amplifiers determine the overall noise performance of the receivers. Very wideband performance has been demonstrated in GaAs and CMOS technologies, respectively (Nosal, 2001; Jung et al, 2006; Xu et al, 2005 & Wang et al, 2005). However, in most cases a noise figure NF>1.0 dB over a frequency range of DC - 10 GHz has been achieved. There is a need to design amplifiers complying with the frequency range of DC - 10 GHz, but exhibiting a noise figure NF < 1.0 dB with an associated gain of G > 30 dB. These parameters are well beyond the state-of-the-art today. There is a need to develop MMIC components that can be used for the assembly of the microwave radiometer system. Figure 5 shows one possible functional scheme of Multi-Channel Microwave Radiometer.

Multi-Channel Microwave Radiometer's development consists of the following stages.

- Designing of Multi-Channel switch.
- Designing of Radiometer's microwave parts
- Designing of radiometer's digital part and analog low-frequency part of feedback circuit.
- Software design for visualization of the measurements and for the radiometer's microcontrollers.

Microwave radiometer consists of an electronic switch, circulator, isolator, low-noise amplifier, filter, amplitude detector and miniature reference noise source with the temperature sensor. All of these components parts must be designed in miniature sizes using MMIC and plastic materials.
There are two critical parameters which define Radiometer's quality:

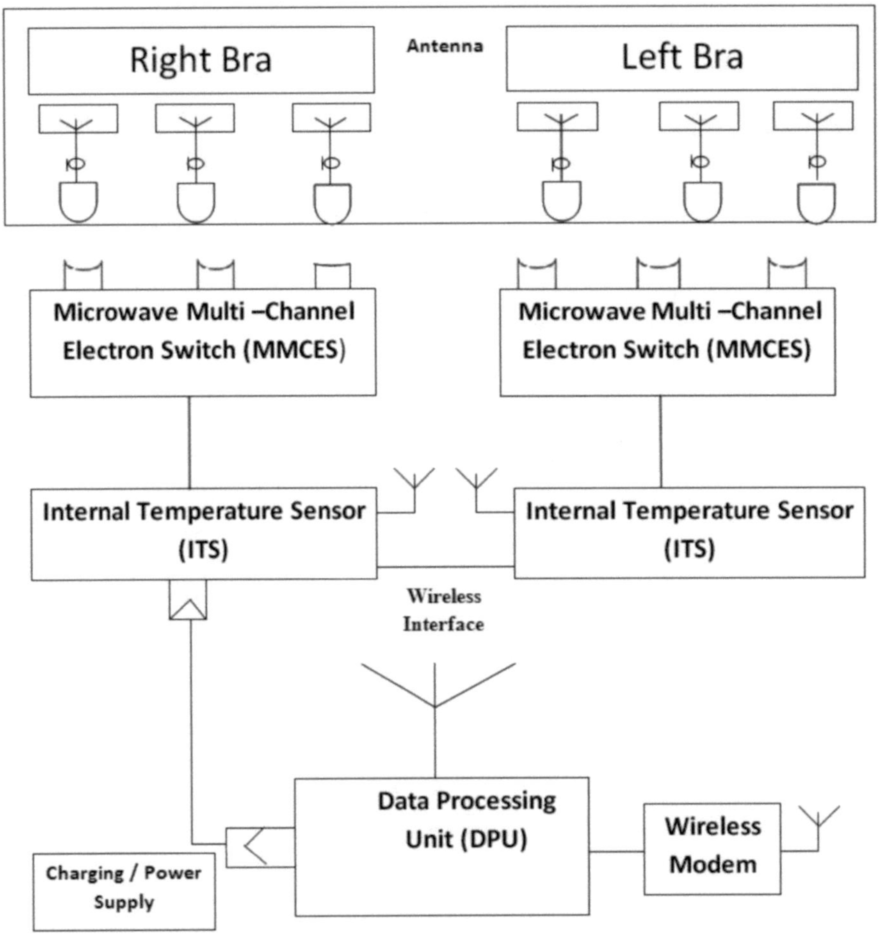


Fig. 5. The functional scheme of Multi-Channel Microwave Radiometer

1. Brightness temperature error when the reflection's coefficient of antenna changes.
2. Brightness temperature error when the environment's temperature changes.

The over arching aim of the research in progress on the development of wearable breast cancer detection system is to deliver a miniaturized microwave technology, Multi-frequency Microwave Radiometry (MFMWR), which is a totally non-invasive and passive method for cancer detection. It is proposed to use microwave radiometry (MWR) to detect the "hot spots" (the cancerous regions) in the breast tissue. This technology was initially used in the field of astrophysics, measuring the minute amounts of microwave energy emitted by stars and planets. The same principle can be used for medical diagnostics (Chaudhary, 1984), as anything that can absorb radiation also emits radiation. In MWR, the power in the microwave region of the natural thermal radiation from body tissues is measured to obtain the brightness temperature of the tissue under observation. The brightness temperature at an antenna centre frequency $f_i$ is,

$$T_{B,i} = \frac{P_i}{k\,df_i} = \frac{(1-R_i)\,P_{tissue,i}}{k\,df_i} = (1-R_i)T_{B,tissue,i} \tag{1}$$

Where $P_{tissue,i}$ is the thermal radiation power emitted by the tissue, $P_i$ is the power received by the antenna in a bandwidth $df_i$ around $f_i$, $R_i$ is the power reflection coefficient at the skin-antenna interface at $f_i$ and $k$ is Boltzmann's constant.
According to the Rayleigh-Jeans law, at microwave frequency $f_i$, the thermal radiation intensity is proportional to the absolute temperature, so that

$$T_{B,i} = \int_{\Omega} W_i T(r)\,dv \tag{2}$$

where $T(r)$ is the absolute temperature in a tissue volume of $dv$ located at $r$, $W_i(r)$ is the receiving antenna's weighting function and the integration is over the antenna's field of view $\Omega$.
It can be seen that (equation 1) that the brightness temperature $T_{B,i}$ is dependent upon the temperature in the tissue $T_{B,tissue,i}$ and the reflection coefficient R. For balance zero radiometer with the compensation of the reflection on the border antenna and tissue the reflection from the tissue is compensated by thermal radiation of the radiometer and the brightness temperature is independent of reflection coefficient R. Therefore, for non-invasive detection of temperature abnormalities it is possible measure the power radiation P from the tissue.
Thus the measured brightness temperature at frequency $f_i$,

$$T_{B,i} = \frac{\int_{\Omega} W_i T(r)\,dv}{1-R_i} \tag{3}$$

The receiving antenna's weighting function depends upon its operating frequency and microwave attenuating properties of the tissues, as well as antenna characteristics. Microwave reflections occur at interfaces between different tissue regions and between these regions and the measuring equipment. Since the attenuation of microwaves in tissue and the antenna characteristics are frequency dependent, the temperature-depth profile within the tissue beneath the antenna can be found using a multi-frequency radiometer and a stable solution to the inverse problem of retrieving the temperature-depth dependence from a set of measured brightness temperatures. The human body's tissues have different permittivities therefore the reflection coefficient of the antenna for diverse people or in different tissues can reach 10%. This fact can decrease noise power at the input on the radiometer. But brightness temperature cannot change in spite of the fact that the brightness temperature is proportional to noise power at the input on the radiometer. This problem can be overcome by balance zero radiometer with sliding scheme of the reflections compensation.
Evidently the temperature of microwave part of the radiometer may change greatly. This leads to noise power change at the input of the radiometer. If the front-end loss of

radiometer is about 1 dB, one degree change in the environment temperature will lead to brightness temperature change in 0.4 degree. This is why the radiometer input circuits temperature is usually stabilized. But this is not feasible for the wearable self-powered detection system because of the power demand. For balanced radiometer it is possible to optimize parameters of input circuit including Multi-Channel Switch and the reference noise source circuit to minimize error due to environment temperature changes. However, if the losses of microwave part of radiometer do not change in time, the error due to environment temperature change can be compensated. For this purpose it is necessary to measure the front-end temperature. This principle was successfully used in industrial single-channel radiometer (RTM-01-RES) and can be applied to the multi-channel radiometer. For this purpose it is important to measure antenna array temperature and to transmit this information to the radiometer. Software is a need for visualisation of the results of the measurements and the database storage in the control centre. It is vital that radiometer should monitor the function of its various components appropriately, estimate the measurement error and transmit this information to the central database by wireless connection. This allows the estimation of the radiometer's accuracy automatically. Fabrication of the breast cancer microwave screening system also requires the development of the hardware for the system.

Microwave thermometry is the detection of microwave radiation from the human body and may be considered as the microwave equivalent of infrared thermography. Infrared thermography typically uses wavelengths of 10 μmetre, whereas in microwave thermometry much longer wavelengths are employed (1 -20 cm). The other major differences between the two modalities can be summarised as following:

- Microwave radiation is capable of penetrating human tissue and therefore the emissions can provide useful thermal signals related to the subcutaneous conditions within the body. On the other hand, infrared radiation is not able to penetrate such depths and therefore is able to detect conditions close to the surface i.e. skin.
- The intensity of microwave emission is linearly proportional to the temperature of the emitter. Therefore a measurement of the emission may be easily related to the temperature of the emitter. Infrared intensity measurements may also be related to the body temperature but this relationship is somewhat nonlinear.
- Microwave emission gives coarser spatial resolution (~ 1cm) than infrared because of its longer wavelength than infrared (~1mm). This supposes that microwave thermography provides information about internal body temperatures. The depth of penetration, and hence the depth from which microwave radiation may escape from the body, depends on the wavelength, the dielectric properties of the tissue, and, most importantly, on the water content of the tissue.

Development of a wearable, self-powered early warning system for breast cancer will also require the production of textile structures that are flexible, comfortable, breathable, light and suitable for integration with the materials developed to perform various functions to operate the cancer detecting devices produced. Conducting fibres and filaments are needed to produce fabrics using a range of mechanical conversion methods, particularly knitting, crochet or braiding to produce the developmental materials. The structures then need to be characterised and optimised. Conducting fabrics can also be prepared using chemical methods, including coating, printing and lamination. Wet chemical methods and dry methods can be employed for this purpose. The integrated textile structures must be tested for their efficiency, durability, launderability, mechanical and comfort properties. Finally, the integrated textiles need to be converted into wearable structures to act as cancer detection devices.

## 4. Conclusions

At present x-ray mammography is the most commonly used breast imaging technique and is the only modality used for routine screening. X-ray mammography has become the "gold standard" for breast imaging. The technique has a high sensitivity and is able to detect very small tumours and calcifications. The main limitations of x-ray mammography are that it has a poor specificity for some tumour types and that it is unsuitable for use on women with dense breasts. In addition, x-ray mammography uses ionising radiation and usually causes considerable discomfort to the patient. Thus there is potential for an alternative technique to replace x-ray mammography or to be used as an additional resource to improve the overall specificity of the diagnosis. As discussed MRI, ultrasound and Nuclear medicine are currently used to provide additional diagnostic information, but all have their limitations and are not alternatives to mammography. Other techniques are currently being investigated such as EIT and infrared thermography but as yet these have severe limitations in resolution and specificity. Thus there still remains a niche for an additional imaging modality to aid in the early detection and diagnosis of breast tissue oncological abnormalities.
Microwave radiometry (MRT) appears to be an attractive alternative modality for breast imaging. MRT can be used effectively in breast cancer investigation. The method has many advantages over the currently used breast cancer detection techniques:

- Oncological changes in tissues could be detected earlier using MRT as compared to the classical methods based on ultrasounds and ionising radiation
- Breast cancer detection is made at a curable stage
- The technique is non-invasive and non-hazardous both to the patient and the device operator.
- MRT is easy to use, cheap and fast
- Involves no risk for patients of any age
- Involves a minimum discomfort for patient, easily accepted by women - is easy to interpret and objective.

The MRT can be used repeatedly to improve cancer detection rates and monitor the progress of cancer treatment. Using microwave radiometry in conjunction with other traditional modalities can significantly improve the diagnosis, especially for the patients with fast growing tumours. Studies show that breast thermometry has the ability to warn a woman that a cancer may be forming many years before any other test can detect the condition. The major gaps in knowledge can be addressed by more robust research on the technologically advanced microwave thermometry devices and large-scale, prospective randomised trials for population screening and diagnostic testing of breast cancer. The MRT system components can be miniaturised and integrated with textiles to produce wearable early warning systems for breast cancer.

## 5. References

Alomainy, A.; Hao, Y.; Parini, C. & Hall, P. (2005). Comparison Between Two Different Antennas for UWB Onbody Propagation Measurements', *IEEE Antennas and Wireless Propagation Letters*, Vol. 4, pp. 31-34

Bardati, D.; Marrocco, G. & Tognolatti, P. (2002). New-born-infant Brain Temperature Measurement by Microwave Radiometry, *Antennas and Propagation Society International Symposium, 2002. IEEE*,Vol.1, pp. 811,

Barrett, A et al, (1980)Microwave Thermography in the Detection of Breast Cancer', *AJR*, Vol.134, pp. 365-368.

Barrett, A. & Myers, P. (1975). Microwave Thermography', *Bibl Radiol,* Vol.6, pp. 45-56

Barrett, A. & Myers, P. (1975). Subcutaneous Temperatures: A Method of Noninvasive Sensing, *Science, Vol.*1 90, pp.669-671

Barrett, A.; Myers, P. & N L Sadowsky, N. (1977). Detection of Breast Cancer by Microwave Radiometry, *Radio Science, Vol.*1 2, pp.167-171

Barrett, A.; Myers, P. & N L Sadowsky, N. (1980), Microwave Thermography of Normal and Cancerous Breast Tissue. *Conference on thermal characteristics of tumors: applications in detection and treatment,* New York, March, 979. Ann NY Acad Sci.

Barter, S & IP Hicks (2000). Electrical Impedance Imaging of the Breast (TranScan TS 2000): Initial UK Experience. *Breast Cancer Res, Symposium Mammographicum 2000.* Vol. 2, (Suppl 2):A11

Behdad, N. (2004). A Wideband Multiresonant Single-Element Slot Antenna. *Antennas and Wireless Propagation Letters,* Vol. 3, pp.5-8

Boyd, N.; Byng, J. & Jong, R. (1995). Quantitative Classification of Mammographic Densities and Breast Cancer Risk. *J. Natl Cancer Inst.,* Vol.87, pp. 670

Burdina, L. et al. (2005).Tikhomirova «Microwave Radiometry in Algorithm Complex Diagnosis of Breast Diseases', *Modern Oncology,* 2005, V6, №1, p.8-9 (in Russian)

Brem, R.; Kieper, D.; Rapelyea, J. & Majewski, S. (2003). Evaluation of a High-Resolution, Breast-Specific, Small-Field-of-View Gamma Camera for the Detection of Breast Cancer. *Nuclear Instruments and Methods in Physics Research A* Vol.497, (2003), pp. 39–45

Catrysse, M. et al (2004). Towards the Integration of Textile Sensors in a Wireless Monitoring Suit. *Sensors and Actuators.* Vol. A114, pp. 302-311, 2004

Chaudhary, S.; R. K. Mishra.; Swarup, A. & Thomas, J. (1984). Dielectric Properties of Normal and Malignant Human Breast Tissues at Radiowave and Microwave Frequencies. *Indian J. Biochem. Biophys.* Vol.21, pp. 76–79

Cheng, X.; Mao, J.; Bush, R.; Kopans, D.; Moore, R. & Chorlton, M. (2003). Breast Cancer Detection by Mapping Hemoglobin Concentration and Oxygen Saturation. *Applied Optics,* Vol.42, pp. 6412-6421

Coosemans, J.; Hermans, B. & Puers, R. (2005). Integrating Wireless ECG Monitoring in Textiles', *International Conference on Solid-State Sensors and Actuators, Transducers 05,* pp. 228-232, June 5-9, 2005

Cutler, M. (1929). Transillumination as an Aid in the Diagnosis of Breast Lesions. *Surg Gynecol Obstet,* Vol. 48, pp. 721-729

Dabrowski, J. et al, 'Design and Performance of Low Noise Cascode IC for Wireless Applications', *15th International Conference on Microwaves, Radar and Wireless Communications,* Vol. 3, pp. 882-885, May 2004

Elmore, J.; Wells, F. & Carol, M. (1994). Variability in Radiologists Interpretation of Mammograms. *NEJM.* Vol. 331, No.22, pp. 1493

Fraseri, S et al. (1987). Microwave Thermography – An Index of Inflammatory Joint Disease. *British Journal of Rheumatology.* Vol. 261, pp. 37-39

Hand, J. Van Leeuwen,G.; Mizushina, G.; Van de Kamer, J.; Maruyama, K.; Sugiura, T.; Azzopardi, D. & Edwards, A. (2001). Monitoring of Deep Brain Temperature in Infants Using Multi-Frequency Microwave Radiometry and Thermal Modelling. Phys. Med. Biol. Vol.46, pp. 1885–1903

Harris, L.; Fritsche, H.; Mennel, R.; Norton, L.; Ravdin, P.; Taube, S.; Somerfield, M.; Hayes, D.; Bast, R (2007). Update of Recommendations for the Use of Tumor Markers in Breast Cancer. *J. Clinical Oncology*, Vol. 25, No. 33, pp. 5287-5312

Hebden, J.; Arridge, S. & Delpy, D. (1997). Optical Imaging in Medicine: I. Experimental Techniques. *Phys.Med.Biol.,* Vol. 42, pp. 825-840

Hermans, B.; Coosemans, J. & Puers, R. (2005). Integration of Sensors and Electronics in Textile for use in Infant Medicine. *European Microlectronics and Packaging Conference and Exhibition*, pp. 588-592, June 12-15, 2005

Jiang, S.; Pogue, B.; McBride, T. & Paulsen, K. (2003). Quantitative Analysis of Near-infrared Tomography: Sensitivity to the Tissue-simulating Precalibration Phantom. *Journal of Biomedical Optics,* Vol.8, pp. 308-315

Jung, J. et al, 'Ultra-Wideband Low Noise Amplifier Using a Cascode Feedback Topology', *IEEE Silicon Monolithic Integrated Circuits in RF Systems*, 2006. pp. 202-205

Keyserlignk, J. & Ahlgren, P (1998). Infrared Imaging of the Breast: Initial Reappraisal Using High Resolution Digital Technology in 100 Successive Cases of Stage 1 and 2 Breast Cancer. *Breast J.* Vol.4, pp.245-251

Klemm, M.; Locher,I. & Troster, G. (2004). A novel circularly polarized textile antenna for wearable applications. *The 34rd European Microwave Conference (EuMC),* pp.11-14, 2004.

Klemm,M.; Kovcs,I.; Pedersen, G. & Troster, G. (2005). *Novel* small-size directional antenna for UWB WBAN/WPAN applications', *IEEE Trans. on Antennas and Propagation.* Vol. 53, No. 12 pp. 3884- 3896

Klemm, M & Troester, G. (2006). EM Energy Absorption in the Human Body Tissues due to UWB Antennas', *Progress In Electromagnetics Research.* Vol. 62, pp.261-280

Klemm, M. & Troster, G. (2005). Integration of Electrically Small UWB Antennas for Body-Worn Sensor Applications. *IEE Wideband and Multi-band Antennas and Arrays*, 2005, pp.141-146.

Lee, J.; Kim, K.; Lee, S.; Eom, S. & Troitsky, R. (2002). A Novel Design of Thermal Anomaly for Mammary Gland Tumor Phantom for Microwave Radiometer', *IEEE Trans. Biomed. Engineering*. Vol. 49, pp.694-699

Leroy, Y. Bocquet, B. & Mamouni, A. (1998). Non-invasive Microwave Radiometry Thermometry. *Physiol. Meas,* Vol.19, pp.127-148

Li, X.; Bond, E.; Van Veen, B. & Hagness, S. (2005). An Overview of Ultra Wide Band Microwave Imaging via Space-Time Beam Forming for Early-Stage Breast Cancer Detection. *IEEE Antennas and Propagation Magazine.* Vol. 47, No. 1, pp. 19-34

Locher, I. (2006). Technologies for System-on-Textile Integration. *PhD Thesis,* ETH Zürich, Zürich, Switzerland, 2006

Lundgren, B. (1981). Observations on Growth Rate of Breast Carcinomas and its Possible Implications for Lead Time. *Cancer.* Vol. 47, pp. 2769

MacDonald, I. (1951) Biological Predeterminism in Human Cancer. *Surg Gaenecol Obstet.* Vol. 92, pp. 443-452

Moskowitz, M. (1983). Screening for Breast Cancer. How Effective are our Tests? *CA Cancer J Clin. Vol.* 33, pp. 26-39

Moskowitz, M.(1995). Breast imaging, In:*Cancer of the Breast*, W.L Donegan & J.S. Spratt, (Eds.), , 206–239, Saunders, New York

Nathanson, S.; Zarbo,R.; Wachna, D.; Spence, C.; Andrzejewski, T. & Abrams, J. (2000). Microvessels That Predict Axillary Lymph Node Metastases in Patients with Breast Cancer. *Arch Surg.* Vol. 135, pp.586-594

Nealon T., Kongho A., Grossi C.(1979). Pathological Identification of Poor Prognosis of Stage I (T.N.M.) Cancer of the Breast. Ann. Surg, 1979:190, 129-32

Nosal, Z. (2001). Simple Model for Dynamic Range Estimate of GaAs Amplifiers', *IEEE-MTTS, Proc. Intern. Microwave Symp.* 2001

Osterman, K.; Kerner, T.; Williams, D.; Hartov, A.; Poplack, S. & Paulsen, K . (2000). Multifrequency Electrical Impedance Imaging: Preliminary In Vivo Experience in the Breast, *J. Phys Meas,* Vol.21, pp. 67-77

Paradiso, R.; Loriga, G. & Taccini, N.(2005). A Wearable Health Care System Based on Knitted Integrated Sensors', *IEEE Tran. Information Technology in Biomedicine.* Vol. 9, No. 3, pp. 337-344.

Reidy, J.(1988). Controversy Over Breast Cancer Detection. Br. Med. J. Vol. 297, pp. 932-3

Scilingo, E.; Gemignani, A.; Paradiso, R.; Taccini, N.; Ghelarducci, B. & De Rossi, D. (2005). Performance Evaluation of Sensing Fabrics for Monitoring Physiological and Biomechanical Variables. *IEEE Tran. Information Technology in Biomedicine,* Vol. 9, No. 3, pp. 345-352

Sickles, E. (1984). Mammographic Features of Early Breast Cancer. *Am J Roentgenol.* Vol.143, pp.461-464

Skou, N & Le Vine, D. (2006). *Microwave Radiometer Systems, Design and Analysis.* Artech House, ISBN 978-1-58053-974-6

Tetlow, R & Hubbard, A. (2000). Preliminary Results of a Pilot Study into the Diagnostic Value of T-scan in Detecting Breast Malignancies. *Breast Cancer Research Breast Cancer Res.,* Vol.2:A13

Thomas, D.; Gao, D.; Self,S.; Allison, C.; Tao, Y.; Mahloch, J.; Ray, R.; Qin, Q.; Presley, R. & Porter, P. (1997). Randomized Trial of Breast Self-Examination in Shanghai. Methodology and Preliminary Results, *J Natl Cancer Inst.* Vol. 5, pp. 355-65.

Van Langenhove, L. et al, 'Textile electrodes for monitoring cardio-respiratory signals', *European Conference on Protective Clothing,* Montreux, Switzerland, CDROM poster no. 27, May 21-24, 2003.

Van Langenhove, L.; Hertleer, C.; Catrysse, M.; Puers, R.; Van Egmond, H. & Matthys, D. (2003). The use of textile electrodes in a hospital environment', *AUTEX - World Textile Conference.* pp. 286-290, ISBN 83-89003-32-5, Gdansk, Poland, June 25-27, 2003

Vaupel, P.; Schlenger, K.; Knoop, C. & Hockel. M. (1991). Oxygenation of Human Tumors: Evaluation of Tissue Oxygen Distribution in Breast Cancers by Computerized $O_2$ Tension Measurements. *Cancer Res. Vol.*51, No.12, pp.3316–22

Vaupel, P.; Thews, O.; Kelleher, D. &. Hoeckel. M.(1998). Current Status of Knowledge and Critical Issues in Tumor Oxygenation, *Adv. Exp. Med. Biol.* Vol.454, pp.591–602

Wade, T. & Kozlowski, P. (2007). Longitudinal Studies of Angiogenesis in Hormone-Dependent Shionogi Tumors. *Neoplasia.* Vol.9, No.7, pp 563–568

Wang, Y.; Duster, J. & Kornegay, K. (2005). Design of an Ultra-wideband Low Noise Amplifier in 0.13m CMOS. *IEEE International Symposium on Circuits and Systems,* May 2005.

Weidner, N.; Folkman, J.; Pozza, F.; Bevilacqua, P.; Allred, E.; Moore, D.; Meli, S. & Gasparini, G. (1992). Tumor Angiogenesis: A New Significant and Independent Prognostic Indicator in Early-Stage Breast Carcinoma. *J. Natl. Cancer Inst.,* Vol. 84, No.24, pp. 1875–87

Xu, J. Woestenburg, B.; Geralt bij de Vaate, J. & Serdijn, W. (2005). GaAs 0.5 dB NF dual-loop negative-feedback broadband low-noise amplifier IC. *IEE Electronics Letters.* Vol. 41, No. 14, pp. 780 - 782

# 22

# Immunophenotyping of the Blast Cells in Correlations with the Molecular Genetics Analyses for Diagnostic and Clinical Stratification of Patients with Acute Myeloid Leukemia: Single Center Experience

Irina Panovska-Stavridis
*University Clinic of Hematology, Skopje*
*Republic of Macedonia*

## 1. Introduction

### 1.1 Acute leukemias

Acute leukemias are a heterogeneous group of malignancies that result from the malignant transformation of immature hematopoietic cells followed by clonal proliferation and accumulation of the transformed cells. They are characterized by aberrant differentiation and maturation of the malignant cells, with a maturation arrest and accumulation of more than 20% of leukemic blast in the bone marrow (Lichtman et al., 2010).

The natural history of acute leukemia and the response to therapy varies according to the type of blast involved in the leukemic process. Although in many instances the lineage assignment of the different types of blast cells may be recognized by simple morphological and cytochemical stains, it is necessary to employ immunological analyses with monoclonal antibodies and cytogenetic or molecular biological techniques to identify their particular differentiation features (Haferlach et al., 2007).

Acute leukemias are primarily characterized according to their differentiation along the myeloid and lymphoid lineage and they are divided into two main groups: acute myeloid leukemia (AML) and acute lymphoblastic leukemia (ALL). In 10% to 20% of patients, the leukemic cells have characteristics of both myeloid and lymphoid cells (Lichtman et al.,2010).

The classification of the acute leukemias underwent many changes in recent years. The French-American-British (FAB) classification of AML and ALL was based on cytomorphological and cytohemistry details only. Since then, the diagnostic of acute leukemias had undergone a complete change and the routine diagnostic work-up incorporated immunophenotyping by multiparameter flow cytometry, classical cytogenetics, molecular cytogenetics (comprising diverse fluorescence in situ hybridization techniques and comparative genomic hybridization) and molecular genetics (mostly polymerase chain reaction (PCR)-based techniques and sequencing) (Bennet et al., 1997; First MIC Cooperative Study Group, 1985; Haferlach et al., 2007).

According to the proceedings in diagnostic methods and the improved understanding of the diversity of acute leukemia subtypes, the latest World Health Organization (WHO) classification of acute leukemias incorporates and interrelates morphology, cytogenetics, molecular genetics and immunologic markers and pays major attention on the importance of genetic events in the classification, prognosis and therapy of the AMLs. Its prognostic relevance is most clearly demonstrated in the AMLs characterized by recurrent chromosome translocation: t(15,17), t(8,21) and inv(16)/t(16,16) which generally have a favorable prognosis when treated with appropriate therapeutic agents. All other genetic events identified among AMLs had strong prognostic meaning but did not influence on the therapeutic decision (Swerdlow et al., 2008).

In the WHO classification of precursor B-cell and T-cell neoplasms, immunophenotying of the malignant cells plays a decisive role in the diagnosis, prognosis and clinical stratification of patients (Swerdlow et al., 2008).

Correct diagnosis of the diverse subtypes of AML and ALL play a central role for individual clinical risk stratification and therapeutic decisions.

### 1.2 Acute myeloid leukemia

Acute myeloid leukemia (AML) is one of the most common types of leukemia in adults. It is characterized by limited myeloid differentiation of the malignant cells. The malignant cells characteristically undergo maturation arrest at the level of the early myloblast or promyelocyte, although varying proportions of mature hematopoietic cells are leukemia derived. The cells that display myeloid markers include morphology, Auer rods (aberrant primary granules), cytochemistry (Sudan black, myeloperoxidase, or nonspecific esterase), and cell surface antigens (Lichtman et al., 2010).

AML encompasses a family of hematologic malignancies that can be categorized according to their cytogenetic and associated genetic abnormalities, which have major prognostic importance. During recent years, considerable progress has been made in deciphering the molecular genetics and epigenetic basis of AML and in defining new diagnostic and prognostic markers. A growing number of recurring genetic changes have been recognized in the new WHO classification of AML. Furthermore, novel therapies are now being developed that target some of the genetic lesions and the treatment increasingly is being individualized by prognostic groups, with a goal of developing treatment tailored to the molecular basis of the patient's malignancy (Swerdlow et al., 2008).

#### 1.2.1 WHO classification of AML

The current WHO classification of AML reflects the fact that an increasing number of new clinico-pathologenetic entities of AML are categorized based upon their underlying cytogenetic or molecular genetic abnormalities (Swerdlow et al., 2008). A number of recurrent genetic abnormalities are adequately defined and are recognized as entities of AML. The subgroup "AML with recurrent genetic abnormalities" is comprised of entities that are defined with seven recurrent balanced translocations and inversions, and their variants. Two entities from this group: "AML with t(8;21)(q22;q22); AML1/ETO" and "AML with inv(16)(p13.1q22) or t(16;16)(p13.1;q22); CBFβ/MYH11" are considered as AML regardless of bone marrow blast counts. In "APL with t(15;17)(q22;q12); PML/RARα," RARα translocations with other partner genes are recognized separately. The former category "AML with 11q23 (MLL) abnormalities" is redefined in "AML with t(9;11)(p22;q23); MLLT3/MLL", and now is a unique entity. Three new cytogenetically defined entities also are incorporated: "AML with t(6;9)(p23;q34);DEK-NUP214", "AML with inv(3)(q21q26.2) or t(3;3)(q21;q26.2); RPN1-EVI1"; and "AML (megakaryoblastic) with t(1;22)(p13;q13); RBM15-MKL1," a rare leukemia most commonly occurring in infants (Vardiman et al., 2008).

Moreover, two new provisional entities defined by the presence of gene mutations between the group of cytogenetically normal AML (CN-AML) were added, "AML with mutated NPM1 (nucleophosmin)," and "AML with mutated CEBPA [CCAAT/enhancer binding protein(C/EBP), alpha]." There is growing evidence that these two gene mutations represent primary genetic lesions (so-called class II mutations), that impair hematopoietic differentiation, and when present alone in AML have favorable prognostic meaning. Mutations in the FMS-related tyrosine kinase 3 (FLT3) gene are found in many AML subtypes and are considered as class I mutations conferring a proliferation and/or survival advantage. AML with FLT3 mutations are not considered as a distinct entity, although determining the presence of those mutations is recommended by WHO because they have prognostic significance. The former subgroup termed "AML with multilineage dysplasia" is now designated "AML with myelodysplasia-related changes." Dysplasia in 50% or more of cells, in 2 or more hematopoietic cell lineages, was the diagnostic criterion for the former subset (Schhlenk et al, 2008; Vardiman et al.,2008)

However, the clinical significance of this morphologic feature has been questioned. AMLs are now categorized as "AML with myelodysplasia-related changes" if (1) they have a previous history of myelodysplastic syndrome (MDS) or myelodysplastic/myeloproliferative neoplasm (MDS/MPN) and evolve to AML with a marrow or blood blast count of 20% or more; (2) they have a myelodysplasia-related cytogenetic abnormality; or (3) if 50% or more of cells in 2 or more myeloid lineages are dysplastic (Swerdlow et al., 2008).

"Therapy-related myeloid neoplasms" has remained a distinct entity; however, since most patients have received treatment using both alkylating agents and drugs that target topoisomerase II for prior malignancy, a division according to the type of previous therapy is not often feasible. Therefore, therapy-related myeloid neoplasms are no longer subcategorized. Myeloid proliferations related to Down syndrome are now listed as distinct entities (Döhner et al., 2010).

A previous FAB classification is recognized in WHO classification as the entity AML, not otherwise specified. In this subgroup one can find the morphologic separation of AML according to the immaturity of leukemic cells as well as according to the hematopoietic lineage involved. This subtype of AML is reserved for the patients without the known cytogenetic or molecular genetic abnormalities. In some of them, there are markers associated with prognostic significance (Swerdlow et al., 2008; Vardiman et al, 2008).

The rare forms of AML and acute leukemia of ambiguous lineage recognized in WHO classification are also associated with poor prognosis (Döhner et al., 2010; Vardiman et al., 2008).

### 1.3 Diagnostic procedures

The diagnosis of the diverse subtypes of AML is a major challenge for modern hematology. Modern therapeutic concepts of AML are based on individual risk stratification in diagnosis and during follow-up. In the 1970s cytomorphology and cytochemistry represented the only available diagnostic tools. Nowadays, the routine diagnostic setting is completely changed and it consists of classic cytogenetics, molecular cytogenetics, molecular genetics and immunophenotyping by multi-parameter flow cytometry (Döhner et al., 2010 ).

### 1.3.1 Cytomorphology

First steps in the diagnostic work-up of a patient with suspected AML is a morphological evaluation of a classical bone marrow aspirate and a peripheral blood smear by using a May-Grunwald-Giemsa or a Wright-Giemsa stain. It is recommended that at least 200 leukocytes on blood smears and 500 nucleated cells on marrow smears to be counted. For a diagnosis of AML, a marrow or blood blast count of 20% or more is required, except for AML with t(15;17), t(8;21), inv(16) or t(16;16), and some cases of erythroleukemia. Myeloblasts, monoblasts, and megakaryoblasts are included in the blast count. Erythroblasts are not counted as blasts except in the rare instance of pure erythroid leukemia (Bennet et al,1997; Döhner et al., 2010; Panovska-Stavridis et al., 2008).

### 1.3.2 Cytochemistry

Lineage involvement could be identified with cytochemistry by using myeloperoxidase (MPO) or Sudan black B (SBB) and nonspecific esterase (NSE) stains. Detection of MPO (if present in > 3% of blasts) indicates myeloid differentiation, but its absence does not exclude a myeloid lineage because early myeloblasts and monoblasts may lack MPO. SBB staining parallels MPO but is less specific. NSE stains show diffuse cytoplasmic activity in monoblasts (usually 80% are positive) and monocytes (usually 20% positive). In acute erythroid leukemia, a periodic acid-Schiff (PAS) stain may show large globules of PAS positivity (Bennet et al,1997; Döhner et al., 2010, Panovska-Stavridis et al., 2008).

### 1.3.3 Immunophenotyping

Application of immunophenotyping together with the cytomorpohology and cytohemistry has a crucial role in the initial diagnosis of all cases with a suspected or proven diagnosis of acute leukemias. Immunophenotyping allows the discrimination of different cell population on the basis of their size, granularity, and antigen expression patterns. Flow cytometry is a powerful technology for characterization and analysis of cells. It simultaneously measures and analyzes multiple physical characteristics of single particles, usually cells, as they move in a fluid stream through a beam of light through an optical and/or electronic detection apparatus. Flow cytometry uses the principles of light scattering, light excitation, and emission of fluorochrome molecules to generate specific multi-parameter data from particles and cells in the size range of 0.5nm to 40nm diameter (Panovska-Stavridis et al., 2008).

The applied methodology detects cell surface antigens in a suspension of viable cells and cytoplasmic and nuclear antigens in previously fixed and stabilized cell suspension with the application of monoclonal antibodies conjugated with different fluorochromes. It permits simultaneous detection (multiparameter analyzes) of more than two membrane and nuclear or cytoplasmic antigens by means of double or multiple immunostaining (Bain et al., 2002; Bene et al., 1995; Döhner et al., 2010; Panovska-Stavridis et al., 2008).

### 1.3.4 Cytogenetics

Chromosome abnormalities are detected in approximately 55% of adult AML. Conventional cytogenetic analyses are part of the standard diagnostic approach of a patient suspected with AML. This allows the identification of genetics entities that deserve targeted treatments like acute promyelocytic leukemia (APL). Also, it allows the distinction of the disease with widely different prognosis. For example AML t(8;21)(q22;q22) with favorable risk versus AML abn 3q26 with adverse risk (Döhner et al., 2010; Grimwade D.,2001).

### 1.3.5 Molecular genetics

Numerous genetic abnormalities that escape cytogenetic detection like gene mutations and gene expression abnormalities are more recently discovered among CN-AML. Molecular diagnosis by reverse transcriptase- polymerase chain reaction (RT-PCR) for the frequent gene fusions, such as AML1/ETO, CBFβ/MYH11, MLLT3/MLL, DEK/NUP214, can also be useful in certain circumstances. RT-PCR, for which standardized protocols are already published, is also an excellent option to detect recurrent cytogenetic rearrangements, if chromosome morphology is of poor quality, or if there is typical marrow morphology but the suspected cytogenetic abnormality is not present. (Gabert et al., 2003; Beillard et al, 2003).

## 1.4 Prognostic factors

Prognostic factors of an AML case may be subdivided into those related to patient characteristics and general health condition and those related to characteristics particular to the AML clone. The former subset usually predicts treatment-related mortality (TRM) and becomes more important as patient age increases while the latter predicts resistance to, at least, conventional therapy.

### 1.4.1 Patient-related factors

Age, comorbidities, performance status and genetic variation in the drug metabolism are the main prognostic factors related to patients with AML. Increasing age is an important independent adverse prognostic factor (Appelbaum et al., 2006). Nonetheless, calendar age alone should not be a reason for not offering potentially curative therapy to an older patient because age is not the most important prognostic factor for either TRM or resistance to therapy. Currently all patients under the age of 60 are candidates to receive standard intensive chemotherapy and according to prognostic factors stem cell transplantation or intensive chemotherapy as postremission therapy. It has to be stressed that age as a factor is not only dependent on so-called „calendar age". Recently many older patients with a good clinical status have been successfully treated with intensive chemotherapy. Attention should be given to a careful evaluation and documentation of comorbidities. Comorbidity scoring is a current field of investigation and should contribute to a better definition of the patient considered "unfit" for intensive chemotherapy (Piccirillo et al., 2004; Sorror et al., 2005).

### 1.4.2 AML-related factors

According to the AML working party of European Leukemia Net, several important and independent prognostic factors have been recognized: white blood cell counts, existence of prior MDS or AML with MDS features, previous cytotoxic therapy for another malignancy, and cytogenetic and molecular abnormalities in leukemic cells (Döhner et al., 2010).

#### 1.4.2.1 Cytogenetics

Chromosome abnormalities are detected in approximately 55% of adult AML. Although, there is a diversity of cytogenetic entities of AML, the karyotype of the leukemic cells is the strongest prognostic factor for response to induction therapy and for survival for AML patients

(Swerdlow et al., 2008). Younger adult patients are commonly categorized into 3 risk groups, favorable, intermediate, or adverse. The favorable group is represented by the reciprocal translocations t(15;17)/PML/RARα, t(8;21)/AML1/ETO, and inv(16)/CBFβ/MYH11, which are associated with a favorable prognosis In contrast, AML associated with t(9;11)(p22;q23) shows an inferior prognosis. These subgroups represent the first hierarchy of the WHO classification of AML, emphasizing that these subtypes represent distinct biologic entities. The second subgroup of AML patients shows a normal karyotype and an intermediate prognosis. However, from molecular aspects, this subgroup is very heterogeneous. Lately, there are emerging data suggesting that two genetics entities from this group, the AML with mutation of NPM1 gene without FLT3 mutations and AML with mutation in CEBPA gene should be moved from the intermediate prognosis group to the favorable group of AML. Those two entities are also added to the new WHO classification (Schlenk et al., 2008). The third (prognostically unfavorable) subgroup includes mostly unbalanced karyotypes characterized by a gain or loss of larger chromosomal regions. Within these, an especially complex aberrant karyotype, which occurs in 10% to 12% of patients and that is defined by ≥3 chromosomal anomalies shows a very unfavorable prognosis. Cytogenetics is further helpful to delineate patients with therapy related AML (t-AML), who are classified as third hierarchy in the WHO classification, and developed either after treatment with alkylating agents often associated with cytogenetic aberrations involving 5q-, −7, or p53 and complex aberrant karyotype or are showing MLL/11q23 or other balanced cytogenetic aberrations which are in frequent association to previous treatment with topoisomerase II inhibitors One striking observation is the increasing incidence of adverse versus favorable cytogenetic abnormalities with increasing age. This, at least in part, contributes to the poorer outcome of AML in older adults. (Byrd et al., 2002; Schlenk et al., 2008, Swerdlow et al., 2008)

#### 1.4.2.2 Molecular genetics

Nowadays, considerable progress has been made in elucidating the molecular pathogenesis of acute leukemias that resulted in identification of new molecular diagnostic and prognostic markers. Gene mutations and deregulated gene expression have been identified that allow us to interpret the genetic diversity within defined cytogenetic groups, in particular the large and heterogeneous group of patients with CN-AML. Risk stratification by molecular markers in patients from the former group of AML plays an increasing role at diagnosis. The most relevant markers, which can be detected alone or in coincidence with other mutation are NPM1 mutations that is detected in approximately 40% of cases, MLL-PTD in 6%, NRAs in 8-10%, CEBPA in 10% and FLT3-TKD mutations in 6% of CN-AML. Thus, a rather of limited number of markers further subclassifies more than 85% of CN-AML. Data from the literature suggest that those markers have different prognosis regarding the outcome of the disease and they all indicate that in the near future molecular screening may allow " targeted allogeneic stem cell transplantation (alloSCT)" in AML patients with normal karyotype (Schlenk et al., 2008; Koreth et al, 2009).

There is a growing list of the new genetic abnormalities with clinical value that are being investigated. These genetic events perturb diverse cellular pathways and functions, and they often confer a profound impact upon the clinical phenotype of the disease and treatment response.

It is anticipated that advances in molecular technology will reveal additional markers that will result in more precise classification of this heterogeneous complex of disorders (Löwenberg B., 2008b; Haferlach T., 2008)

### 1.5 Treatment

The parallel progress of the development of the diagnostic techniques improvement of the classification and therapeutical approach lead acute leukemia which were for the first time described before 150 years, and in the 1970s were still fatal disease nowadays to have overall 5 years survival rates of up to 40%. (Appelbaum et al, 2001).

Despite heterogeneity of the disease, with the exception of acute promyelocytic leukemia, this disease has been treated with a "one size fits all" approach. Although, the vast majority of AML patients can be individually characterized on the basis of the distinct chromosomal aberrations and molecular markers, treatment of AML is still based on quite unspecific cytotoxic therapy. For almost 40 years, the use of continuous infusion of cytarabine combined with another agent, usually an anthracycline, the "3+7" regimen, has been the mainstay of therapy (Yates et al, 1973). Response rates for induction with standard chemotherapy ranged from 70% to 80% for adults aged less than 60years which are enrolled in clinical trials and average in 50% for patients older than 60 years (Lichtman et al.,2010) .

Alternative consolidation therapies by applying additional chemotherapy, autologous stem cell transplantation (autoSCT) or alloSCT based on the initial cytogenetic and molecular studies are available (Cornelissen J.J.et al.(2007); Fernandez H.F.,2010; Koreth et al, 2009)

As more sophisticated molecular techniques have become available, it is clear that it is still possible to detect residual disease when all morphological and functional criteria for remission are met. Techniques such as "real–time"-quantitative polymerase chain reaction (RQ-PCR) are capable of detection at a level of 1 in $10^4$ or 1 in $10^5$ residual cells, but such markers are available for only a minority of cases in which the molecular lesion has been characterized(Freeman et al., 2008).

AlloSCT is the most effective antileukemic modality that is characterized by immune mediated graft-versus-leukemia effect of the transplanted cells that reduce the risk of relapse considerably and improve the relapse-free survival but also is associated with the increased risk of death and morbidity. Therefore, the alloSCT advantage has to be carefully balanced against the excess mortality (ranging between 10% and 40%) and morbidity due to transplant-related complications, such as infection and graft-versus-host disease that are typically connected with alloSCT and can diminish all of the benefit of a reduced risk of relapse. (Cornelissen et al., 2007). For this reason, allogeneic stem cell transplantation is usually avoided in a type of AML that has a pattern of cytogenetics with a relatively favorable prognosis, such as AML with the chromosomal translocations t(8;21) or inv(16)/t(16;16)(Marcucci et al., 2000; Perea et al.,2006). In the latter subtypes the risk of relapse is in the order of 35% to 40% or less. By contrast, a transplant is treatment of choice for all other patient whose leukemia cells bear a cytogenetic or molecular abnormality that predicts a high or intermediate risk of relapse after chemotherapy (Löwenberg et al., 2008b; Koreth et al, 2009). Exception could be done for two additional genotypically defined subsets of AML that are categorized as low-risk within the large category of CN-AML. Each of those entities has a risk of relapse of about 35%. The first genotype is defined by the presence of 'favorable' mutations in *NPM1* and the absence of concurrent 'unfavorable' *FLT3*-internal tandem duplications (*NPM1*mut /*FLT3*-ITDneg).61 This genotype accounts for approximately 16% of all newly diagnosed patients younger than 60 years old. There is no demonstrable benefit from transplantation in patients with *NPM1*mut/*FLT3*-ITDneg AML. The second subset of AML with 'favorable' mutations in the transcription factor gene *CEBPA* (*CEBPA*mut) could not be analyzed in this way because of a lack of statistical power due to a limited number of cases. The latter low-risk subtype *CEBPA*mut accounts for 8% of all AML. Nevertheless, the available body of evidence suggests that these AMLs are unlikely to profit from an alloSCT (Schlenk et al., 2008).

Thus, it could be concluded that patients with AML with t(8;21), AML with inv(16)/t(16;16), AML with *NPM1*mut/ *FLT3*-ITDneg and AML with *CEBPA* mutations should not considered for alloSCT. Nevertheless, it is important to stress that sufficient evidence so far exist only for the AML with recurrent cytogenetic abnormalities and the benefits for the two additional genetic low-risk AML entities should be validated in the larger studies in the future (Schlenk et al., 2008).

In the near future these results will also need to be considered more specifically in the light of the extended scale of allogeneic stem cell transplantation strategies with respect to reduced-intensity conditioning regimens and in relationship to different transplant sources and donor types (matched unrelated and haploidentical donors, umbilical stem cell grafts).(Löwenberg et al, 2008a)

## 2. Motivation and aim of the study

Correct diagnosis of the diverse subtypes of acute myeloid leukemia (AML) and acute lymphoblastic leukemia (ALL) play a central role for individual clinical risk stratification and therapeutic decisions. Modern therapeutic concepts of AML are based on individual risk stratification at diagnosis and during follow-up. The ultimate test of any disease diagnostic algorithm approach is its usefulness in guiding the selection of effective treatment strategies. (Haferlach et al., 2007, Löwenberg et al, 2008b) As discussed above, cytogenetic as well as various genomic markers (gene mutations, gene overexpression) may provide input for algorithms for remission induction and post-remission treatment decisions. At the same time, it remains appropriate to realize that prognostic factors in fact remain a moving target and they are only relevant to therapies available at a given time. Algorithms that provide a basis for risk-adapted therapeutic choices may include immunological markers, cytogenetic factors, molecular markers as well as clinical parameters (e.g., age, attainment of an early or late complete remission) and hematological determinants (e.g., secondary AML, white blood cell count at diagnosis).

On the other hand, the more carefully AML is studied, the clearer it becomes that there is considerable heterogeneity between cases with respect to morphology, immunological phenotype, associated cytogenetic and molecular abnormalities and, more recently, patterns of gene expression. This is reflected in the substantially different responses to treatment. Some entities are becoming so distinct that they are regarded as different diseases with specific approaches to treatment.

In order to improve and simplify the diagnosis and management of AML patients that are diagnosed and treated at the at the University Clinic of Hematology-Skopje we conducted a prospective study to establish and standardize a diagnostic algorithm based on minimal screening tests which will facilitate risk adapted therapy for each single AML patient. The aims of our study were: first, to establish the correct lineage assignment of the blast cells, second, to evaluate the incidence of the favorable genetic markers PML/RARα, AML1/ETO and CBFβ/MYH11 among the AML cases, then to correlate the obtained results with the patient age, comorbidities, and performance status and consecutively to select the effective treatment strategy for each single acute leukemia patient.

## 3. Material and methods

### 3.1 Patients and samples

A total of 76 adult (>15 years) patients (from initially 77 tested) with acute leukemia who were consecutively admitted at the Clinic of Hematology-Skopje from January through December 2008 were enrolled in this study. The median age of the patients (41 men, 35 women) was 52 $\pm$ 18.66 years (range 16-80), and most of the patients 37 (48.7%) were between 55 and 75 years old. The diagnosis was made by standard morphological examination and cytochemical analyses of bone marrow smears according to the criteria established by the FAB Cooperative Study Group (Bennet et al, 1997) and confirmed by immunophenotyping of bone marrow aspirates and/or peripheral blood samples (Bain et al., 2002; Bene et al., 1995 ) following the criteria of the European Group for the Immunological Classification of leukemias (EGIL) and the British Committee for Standards in Hematology (BCSH) (Bain et al., 2002; Bene et al., 1995). Consecutively, patients were further stratified in the adequate genetic AML entities according to the results of the molecular analyses. The samples contained more than 20% of blast cells (most of which had more than 50%). All patients were tested for the presence of the fusion transcript of the mayor recurrent cytogenteic abnormalities in AML (PML/RARα, AML1/ETO, CBFβ/MYH11) by RT-PCR, according to standard procedures. (Gabert et al.2003; Beillardet al, 2003).

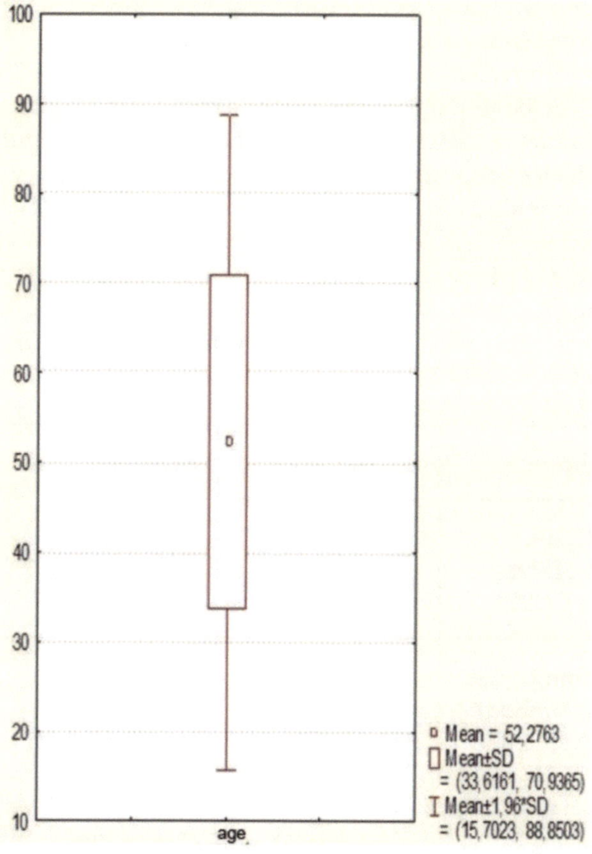


Fig. 1. Average age of the patients in the study group

### 3.1.1 Clinical data from the patients

Clinical data from the patients were collected according the internal protocol that was approved by the University Clinic of Hematology Institutional Review Board. All included patients had to sign a written consent.

## 3.2 Morphology

The morphology was analyzed by microscopic examination of >500 nonerythroid cells on May Gruenwald Giemza stained air-dried bone marrow smears (Bennet et al,1997; Döhner et al., 2010; Panovska-Stavridis et al., 2008).

## 3.3 Cytochemical analysis

Air-dried bone marrow smears were stained for MPO, non specific esterase (NSE) and periodic acid-Schiff (PAS) according to the manufacturers guidelines. The percentage of positive cells for either stain was assessed by microscopic examination of 200 nonerythroid cells (Bennet et al, 1997; Döhner et al., 2010; Panovska-Stavridis et al., 2008).

## 3.4 Immunophenotyping

The muliparameter flow cytometry (MPF) was performed at the beginning at the Institute for Immunobiology and Human Genetics, Faculty of Medicine-Skopje and then continued at the University Clinic of Hematology-Skopje. Immunophenotyping was done first, by using Cytomation (DAKO-Cytomation) flow-cytometer and than by BD FACSCanto™ II analyzer, on whole blood and/or bone marrow specimens using lysing solutions (BD-Biosciensies, San Jose.CA. USA)(Bain et al., 2002). We prepare the samples for simultaneous detection of three cytoplasmic/nuclear and membrane antigens. The first step involved immunostaining of cell suspension with multiple panels of tree monoclonal antibodies (McAb) labeled with fluorescein (FITC), phycoerythrin (PE) and phycoerythryn-Cy5 tandem complex (Pe-Cy5) as third color (Panovska-Stavridis et al., 2008). The slightly modified panel of monoclonal antibodies (McAb) against myeloid- and lymphoid-associated antigens as suggested by the EGIL was utilized (Bain et al., 2002; Panovska-Stavridis et al., 2008). The antibodies and their manufacturers are listed in Table 1.

| | B-lineage | T-lineage | Myeloid markers | Non-lineage restricted |
|---|---|---|---|---|
| First line | CD19, cyt CD79b, cyt CD22 | CD 2, CD7, cyt CD3 | CD117,CD13, CD33,CD14, CD15, anti-MPO, anti-lisosyme | TdT, CD34, HLA-DR, CD 56 |
| Second line | SmIg (kappa/lambda)**, cytIgM[2],CD138 | CD1a,mCD3[1], CD4,CD5,CD8, anti TCR $\alpha/\beta$, anti TCR $\gamma/\delta$*** | CD41, CD61, CD42,CD71 Anti-glycophorin A | CD38 |

All markers were manufactured by BD-Biosciences, except antilysozyme (DAKO); 1.cyt: cytoplasmic; 2.m: membrane *MPO: myloperoxidase;** SmIg:surface immunoglobulin;*** TCR:T cell receptor

Table 1. Panel of monoclonal antibodies (McAb) for diagnosis of acute leukemias

For the detection of cytoplasmic and nuclear antigens we used commercially available permeabilization/fixation solutions (FACS Permeabilization solution BDBiosciencies;San Jose.CA.USA) ((Bain et al., 2002).
We incubated 100ml of specimens (peripheral blood or bone marrow) and appropriate McAb for 15min at room temperature, than added the permeabilization solutions and/or lysing solution and repeated the incubation procedure. After the incubation we washed the samples three times with PBS-A, than re-suspended the cell with isotones solution and acquired the data. As control we used a lysed, but unstained sample (Panovska-Stavridis et al., 2008)
Acquired data were analyzed with software by using CD45 gating strategy (Borowitz et al, 1993). This technique involves incubation of all samples with fluorochrome - labeled CD45 McAb and with the McAb for which reactivity needs to be established with an alternative fluorochrome). In the initial step of the analyses, gating was set up on a CD45-positive versus light side-scatter dot plot. The procedure allowed the discrimination between the blast cell population and normal cells and the exclusion of platelets and debris. Thereafter, if necessary, it was possible to perform another gating, to separate the cells positive with the McAb under study (Borowitz et al, 1993). Leukemias were first screened by the primary panel and, if necessary, further characterized by the McAb of the secondary panel (Bain et al., 2002).
Antigen expression was considered positive if 20% or more blast cells reacted with a particular antibody, except reactivity of blasts cells with MPO. It was considered positive if 10% or more of mononuclear cells were MPO positive (Bain et al., 2002; Döhner et al., 2010).

### 3.5 Molecular analysis

Mononuclear cell preparation, RNA isolation, and cDNA synthesis were performed at the Department of Molecular Biology, Immunology and Pharmacogenetics, Faculty of Pharmacy-Skopje, according to standard procedures. Aliquots of 5 µL of cDNA (100 ng RNA equivalent) were used for Real-time Quantitative polymerase chain reaction (RQ-PCR) with primers and dual-labeled probes as described by Gabert et al. Positions and nucleotide sequences of the primers and probes are shown in Table 2.
The RQ-PCR reaction was performed in a 25-µl reaction volume using 12.5 µl (1x) Master Mix (Applied Biosystems), 300nM primers and 200nM probes on a Mx3005P(TM) QPCR System (Stratagene) under the following conditions: 95°C for 10min, followed by 50 cycles of 95°C for 15s, 50°C for 1min. In order to correct variations in RNA quality and quantity and to calculate the sensitivity of each measurement, a control gene (CG) transcript was amplified in parallel to the fusion gene (FG) transcript. Since ABL (Abelson) gene transcript expression did not differ significantly between normal and leukemic samples, ABL was used as a control gene in this study (24). Positions and nucleotide sequences of the primers and probe are shown in Table 2.

### 3.6 Statistical analysis

Statistical analyses were performed by using the statistical analyses software SPSS 18.0 and by applying the Descriptive statistics (cross tabulation, frequencies, descriptive ratio statistics), bivariate statistics (means, t-test, correlation (bivariate, partial, distances), nonparametric tests and linear regression statistical methods. The Level of probability for obtaining the null hypothesis, in accordance with the international conventions for bio-medical sciences was 0.05 or 0.01 (Armitage et al., 2002).

| Transcript | EAC code[a] | Primer/probe localization, 5'–'3' position (size) | Sequence |
|---|---|---|---|
| AML1 /ETO | ENF701 | AML1, 1005–1026 (22) | 5'-CAC CTA CCA CAG AGC CAT CAA A-3' |
| | ENR761 | ETO, 318–297 (22) | 5'-ATC CAC AGG TGA GTC TGG CAT T-3' |
| | ENP747 | AML1, 1049–295 (30) | FAM 5'-AAC CTC GAA ATC GTA CTG AGA AGC ACT CCA-3' TAMRA |
| PML /RARα | ENF905 | PML, 1198–1216 (19) | 5'-CCG ATG GCT TCG ACG AGT T-3' |
| | ENF906 | PML, 1642–1660 (19) | 5'-ACC TGG ATG GAC CGC CTA G-3' |
| | ENF903 | PML, 1690–1708 (19) | 5'-TCT TCC TGC CCA ACA GCA A-3' |
| | ENR962 | RARA, 485–465 (21) | 5'-GCT TGT AGA TGC GGG GTA GAG-3' |
| | ENR942 | RARA, 439–458 (20) | FAM 5'-AGT GCC CAG CCC TCC CTC GC-3' TAMRA |
| CBFβ /MYH11 | ENF803 | CBFB, 389–410 (22) | 5'-CAT TAG CAC AAC AGG CCT TTG A-3' |
| | ENR862 | MYH11, 1952–1936 (17) | 5'-AGG GCC CGC TTG GAC TT-3' |
| | ENR863 | MYH11, 1237–1217 (21) | 5'-CCT CGT TAA GCA TCC CTG TGA-3' |
| | ENR865 | MYH11, 1038–1016 (23) | 5'-CTC TTT CTC CAG CGT CTG CTT AT-3' |
| | ENPr843 | CBFB, 434–413 (22) | FAM 5'-TCG CGT GTC CTT CTC CGA GCC T-3' TAMRA |
| ABL | ENF1003 | ABL, 372–402 (31) | 5'-TGGAGATAACACTCTAAGCATAACTAAAGGT-3' |
| | ENF1063 | ABL, 495–515 (21) | 5'-GATGTAGTTGCTTGGGACCCA-3' |
| | ENF1043 | ABL, 467–494 (28) | FAM 5'-CCA TTT TTG GTT TGG GCT TCA CAC CAT T-3' TAMRA |
| [a]ENF = forward primer, ENR = reverse primer, ENP = TaqMan probe | | | |

Table 2. Sequences and positions of the RQ-PCR primers and probes

## 4. Results

In the period of twelve months, between January and December 2008, 77 patients were submitted and tested for acute leukemia at the University Clinic of Hematology-Skopje. Cyto-morphological analyses showed that the average rate of the blast cells in the differential blood counts and in the bone marrow was 54.6%(3-99.0%) and 73,5%(20-98.0%) respectively. In 7 patients blast cells were not detected initially.

**4.1 Results from the cytochemical analyses**

Results from the cytochemical analyses and the images of peripheral smears with positive examples from different cytochemical staining are presented at Figure 2 and Photo 1 respectively.

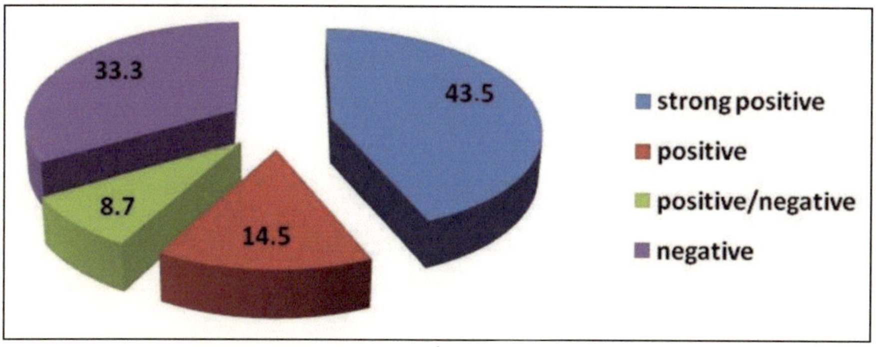


A

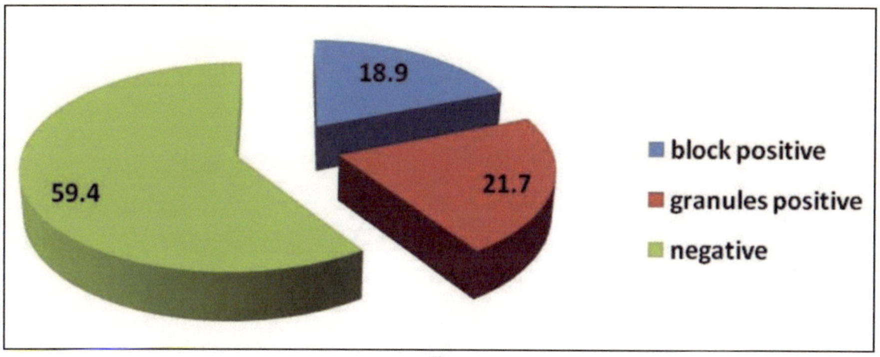


B

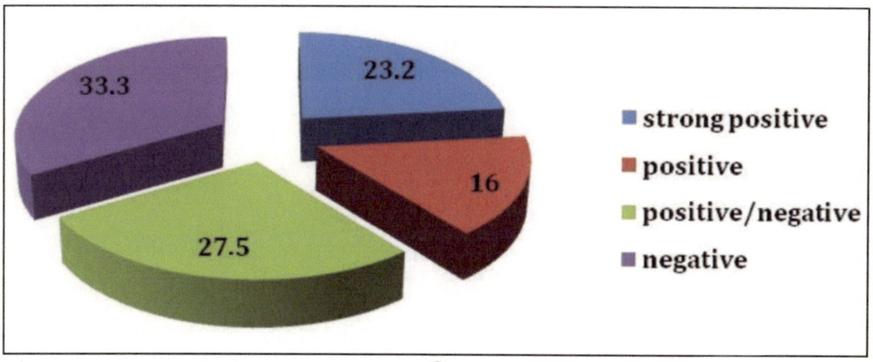


C

Fig. 2. Distribution of patients according to reactivity with different cytochemial staining. A:Patient distribution according to MPO reactivity of the blasts cells. B: Patient distribution according to PAS reactivity of the blasts cells. C: Patient distribution according to NSE reactivity of the blasts cells.

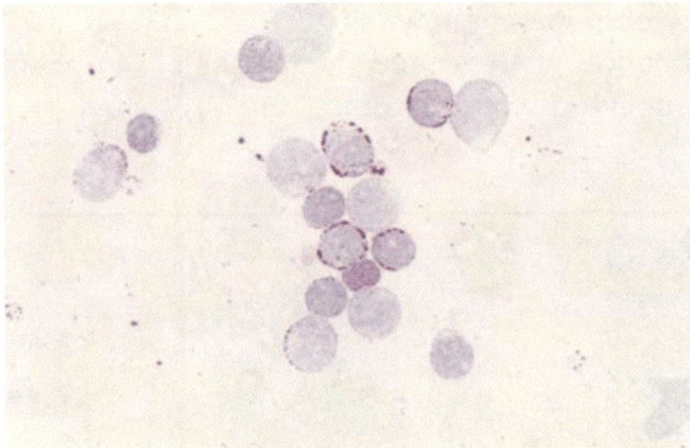

A

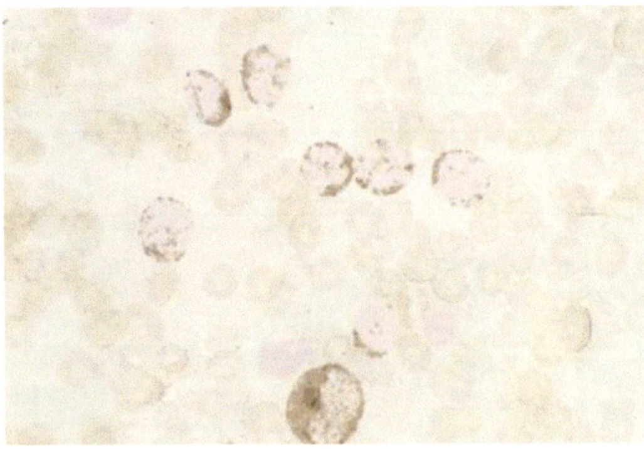

B

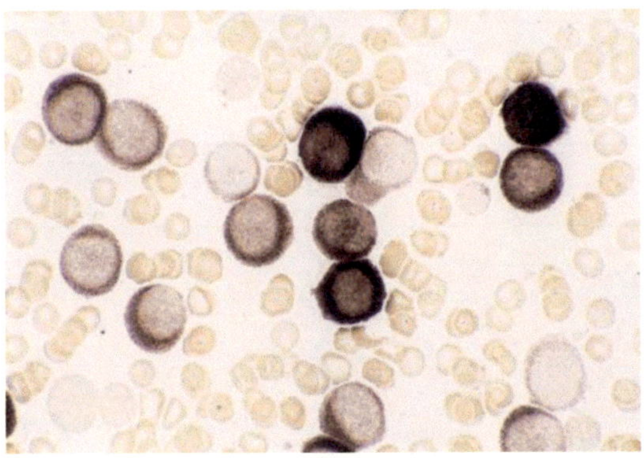

C

Photo 1. Images from positive reactivity of peripheral blast cells with different cytochemical staining , A: PAS reactivity, B: POX reactivity, C: NSE reactivity

Statistical analyses showed that there is a statistically significant correlation between the AML and MPO positivity ($X^2$ with Yates's correction=16.628 $p<0.01$)(Figure 2A). According to cross reaction ratio, MPO positivity presents statistically significant risk which improves the chance of AML diagnosis for 39 times (OR=392.1603 ($4.177<0R<305.9796$, CI 95%)). Also, a statistically significant correlation was noted between the PAS positivity and ALL ($X^2$ with Yates's correction=5.514 $p<0.01$)( Figure 2B). Strong PAS positivity was registered in 75% of ALL cases. Regarding the cytochemical stain NSE and AML no statistical correlation was observed ($X^2$ with Yates's correction=2.456 p=0.117), expect for AML M4 and M5 entities which showed statistically significant correlation (p<0, 05) (Figure 2C).

Morphology and cytochemistry established myeloid lineage in 57 (74.0%) cases and lymphoid differentiation in 11 (14.3%) cases (Figure 2). Morphology and cytochemistry did not establish lineage involvement in 9 (11.7%) cases. Basic morphological and cytochemical analyses established the lineage assignment of the blasts cells in 68 (88.3%) patients.

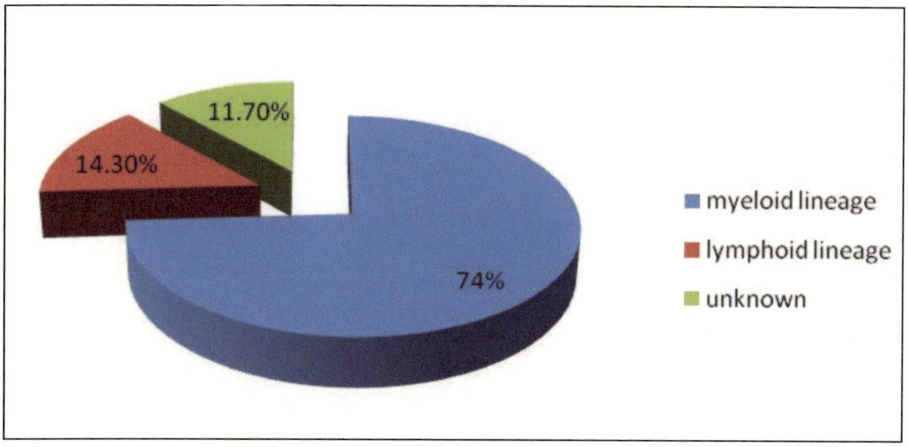


Fig. 3. Distribution of cases based on lineage assignment of blasts cells detected with basic morphological and cytochemial analyses

### 4.2 Results from the immunological analyses

Immunological analyses with multi-parameter flow-cytometry were performed in all 77 patients. Further immunological analyses of cases in which lineage could not be assigned based on morphology and cytochemistry established myeloid lineage in 4 patients, (AML-M0) and one case indicated nonhematopoietic malignancy. In this case, immunophenotype of the malignant cells (CD45-/CD56+/CD9+) indicated a neuroectodermal origin of the malignant cells (Bain et al., 2002). Later neuroblastoma was diagnosed in this patient. Immunological analyses change the assigned lineage based on morphology and cytochemistry in 3(3.8%) of the patients from lymphoid to myeloid. The results of our study showed that routine immunophenotyping improved diagnosis in 12 (15.5%) cases.

Consequently, based on FAB and immunologic criteria of EGIL and BTSH 64 acute leukemias were classified as myeloid. Correlation between the antigen expressions with FAB morphology of AML cases which confirmed the AML diagnosis in 83. 1% of the cases is presented at Table 3. According to FAB criteria, the leukemias were classified as M0 (n=4), M1 (n=8), M2 (n=20), M3 (n=5), M4 (n=17), M4-Eo (n=1), M5 (n=8), M6 (n=1).

Multivariate Cox-proportional regression analyses showed that in 89.7% of AML cases lineage assignment is defined with the following five markers: CD13, CD33, CD117, HLA-DR and anti-MPO. Most frequently detected maturation myeloid marker which was expressed in 42.9% of AML case was CD15. Twenty three (35.9 %) of AML patients showed expression of lymphoid antigens. Co-expression of two lymphoid markers was detected in eleven (17.1%) cases, and most frequently co-expressed lymphoid marker was CD7 and was detected in 28.5% of the cases.

| | CD45 | CD117 | CD13 | CD14 | CD15 | CD33 | CD10 | CD34 | HLA-DR | MPO | Lysosime | TdT | CD2 | CD7 | CD19 | CD56 |
|---|---|---|---|---|---|---|---|---|---|---|---|---|---|---|---|---|
| Number of tested patients | 64 | 64 | 64 | 64 | 64 | 64 | 64 | 64 | 64 | 64 | 64 | 64 | 64 | 64 | 64 | 64 |
| Number of positive patients (%) | 63 (98.4) | 53 (82.8) | 57 (89.2) | 17 (26.7) | 28 (43.7) | 57 (89.2) | 5 (7.8) | 40 (62.5) | 55 (85.9) | 46 (71.8) | 30 (46.8) | 8 (12.5) | 10 (15.6) | 18 (28.1) | 3 (4.6) | 15 (23.4) |
| FAB morphology | | | | | | | | | | | | | | | | |
| M0 | 4 | 2 | 1 | 0 | 0 | 2 | 0 | 4 | 4 | 4 | 0 | 2 | 0 | 1 | 0 | 0 |
| M1 | 8 | 7 | 7 | 0 | 0 | 8 | 2 | 6 | 7 | 6 | 0 | 3 | 1 | 4 | 0 | 1 |
| M2 | 21 | 20 | 19 | 1 | 6 | 18 | 1 | 16 | 17 | 18 | 6 | 1 | 0 | 0 | 2 | 7 |
| M3 | 4 | 4 | 4 | 0 | 4 | 4 | 0 | 2 | 1 | 4 | 4 | 0 | 1 | 2 | 0 | 2 |
| M4 | 17 | 14 | 15 | 8 | 8 | 16 | 4 | 9 | 16 | 12 | 12 | 0 | 5 | 6 | 0 | 3 |
| M4E-0 | 1 | 1 | 1 | 1 | 1 | 1 | 0 | 0 | 1 | 1 | 1 | 2 | 0 | 1 | 1 | 0 |
| M5 | 9 | 4 | 7 | 7 | 9 | 7 | 1 | 2 | 8 | 1 | 7 | 0 | 3 | 4 | 0 | 2 |
| M6 | 0 | 1 | 1 | 0 | 0 | 1 | 0 | 1 | 1 | 0 | 0 | 0 | 0 | 0 | 0 | 0 |

Table 3. Correlation between the antigen expressions with FAB morphology of AML cases

### 4.3 Results from the molecular analyses

Molecular evaluation of AML cases demonstrated presence of the three major recurrent genetic abnormalities as follows: 5 patients were positive for the fusion transcript PML/RAR α (Figure 5), 3 patients were positive for AML/ETO1 and 7 for the fusion transcript CBFβ/MYH11 (Figure 4).

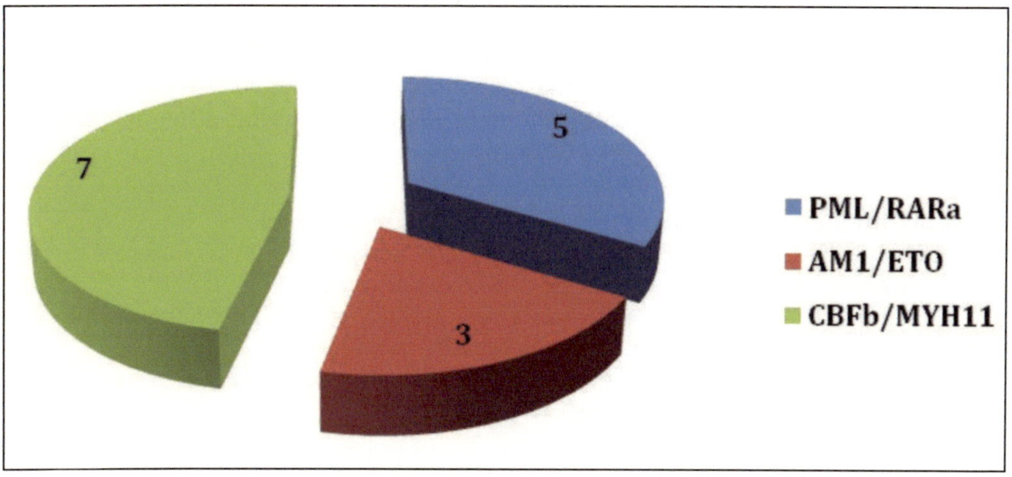


Fig. 4. Distribution of molecular abnormalities detected with the RQ-PCR assay in the group of AML patients;

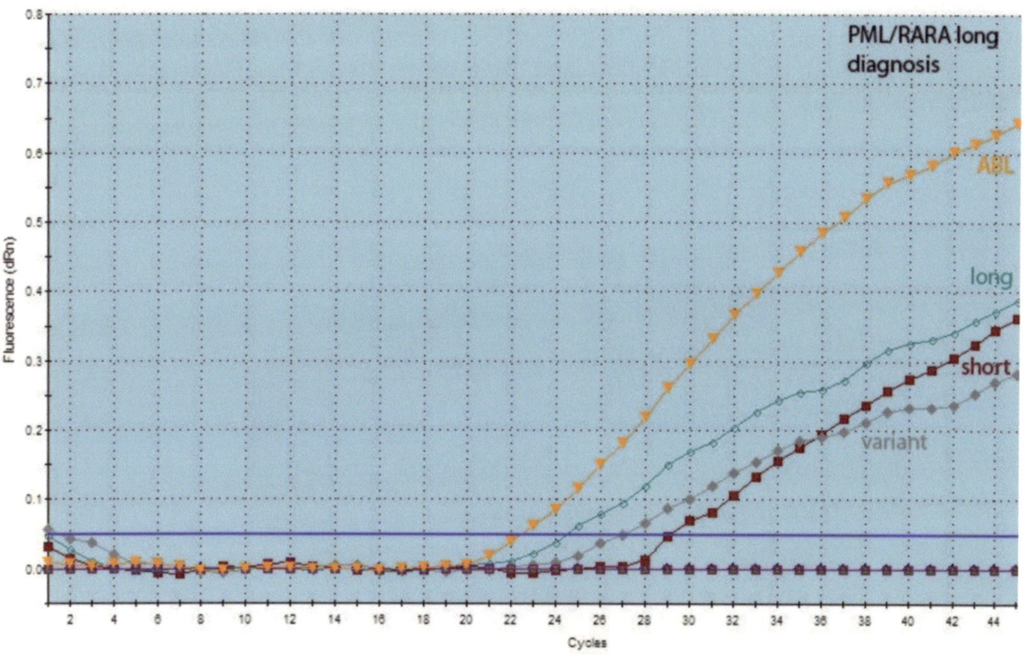


Fig. 5. Detection of fusion transcript PML/RARα using the RQ-PCR method

In 5 of the AML case PML/RARα fusion transcript was detected. Four of those patients had morphology and immunophenotype that correlate with AML-M3 diagnosis. The five patients were first diagnosed as AML-M2 and only after the positive result for PML/RARα the diagnosis was revised as AML-M3. In all those five patients target therapy with ATRA was initiated.
RT-PCR analysis also detected molecular abnormalities in the Core binding factor (CBF) in 10 AML patients; the presence of the AML/ETO1 fusion gene was confirmed in 3 patient and CBFβ/MYH11 in 7 patients.
Molecular analyses enabled 23.7% of the cases from our study to be classified in the adequate genetic entities of AML with different prognosis requiring different therapeutic approach.

### 4.4 Results from the analyses of the clinical data of the patients

We evaluate the distributions of the patients from our study group in the different grades of the Eastern Cooperative Oncology Group (EKOG) performance status scale (Oken et al. 1982)(Figure 6). All the patients with EKOG performance status higher than grade 2 and patients with serious co morbidities were not suitable candidates for alloSCT.
Furthermore, all the obtained results were correlated and consecutively effective treatment strategy for each single acute leukemia patient was selected.

## 5. Discussion

Modern diagnostic approach for acute leukemias combines cytomorphology, cytochemistry, multiparameter flow cytometry, chromosome banding analysis, accompanied by diverse fluorescence in situ hybridization techniques, and molecular analyses. The correct diagnosis is essential for classification of this heterogeneous complex of disorders and plays a central role for individual risk stratification and therapeutic decisions (Haferlach et al., 2007; Lichtman et al., 2010)

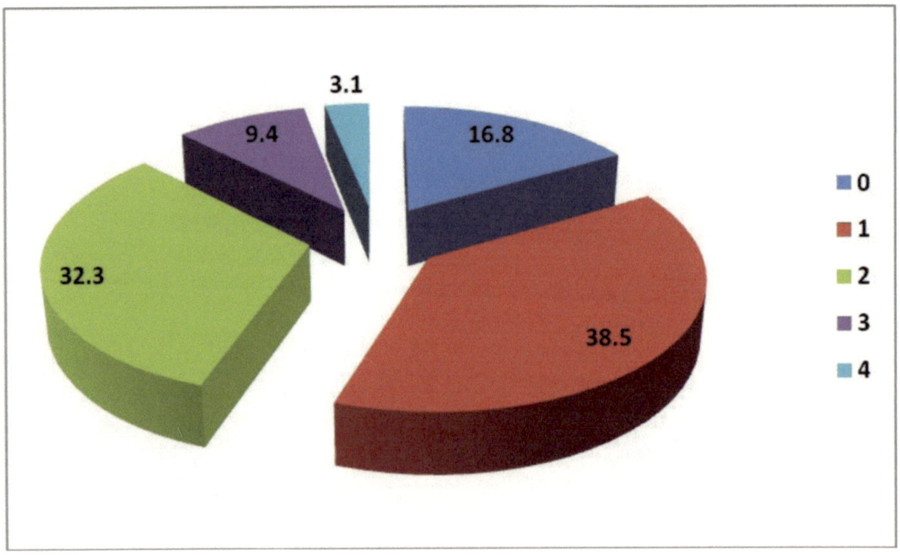


Fig. 6. Distribution of patients according to the grades of the EKOG performance status

### 5.1 Immunophenotyping in modern diagnosis of AML

Assignment of lineage is critical in the diagnostic evaluation of acute leukemia, as treatment for AML and ALL markedly differs. Myeloid and lymphoid lineage may be distinguished based on cellular morphology, cytochemical staining, and expression of lineage-specific antigens (Döhner et al., 2010). Analyses of diagnostic evaluation of acute leukemia in our study showed that immunophenotyping was necessary for lineage assignment in 4 (8.9%) cases that were morphologically and cytochemically undifferentiated, and also for correction of the lineage that was assigned based on morphology and cytochemistry in 3(3.8%) additional cases.

Flow cytometric immunophenotyping is a powerful technological tool that aids in the diagnosis, classification and monitoring of hematological malignancies. It is essential in the diagnosis of AML, as it demonstrates a particular lineage involvement and has a prognostic significance in the majority of AML cases. We used the panel based on the recommendation of the EGIL group and BTSH. Our analyses comprised of a two step process with the first panel of markers being applied to all cases of acute leukemia and the second only in patients with AML that did not demonstrate a clear myeloid commitment. We also evaluated further lymphoid antigen positive AML cases by using the second panel of McAb (Stelzer & Goodpasture, 2000).

The second panel of McAb was aimed at identifying uncommon types of AML, such as those with megakaryocytic or elytroid differentiation and the exclusion or conformation of diagnosis of non-hematological malignancy. In our study, we applied the second AML panel in 27 cases; 4 which did not demonstrate clear myeloid commitment and 23 cases with lymphoid antigen positive AML cases. With our primary McAb we were able to differentiate AML form ALL in 96.8% of cases. Only in one patient (AML-M6-1.5%) lineage differentiation was assigned after staining with the secondary McAB panel and one case of non-hematological malignancy was confirmed.

Immunophenotyping was crucial in all cases of poorly differentiated myeloid leukemia (AML-M0), megakaryoblatstic leukemia (AML-M7) and in some case of monoblastic leukemia (AML-M5) and those with primitive erythroid cells as predominant leukemic cells (AML-M6). This is also important for recognizing an AML case that co-expresses lymphoid-associated antigens. In addition, immunophenotyping enables recognition of unusual forms of acute leukemia: designated acute biphenotypic or acute mixed lineage leukemia. The leukemia associated immunophenotype (LAIP) of the blast cells is a useful tool for detection of minimal residual disease in AML cases (Döhner et al., 2010; Stelzer & Goodpasture, 2000; Swerdlow et al., 2008).

In order to classify AML cases in the different AML entities we correlated the immunological data from immunophenotyping with the FAB morphological and cytochemical classification. One of the difficulties in knotting the flow cytometric data with traditional morphology is the lack of routine flow cytometric data analyses that would ensure correlation of the immunophenotyping data to abnormal morphologic counterpart. Our approach was based on the fact that complete eight-part differential of the myeloid lineage in the normal bone marrow could be done with correlations of the expression of CD45 expression versus light side scatter (SSC) characteristics of the cells. Extension of this technique to the analyses of leukemias allows abnormal cell to be recognized as independent clusters in CD45/SSC histograms with pattern of CD45 and SSC expression that correlate to the same pattern of the morphologically similar cells in normal bone marrow. Flow-cytometric analyses by using CD45 gating strategy reveled that leukemic myeloblasts demonstrate very similar CD45/SSC characteristics to normal myeloblasts, especially the early myeloblasts. In fact, leukemic cells generally demonstrate CD45/SSC characteristics that closely resemble their nearest normal morphological counterparts in the bone marrow. In the histograms the leukemic cells can be easily recognized as an abnormal cluster of cells in CD45/SSC „space" which is usually occupied by normal myeloid blasts. Using this method we define in our study group each category of AML as defined by FAB system (Stelzer & Goodpasture, 2000). Early myeloblasts are presented at Figure 6. Flow cytometric analyses show that those leukemic cells demonstrate low light forward and side scatter (FSC&SSC), which means that those cells are small and don't contain any granules. They also have low CD45 expression.

The predominant immunophenotype characteristics of early myeloblasts are an expression of all pan-myeloid antigens: CD13, CD33, CD117 and HLA-DR and lack expression of more mature myeloid antigens such as CD15 and CD14. Also, high proportion of the leukemic cells expresses CD34. With the maturation process of the blast cells, CD34 expression becomes more heterogeneous and weaker. The densest is at AML-M0 blasts, which typically express only one myeloid-associated antigen plus. Myeloid blasts that arise as a result of the genetic change in more mature myeloid progenitor lose the characteristics of the early myeloblasts. For example, AML-M3 blasts usually lack the expression of CD34 and HLA-DR.

At Figure 7 are presents more mature myeloblasts, M5 blast. It is obvious that they are bigger when compared with the AML-M1 blasts presented on Figure 6, and contain some more granules (have higher FSC&SSC). Immunophenotypically, they are characterized with expression of some more mature myeloid markers as CD14 and CD15, and in most of the case with lost CD34 expression.

The results from our study showed that routine immunophenotyping improved the diagnosis in 12 (15, 5%) cases with acute leukemia which was essential for more appropriate individual clinical stratification of the patient with acute leukemia. Our data demonstrate that flow cytometry in correlation with the morphological classification criteria for each subtype of AML can be used for initial classification of each FAB AML entities and and justify routine implementation of flow cytometry analyses in the diagnostic evaluation of AML cases.

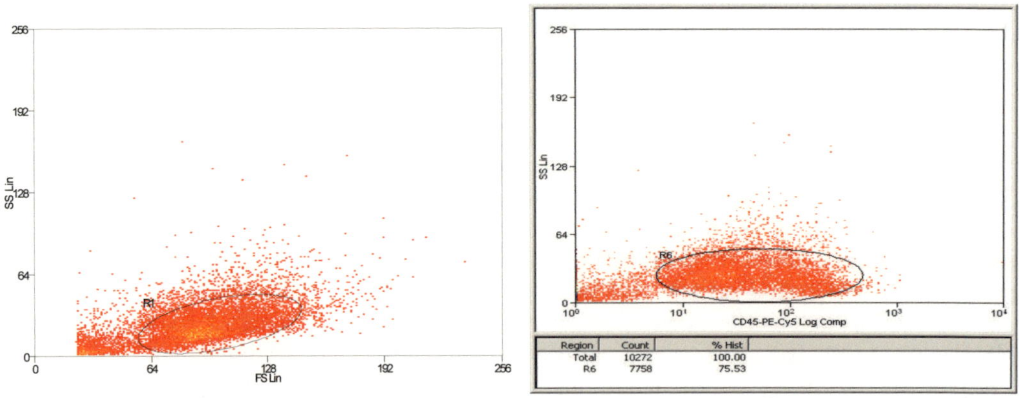


A B

Fig. 6. Histogram analyses of early M1 myeloblasts ; A: Blast cells demonostrate low FSC&SSC, B:Blast cells have low CD45 expression

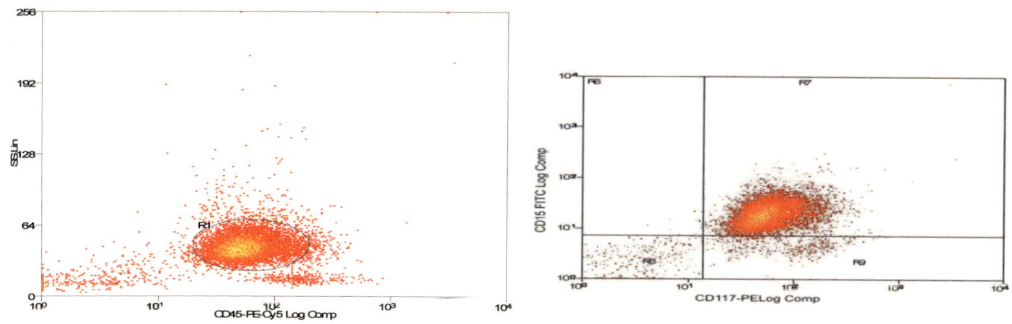


A B

Fig. 7. Histogram analyses of M5-myloblasts; A: Blast cells are biger and more granular and have higher CD45,B: Blasts cells express CD117 and the myeloid expression maturation marker CD15

### 5.2 Molecular analyses in the modern diagnosis of AML

Results from the immunophenotying guided us to perform exact molecular analyses and further define some specific genetic entities of AML. We tested our AML patients for the presence of PML/RARα, AML1/ETO and CBFβ/MYH11 fusion transcripts, by using RT-PCR method. Results from those analyses additionally improved the exact classification of the AML subtypes and made target and specific therapy available for some of the specific AML subtypes (Marcucci et al., 2000; Perea et al.2006; Wang et al., 2008)

Nonrandom chromosomal abnormalities are identified at the cytogenetic level in approximately 55% of all adult primary or de novo AML patients and have long been recognized as important independent prognostic indicators for achievement of complete remission (CR), duration of first CR, and survival after intensive chemotherapy treatment. Two of the most prevalent cytogenetic subtypes of adult primary or de novo AML are t (8; 21) (q22; q22) and inv (16) (p13q22). These abnormalities result in the disruption of genes encoding subunits of the CBF, which is a αβ heterodimeric transcriptional factor involved in the regulation of normal hematopoiesis and are collectively referred as CBF-AML. At the molecular level, t(8;21)(q22;q22) and inv(l6)(p13q22) result in the creation of novel fusion genes, AML1/ETO and CBFβ/MYH11.Detection of t(8;21)(q22;q22) or inv(16)(p13q22) in adult patients with primary AML is a favorable independent prognostic indicator for achievement of cure after intensive chemotherapy or bone marrow transplantation, and may serve as a as a paradigm of the risk-adapted treatment in AML (Döhner et al. 2010& Marcucci et al., 2000).

In almost all studies of adult primary AML, the highest CR rate (approximately 90%) and the longest disease free survival (DFS) at 5 years (approximately 50%) have been associated with CBF-AML cases. It has been suggested that the superior outcome of AML patients with CBF gene rearrangements compared with other AML patients may be attributed to an increased sensitivity of the leukemic blasts to cytarabine that in combination with anthracyclines represents the backbone of AML treatment. The collective analysis of all data regarding the treatment of CBF-AML indicates that incorporation of multiple courses of high dose of cytarabine as consolidation therapy should be considered as the therapeutic standard for primary adult CBF-AML (Marcucci et al., 2001; Perea et al.2006).

The prognostic impact of the CBF gene rearrangements appears equally significant in the setting of BMT of AML patients in first CR. However, the iatrogenic morbidity and mortality of BMT suggest that patients with CBF-AML should not receive this therapeutic modality as initial treatment. The collective analysis of all data regarding the implementation of all SCT in AML treatment suggest that although allo SCT and auto SCT may have a potential role in the initial management of AML other than CBF-AML, the treatment-related morbidity and mortality of SCT represent a therapeutic limitation for treatment of CBF-AML patients. Considering the high probability of cure that these patients can achieve with intensive chemotherapy, it is reasonable to spare them the toxicity of SCT as consolidation in first complete remission (Löwenberg et al., 2008a; Koreth et al, 2009; Marcucci et al., 2000; Marcucci et al., 2001 & Perea et al.2006).
APL or AML-M3 is a distinct subtype of AML which is characterized by a t(15;17) translocation leading to a *PML-RARA* fusion gene. Historically, recognition of this form of AML as a separate entity was important for the clinicians, not because the chemotherapy used as treatment differed substantially from that used for the other subtypes of AML, but because the relatively common occurrence of life-threatening coagulopathy mandated special supportive maneuvers, including the use of low-dose heparin and aggressive blood product support. In the past, induction mortality was often significant, with some older series reporting an incidence approaching 50%. APL was typified with the worst features associated with leukemia: a fulminant disorder that struck primarily young people, had devastating effects on an individual's life, and resulted in death for a large number of patients during the initial phases of treatment. The last two decades have seen a fundamental shift from this paradigm, with APL now recognized as one of the most curable forms of acute leukemia. Introduction of the differentiation therapy with ATRA into the treatment of APL completely revolutionized the management and outcome of this disease, and presents the first model of targeted therapy for cancer. This agent represents one of the most spectacular advances in the treatment of human cancer, providing the first paradigm of molecularly targeted treatment. Treatment of APL with ATRA combined with anthracycline-based chemotherapy yields a CR rate of approximately 90% for newly diagnosed APLs. The relapse rate is approximately 20%, and with the development of new molecular target therapies such as arsenic trioxide, a cure can now be expected even for relapsed patients. After the advent of ATRA, the introduction of arsenic trioxide (ATO), probably the most biologically active single drug in APL has provided a valuable addition to the armamentarium and may have contributed to further improvements in the clinical outcome of this disease. Several treatment strategies using these agents, usually in combination with chemotherapy, have provided excellent therapeutic results with survival rates exceeding 70% in multicenter clinical trials. Cure of patients with APL depends not only on the effective use of combination therapy involving differentiating and classical cytotoxic agents, but also, critically, upon supportive care measures that take into particular account the biology of the disease and the complications associated with molecularly targeted therapies. Moreover, it is important to consider diagnostic suspicion of APL as a medical emergency (uncommon in AML) that requires several specific and simultaneous actions, including immediate commencement of ATRA therapy, prompt genetic diagnosis, and measures to counteract the coagulopathy (Grimwade et al., 2002; Wang et al., 2008).

### 5.2.1 Why we used RT-PCR method for detection of the genetic abnormalities?

RT-PCR methods for detecting the PML/RARα fusion transcript also provide the "gold standard" approach for confirming a diagnosis of APL. In addition to its high specificity and sensitivity, it is essential for defining PML breakpoint location thereby establishing the target for reliable monitoring of the minimal residual disease (MRD).

Standard cytogenetic analysis is currently the most common method for identifying the most common recurrent cytogenetic abnormalities t(8;2l)(q22;q22) and inv( 16)(pl3q22) or t(16;16)(p13;q22) in AML patients. This technique also allows detection of secondary chromosomal abnormalities such as del (9q),-X and -Y which are frequently associated with t(8;21)(q22;q22), or +8 and +22 more often found with inv(16)(p13q22). Still, despite the recent improvements in the cytogenetic methodology and the use of complementary techniques such as fluorescence in situ hybridization and comparative genomic hybridization to increase the rate of successful karyotyping, the possibility that subtle structural chromosomal aberrations are missed remains (Marcucci et al., 2000). In t(8;21) (q22;q22) or inv(16) (p13q22), failure to detect submicroscopic (cryptic) rearrangements of the involved genes leads to false-negative results that may ultimately impact the correct stratification of this patient population in prognostic and risk-adapted therapy groups. Sensitive molecular methodologies such as RT-PCR have been successfully used to detect cryptic CBF abnormalities in diagnostic samples of AML patients with karyotypes that are otherwise negative for t(8;21)(q22;q22) or inv(16)(p13q22). Andrieu et al.,1997 reported detection of AML1/ETO fusion transcripts by RT-PCR in cases with unsuccessful cytogenetic studies, normal karyotypes, or karyotypes other than t(8:2 l)(q22;q22) such as del(8q), i(8)(q10) or del(9q). Langabeer et al., 1997 used a two-step RT-PCR to screen for the AMLI/ETO and CBFβ/MYHll fusion transcripts in AML patients entered into the U.K. MRC AML 10, 11, and 12 trials and compared the results with conventional cytogenetics. All patients with cytogenetic evidence of t(8;21)(q22;q22) or inv(16)(pl3q22) were positive by RT-PCR for the corresponding fusion transcripts. RT-PCR was also positive in 31 cases (19 cases of AML1/ETO and 12 cases of CBFβ/MYH11) without CBF cytogenetic abnormalities, increasing the overall detection rate of "t(8;21)(q22;q22)" and "inv(16)(p13q22)" from 8.1% to 12.9% and from 6.5% to 10.3%, respectively. The authors of these studies concluded that all primary AML should be routinely tested for the presence of the CBF fusion genes by molecular screening to improve genomic stratification of AML patients in risk-related treatment groups (Marcucci et al., 2000).

Although patients with CBF-AML have a relatively good prognosis, a substantial number of them relapse and eventually die of their disease. Because relapse after intensive treatment is likely to occur as the result of failure to completely eradicate the leukemic blasts, evaluation of MRD by a sensitive molecular technique such as PCR based techniques has been proposed to detect persistence of malignant clones and predict disease relapse in AML patients in CR. This strategy has been successful in CML (Radich et al.,1995) and acute promyelocytic leukemia (Grimwade et al., 2002; Wang et al., 2008), but its clinical applicability to other subgroups of acute leukemia remains controversial.

RQ-PCR provides the most sensitive parameters for AML with reciprocal gene fusions PML/RARα, CBFβ-MYH11, AML1-ETO (Haferlach et al., 2007). The score of gene expression of the respective fusion transcripts after consolidation therapy in relation to gene expression at diagnosis correlates significantly with prognosis [Haferlach et al., 2007]. The

prognostic value of quantitative PCR in MRD diagnostics in these subgroups was demonstrated in several studies. Patients with an MRD level<1% after induction chemotherapy in relation to initial diagnosis had a relapse rate of 8% in contrast to 91% in the patients with MRD levels of ≥1% in the investigation on the CBF-leukemias by Krauter et al.,2003. Marcucci et al, 2000, were able to define a distinct transcript copy number in inv(16)/CBFB/ MYH11 below which relapse was unlikely and above which relapse occurred with high probability. A Gruppo Italiano Malattie Ematologiche Maligne dell' Adulto (GIMEMA) trial showed that molecular switch from CR to PML/RARα positivity was followed by hematologic relapse after a median time of 3 months in 95% of all APL cases (Diverio et al. 1998). Data from different studies indicate that of all AML subtypes, quantitative PCR monitoring could be best established for the reciprocal gene fusions.
Molecular analyses enabled 23.7% of the cases of our study to be classified in the adequate genetic entities of AML with different prognosis requiring different therapeutically approach.

### 5.3 Analyses of the clinical characteristics of the patients in the era of modern diagnosis of AML

#### 5.3.1 Analyses of the EKOG performance status

Several studies support the use of the ECOG performance status as a measure of physical functioning and prognosis in patients with AML (Oken et al. 1982). A retrospective study of data from five Southwestern Oncology Group (SWOG) trials that included 968 patients with AML found that the mortality rate within 30 days of initiation of induction therapy is dependent upon both the patient's age and ECOG performance status at diagnosis. A second retrospective analysis of 998 patients age 65 or greater (range 65 to 89; median 71 years) who underwent intensive induction chemotherapy reported eight-week mortality rates of 23, 40, and 72 percent for patients with ECOG PS of zero to 1, 2, and 3 to 4, respectively. One-year overall survival rates for the same groups were 35, 25, and 7 percent, respectively. A third retrospective study of 2767 patients with non-APL AML from the Swedish acute leukemia registry also reported that older patients with an ECOG PS of zero to 1 had 30 day death rates after intensive chemotherapy of less than 15 percent, while patients with a PS of 3 or 4 had higher early death rates regardless of patient age ranging from 26 to 36 percent. Seventy percent of patients up to age 80 years had a PS of zero to 2. A prospective trial of induction chemotherapy with cytarabine plus daunorubicin in 811 older adults (median age 67 years, range 60 to 83 years) with ECOG PS of zero to 2 reported a 30-day mortality rate of 11 percent (Appelbaum et al, 2006). We used the EKOG performance status score in initial randomization of our AML patients for different induction and consolidation approaches, in order to avoid intensive induction and consolidation treatment for patient with EKOG performance status higher than 2. Only 8 (12.5%) patients from our study group have EKOG performance status higher than 2, but only 3 of those patients were younger than 60 years of age.

#### 5.3.2 Analyses of the comorbidities

Comorbidity is an also a distinct additional clinical entity that exists or may occur during the clinical course of patient with a primary disease (i.e. AML). Comorbid conditions are poor prognostic factors especially in older patients with AML. Patients with age-related chronic cardiac, pulmonary, hepatic or renal disorders or diabetes suffer greater acute toxicity from chemotherapy. Older patients may also have decreased bone marrow regenerative capacity, even after successful leukemia cytoreduction. Inability to tolerate long periods of pancytopenia and malnutrition or the nephrotoxicity of drugs such as amino glycosides or amphotericin remains a major barrier to successful treatment (Piccirillo et al.2004; Sorror et al, 2005). Six 6(9,3%) patients from our study had seriouos comorbidities which limited the aplication of intensive chemotherapy in their treatment. Five of them were older than 60years.

### 5.4 Approach to AML diagnostic algorithms

Modern diagnostic approaches in the AML should be created as integral and basic parts of optimized treatment concepts for the benefit of the each individual patient. The ultimate test of any disease diagnostic algorithm approach is its usefulness in guiding the selection of effective treatment strategies. Algorithms that provide a basis for risk-adapted therapeutic choices may include immunological markers, cytogenetic factors, molecular markers as well as clinical parameters (e.g., age, attainment of an early or late complete remission) and hematological determinants (e.g., secondary AML, white blood cell count at diagnosis) (Haferlach et al., 2007).

A comprehensive approach in diagnosis, classification, and treatment follow-up in patients with acute leukemias can, therefore, be suggested by diagnostic algorithms, which also show the relationship and the hierarchy between single methods. These standard guidelines for AML mostly result from a combination of different methods and intend to add prognostic information (Lowenberg 2008).

Our diagnostic algorithm for AML (as shown in Fig. 8) starts with cytomorphology and cytochemistry. These methods should be performed in combination: cytomorphology and cytochemistry allow rapid classification of the acute leukemias and further enables the choice of the antibody panel for flow cytometric analyses. In case cytomorphology gives indices for characteristic aberrations—in the FAB subtypes M3/M3v for t(15;17)/PML/RARα, in FAB M4eo for inv(16)/CBFβ/MYH11, or in M1/2 with the characteristic long Auer rods for the t(8;21)/AML1/ETO, PCR analyses for these rearrangements should be promptly applied.

Especially in case of suspicion for APL due to clinical symptoms or due to the morphological findings, RT-PCR for PML/RARα should be initiated as soon as possible (Schoch et al., 2002). We think that, regardless of the morphological, cytochemical and immunological futures of the blast cells, RT-PCR for the fusion oncogene PML/RARα are recommendable in all AML cases. The RT- PCR method is the most sensitive and rapid technique for detection of this oncogene and provides an optimal basis for MRD analyses. Further we suggest all AML cases which are PML/RARα negative to be tested for the presence of the reciprocal fusions genes that describe CBF-AML, AML1/ETO and CBFβ/MYH11.Those analyses provides the basis for sub-classification of the AML cases in prognostically relevant subclasses. This is the prerequisite for adequate individual clinical risk stratification and therapeutic decisions.

Moreover, we correlated the obtained result for the applied multimodal diagnostic approach with the patient age, EKOG performance status and comorbidities, which allowed us to optimize the individual risk stratification for each AML patient.

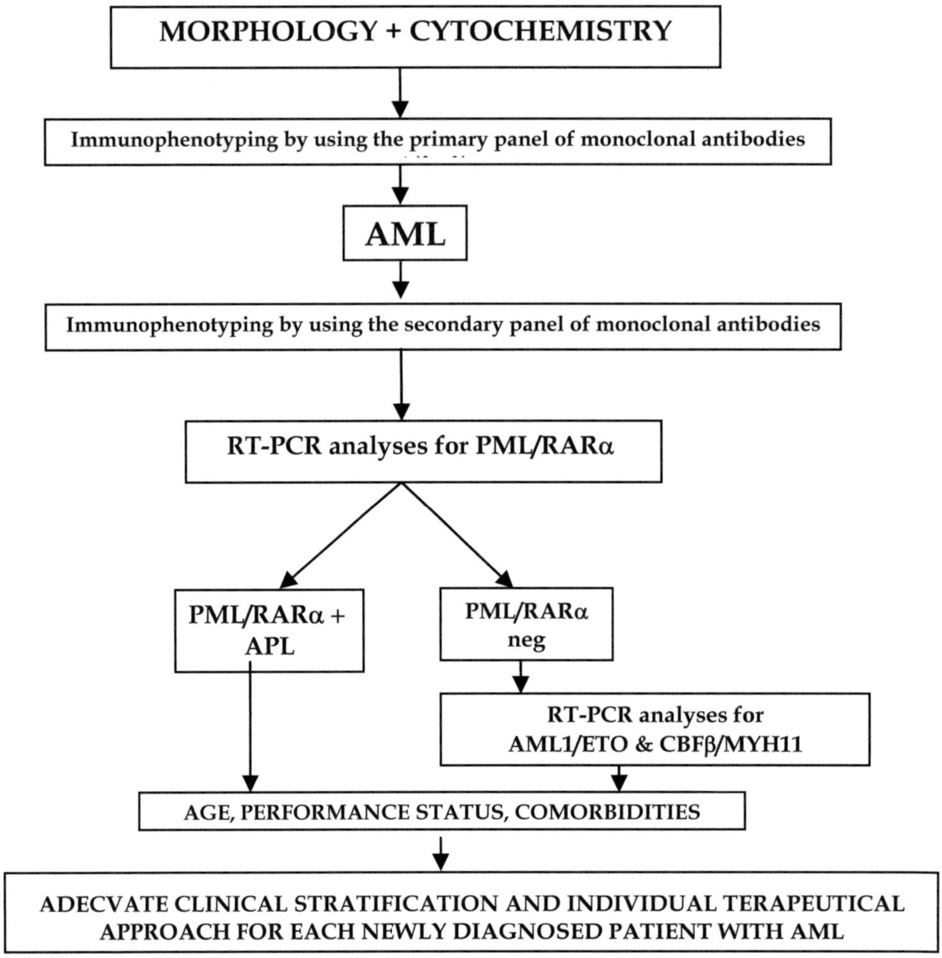


Fig. 8. Diagnostic algorithm and algorithm for risk adapted therapy in AML patients

## 6. Conclusions

A basis for every therapeutic decision in AML cases should be provided by a multimodal diagnostic approach. The optimal therapeutic conditions are based on exact classification and prognosis of the AML subtype at diagnosis and to delineation of sensitive markers for MRD studies during the complete hematologic remission. MRD methods have many potential applications in the clinical management of patients with acute leukemia. Today, a multimodal diagnostic approach which combines different diagnostic techniques is needed to meet these requirements. The diagnostic process is becoming more demanding with respect to experience, time and costs due to the expansion of methods and algorithms, which guide the diagnostic procedure from basic to more specific methods and which finally lead to results that are essential for modern diagnostics and therapeutic concepts. There are numerous overlaps between different diagnostic methods. These can be used for optimal pathways in the complex diagnostic proceedings and for validation of the results of single methods, which can be summarized in diagnostic algorithms. Basic morphological and cytochemical analyses performed in our study group established the lineage assignment of the blasts cells in 68 (88.3%) patients. Routine immunophenotyping improved the diagnosis in 12 (15.5%) more cases. Molecular analyses enabled 23.7% of the cases from our study to be classified in the adequate genetic entities of AML with different prognosis requiring different therapeutical approach.

The applied multimodal diagnostic approach consisted of minimal number of cytomorphological, cytochemistry, immunological and molecular analyses enables improved and more precise diagnosis and clinical stratification in 38.2% acute leukemia patients from our study. Moreover, when we correlate those results with the results obtained from the analyses of the EKOG performance status and the incidence of the serious comborbidities in our study group, an additional 12.5% of the patients were stratified to a different risk adapted therapy.

Our initial results are consistent with literature data and indicate that our applied multimodal diagnostic approach improved the diagnosis of the specific genetic entities of AML in which specific treatment approach is indicated and allows individual clinical stratification in treatment protocols of the patients.

## 7. References

Andrieu, V., Radford-Weiss, I., Troussard, X., Chane, C., Valensi, F., Guesnu, M., Haddad, E., Viguier, F., Dreyfus, F.; Varet, B.; Flandrin, G.; & Macintyre, E. (1997). Molecular detection of t(8;2 I)/AMLI-ETO in AML MI/M2: Correlation with cytogenetics, morphology and immunophenotype. *Br J Haematol,* Vol.4, No.92,(March 1996), pp. 855-865, ISSN 0007-1048

Appelbaum, F.R., Rowe, J.M., Radich, J., & Dick, J.E. (2001). Acute myeloid leukemia. *Hematology (Am Soc Hematol Educ Program),*(November 2001), pp. 62-86, ISSN 1520-4391

Appelbaum, F.R., Gundacker, H., Head, D.R., Slovak, M.L., Willman, C.L., Godwin, J.E., Anderson, J.E.,& Petersdorf, S.H. (2006). Age and acute myeloid leukemia. *Blood,*Vol. 107, No.9, (May 2006), pp.3481–3485,ISSN0006-4971

Armitage P., Berry G., & Matthews J.N.S.(2002) *Statistical Methods in Medical Research* (4th edition),Blackwell ISBN:978063052578,Oxford,UKBain, BJ, Barnet, D, Linch, D, Matutes, E, & Reilly, J.T. (2002).Revised guidelines on immunophenotyping in acute leukemias and chronic lymphoproliferative disorders. *Clin Lab Hem,*Vol. 24,(2002),pp.1-13, ISSN 0141-9854

Beillard, E., Pallisgaard, N., van der Velden, V.H., Bi, W., Dee, R., van der Schoot E., Delabesse E., Macintyre E., Gottardi E., Saglio G., Watzinger F., Lion T., van Dongen, J.J., Hokland, P., & Gabert, J.(2003). Evaluation of candidate control genes for diagnosis and residual disease detection in leukemic patients using 'real-time' quantitative reverse-transcriptase polymerase chain reaction (RQ-PCR) - a Europe against cancer program. *Leukemia,* Vol. 17, No. 12,( December 2003), pp 2474-2486, ISSN 0887-6924

Bene, M.C., Castoldi, G., Knapp, W., Ludwig, W.D., Matutes, E., Orfao, A., & van't Veer, M.B. (1995). Proposals for the immunological classification of acute leukemias. European Group for the Immunological Characterization of Leukemias (EGIL). *Leukemia,* Vol. 9, No. 10, (October 1995), pp.1783-1786, ISSN 0887-6924

Bennett, J.M., Catovsky, D., Daniel, M.T., Flandrin, G., Galton, D.A., Gralnick, H.R., & Sultan, C.(1976). Proposals for the classification of the acute leukaemias. French–American–British (FAB) Cooperative Group. *Br J Haematol,*Vol.33, No.4 (August 1976), pp.451–458, ISSN 0007-1048

Borowitz, M.I., Guenter, K.I., Shults, K.E., & Stelzer, G.T. (1993). Immunophenotyping of acute leukemia by flow cytometry analysis. Use of CD45 and right-angle light scatter to gate on leukaemic blasts in three colour analysis. *Am J Clin Pathol,* No.100,(November 1993), pp.534-540,ISSN 0002-9173

Byrd, J.C., Mrózek, K., Dodge, R.K., Carroll, A.J., Edwards, C.G., Arthur, D.C., Pettenati, M.J., Patil, S.R., Rao, K.W., Watson, M.S., Koduru, P.R., Moore, J.O., Stone, R.M., Mayer, R.J., Feldman, E.J., Davey, F.R., Schiffer, C.A., Larson, R.A., & Bloomfield, C.D.; Cancer and Leukemia Group B (CALGB 8461). (2002). Pretreatment cytogenetic abnormalities are predictive of induction success, cumulative incidence of relapse, and overall survival in adult patients with de novo acute myeloid leukemia: results from Cancer and Leukemia Group B (CALGB 8461).*Blood,* Vol. 100, No.13, (December 2002), pp. 4325-4336, ISSN 0006-4971

Cornelissen, J.J., van Putten, W.L., Verdonck, L.F., Theobald, M., Jacky E., Daenen, S.M., van Marwijk-Kooy, M., Wijermans, P., Schouten, H., Huijgens, P.C., van der Lelie, H., Fey, M., Ferrant, A., Maertens, J., Gratwohl, A.,& Lowenberg, B. (2007). Results of a HOVON-SAKK donor versus donor analysis of myeloablative HLA-identical sibling stem cell transplantation in first remission acute myeloid leukemia in young and middle aged adults: benefits for whom? *Blood,* Vol.109, No. 9, (May 2007), pp. 3658-3666,ISSN 0006-4971

Diverio D., Rossi V., Avvisati G., De Santis S., Pistilli A., Pane F., Saglio G., Martinelli G., Petti M.C., Santoro A., Pelicci, P.G., Mandelli, F., Biondi, A., & Lo Coco, F.(1998). Early detection of relapse by prospective reverse transcriptase-polymerase chain reaction analysis of the PML/RAR alpha fusion gene in patients with acute promyelocytic leukemia enrolled in the GIMEMA-AIEOP multicenter "AIDA" trial. GIMEMA-AIEOP Multicenter "AIDA" Trial. Blood, Vol. 92, No.3, (August 1998), pp.784-789, ISSN 0006-4971

Döhner, H., Estey, E.H., Amadori, S., Appelbaum, F.R., Büchner, T., Burnett, A.K., Dombret, H., Fenaux, P., Grimwade, D., Larson, R.A., Lo-Coco, F., Naoe, T., Niederwieser, D., Ossenkoppele, G.J., Sanz, M.A., Sierra, J., Tallman, M.S., Löwenberg, B.,& Bloomfield, C.D.; European Leukemia Net. (2010). Diagnosis and management of acute myeloid leukemia in adults: recommendations from an international expert panel, on behalf of the European Leukemia Net. *Blood,* Vol.115, No.3, (January 2010), pp.453-474, ISSN 0006-4971

Fernandez, H.F. (2010). New Trends in the Standard of Care for Initial Therapy of Acute Myeloid Leukemia. *Hematology (Am Soc Hematol Educ Program),* (November 2010), pp. 62-86, ISSN 1520-4391

First MIC Cooperative Study Group. (1986). Morphologic, immunologic, and cytogenetic (MIC) working classification of acute lymphoblastic leukemias: report of the workshop held in Leuven, Belgium, April 22-23, 1985. *Cancer Genet Cytogenet,* Vol. 23, No.3, (November 1986), pp.189-197, ISSN 0165-4608

Freeman, S.D., Jovanovic, J.V., & Grimwade, D. (2008). Development of minimal residual disease-directed therapy in acute myeloid leukemia. *Semin Oncol,* Vol. 34, No.4, (August 2008), pp.388-400, ISSN 0093-7754

Gabert, J., Beillard, E., van der Velden, V.H., Bi, W., Grimwade, D., Pallisgaard, N., Barbany, G., Cazzaniga, G., Cayuela, J.M., Cavé, H., Pane, F., Aerts, J.L., De Micheli, D., Thirion, X., Pradel, V., González, M., Viehmann, S., Malec, M., Saglio, G., & van Dongen, J.J. (2003). Standardization and quality control studies of 'real-time' quantitative reverse transcriptase polymerase chain reaction of fusion gene transcripts for residual disease detection in leukemia - A Europe Against Cancer Program. *Leukemia,* Vol.17, No.12, (December 2003), pp.2318–2357, ISSN 0887-6924

Grimwade, D. (2001). The clinical significance of cytogenetic abnormalities in acute myeloid leukaemia. *Best Pract Res Clin Haematol,* Vol. 14, No. 3, (September 2001), pp. 497-529, ISSN 1521-6926

Grimwade, D. & Lo Coco, F. (2002). Acute promyelocytic leukemia: a model for the role of molecular diagnosis and residual disease monitoring in directing treatment approach in acute myeloid leukemia. *Leukemia,* Vol.16, No.10,( October 2002), pp:.1959–1973, ISSN 0887-6924

Haferlach, T., Bacher, U., Kern, W., Schnittger, S., & Haferlach, C. (2007). Diagnostic pathways in acute leukemias: a proposal for a multimodal approach. *Ann Hematol,* Vol. 86, No. 5, (May 2007), pp.311–327, ISSN 0939-5555

Haferlach, T. (2008). Molecular Genetic Pathways as Therapeutic Targets in Acute Myeloid Leukemia. *Hematology (Am Soc Hematol Educ Program),*(November 2008), pp.401-411, ISSN 1520-4391

Koreth, J., Schlenk, R., Kopecky, K.J., Honda, S., Sierra, J., Djulbegovic, B.J., Wadleigh, M., De Angelo, D.J., Stone, R.M., Sakamaki, H., Appelbaum, F.R., Döhner, H., Antin, J.H., Soiffer, R.J.,& Cutler, C. (2009). Allogeneic stem cell transplantation for acute myeloid leukemia in first complete remission: systematic review and meta-analysis of prospective clinical trials. *JAMA,* Vol. 301, No. 22, (June 2009), pp.2349-2361, ISSN 0098-7484.

Krauter, J., Gorlich, K., Ottmann, O., Lubbert, M., Dohner, H., Heit, W., Kanz, L., Ganser, A., & Hei,l G. (2003). Prognostic value of minimal residual disease quantification by real-time reverse transcriptase polymerase chain reaction in patients with core binding factor leukemias. *J Clin Oncol,* Vol. 21, No.23, (December 2003), pp.4413-4422, ISSN 0002-9173

Langabeer, S.E., Walker, H., Rogers, J.R., Burnett, A.K., Wheatley, K., Swirsky, D., Goldstone, A.H., & Linch, D.C. (1997). Incidence of AMLl/ETO fusion transcripts in patients entered into the MRC AML trials. *Br J Haematol,* Vol. 99, No. 4, (December 19970), pp.925-928, ISSN 0007-1048

Langabeer, S.E., Walker, H., Gale, R.E., Wheatley, K., Burnett, A.K., Goldstone, A.H., & Linch, DC.(1997). Frequency of CBFβ/MYHII fusion transcripts in patients entered into the UK MRC AML trials. The MRC Adult Leukaemia Working Party.*Br J Haematol,* Vol. 96, No. 4, (March 1997), pp. 736-739, ISSN 0007-1048

Lichtman, M.A.; Kipps, T.J.; Seligsohn, U.; Kaushansky, K.; & Prchal, J.T. (2010). *Williams Hematology,* Eighth Edition, The McGraw-Hill Companies, Inc., ISBN 978-0-07-162144-1, China

Löwenberg, B. (2008a). Diagnosis and prognosis in acute myeloid leukemia: the art of distinction. *N Engl J Med,* Vol. 358, No. 18, (May 2008), pp. 1960-1962, ISSN 0028-4793

Löwenberg, B. (2008b). Acute Myeloid Leukemia: The Challenge of Capturing Disease Variety. *Hematology (Am Soc Hematol Educ Program),* (November 2008), pp.1-11, ISSN 1520-4391

Marcucci, G., Caligiuri, M.A., Döhner, H., Archer, K.J., Schlenk, R.F., Döhner, K., Maghraby, E.A., & Bloomfield, C.D. (2001).Quantification of CBF beta/MYH11 fusion transcript by real time RT-PCR in patients with inv(16) acute myeloid leukemia. *Leukemia,* Vol. 15, No.7, (July 2001), pp. 1072–1080, ISSN 0887-6924

Marcucci, G., et al. (2000). Molecular and Clinical Advances in Core Binding Factor Primary Acute Myeloid Leukemia: A Paradigm for Translational Research in Malignant Hematology. *Cancer Investigation,* Vol.18, No. 8, (2000), pp.768-780, ISSN 0735-7907

Oken, M.M., Creech, R.H., Tormey, D.C., Horton, J., Davis, T.E., McFadden, E.T., & Carbone, P.P. (1982). Toxicity And Response Criteria Of The Eastern Cooperative Oncology Group. *Am J Clin Oncol,* Vol.5, No.6, (December 1982), pp.649-655, ISSN 0002-9173

Panovska-Stavridis, I., Cevreska, L., Trajkova, S., Hadzi-Pecova, L., Trajkov, D., Petlickovski, A., Srbinovska, O., Matevska, N., Dimovski, A., & Spiroski, M. (2008). Preliminary results of introducing the method multiparameter flow cytometry in patients with acute leukemia in the Republic of Macedonia. *Macedonian Journal of Medical Sciences,* No.1(2), pp:36-43, ISSN 1857-5749

Perea, G., Lasa, A., Aventín, A., Domingo, A., Villamor, N., Queipo, de Llano, M.P., Llorente, A., Juncà, J., Palacios, C., Fernández, C., Gallart, M., Font, L., Tormo, M., Florensa, L., Bargay, J., Martí, J.M., Vivancos, P., Torres, P., Berlanga, J.J., Badell, I., Brunet, S., Sierra, J., & Nomdedéu, J.F.; Grupo Cooperativo para el Estudio y Tratamiento de las Leucemias Agudas y Miel.(2006). Prognostic value of minimal residual disease (MRD) in acute myeloid leukemia (AML) with favorable cytogeneticst(8;21) and inv(16)]. *Leukemia,* Vol. 20, No.1, (January 2006), pp.87-94, ISSN 0887-6924

Piccirillo, J.F., Tierney, R.M., Costas, I., Grove, L., & Spitznagel, E.L. Jr.(2004). Prognostic importance of comorbidity in a hospital-based cancer registry. *JAMA,* Vol. 291, No. 20, (May 2004), pp.2441-2447, ISSN 0098-7484

Radich, J.P., Gehly, G., Gooley, T., Bryant, E., Clift, R.A., Collins, S., Edmands, S., Kirk, J., Lee, A., Kessler, P., et al. (1995). Polymerase chain reaction detection of the BCR-ABL fusion transcript after allogeneic marrow transplantation for chronic myeloid leukemia: Results and implications in 346 patients. *Blood,* Vol. 85, No. 9, (May 1995), pp.2632-2638, ISSN 0006-4971

Schlenk, R.F., Döhner, K., Krauter, J., Fröhling, S., Corbacioglu, A., Bullinger, L., Habdank, M., Späth, D., Morgan, M., Benner, A., Schlegelberger, B., Heil, G., Ganser, A., & Döhner, H.; German-Austrian Acute Myeloid Leukemia Study Group. (2008). Mutations and treatment outcome in cytogenetically normal acute myeloid leukemia. *N Engl J Med.* Vol. 358, No. 18, (May 2008), pp.1909–1918, ISSN 0028-4793

Schoch, C., Schnittger, S., Kern, W., Lengfelder, E., Löffler, H., Hiddemann, W., & Haferlach, T. (2002). Rapid diagnostic approach to PML-RAR alpha-positive acute promyelocytic leukemia. *Hematol J* ,Vol.3, No.5, (2002), pp.259–263, ISSN 1466-4860

Sorror, M.L., Maris, M.B., Storb, R., Baron, F., Sandmaier, B.M., Maloney, D.G., Storer, B.(2005). Hematopoietic cell transplantation (HCT)-specific comorbidity index: a new tool for risk assessment before allogeneic HCT. *Blood.* Vol. 106, No.8, (October 2005), pp.2912-2919, ISSN 0006-4971

Stelzer, G.T., & Goodpasture, L. (2000). Use of multiparameter flow cytometry and immunophenotyping for the diagnosis and classification of acute myeloid leukemia, In *Immunophenotyping,* Stewarat C,S & Nicholson J.K.A.,pp.215-238,Wiley-Liss, ISBN 0-471-23957-7, United States of America

Swerdlow, S.H.; Campo, E.; Harris, N.L.; Jaffe, E.S.; Pileri, S.A.; Stein, H.; Thiele, J.; Vardiman, J.W. (2008). *WHO Classification of Tumours of Haematopoietic and Lymphoid Tissues,* Fourth Edition, IARC, WHO Press, ISBN 9789283224310, Geneva, Switzerland

Vardiman, J.W., Thiele, J., Arber, D.A., Brunning, R.D., Borowitz, M.J., Porwit, A., Harris, N.L., Le Beau, M.M., Hellström-Lindberg, E., Tefferi, A., & Bloomfield, C.D.(2009). The 2008 revision of the WHO Classification of Myeloid Neoplasms and Acute Leukemia: rationale and important changes. *Blood,* Vol. 114, No.5, (July 2009), pp. 937–951, ISSN 0006-4971

Wang, Z.Y., & Chen, Z. (2008). Acute promyelocytic leukemia: from highly fatal to highly curable. *Blood,* Vol. 111, No. 5 (March 2008), pp.2505-15, ISSN 0006-4971

# 23

# Prospective Applications of Microwaves in Medicine

Jaroslav Vorlíček, Barbora Vrbova and Jan Vrba
*Czech Technical University*
*Czech Republic*

## 1. Introduction

Research of interactions between Electromagnetic (EM) Field and biological systems is of growing interests elsewhere. In this area of research very important activity are studies of prospective medical applications of microwaves (i.e. a possibility to use microwave energy and/or microwave technique and technology for treatment purposes) are a quite new and a very rapidly developing field. Microwave thermotherapy is being used in medicine for the cancer treatment and for some other diseases since early eighties. Most common methods used for treatment of cancer are radiotherapy and chemotherapy. These therapeutic methods have many undesirable effects, such as usage of ionizing radiation. Another method used for treatment of cancer is hyperthermia. This method is based on the principle of destruction of malignant cells by artificially increased temperature in the temperature range between 41 and 45 °C fails self-protective mechanism of malignant cells. In contrast with chemotherapy and radiotherapy, hyperthermia is not limited by the number of doses of radiation.

## 2. Prospective applications of microwaves in medicine

In the following text we would like to outline scope and new trends in medical applications of microwaves. We can divide these results and new trends into two major groups:

- clinical results and trends,
- technical results and trends.

### 2.1 Clinical results and trends

Applications of microwaves in medicine is a quite a new field of a high interest in the world (since early 80's). It is necessary to mention one of the most important trends in the research of medical applications of microwaves, i.e. the thermal effects of EM field (since early 80's a microwave thermotherapy is used for cancer treatment, Benign Prostate Hyperplasia (BPH) treatment and for some other areas of medicine; it can be used in combination with other complementary treatment methods also.

To give a basic overview, we can divide medical applications of microwaves in following three basic groups according to purpose, how are microwaves used:

- Microwave energy and/or technique used for the **treatment of patients** (with the use of either thermal or non-thermal effects – sometimes both of these types of effects can play its role).

- Microwave energy and/or technique used for **diagnostics of diseases** (e.g. by aid of permittivity measurements, attenuation measurements and very prospective in the near future can be a microwave tomography).
- Microwave energy and/or technique used as a **part of a treatment or diagnostic system** (e.g.linear accelerator).

As is given above, until now medical applications of microwaves are above all represented by the treatment methods based on thermal effect – i.e. we can speak about the Microwave thermotherapy, which can be further divided into three different modalities distinguished according to the goal temperature level or interval:

- diathermia: heating up to 41 C (applications in physiotherapy)
- hyperthermia: heating into the interval of 41-45 C (applications in oncology)
- thermodestruction / thermoablation: over 45 C (applications in urology)

First three of the following list of thermotherapeutical applications are just largely used in many countries around the world, last three instead are in this moment in the phase of very promising projects:

- Oncology - cancer treatment.
- Physiotherapy - treatment of rheumatic diseases.
- Urology - BPH treatment.
- Cardiology - heart stimulations.
- Surgery - growing implants.
- Ophthalmology - retina corrections.

E.g. in cancer treatment is thermotherapy usually used in the combination with some of other modalities used in the clinical oncology (e.g. radiotherapy, chemotherapy, immunotherapy or chirurgical treatment). It is used in USA, Japan and in many countries in European Union (EU), including the Czech Republic, from early 80s. Up to now local microwave hyperthermia for cancer treatment and thermotherapy of BPH are the most important applications of microwaves in medicine. In the Czech Republic we have treated more than 500 patients. Results of our treatments are given the following table:

| | |
|---|---|
| Complete response of the tumor | 52.4 % |
| Partial response of the tumor | 31.7 % |
| Without response | 15.9 % |

Table 1. Clinical results of cancer treatment by radiothermotherapy

Successful treatment thus has been indicated in the case of 84 % of patients. This corresponds very well to the results published in EU and USA. Actual scientific information about microwave thermotherapy and its new developments is possible to get from „International Journal of Hyperthermia" issued by European Society for Hyperthermia Oncology (ESHO) together with North American Hyperthermia Society (NAHS) and Asian Society of Hyperthermia Oncology (ASHO). On the following series of photographs (Fig. 1) there is example of the typical 4 phases of the treatment of one of our patients obtained by radio-thermo-therapy (i.e. combination of microwave hyperthermia with significantly reduced doses of radiotherapy).

Very interesting results for the near future can give us the research of microwave medical applications based on so called non-thermal effects. In the literature it is possible just now to identify research projects on:

- to reduce pain feeling (analogically to analgesics),
- to increase of reaction capabilities of a human being,
- to examine the teaching capabilities, etc.

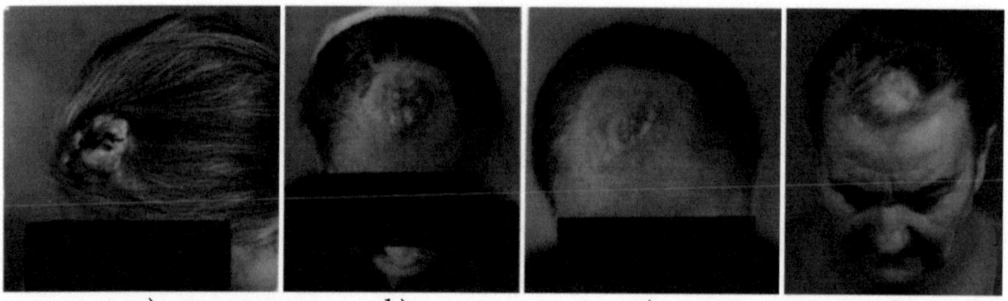

a) b) c) d)

Fig. 1. Typical example of 4 phases of the patient treatment: a) Patient before the treatment. b) At the end of the treatment. c) Two months after treatment. d) One year after treatment.

### 2.2 Technical results and trends

Our work is focused on the design, optimization and tests of the microwave applicators for medical applications, above all for hyperthermia cancer and BPH treatment. This means to design a microwave structure capable to:

- transfer EM energy into the biological tissue without power reflections back to the microwave generator,
- guarantee the best possible approximation of the area to be treated by the 3D distribution (coverage) of Specific Absorption Rate (SAR).

Our applicators (working at 434 MHz and at 2450 MHz) were used for the treatment of more than 500 patients with superficial or subcutaneous tumour. Now, following new trends in this field, we continue our research in the important directions of deep local and regional applicators. Most important technical fields of microwave thermotherapy development (covered also by our activities) can be specified as:

- Applicators: development and optimization of new applicators for more effective local, intracavitary and regional treatment,
- Treatment planning: mathematical and experimental modelling of the effective treatment
- Non-invasive temperature measurement: research of the possibilities of new techniques like Magnetic Resonance Imaging (MRI) and Ultrasound (US) for exact non-invasive measurements.
- Microwave medical diagnostics - e.g. Microwave Tomography (MT).

## 3. Applicators for microwave thermotherapy

Simulations of SAR distribution obtained by array of microwave applicators radiating at frequency 434 MHz will be described here. We will compare here the SAR distribution in a homogeneous agar phantom (which has similar dielectric characteristics to muscle tissue) and in an anatomical based biological model, which has been developed from a Computer Tomography (CT) scan.

### 3.1 Waveguide applicators

Wave guide applicators are based on microwave waveguide technology. Major advantage of waveguide applicator is that EM field in theirs aperture is roughly at 50% of its area very near to the case of EM plane wave, which is the wave with the best homogeneity and gives us the deepest penetration into the treated area.

Mostly rectangular and circular waveguides are being used to build microwave thermotherapy applicator. Examples of mentioned applicators are given in the Fig. 2. Typically they are operating at 434 MHz (depth of efficient treatment is between 4 and 6 cm), in case of deeper treatment lower frequency must be selected . Waveguide applicators displayed in Fig. 2a. are filled by dielectric material in order to decrease their cut off frequency. Air filled Evanescent mode applicator (Fig. 2b.) is excited under its cut-off frequency.

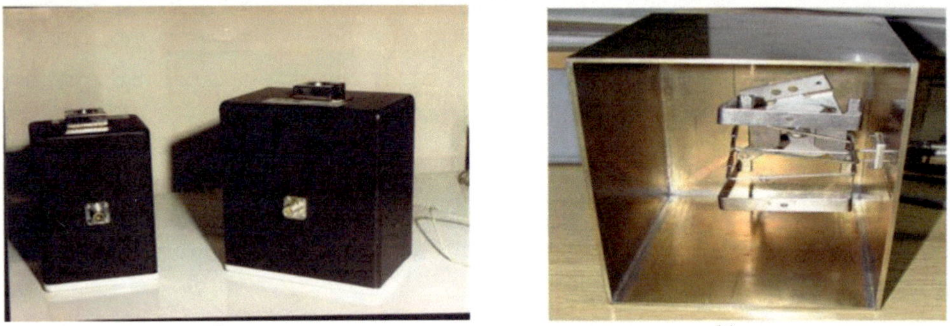

a) b)

Fig. 2. a) Dielectric filled waveguide applicator, b) air filled Evanescent mode applicator.

On the next picture (Fig. 3.) there is a sketch of evanescent waveguide mode applicator working at 70 MHz, including its SAR distribution. There is a water bolus between aperture of the applicator and the agar phantom mimicking the biological tissue.

Interesting possibility how to achieve relatively sharp beam from external applicator is to use a focusing principle. The aperture of a standard rectangular waveguide applicator is then divided into 3 or 5 sectors with shifted excitation (i.e. different amplitude and phase). Another way how to focus microwave power is to use an array of external applicators, where amplitudes and phases of excitation of single applicators can be used for electronic steering of the focus area.

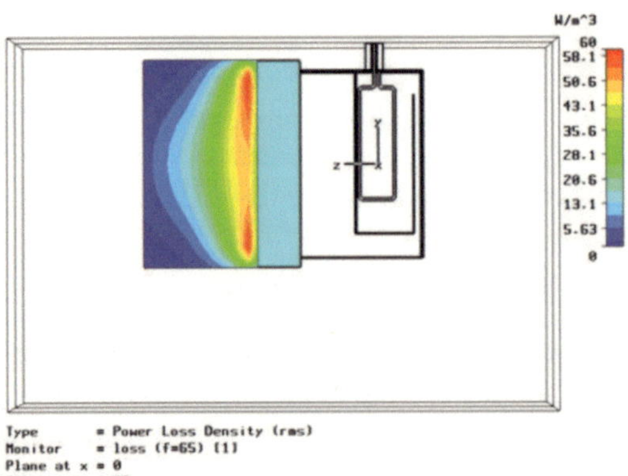


Fig. 3. Evanescent mode applicator and its calculated SAR pattern

### 3.2 Microwave stripline TEM applicators

Microwave stripline applicator with TEM (Transversal Electromagnetic Mode) is being described in the following. The TEM wave propagation depends on dielectric parameters, such as permittivity ε and permeability μ. The upper and bottom part of applicator consists of high conductivity material (copper). Transversal dimensions of the described applicator are 50 x 30 mm. Distance of exciting probe from short circuited section is 15 mm. Lateral sides of applicator are made from dielectric material, from acrylic glass, which is 2 mm thick. The second part of applicator consists of stripline horn. Dimensions of the horn aperture are 120 x 80 mm and length of applicator equals to two wavelengths. Wavelength depends on permittivity of environment (in our case $\varepsilon_{H20}$ = 78). Whereas 70% of human body consists of water, applicator is filled with water. Advantage of this is better transfer of EM energy into human body and smaller dimensions of the applicator. This applicator was designed by the Finite Difference Time Domain (FDTD) simulator EM Field simulator (e.g. SEMCAD X).

### 3.3 Deep local heating applicators

Waveguide type applicators are very suitable for the deep local thermotherapy treatment based either on the principle of dielectric filled waveguide or on the principle of evanescent modes (i.e. waveguides excited below its cut-off frequency) - which is our specific solution and original contribution to the theory of microwave hyperthermia applicators. Technology of evanescent mode applicators enable us to design applicators with as small aperture as necessary also for relatively low frequencies e.g. from 10 to 100 MHz, needed for deep penetration into the biological tissue (i.e. up to 10 centimetres under the body surface). In theoretical and experimental evaluation, the grade of homogeneity of the temperature distribution in the target area has been tested, see the Fig. 4. Our mathematical approach is based on idea of waveguide $TM_{01}$ (Transverse Magnetic) mode excited in the agar phantom under the given conditions (see the dashed lines). Measurement of SAR (full lines) has been done on agar phantom of the muscle tissue.

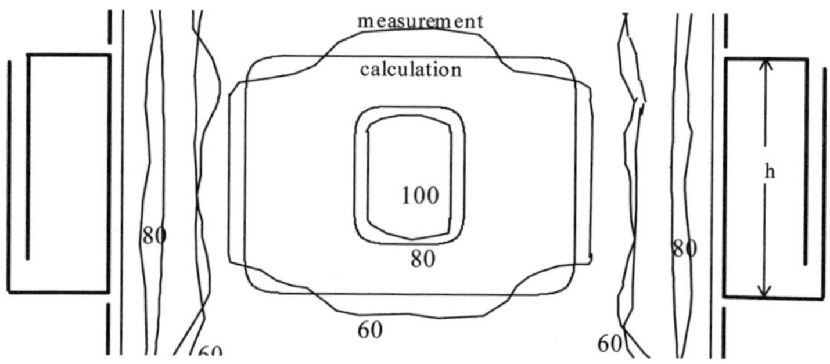


Fig. 4. Normalized SAR distribution (both calculated (full line) and measured (dashed line)) in the agar phantom.

### 3.4 New principles for the regional applicators

Goal of this work is the development of the new applicators with higher treatment effects. Methodological approach for the solution of the problem will be theoretical and experimental study of the new types of regional applicators. Our aim is to improve the present theoretical model to optimize the temperature distribution in the treated area.

We can design the regional applicators on the basis of the analytical description of the excited electromagnetic field for the case of simplified homogeneous model of the treated biological tissue. For a more realistic case of the non-homogeneous dielectric composition of the biological tissue the analytical calculation does not guarantee enough exact results. Therefore we would need to build the equipment for experimental tests of the applicators and we will study the possibilities of its numerical mathematical modelling.

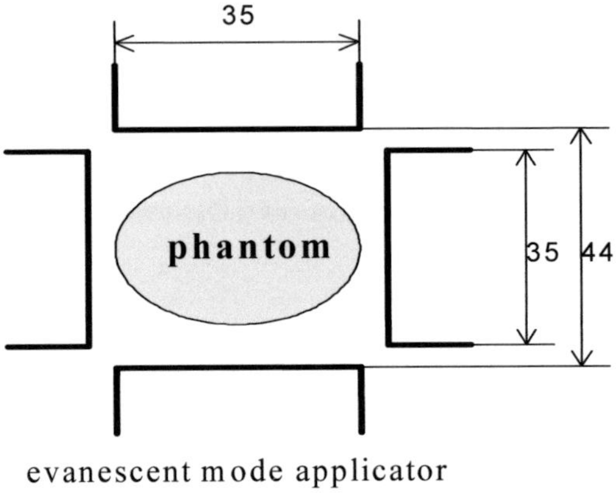


Fig. 5. Set up of proposed regional applicator (4 evanescent mode waveguides applicators)

Applicators must have perfect impedance matching for good protection of microwave generator against reflected power. For measurement of impedance matching a reflection parameter $s_{11}$ is mostly used. This parameter shows, how much electromagnetic power is reflected back to generator. Electromagnetic field is inside discussed applicator excited at frequency of 434 MHz.

### 3.5 Anatomical model

To verify basic functionality of created applicator we can use a homogeneous agar phantom. This homogeneous phantom represents only one type of tissue in human body – in our case it represents muscle tissue. For further discussion we will use cylindrical agar phantom with diameter 8 cm, which can basically represent a human limb. In reality human body is very inhomogeneous, and therefore it is for hyperthermia treatment planning necessary to use anatomical precise 3D models with all types of biological tissues taken into account. 3D model thus can be created from segmentation of series of several scans from CT or MRI. Such scans are 2 dimensional transversal gray – scale cuts. After then is created 3D model imported to the program, which is used for hyperthermia treatment planning. This program must both cooperate well with a segmentation program and in the same moment to enable calculation of SAR distribution.

We can choose e.g. woman's calf (Fig. 6.) as an example to demonstrate EM simulations potential. Given anatomical model was created by segmentation program 3D – DOCTOR (vector-based 3D imaging, modelling and measurement software (Able Software Corp., 2011)). We should have available DICOM scans from CT (MRRF, 2010). DICOM scans hold the original quality of data. Model of woman's calf has resolution of 1 mm and mean voxel size is 1 x 1 x 1 mm.

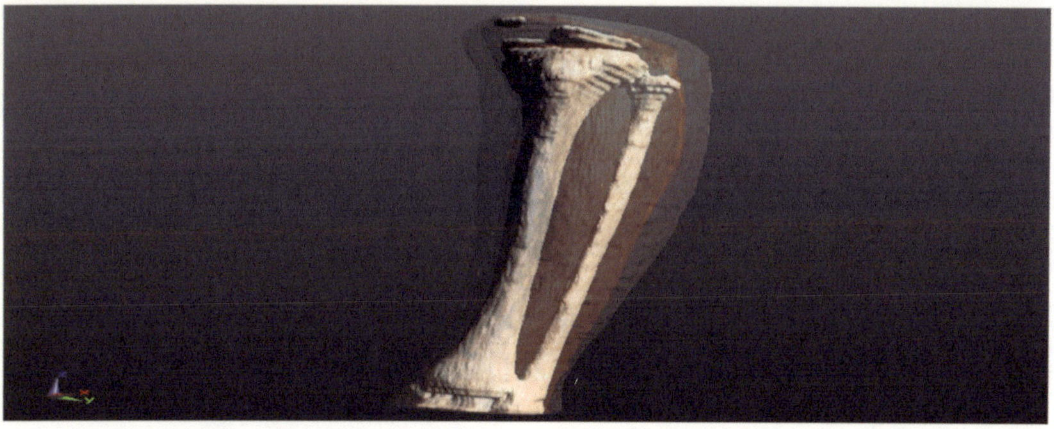

Fig. 6. 3D anatomical model of woman's calf

Each voxel was assigned to one of 3 different types of biological tissue, such as bone, muscle and fat with dielectric parameter shown in table (Table 1.).

| Name | Conductivity [S/m] | Relative Permittivity [-] |
|---|---|---|
| Agar | 0.80 | 54.00 |
| Bone Cortical | 0.09 | 13.07 |
| Muscle | 0.80 | 56.86 |
| Fat | 0.04 | 5.56 |

Table 2. Dielectric properties at frequency 434 MHz

### 3.6 Array of applicators

EM behaviour of arrays of 2, 3 and 4 stripline type applicators coupled to homogeneous cylindrical agar phantom and consequently on 3D anatomical model of woman's calf. Cylindrical agar phantom represents muscle tissue of human limb. In our case we simulated muscle tissue of woman's calf with diameter of 8 cm. The 3D anatomical model consists of 3 various types of tissue of woman's calf created from CT scans. All of here discussed arrays of applicators were simulated by FTDT program SEMCAD X.

#### 3.6.1 Array of 2 microwave stripline applicators

Case of array of 2 applicators on cylindrical agar phantom coupled to 3D anatomical model of woman's calf is shown on following picture (Fig. 7.). From both normalized SAR distributions (Fig. 8.) it follows that this array of 2 applicators is suitable for treatment of tumor, which cover larger area near to surface of human limb.

#### 3.6.2 Array of 3 microwave stripline applicators

The other possible configuration is array of 3 applicators coupled to homogeneous cylindrical agar phantom (Fig. 9a.). Consequently, we studied simulations of 3 applicators coupled to the 3D anatomical model (Fig. 9b.).

Another interesting case is shown on Fig. 10. –in this picture there are displayed interesting shapes of SAR distribution by change of phases of applicators and change of amplitude of one type of applicator located in the middle of all applicators.

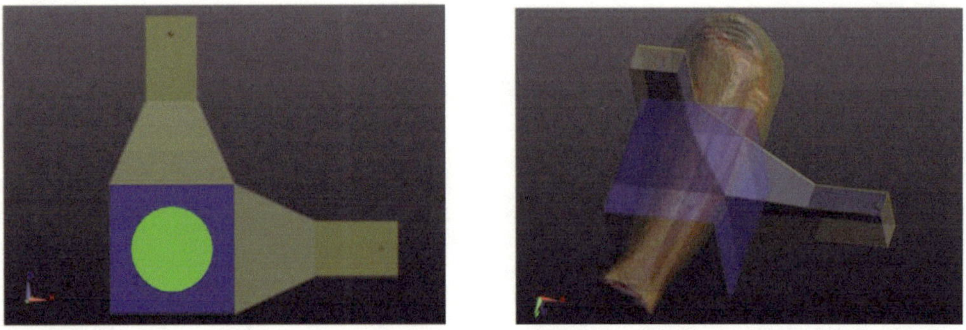

a) b)

Fig. 7. Array of 2 applicators a) on cylindrical agar phantom, b) on anatomical model

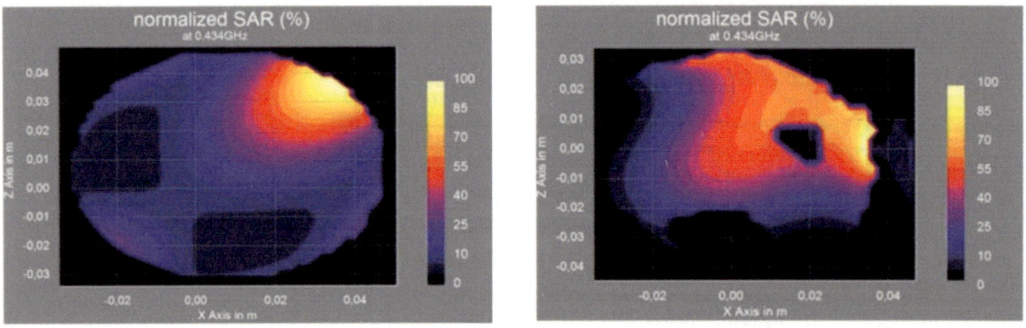


a) b)

Fig. 8. Normalized SAR a) in agar phantom, b) in anatomical model

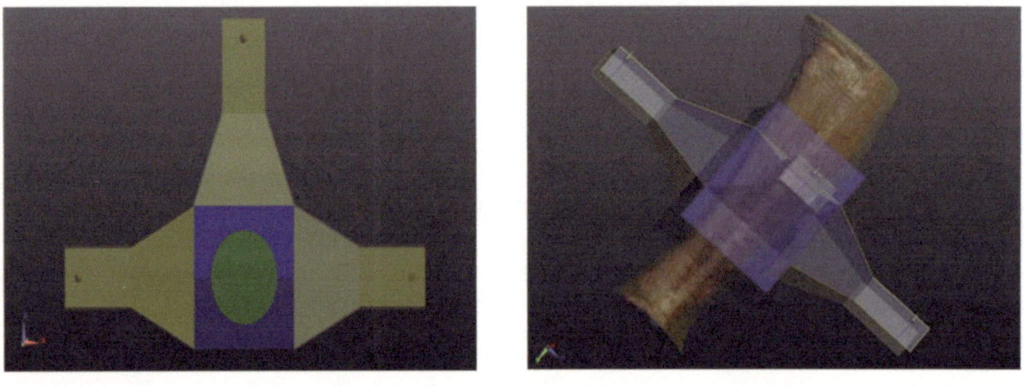

a) b)

Fig. 9. Composition of 3 applicators a) on cylindrical agar phantom, b) on anatomical model

In homogeneous phantom were created 3 maxima, instead in anatomical model we can observe only one maximum of SAR distribution - that demonstrates very nice example of focussing possibilities. By setting of phases and/or amplitude of applicators we can accomplish required shape of SAR.

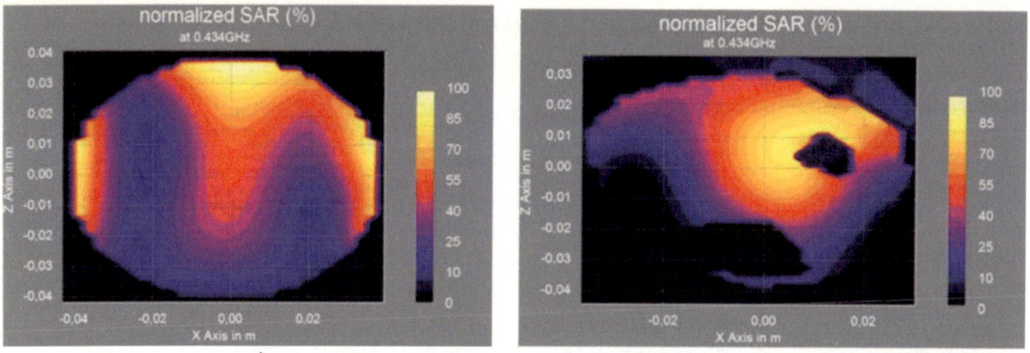


a) b)

Fig. 10. Normalized SAR a) in agar phantom, b) in normalized SAR in anatomical model

### 3.6.3 Array of 4 microwave stripline applicators

By using 4 applicators we can see in following picture (Fig. 11.), that in both cases there is a very good focusing effect of SAR distribution near to the cylindrical axis.
By alternation of phases of several applicators we achieved better focusing in the middle of both homogeneous agar phantom and 3D anatomical model (Fig. 12.). Such array of 4 applicators could be used for treatment tumors located in the middle of human limb.

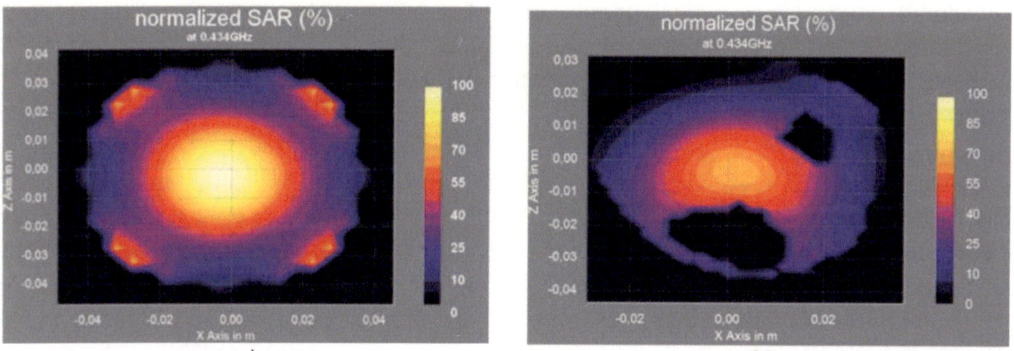


a) b)

Fig. 12. Normalized SAR a) in agar phantom, b) in anatomical model

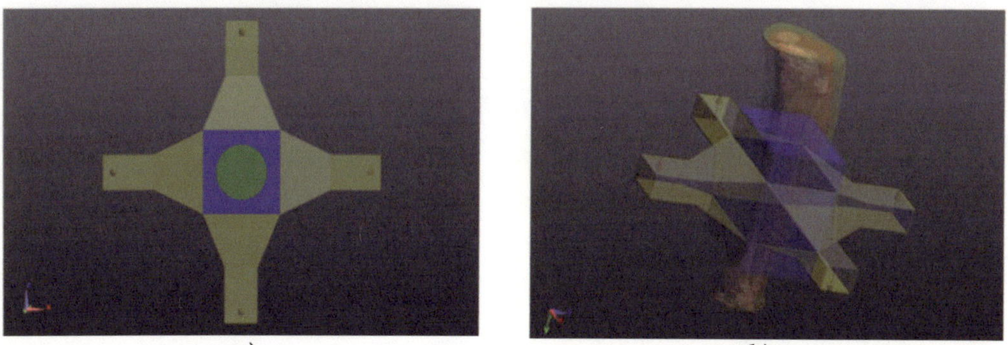

a) b)

Fig. 11. Array of 4 applicators a) on cylindrical agar phantom, b) on anatomical model

## 4. Microwave applicators for „BPH" thermotherapy

In all above mentioned key activities we need to do numerical simulations of SAR and temperature 3D distribution. Temperature distribution inside area of biological tissue heated by microwave energy can be calculated from well known formula:

$$\rho_t c_t \frac{\partial T}{\partial t} = \gamma_t \Delta T - \chi(\mathrm{T} - \mathrm{T_b}) + \mathrm{q} \qquad (1)$$

where t is the time.
$q = q(x,y,z,t)$ is energy delivered by EM field,
$T = T(x,y,z,t)$ is designates the temperature,
$Tb = Tb(x,y,z,t_o)$ is the temperature of blood,
Physical meaning and values of the here used constants for the case of high water contents tissue are:
$r_t = 0.965$ [g/cm3] is density of biological tissue (BT).
$c_t = 3\,586$ [mJ/g/C] is specific heat of BT.
k = 5.45 [mW/cm3/C] is blood flow and temperature capacity of BT.
$g_t = 5.84$ [mW/cm/C] is spec. temp. conductivity of BT.
Possibilities of analytical solution of this equation are very limited to only a few cases - like e.g. "one dimensional" case of plane wave penetrating in homogeneous phantom. Therefore computers are to be used to solve this equation to obtain the temperature *T(x,y,z,t)* time dependence and space distribution. For the treatment planning of microwave thermotherapy we use software product SEMCAD. Fig. 13 gives basic idea about SAR calculated for the case of the monopole intracavitary applicator.

### 4.1 Applicators for „BPH" treatment

We have investigated basic types of microwave intracavitary applicators suitable for BPH treatment, i.e. monopole, dipole and a helical coil structures. These applicators are designed to work either at 915 or at 434 MHz. We would like to discuss its effective heating depth, based on the comparison of the theoretical and experimental results. Basic mechanisms and parameters influencing (limiting) heating effective depth are described and explained in ref. (Vrba et al., 1996, 1999).

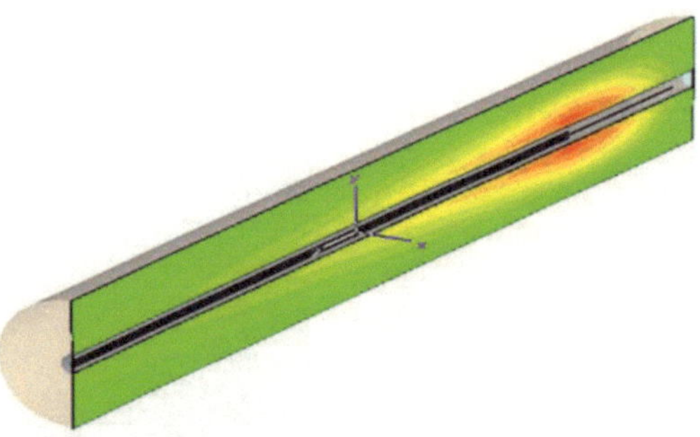

Fig. 13. Calculated SAR of BPH applicator

The basic type of intracavitary applicator is a monopole applicator. The construction of this applicator is very simple, but calculated and measured SAR distribution along the applicator is more complicated, than has been the first idea. SAR can be measured either in water phantom or by infrared camera.

### 4.2 Evaluation of BPH applicators

One of our tools for experimental evaluation of microwave applicators is the apparatus, which enable us to do 3D measurements of SAR distribution. It can be used for both local external and intracavitary applicators.

The basic part of this apparatus is big salt water phantom (water with 0.3% to 0.6% NaCl) and the measurement probe with the possibility of 3D scan around the applicators. As probes we use a Light Emitting Diodes (LED) with a fibber optic link connection to interface of the computer. The purpose of this link is to reduce influence of the metallic (i.e. conductive) components from the measured electromagnetic field. The schematics of the apparatus for 3D measurements of SAR distribution is shown in Fig. 14.

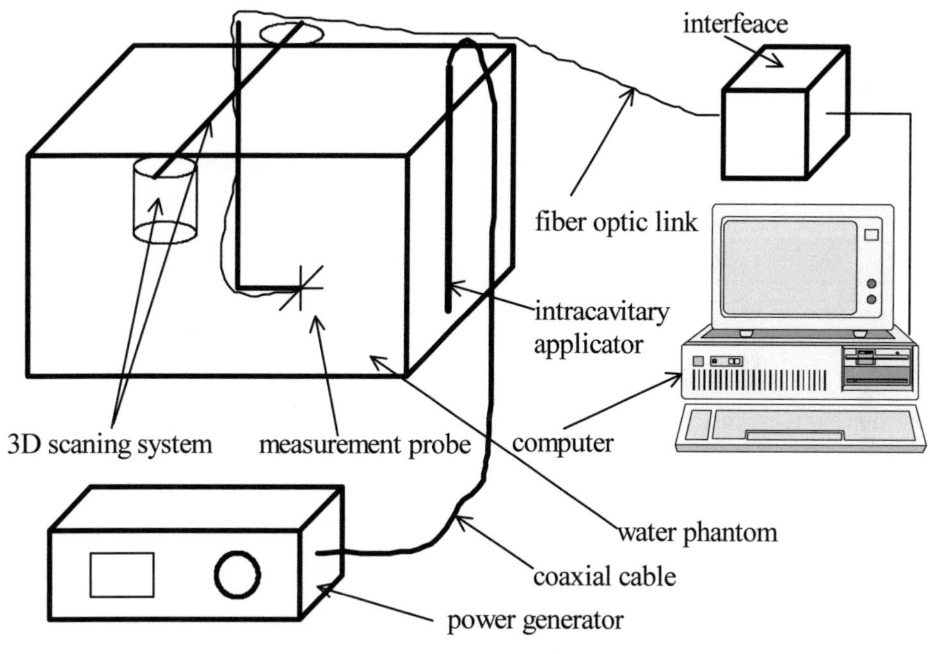


Fig. 14. Apparatus for 3D SAR measurements

During measurements of SAR along the applicator we have found, that typically there is not only a one main SAR maximum (first from the right side), but also a second and/or higher order maxima can be created, being produced by outside back wave propagating along the coaxial cable, see Fig. 15a. In Fig. 15b. SAR distribution improvement (i.e. reduction of second maximum) can be noticed for the case of dipole like applicator. To eliminate this second maximum and optimise the focusing of SAR in predetermined area of biological tissue needs to use the helical coil antenna structure.

After coil radius and length optimisation we have obtained very good results of SAR distribution, see Fig. 16a,b. Some problems can be with the antenna self-heating, but it can be reduced by cooler at the end of applicator tip.

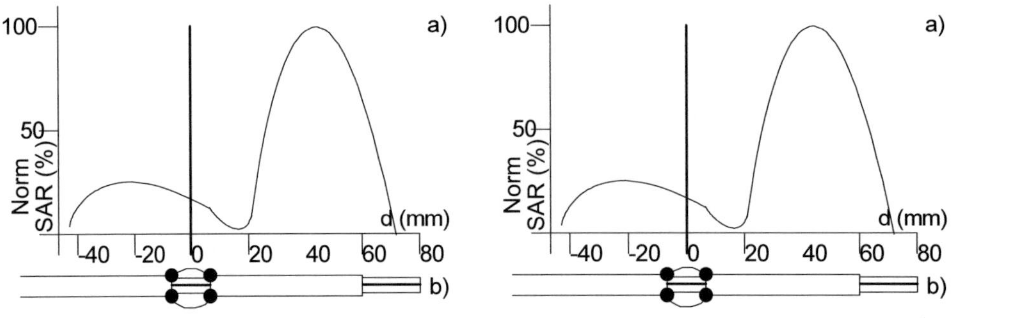


a) b)

Fig. 15. a) Monopole applicator, b) Dipole applicator

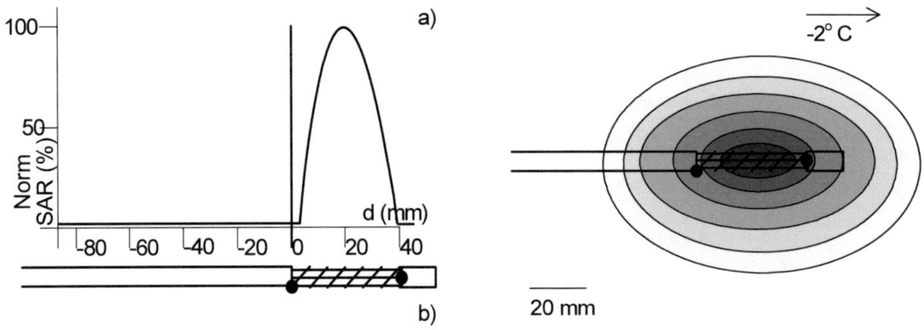


a) b)

Fig. 16. a) Helical coil applicator, b) Temperature field around the helix

### 4.3 Effective treatment depth

We have studied the theoretical limits of intracavitary applicator heating depth. We have found the basic relation for determination of the limit of maximum heating depth for the case of "very long" intracavitary applicator. We suppose excitation of an ideal radial wave around radiating applicator.

Mentioned results can be simply interpreted by following figure, where on the horizontal axis is the working frequency of thermotherapy apparatus and on vertical axis there is effective depth of electromagnetic wave penetration. As a third parameter playing an important role there is a diameter of a discussed intracavitary applicator.

Very important is that in this case we are dealing with a radial wave, not the plane wave, and that's why the penetration depth is smaller than penetration depth of plane wave. Some works published in this field give too optimistic results. Measurements discussed without theoretical analysis can give results influenced by thermal conductivity of mostly used agar phantom of muscle tissue. As the real heating depth is typically a few millimetres (in the best case up to approx. 1 cm under the surface of the cavity), thermal conductivity of the phantom material can easily cause errors of several tenth of percents.

Ideal intracavitary applicator irradiates an ideal cylindrical wave into the biological tissue surrounding the cavity. According to our experience Fig. 17. gives very good approximation, i.e. the results with accuracy better than 5 % for higher frequencies (f >100 MHz) and/or bigger radii (R > 3mm). For lower frequencies (up to 100 MHz) combined with small radius of the cavity (R < 2 mm) the accuracy is cca 10 %. It is not possible to achieve a heating penetration depth (i.e. 50 % decrease) higher than *R* at any frequency and in any propagation medium. The small cavity radius plays a dominant role in the penetration depth.

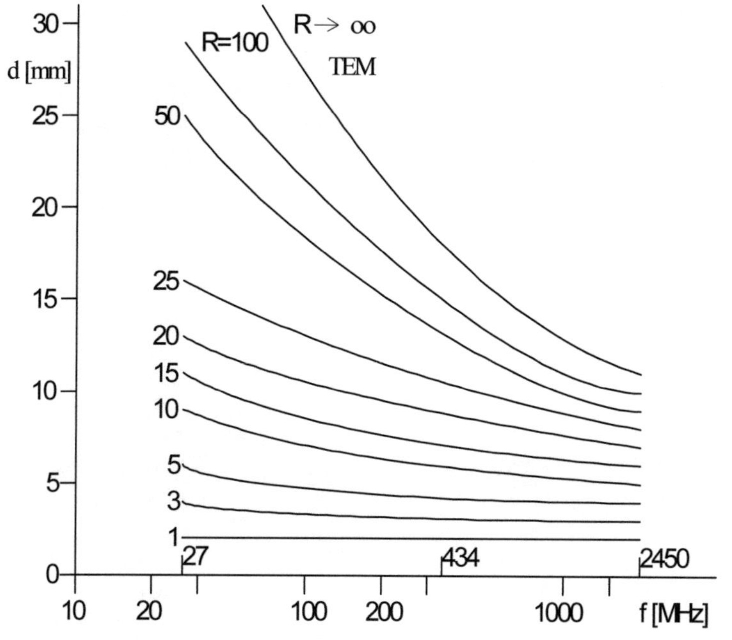


Fig. 17. Effective depth of heating d with respect to frequency f [MHz] and radius R [mm]

### 4.4 SAR measurements by infrared camera

Infrared camera is according to our experiences a very efficient tool for "SAR" measurements of microwave intracavitary applicators. In Fig. 18. there is the typical measured heating pattern of monopole (a), dipole (b), and helical coil antennas (c). This pattern can be obtained by heating suitable phantoms of biological tissue - mimicring the dielectric and thermal properties of the prostate tissue. Such phantoms can be made on the basis of agar or so called superstuff material. The pattern is colour-coded according to a linearly decreasing scale of white-yellow-red, where white is the maximum temperature. A diagrammatic catheter is inserted in each figure; the orientation of the bladder neck in a patient is indicated by a dashed line. Note the long back heating tails with a monopole antenna (Fig. 18a.) which is caused by microwave currents that flow backwards along the cable and cause the feeding cable to radiate. The radiation pattern from a dipole antenna (Fig. 18b.) is generally well confined without any excessive back heating. The dipole antenna is suitable for prostates with axial length > 40 mm. The helical coil antenna (Fig. 18c.) has the shortest and most focussed heating and would be the choice for small prostates, 25 – 40 mm in length.

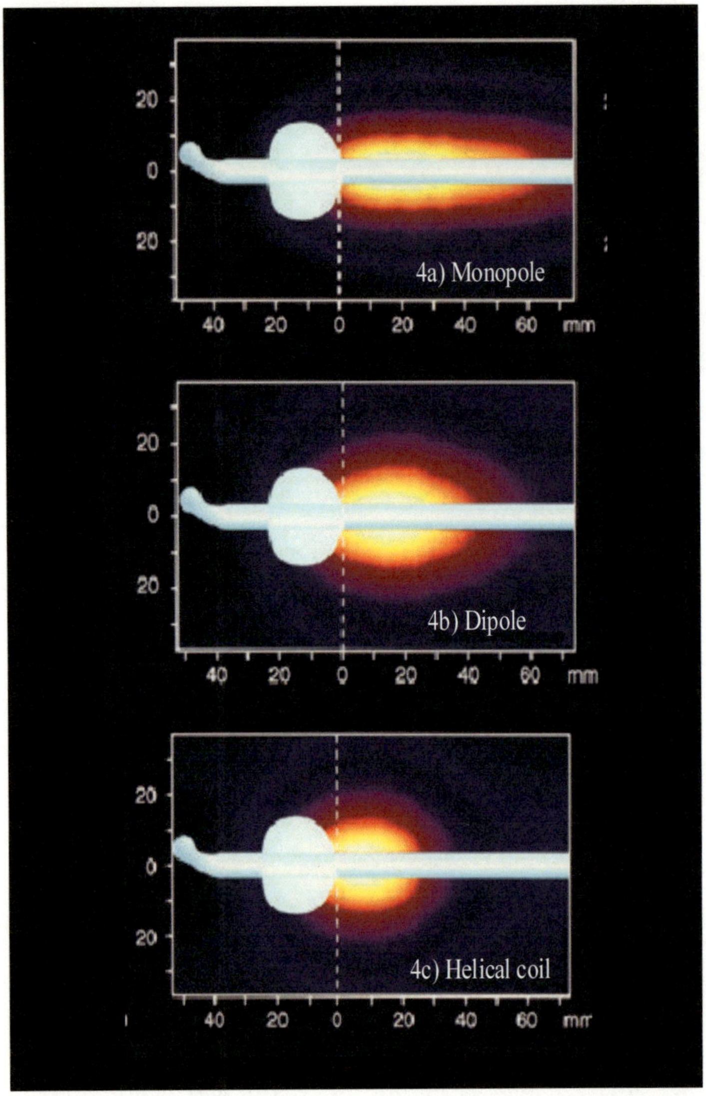


Fig. 18. The heating pattern for different antennas: a) the monopole, b) the dipole, c) the helical coil.

The pattern is colour-coded according to a linearly decreasing scale of white-yellow-red , where white is the maximum temperature. A diagrammatic catheter is inserted in each figure; the orientation of the bladder neck in a patient is indicated by a dashed line.
The pattern is colour-coded according to a linearly decreasing scale of white-yellow-red , where white is the maximum temperature. A diagrammatic catheter is inserted in each figure; the orientation of the bladder neck in a patient is indicated by a dashed line.
Moreover, by using infra-red camera we can follow a lot of other properties resp. behaviour of intracavitary applicators itself, like e.g. standing waves along feeding coaxial cable (i.e. the risk of existence of unwanted SAR and/or temperature maxima), possible overheating of some specific parts of tested applicator itself etc.

## 5. Technical equipment for research of biological effects of EM field

In present time four research institutions here in the Czech Republic run research projects focused on studies of interactions between EM field and biological systems. These institutions are technically supported by Dept. of EM Field of the Czech Technical University in Prague. In this contribution we would like to give more details about that projects and obtained technical results (i.e. description of developed exposition systems).
Three of discussed projects (1 in Germany and 2 here in Czech Republic) are basic research for simulation of the microwave hyperthermia treatment. Other two projects (both in Czech Republic are focused on simulation of the case of exposition by mobile phone.
In the modern view, cancer is intended as a complex illness, involving the cells that undergo to transformation, their environment, and the general responses at biochemical and biological levels induced in the host. Consequently, the anti-cancer treatment protocols need to be multi-modal to reach curative effects. Especially after the technical improvements achieved in the last 15 years by bio-medical engineering, microscopy devices, and molecular biology methods, the combinations of therapeutic procedures are growing in interest in basic and clinical research.
The combination of applied biological research together to the physical sciences can offer important perspectives in anticancer therapy (e.g. different methodologies and technical devices for application of energies to pathological tissues).
The modern bioengineering knowledge applied to traditional tools, as the microscopy, has largely renewed and expanded the fields of their applications (e.g.: in vivo imaging), pushing the interest for direct morpho-functional investigations of the biomedical problems.

### 5.1 Waveguide applicator

Very good results of EM field expositions in biological experiments can be obtained by simple but efficient waveguide applicators see example in Fig. 19. Waveguide offer a very big advantage - in approximately of fifty percents of its aperture the irradiated electromagnetic field is very near to a plane wave, which is basic assumption for good homogeneity of the heating and optimal treatment penetration.
Here described system is being used (shared) for research projects by two institutions (Institute of Radiation Oncology in Prague and Institute of Microbiology of the Czech Academy of Sciences).

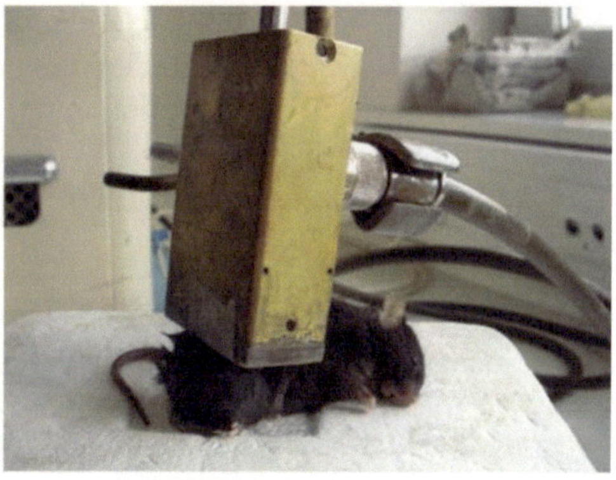

Fig. 19. Waveguide applicator for biological experiments

Aperture of this waveguide is 4.8 x 2.4 cm and it is excited at frequency 2.45 GHz. Effective heating is in the middle of the real aperture - its size is approximately 2.4 x 2.4 cm. Waveguide is filled by teflon to reduce its cut-off frequency. Power from generator is possible to control from 10 to 180 W, in these experiments we work between 10 and 20 W mostly.

### 5.2 Evaluation of waveguide applicator

To evaluate this applicator from technical point of view we made a series of experiments, see e.g. Fig. 20, where you can see example of measurement of temperature distribution by IR camera.

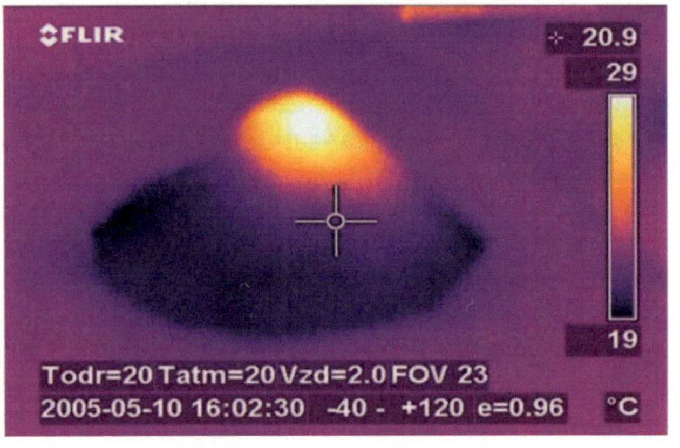


Fig. 20. Temperature distribution obtained on surface of a model of mouse

Here you can see temperature distribution obtained on surface of a model of mouse made from agar - with a simulated tumour on mouse back. Experiment has been done by heating phantom during 2 minutes delivering a power of 10 W. Maximum of temperature increase has been found approximately 10 °C. Similar results with different increase in temperature we have got also in other technical experiments on phantom or live mouse when power or heating time was changed.

Next Fig. 21. gives example of temperature increase on the surface of the phantom and 1 cm in that phantom. Temperature was measured by our 4-chanel thermometer. In this case with two thermo probes. Heating here is scheduled to 9 times repeated 30 s of heating and 30 s pause. Difference in temperature on the surface and under it is on the level of 1 °C. That means very good homogeneity of temperature distribution in the treated area during planned biological experiments.

### 5.3 Array applicator

The main goal of the planned biological experiment is a hyperthermia treatment of the experimentally induced pedicle tumours of the rat to verify the feasibility of ultrasound diagnostics and magnetic resonance imaging respectively to map the temperature distribution in the target area of the treatment. That means to heat effective volume of approximately cylindrical shape (diameter approx. 2 cm, height approx. 3 cm). Temperature to be reached is 41 °C or more (i.e. temperature increase of at least 4 °C from starting point 37 °C), time period of heating is 45 minutes.

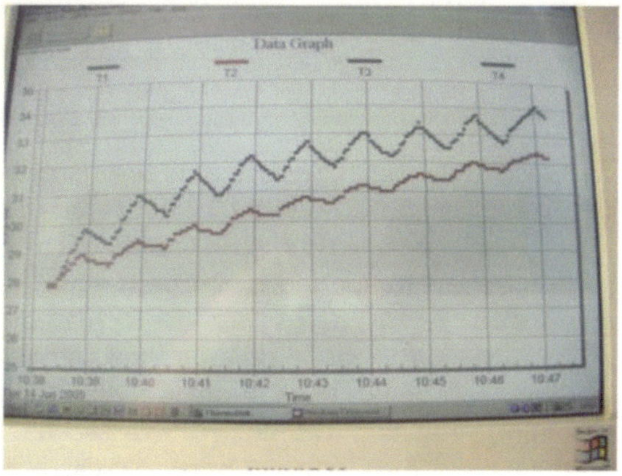

Fig. 21. Temperatures during experiments

Considering the necessary effective heating depth for the planned experiments, we have found 915 MHz to be suitable frequency. As an excellent compatibility of the applicator with non-invasive temperature measurement system (ultrasound or NMR) is a fundamental condition for our project, we should have to use non-magnetic metallic sheets of minimised dimensions to create the conductive elements of the applicator. Therefore the applicator itself (see Fig. 22.) is created by two inductive loops tuned to resonance by capacitive elements (Vrba, 1993). Dimensions of these resonant loops were designed by our software, developed for this purpose. Coupling between coaxial feeder and resonant loops (not shown in Fig. 22.) as well as a mutual coupling between resonating loops could be adjusted to optimum by microwave network analyser.

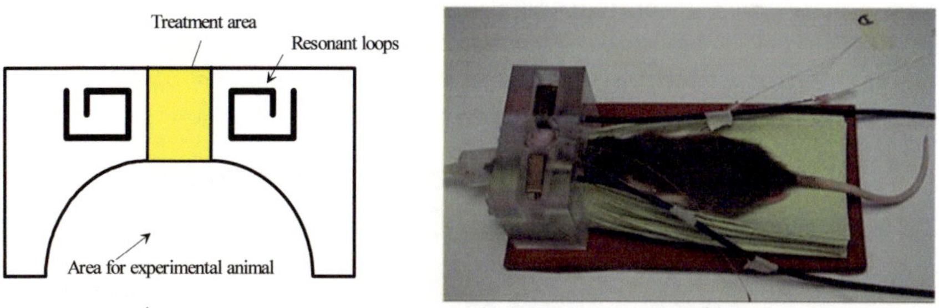


a) b)

Fig. 22. a) Arrangement of discussed microwave hyperthermia applicator, b) Photograph of the discussed applicator

The position of the loops is fixed by perspex holder. There is a special cylindrical space for experimental animal in lower part of this perspex holder. As the heated tissue has a high dielectric losses, both loops are very well separated and so no significant resonance in heated area can occur. From this follows, that either the position of the loops with respect to heated area or the distance between the loops is not very critical.

First measurements to evaluate the basic properties of the discussed applicator were done on agar phantom of muscle tissue:

- evaluation of basic microwave properties (transfer of EM energy to the tissue, reflections),

- evaluation of compatibility with US and NMR,
- calculation and measurement of SAR and temperature distribution and its homogeneity.

Exact tuning of the resonant loops to frequency 915 MHz has been easy and we could optimise the coupling between the coaxial feeders and resonant loops as well, reflection coefficient less than 0.1. We have tested the power to be delivered to the applicator to obtain sufficient temperature increase (approximately 4 °C in less than 5 minutes is required). With power 10 W delivered to each loop for period of 2 minutes we succeeded to obtain the temperature increase of approximately 7 °C. To keep the increased temperature for a long time, 2 W in each loops were sufficient. Similar values were obtained during first experiments on rats also. Even with higher level of delivered microwave power we did not observe the change of resonant frequency (caused by increased temperature of the loops). This applicator has been developed for German Cancer Research Institute in Heidelberg. And it is being used there for a series of animal experiments to study effect of hyperthermia on tumours and possibility to combine hyperthermia with chemotherapy etc.

Compatibility of this applicator with a Magnetic resonance unit (MR) has been studied and it has been demonstrated. We have tested the influence of the applicators on US diagnostics and NMR imaging and the result of this evaluation shows very good compatibility. Only a negligible deterioration of the US images has been observed when the incident power was kept under 100 W.

Details about influence of microwave power on MR imaging are given in Fig. 23. We can see here a sequence of images of the discussed applicator made by MR unit for four different cases. First case (upper left) is image for the case without power excitation of the applicator. Second case (left down) a power of 10 W has been delivered to each loop. We can see quite clear configuration of the applicator set-up. Third case (upper right) gives situation when 20 W has been delivered to each loop. Slight noise but still quite a clear configuration of the applicator set-up can be observed. Fourths case (right down) gives situation when 40 W has been delivered to each loop. In this case noise disturbed the possibility to observe the configuration of the applicator.

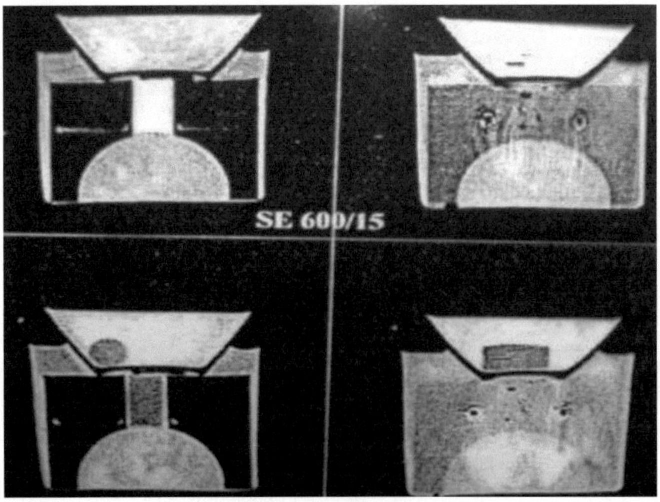


Fig. 23. MR images of the discussed applicator

In Fig. 25. we can see temperature vs. time measurement in the case of agar phantom inserted in the studied applicator. Next Fig. 26. shows experimental setup of applicator and simple exposure chambers installed at Medical Faculty of Charles University in Pilsen. 3D distribution of SAR distribution was verified numerically (Fig. 24).

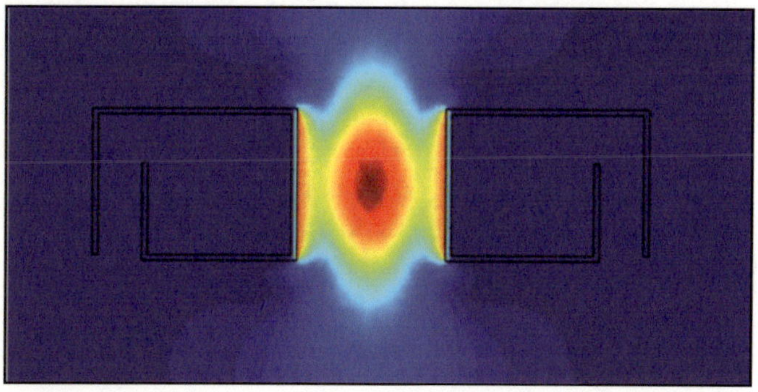

Fig. 24. Numerical SAR analysis.

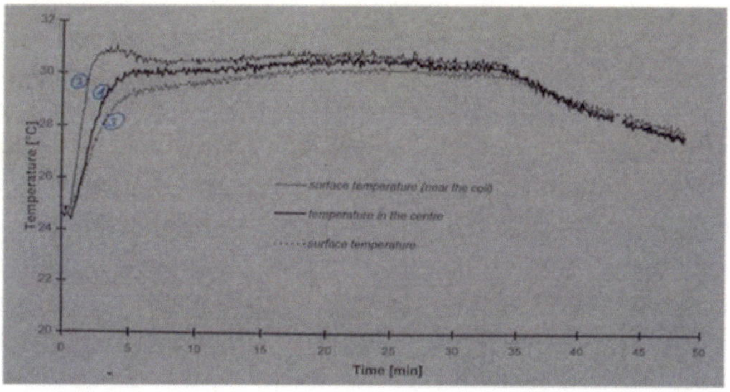


Fig. 25. Temperature measurements

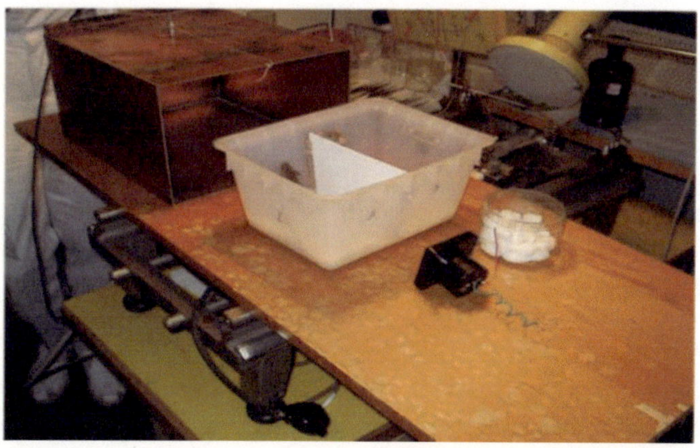

Fig. 26. Exposure system for research of electromagnetic field and biological system interactions

## 6. Measurement of the complex permittivity of the biological tissue as the possible imaging method

### 6.1 Introduction

This sub-chapter describes and evaluates a method for determining complex permittivity, and presents results of permittivity measurement of inhomogeneous agar phantom and living tissue. There are described different approaches for measurement of complex permittivity, in particular the non-invasive method of measuring complex permittivity at the end of the coaxial cable. Vector measurement of the reflection coefficient on the interface between probes and measured samples is performed with the aid of network analyzer in the frequency range from 300 kHz to 2 GHz. The results indicate that using the coaxial probe with dimensions of SMA (subminiature version A) connector is suitable in the frequency range approximately from 300 MHz to 10 GHz. In order to demonstrate the diagnostic potential of this method, measurements were first conducted on artificially created inhomogeneous agar phantom with added mixture of various dielectrics, followed by measurement of living biological tissue.

### 6.2 Complex permittivity

Relative permittivity, loss factor and conductivity are basic parameters for electromagnetic field modeling and simulations. Although these parameters could be found in the tables for many materials, their experimental determination is very often necessary (Hippel, 1954). Dielectric properties of biological tissues are determining factors for the dissipation of electromagnetic energy in the human body and therefore they are useful in hyperthermia cancer treatment. Measurement of the dielectric parameters of biological tissues is also a promising method in the medical diagnostics and imaging. Knowledge of the complex permittivity in an treated area, i.e. knowledge of the complex permittivity of healthy and tumor tissue, is very important for example in the diagnosing of tumor regions in the human body (Choi et al., 2004) or in the design of thermo-therapeutic applicators which transform electromagnetic energy into thermal energy in the tissue (Williams et al., 2008). Permittivity is known as

$$\varepsilon = \varepsilon_0 \varepsilon_c \tag{2}$$

where $\varepsilon_0$ is free space permittivity and $\varepsilon_c$ is complex relative permittivity. Complex relative permittivity can be written as

$$\varepsilon_c = \varepsilon_r - j\varepsilon_r \tan\delta \tag{3}$$

where $\varepsilon_r$ is real part of complex relative permittivity and $\tan\delta$ is loss factor.

### 6.3 Methods of complex permittivity measurement

The most commonly used method for measuring the complex permittivity is a method of measuring dielectric inserted into a dielectric waveguide. This method is very accurate, but unfortunately requires irreversible changes in the measured material. Another method used for measurement of complex permittivity is RLC measuring bridge. This method is very accurate but there are a few requirements on the quality of the interfaces of the measured material and the capacitor plates (Thompson, 1956). In most cases, this method is used as narrowband. The method of measurement in free space has its limitations in the demand for high-loss dielectrics measured. Electromagnetic wave through the material must be attenuated by at least 10 dB. Otherwise, standing waves will be created, which contribute significantly to the inaccuracy of this method. The method of measurement in cavity resonators gives us results with good accuracy. On the other hand, it is difficult to produce precise machining of the resonator and the measured material inserted inside (Ramachandraiah et al., 1975). Latest often used method for measuring complex permittivity measurement method is the open end of the waveguide, in our case, the coaxial cable. This method can be considered as very accurate. Moreover, we can achieve a good repetition of the results when we maintain the phase stability of the measuring coaxial cable (Tanaba & Joines, 1976). In this work, this application was selected for the main method for measuring complex permittivity of biological tissues because of its non-invasive nature.

### 6.3.1 Principle of reflection method

The reflection method represents measurement of reflection coefficient on the interface between two materials, on the open end of the coaxial line and the material under test. It is a well-known method for determining the dielectric parameters (Tanaba & Joines, 1976). This method is based on the fact that the reflection coefficient of an open-ended coaxial line depends on the dielectric parameters of material under test which is attached to it. For calculating the complex permittivity from the measured reflection coefficient, it is useful to use an equivalent circuit of an open-ended coaxial line. The probe translates changes in the permittivity of a material under test into changes of the input reflection coefficient of the probe. The surface of the sample of material under test must be in perfect contact with the probe. The thickness of a measured sample must be at least twice of equivalent penetration depth of the electromagnetic wave. This assures that the waves reflected from the material under test interface are attenuated (Stuchly et al., 1994).

### 6.4 Measurement probes

For measurement probes, we have adapted the standard N and SMA RF connectors from which the parts for connecting to a panel were removed. The measurement probes can be described by the equivalent circuit consisting of the coupling capacitance between the inner and outer conductor out of the coaxial structure and radiating conductance which represents propagation losses (Popovic el al., 2005). These capacitance and conductance are frequency and permittivity dependent.

### 6.4.1 N probe

Probe for measuring the complex permittivity of biological tissues has been adapted from a standard RF connector for coaxial cable N-type connector, see Fig. 27. The original proposed range of application was $f_{BW} = 1$ GHz, which together with the development of microwave technology is extended until today's $f_{BW} = 12$ GHz. N connector used in the construction of the probe is standard N 50Ω connector that can be used up to frequency $f = 5$ GHz. The measurements were kept with a high degree of the accuracy and repeatability. The measurement probe based on N connectors had significantly less bandwidth, and $f_1 = 100$ MHz and $f_2 = 1$ GHz.

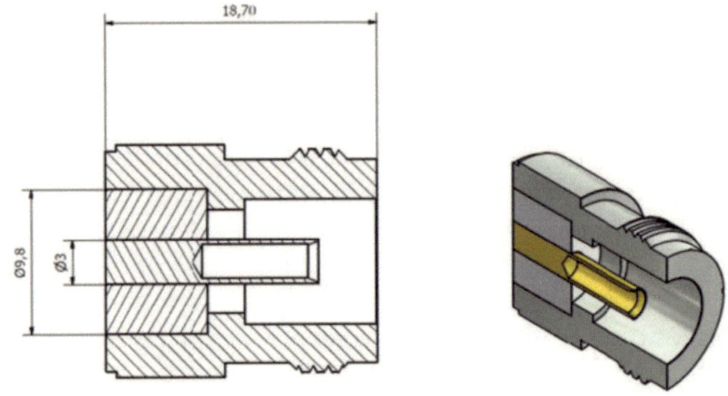


Fig. 27. Basic scheme of the N probe's dimensions

### 6.4.2 SMA probe

Probe for measuring the complex permittivity based on the SMA-connector was adapted from a standard 50 Ω SMA connector which was developed around 1960 when it was required to create a miniaturized version of the N connector with a higher frequency range of application. Today SMA connectors operate in the band up to f = 18 GHz. SMA connector used for the production of SMA probes, Fig. 28. shows low-cost, standard RF connectors with a usable bandwidth up to f = 12 GHz. This solution is appropriate for the purposes of our measurements because the highest frequency measured is equal to f = 2 GHz.

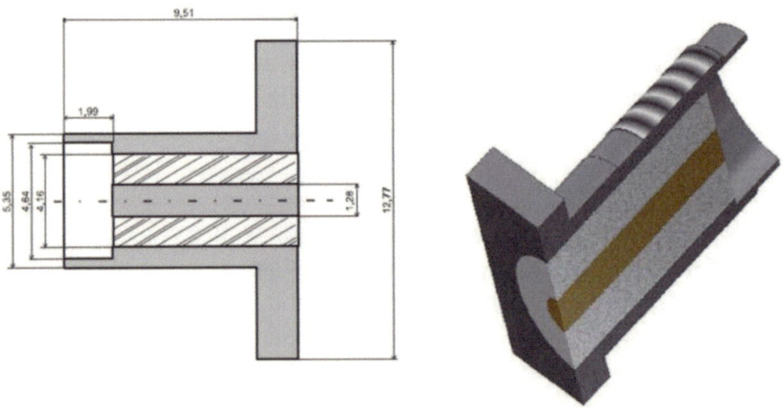


Fig. 28. Basic scheme of the SMA probe's dimensions

### 6.5 Measurement setup

A typical measurement setup using the reflection method on an open-ended coaxial line consists of the network analyzer, the coaxial probe and software. Our measurements were done with the aid of Agilent 6052 network analyzer in the frequency range from 300 MHz to 3 GHz. First the calibration of the vector network analyzer is performed. Then the calibration using a reference material is done. Finally, the reflection coefficient of material under test is measured. The complex permittivity of material under test is evaluated by the MATLAB.

### 6.5.1 Measurement on inhomogeneous agar phantom

The initial measurements on the inhomogeneous agar phantom were performed (Fig. 29.). As the simulations shows that the effective penetration depth in both cases, for N probe and SMA probe, is an interval of 4 mm to 2 mm depending on the frequency of measurement. Therefore, in this model of inhomogeneous agar phantom, strange dielectric immersion depths lies in the range from 4 mm to 1 mm. Thus, the purpose of this measurement was to detect strange dielectrics that are covered with an agar layer in terms of simulating the electrical parameters of human skin and soft tissue. Inhomogeneous agar phantom was covered with a regular square grid (30 points x 30 points), with the 900 points of measurement. Subsequently, measurements were taken at these points by the N probe and SMA-probe.

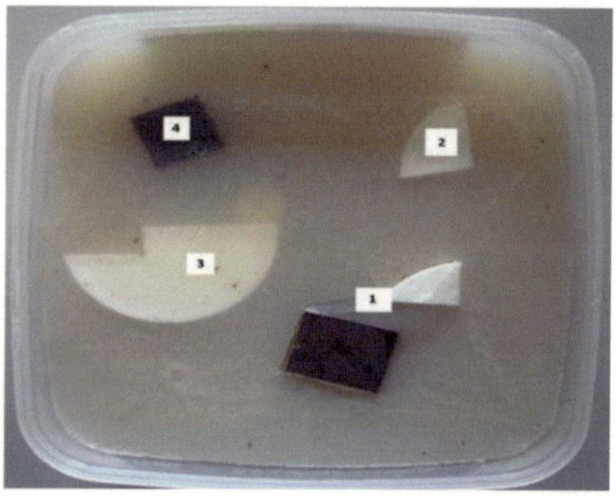

Fig. 29. Inhomogeneous agar phantom setup, the number shows the depth of strange dielectrics submersion

### 6.5.2 Measurement on biological tissue

The final verification of each experiment is necessary for practical usage. In our case, the experiment consisted of measuring the real biological tissue - the left upper limb of the first author (Fig. 30.). For this measurement, the SMA probe was used due to its ability to operate in higher bandwidth, and also because of its smaller size, and therefore a higher lateral resolution. The author's arm was marked with equidistant grid of measuring points, which then for-SMA probe measurements were carried out over a bandwidth of $f_{MIN}$ = 300 MHz to $f_{MAX}$ = 2 GHz. Measurements were carried out very quickly with a delay of 1s and 2s at each measuring point. The data was saved (with the help of an assistant) in CSV data format in the flash drive connected to the vector analyzer. Frequency sweep was set at 1600 points at a bandwidth of $f_{MIN}$ = 300 MHz to $f_{MAX}$ = 2 GHz and averaging was set to 16 in order to eliminate unwanted noise.

### 6.6 Results

The data presented here, obtained from measurements of the inhomogeneous phantom agar, are interpreted as a contour graph. Then there is the measurement on the left upper extremity of the author, which is displayed as contour graphs. All measurements were made in the band $f_{MIN}$ = 300 MHz to $f_{MAX}$ = 2 GHz, from whom were selected three representative frequencies $f_1$ = 500 MHz, $f_2$ = 1 GHz and $f_3$ = 2 GHz.

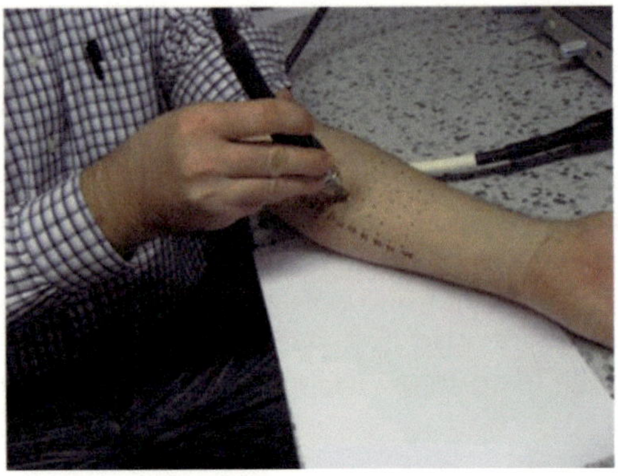

Fig. 30. Measurement on real biological tissue

### 6.6.1 Results of measurement on inhomogeneous agar phantom

For the measurement on inhomogeneous agar phantom was designed with a submerged object of Teflon $\varepsilon_r = 2.1$ and Bakelite $\varepsilon_r = 4.1$, immersed in a variable depth of 4 mm to 1 mm into the agar phantom. After solidify of the agar surface was applied spatially equidistant grid (30 x 30) with 900 data points.

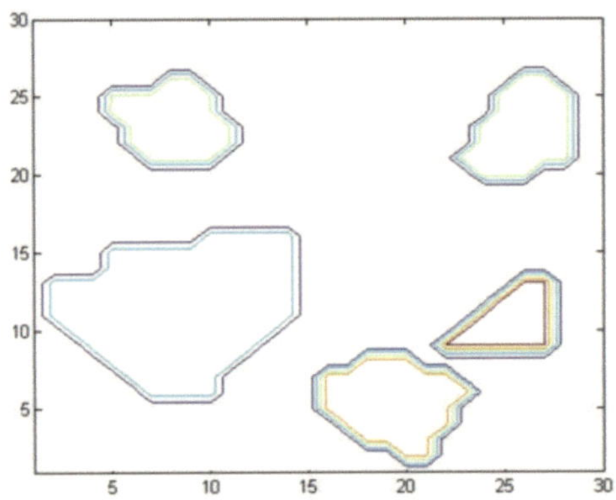


Fig. 31. Results of the measurement on inhomogeneous agar phantom (contour graph of real part of complex permittivity on frequency f = 500 MHz)

Measurements were performed by the SMA probe. Obtained values of the real part of complex permittivity have been rewritten into MATLAB and displayed as a contour graph image, see Fig. 31. The results of the measurement on the inhomogeneous agar phantom have shown the potential of imaging usability of this method for further investigations on real living tissue.

### 6.6.2 Results of measurement on biological tissue

Testing the imaging potential for complex permittivity measurement of biological tissue was finally performed on the left upper extremity of the author, see Fig. 30. SMA probe was used for this measurement. For a small separation of complex permittivity of biological tissue, these data are displayed only in the contour graph. It is very difficult to assess tissue formations without further visual assessment, using MRI and subsequent processing of data segmentation algorithms, but the Fig. 32a,b. shows that contours of real part of complex permittivity during the various measurements still occur in the same places. Among the limitations of the method, we can mention a small depth of penetration shown in Fig. 32c) at frequency f = 2000 MHz; as a result, we can register only the layer of skin. The actual depth of penetration can be improved by using of probes based on the waveguide thus having a greater radiating aperture that would better achieve the quasi-plane waves, but the loss of lateral resolution of the probe. Overcoming this eternal compromise can be achieved through a combination of two probes for a single measurement, one with an emphasis on greater penetration depth and the second for acceptable lateral resolution. When comparing the results of this measurement shown in Fig. 32., we can find among them a high degree of correlation pointing out that in real biological tissue this measuring method will able to detect coherent tissue structure having the same value of the real part of complex permittivity.

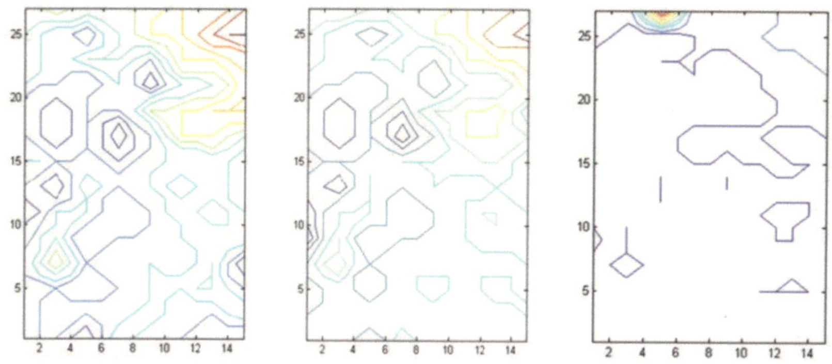

a) b) c)

Fig. 32. Results of the measurement on real biological tissue (contour graph of real part of complex permittivity on frequency a) f1 = 500 MHz, b) f2 = 1 GHz, c) f3 = 2 GHz

### 6.7 Evaluation

Measurements on inhomogeneous agar phantom showed the potential of this imaging method, because the strange dielectrical materials were detectable beneath the surface of agar. Based on this result, the measurement of the left upper extremity of the author was performed, and the contour map of the real part of complex permittivity shown the detectable difference between the tissues. The contour graphs of the real part of complex permittivity of biological tissue give us the hope for the future development that this method may be used as a imaging method. After proving more interaction on the pathological changes in tissues, such as growth of tumor tissue, we can consider this method for diagnostic purposes.

## 7. Conclusions

Research described

## 8. Acknowledgment

Research described in this chapter was supported by Grant Agency of the Czech Republic, projects: 102/08/H081:„Non-standard application of physical fields - analogy, modelling, verification and simulation" and P102/11/0649: „Research and measurements of signals generated by nanoparticles". Further by research program MSM6840770012: "Transdisciplinary Research in the Area of Biomedical Engineering II" of the CTU in Prague, sponsored by the Ministry of Education, Youth and Sports of the Czech Republic.

## 9. References

Able Software Corp. (2011). 3D-DOCTOR, 3D Imaging, Modeling, Rendering and Measurement Software, Available from: http://www.ablesw.com/3d-doctor

Bolmsjö, M.; Wagrell, L.; Hallin, A.; Eliasson, T.; Erlandsson, B.E. & Mattiasson, A. (1996). The heat is on - but how? A comparison of TUMT devices. *The Journal of Urology*, Vol.78, pp. 564-572

Choi, J.; Cho, Y. Lee, J. Yim, B.; Kang, K. & et al. (2004). Microwave detection of metastasized breast cancer cells in the lymph node, potential application for sentinel lymphadenectomy, In: Breast Cancer Research and Treatment, Vol.86, No.2, pp. 107-115, Springer, ISSN 0167-6806

De la Rosette, J.; D'Ancona, F. & Debruyne, F. (February 1997). Current status of thermotherapy of the prostate, *The Journal of Urology*, Vol.157, pp. 430-438

Franconi, C.; Vrba, J. & Montecchia, F. (1993). 27 MHz Hybrid Evanescent-Mode Applicators. *International Journal of Hyperthermia*, Vol.9, No.5, pp. 655 - 673

Hand, J. & James, J. R. (1986). *Physical Techniques in Clinical Hyperthermia*. Wiley, New York

Hippel, A. (1954). Dielectric Materials and Applications. Technology Press of MIT, Cambridge, 1954, pp. 71-75

Popovic, D.; McCartney, L.; Beasley, C.; Lazebnik, M.; Okoniewski, M.; Hagness, S.C. & Booske, J.H. (2005). Precision open-ended coaxial probes for in vivo and ex vivo dielectric spectroscopy of biological tissues at microwave frequencies. *IEEE Transactions on Microwave Theory and Techniques*, Vol.53, No.5, pp. 1713-1722, ISSN 0018-9480

Ramachandraiah, M. S. & Decreton, M. C. (December 1975). A Resonant Cavity Approach for the Nondestructive Determination of Complex Permittivity at Microwave Frequencies. *Instrumentation and Measurement, IEEE Transactions on Instrumentation and Measurement*, Vol.24, No.4, pp.287-291, ISSN 0018-9456

Tanaba, E. & Joines, W. T. (1976). A nondestructive method for measurement of the complex permittivity of dielectric materials at microwave frequency using an open-ended coaxial line resonator. *IEEE Trans. on Measurement and Instrumentation*, Vol.25, pp. 222-226, ISSN 0018-9480

Thompson, A. M. (November 1956). A bridge for the measurement of permittivity. *Proceedings of the IEE - Part B: Radio and Electronic Engineering*, Vol.103, No.12, pp. 704-707

Vrba, J.; Franconi, C. & Lapeš, M. (1996). Theoretical Limits for the Penetration Depth of the Intracavitary Applicat. *International Journal of Hyperthermia*, No.6., pp.737 - 742

Vrba, J.; Franconi, C.; Montecchia, F. & Vannucci, I. (May 1993). Evanescent-Mode Applicators for Hyperthermia. *IEEE Trans.on Biomedical Engineering*, Vol.40, No.5, pp. 397-407

Vrba, J.; Lapeš, M. & Oppl, L. (1999). Technical aspects of microwave thermotherapy. *Bioelectrochemistry and Bioenergetics*, Vol.48, pp. 305 - 309

Williams, T. C.; Sill, J.M. & Fear, E.C. (May 2008). Breast surface estimation for radar-based breast imaging systems. *IEEE Transactions on Biomedical Engineering*, Vol.55, No.6, pp. 1678-1686, ISSN 0018-9294

24

# Photon Total Body Irradiation for Leukemia Transplantation Therapy: Rationale and Technique Options

Brent Herron, Alex Herron, Kathryn Howell,
Daniel Chin and Luann Roads
*PSL Medical Center, Denver*
*USA*

## 1. Introduction

Leukemia is a classification of disease in which the two major defects are unregulated proliferation and incomplete maturation of the hemopoietic progenitors (Scheinberg, Maslak, & Weiss, 2001). Leukemia originates in the marrow, although leukemia cells may infiltrate lymph nodes, liver, spleen, and other tissues. Scheinberg et al. (2001) describe the principal clinical manifestation is the decrease of red cells and platelets as a result of the suppression of normal hemopoiesis or turnover and repopulation of blood components. In the chronic leukemias, unregulated proliferation of leukemia cells and elevated white cell count dominate. Differentiation and maturation of the leukemia cells may be largely preserved. Scheinberg further characterizes acute leukemias with unregulated proliferation also, but the maturation of the leukemia progenitors is profoundly impaired.

Transplantation of blood products, in particular stem cells, has become a common treatment procedure for various types of leukemias since the early 1990's (Scheinberg, Maslak, & Weiss, 2001). Cells void of leukemia are transplanted into the leukemia patient. The purpose of the transplant is the repopulation of the non-cancerous cells. Urbano-Ispizua et al. (2002) describes the current practice of stem cell transplantation for hematological diseases, solid tumors and immune disorders. Definitions, abbreviations and classifications described in this review are summarized here.

Hemopoietic stem cell transplantation (HSCT) refers to any procedure where hemopoietic cells of any donor type and any source are given to a recipient with the intention of repopulation/replacing the hemopoietic system of the recipient in total or in part (Urbano-Ispizua et al., 2002). Human Leukocyte Antigen (HLA) matching is a six point scoring system that identifies antigens and antibodies for both donor and recipient. Allogenic and autologous implants are also characterized by Urbano-Ispizua, et al (2002). Allogenic implants are procedures in which the recipient receives stem cells from a related or unrelated donor whose HLA score is identical (HLA score=6) or nearly identical (HLA score=5) to the recipient. Autologous implants refer to procedures in which the recipient receives stem cells from a collection performed while the patient is in remission or leukemia-free.

Bone marrow and cerebral spinal fluid peripheral cells are standard sources of hemopoietic stem cells (Urbano-Ispizua et al, 2002). For autologous HSCT, peripheral blood has become the preferred choice in view of its more rapid hemopoietic reconstitution. For allogenic HSCT, both sources are used. Both methods have their specific advantages and disadvantages. There are marked differences in toxicity concerning the donors. For recipients, the final issue concerning long-term outcome remains open. Peripheral blood is associated with more rapid engraftment or repopulation in the recipient. Urbano-Ispizua (2002) warns of a major concern with allogenic transplantation with peripheral blood is the high incidence of chronic graft-versus-host disease. That is, the recipient's immune system rejects the donor cells. In general, cord blood transplantation is recommended when patients require allogenic transplantation and do not have an HLA identical or a one-antigen mismatched donor.

Both allogenic and autologous implants are performed subsequent to subjecting the leukemia patient to intensity conditioning regimens (Shank, 1998). Despite the classification of the patient as in remission or disease-free, there is still significant opportunity that undetected leukemia cells are still present and will repopulate along with the transplanted stem cells. Shank describes the conditioning regimen's intent is to reduce the likelihood of the leukemia cell re-growth. Conditioning regimens include intense chemotherapy or radiation therapy or a combination of both. The intensity of these treatments is severe. Shank cautions of the fine balance between transplant-related mortality and the risk of relapse or repopulation of the leukemia cells.

The role of radiation therapy in the preparation of patients for bone marrow transplantation is the primary focus of this chapter. The primary utilization of radiation in oncology management is the use of small (less than 100 sq.cm) beams or fields directed at localized solid tumors (Bentel, 1992). Since leukemia cells are present throughout the body, large fields encompassing the entire body are necessary. This type of radiation treatment is referred to as Total Body Irradiation (TBI) or sometimes as Magna Field Irradiation (Shank, 1998). In her review article, Shank cites sole use TBI did not eradicate all leukemia cells. The addition of chemotherapy such as cyclophosphamide (CY) provides a reduced recurrence rate. Shank notes that although a large number of regimens now combine chemotherapeutic agents with and without TBI for marrow ablation, combined therapy of CY and TBI remains the standard for comparison.

Irradiation holds several advantages over chemotherapy as a systemic agent (Shank, 1998). These advantages include a lack of crossreactivity with other agents, dose homogeneity independent of blood supply, no requirements for detoxification and excretion, and the ability to tailor dose distribution within the body by shielding areas of greater sensitivity or boosting the radiation dose in areas that may contain additional disease. This discussion will focus primarily on the clinical aspects of TBI. Technical aspects of providing these large fields will also be addressed..

## 2. Total body irradiation: Criteria and nuances

Bentel (1992) describes standard methodology of radiation oncology treatments. Standard radiation therapy treatments are provided utilizing a linear accelerator with x-ray energies approximately 100 times greater than conventional machines used for chest or dental x-rays. The accelerator is capable of rotating 360 degrees about a patient with the center of rotation placed within the tumor volume. Typically, 2-6 fields or beams are directed at the tumor volume from various angles. A criterion for field arrangement is accounting for dose uniformity within the tumor volume. That is, large variations in dose throughout the tumor are rarely acceptable. Bentel continues by specifying that additional beams will aid with dose uniformity. Beam angulation is determined by the desire to "spare" or reduce the radiation dose to non-malignant or non-cancerous tissue or organs. In most cases, the delivered radiation dose to the tumor is limited by normal tissue or organ tolerance in areas surrounding or close to the tumor volume (Bentel, 1997). Radiation doses are expressed in units of centigray (cGy) which is equivalent to the more common unit rad. Typical dose levels for standard non-TBI treatments are 4500-7000 cGy. Field dimensions are usually 100-200 sq.cm therefore; the fields are roughly 5 inches by 5 inches. Dose uniformity criteria is typically +/- 5%. The standard treatment distance from the housing of the accelerator is 100cm.

Van Dyk (2000) addresses the degree of accuracy required for total body irradiation treatments. As the specification of dose becomes less certain, disease control can be affected. In addition, undesirable radiation induced side effects can be pronounced. Van Dyk cites research that a 5% change in dose could result in a 20% change in the incidence of radiation pneumonitis. Under such circumstances, it is difficult to argue that +/- 5% accuracy is sufficient. Conversely, if the prescribed dose is well below the onset of radiation pneumonitis and if the dose is sufficient for adequate tumor control, then perhaps the guideline of +/- 5% accuracy can be relaxed and +/- 10% or even +/- 15% may be sufficiently accurate. The beam arrangement for total body irradiation is typically chosen with +/- 10% accuracy and uniformity criteria.

For large field radiotherapy, the delivery of a uniform dose of radiation over the entire target volume is not a trivial task. The irradiation method must be devised to produce radiation fields large enough to cover the entire body adequately. With this larger field size requirement, the patient is positioned further from the linear accelerator than the standard 100cm treatment distance. The increased distance takes advantage of the spread or divergence of the radiation field from the accelerator. The treatment distance can vary depending on the accelerator vault size, but is typically 350 to 500cm. The treatment distance for the TBI procedure represents a few additional problems (Lindsey & Deeg, 1998). These distances can be difficult to achieve in some linear accelerator vaults. Counter tops or other equipment will need to be removed. Since the patient will not be on the standard treatment couch at this extended distance, another adjustable patient support table must be acquired or fabricated.

Dose uniformity is a major concern for the TBI process and the technique option chosen (Bradley et al., 1998). Bentel (1992) describes the principle of radiation absorption. The absorption of radiation is exponentially proportional to the thickness of the different body sections of the patient. The variance between absorption and dose between thinner and thicker body sections is more pronounced as the x-ray energy is decreased. Therefore, higher x-ray energy aids the dose uniformity criteria. Fletcher describes a negative side to the use of higher x-ray energy. Unfortunately, higher x-ray energies provide decreased entrance dose with the first 2cm of the patient. That is, high energy x-rays will provide a more uniform dose in tissue only after the first 2cm. Therefore, the use of a x-ray energy greater than 4MV require the addition of an acrylic sheet placed in close proximity to the patient (Bradley et al., 1998). This acrylic sheet serves as a "beam spoiler" and produces scatter radiation that allows the entrance 2cm of tissue to receive a higher and more adequate dose.

Even with the use of high-energy x-rays and beam spoilers, the dose uniformity across the patient and from thicker to thinner body sections may not meet the +/- 10% criteria (Bredeson et al., 2002). Dose uniformity will improve if opposed beams are used. As shown and described in Figure 1, the beam can be directed from different sources (item d) or by changing the patient position from supine to prone. If a two-beam arrangement is utilized, half of the radiation dose is provided by one beam. The patient is rotated or the source of radiation is moved and the remaining dose is provided. Typically, two fields are adequate to provide acceptable dose homogeneity for TBI treatments (Bredeson et al., 2002).

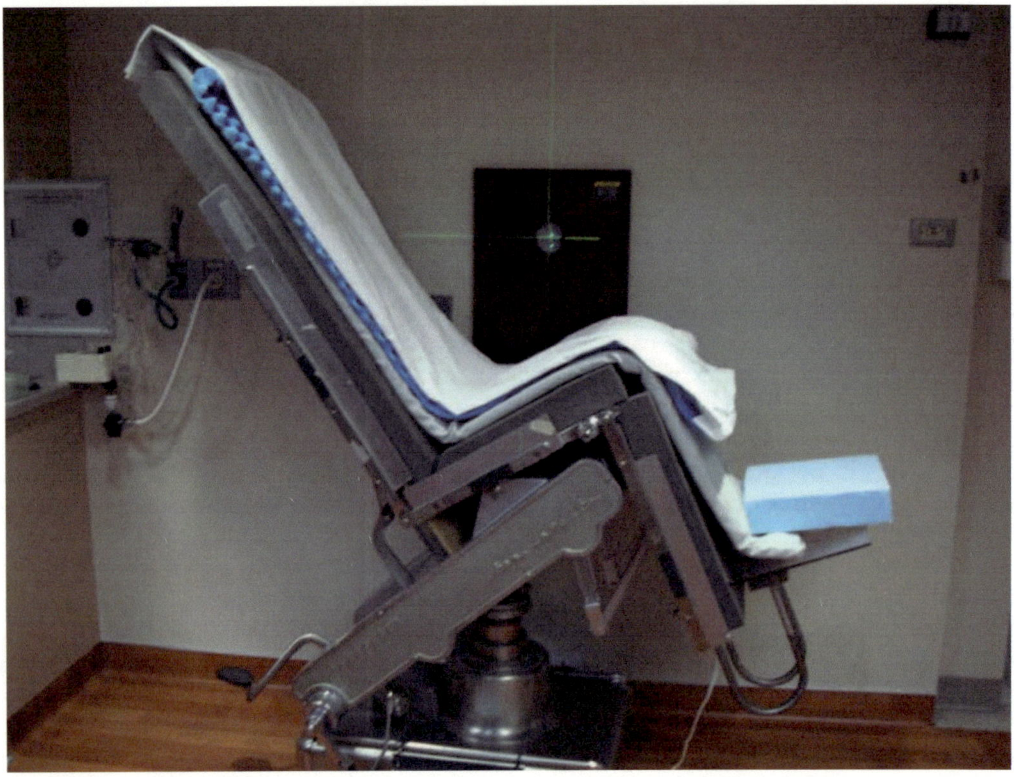

Fig. 1. Front view of TBI table used for opposed lateral treatments with couch sections angled at 45°.

Large variations in patient thickness, e.g. head thickness compared to shoulder thickness, pose problems with dose uniformity that multiple fields cannot resolve (Bredeson et al., 2002). Galvin and D'Angio and Walsh (2000) and Lin and Chu (2001) have described methods for compensating for the lack of patient thickness in certain areas such as the head or feet. The addition of rice bags or water-filled bags serves as adequate substitutes in these areas of decreased thickness. Rice or water exhibits the same attenuation characteristics as human tissue. Therefore, packing the patient or filling voids with these materials presents the patient as a uniform thickness. Therefore absorption variations are minimized.

The parameters used to characterize the x-ray beam at the standard 100cm distance will not necessarily apply to the extended distance (Van Dyk, 2000). Beam profiles and output calibration of the linear accelerator at the treatment position will need to be measured.

Verification of the attenuation of the beam should be made with anthropomorphic or tissue equivalent phantoms. Scatter radiation from other components within the room, such as walls and equipment, will apply to this extended distance large field treatment and should be accounted.

One of the major complications of large field radiotherapy is radiation pneumonitis (Corns et al., 2000). For total lung radiation, this syndrome is lethal in 80% of the patients who develop it. Because of this effect, Corns et al. (2000) warns that it is imperative that the dose to the lung be precisely controlled to ensure the probability of its occurrence is minimal. Even in standard radiation treatments, a calculation of the lung dose requires density corrections to the standard attenuation data (Bentel, 1992). The lower density lungs will transmit more radiation than regular more dense tissue. Several methods have been developed to correct for the lower density lung tissue and provide an accurate accounting of dose in this region (Bentel, 1992). Unfortunately, these calculations vary in ease of use as well as in the resulting correction factor. Van Dyk (2000) has calculated the correction factor from four of the most popular methodologies and observed a +/-12% variation. Despite this variation in accounting accuracy, methods of lung dose reduction is often required (Van Dyk, 2000).

When a prescribed tumor dose is well above lung tolerance, the dose to lung will have to be reduced to minimize the probability of lung complication. Several methods can be used to reduce the dose. The techniques vary in complexity of design and application. All techniques incorporate one common concept: the use of an attenuator (Van Dyk, 2000). The attenuator absorbs radiation prior to delivering dose to the lungs. The decreased dose delivered to the lungs coupled with the increased transmission of dose within the lungs because of their lower density provides a dose comparable to rest of the body. Van Dyk describes several methods for the design of these attenuators. These methods vary from shielding the lungs with arm positioning to full or partial-transmission shielding blocks based on Computerized Tomography scans.

## 3. Representative Total Body Irradiation program

A representative TBI program is described here as an aid to the development of similar programs. Room modifications, technique selection, energy choice, and equipment necessary to achieve adequate dose uniformity in a comfortable setting are included in this discussion.

### 3.1 Accelerator room

TBI treatments should be performed with a high energy accelerator capable of providing photons of 15MV or greater. Lower x-ray energies can be utilized, but as the energy is decreased, dose homogeneity becomes more difficult to achieve with opposed fields. The distance to the closest wall with the gantry angled at 90 or 270 degrees will dictate the maximum field size to encompass the patient. Offset of the isocenter in the treatment vault design may allow for a greater treatment distance. Unfortunately, the desire to add TBI to the radiation therapy services may occur after a vault has been constructed. Most vaults are configured with a 20 foot width. Without an isocenter offset, this room width provides a source-wall distance of approximately 4m. Our institution's vault design provided a source-wall distance of slightly less than 4m. A 40x40 $cm^2$ field at 1m projects to 1.58$m^2$ without collimator rotation and 2.2$m^2$ with a 45° collimator rotation. Only a minor room modification may be necessary to provide audio and visual communication with a patient positioned at this location.

### 3.2 Opposed lateral field TBI table

A portable surgical couch was obtained from a medical equipment reclamation firm. This modified couch is utilized for providing TBI treatments with opposed lateral fields. It is the technique of choice where treatment goals include dose uniformity without specific organ blocking. Figure 1 is a front view schematic of the couch arrangement. The effective length of the patient was reduced as sections of the couch are angled 45°. Four inch urethane foam cushions are used to separate the patient from any metal located on the couch. An additional egg crate cushion is provided for patient comfort. The couch height is adjusted vertically to coincide with the isocenter height of 1.3m.

After patient positioning, four beam spoiler plates constructed of ¼" lexan polycarbonate are inserted into aluminum slots added to the couch. The width of the treatment table including the lexan polycarbonate plates is 52cm. Factoring in couch clearance to the wall, the source-tray distance for these lateral treatments is 374 cm. Our wall choice required a gantry angle selection of 270° (IEC). A collimator position of 20° and 340° is used for right lateral and left lateral fields, respectively.

Prior to treatment, a head and neck missing tissue compensator is positioned. An acrylic compensator is secured to a tray and supported with the accelerator hand support which is affixed to the accelerator couch rail (Fig. 2). The compensator angle position can be pivoted on the tray to match each patient. The compensator tray is rotated for the opposing lateral treatment and the couch longitudinal position is adjusted accordingly. The compensator bottom is curved to match the alignment between the patient neck and shoulders.

Tissue-equivalent rice bolus is used for additional missing tissue compensation for the body below the patient neck level. Figure 3 demonstrates the bolus placement. Since the patient's torso represents the widest section of the patient, bolus is typically only provided below the waist level between and around the legs and feet. The rice bag placement essentially makes the patient separation constant below the neck level and matching the maximum torso separation. Since the dose prescription point is typically at mid-depth at the umbilicus level. Tubes of rice and smaller individual plastic bags of rice with disposable outer covering are used for this aspect of patient preparation.

This treatment assumes that the treatment goal is to provide the same dose to the lungs as provided at the mid-umbilicus level. Prior to treatment, a lateral separation is determined at the nipple level. Previous chest x-ray review for over 50 patients revealed a relationship between this separation and the lateral width of the lungs. Of the lateral tissue separation, 77-83% of the tissue was comprised by the lower density lungs. Rather than measuring the lung width with a chest x-ray on each patient, we calculate the lung thickness as 80% of the full tissue thickness and assume a lung physical density of 0.35g/cm$^3$. An effective thickness at this level is determined.

The arms are positioned at the patient's side thus adding higher density thickness to the chest area (Fig. 3.). The arm separation is determined and added to the effective thickness. This total is compared to umbilicus separation. If additional thickness is needed at the arm level to meet the thickness uniformity criterion of +/-1cm, additional "bolus with skin" (CIVCO, Orange City, IA) is added around the arm in 0.5cm increments until this criterion is met. A simple spreadsheet is used to perform these calculations as well as print setup instructions.

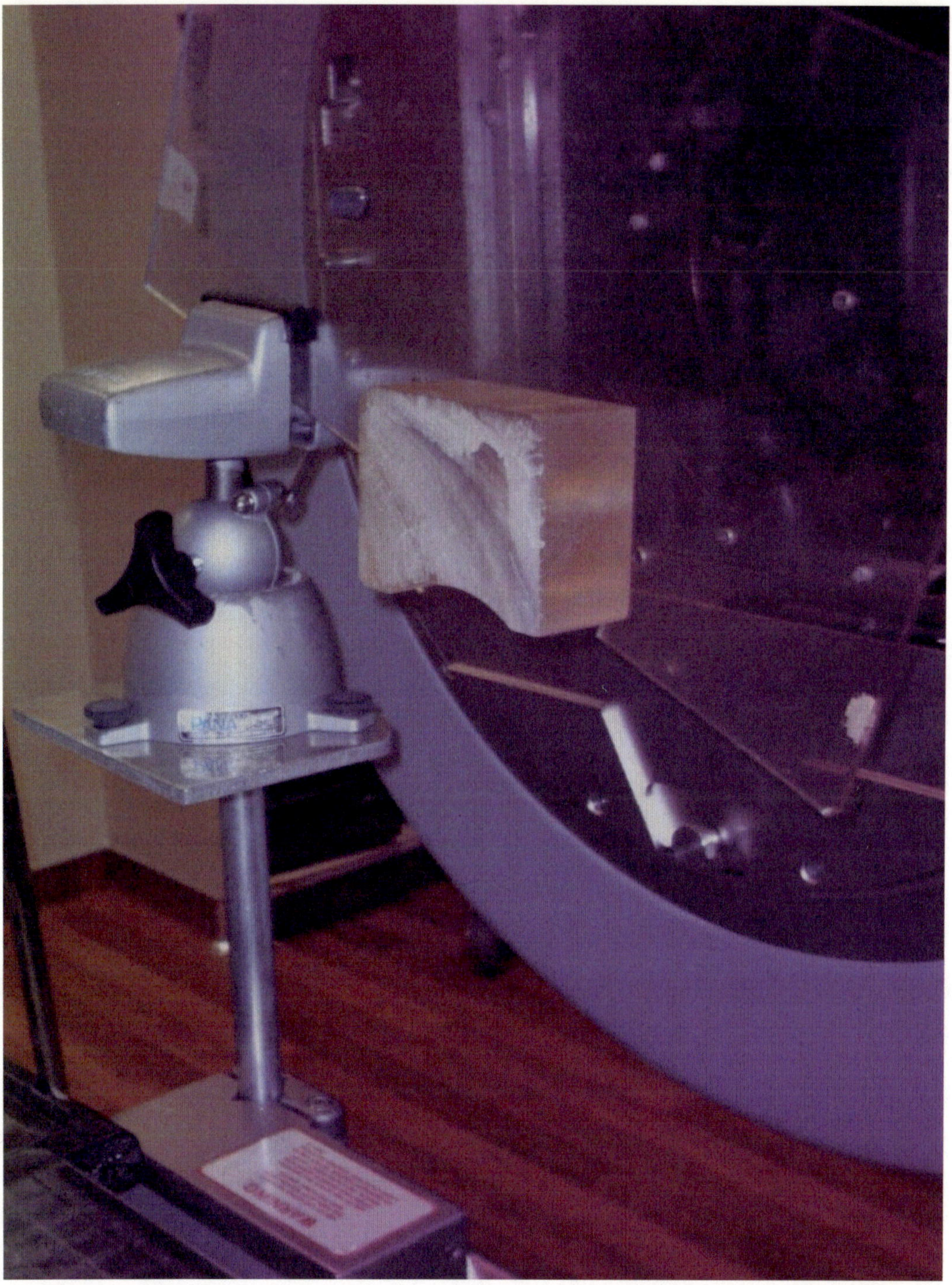

Fig. 2. Acrylic head and neck compensator mounted on post connected to accelerator couch rail arm support.

Monitor unit settings are calculated for the mid-depth at the umbilicus level. In-vivo entrance and exit dosimeters are placed at the head, neck, nipple, umbilicus, knee and ankle levels. After delivery of one half of the fractional dose, the patient remains positioned and the table is rotated 180°. The collimator is rotated to correspond to the new lateral orientation. The head and neck compensator is repositioned. The remainder of the treatment is provided. The dose rate from the accelerator is reduced between 100-200MU/min at isocenter. This machine dose rate reduction, the measured distance correction output factor, and attenuation will provide a dose delivery near 7cGy/minute. Dose rate has been determined to have a significant effect on lung toxicity. Most treatment protocols require dose delivery less than 10cGy/minute. Treatment times are approximately 15 minutes per field. This method of TBI delivery offers a uniform dose, easy and reproducible field arrangement, and a comfortable patient setup.

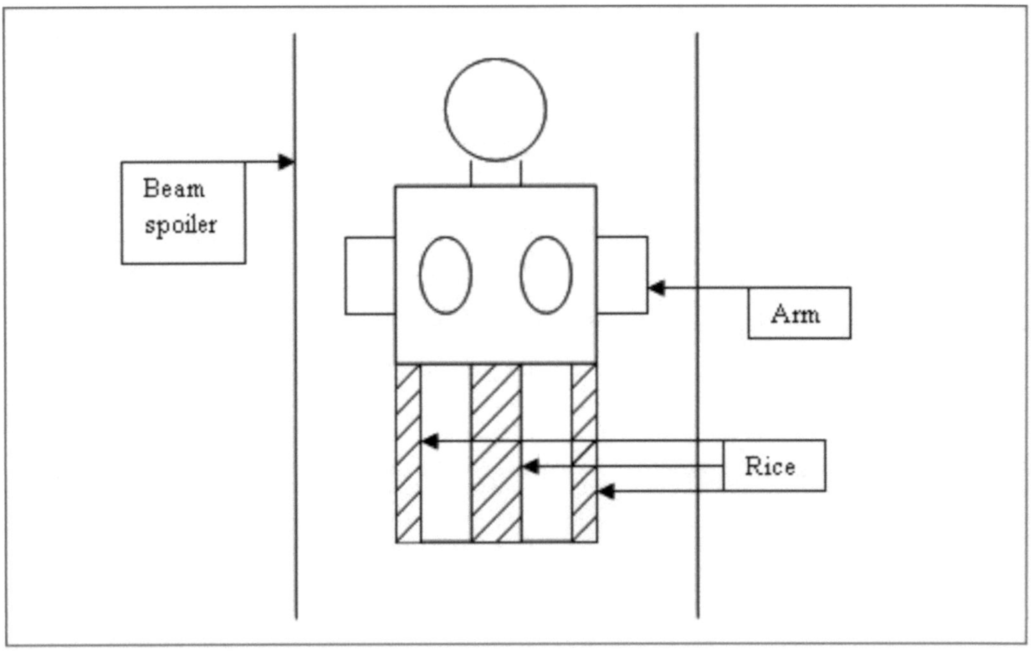


Fig. 3. Schematic of patient on TBI table with beam spoilers and rice bolus in place.

### 3.3 AP/PA TBI treatment stand

The opposed lateral field TBI table method does not allow for partial transmission blocking of the lung or liver as required by various protocols. Towards this goal, an alternative stand was developed to accommodate AP/PA field arrangement, cerrobend blocking, and verification of block placement in a reproducible and comfortable environment for the patient. The initial design of this stand utilized specifications described previously.[6,7] Over the years, significant modifications to these designs have been made largely to accommodate weak patients who had difficulty standing for lengthy periods. The majority of patients presenting for TBI have received a chemotherapy regimen as a complementary preparation before the transplant.

The current version of the AP/PA TBI stand is pictured in Figure 4. Detailed drawings describing the construction of this stand are available from the authors to aid in duplicating this construction. The stand begins with a 29"(w)x29"(l)x27"(h) wooden platform. This height allows field coverage at the treatment distance with the accelerator gantry positioned at 272° and a collimator rotation of 45°. A patient rehabilitation walker was affixed to the platform after wheel removal. The cushioned arm supports can be positioned at varying levels to accommodate different patient heights.

A fabric harness is attached around the patient's waist and thighs. This harness is then attached with plastic buckles to the frame of the walker support. The harness system provides the patient significant stability and tolerance for the required lengthy standing time for this procedure. Patients have experienced episodes of significant weakness or even fainting and the harness system allowed potential injury to be avoided before care could be offered to the patient.

Additional patient support and comfort is provided by an adjustable bicycle seat attached to a slide affixed to the platform. The current seat arrangement represents the evolution from a seat supported from the platform rear to a single post from the platform middle. Other stools were investigated and rejected due to adjustment restrictions or beam attenuation.

The blocking support is attached to a portable beam spoiler (Fig. 5). The plastic spoiler is fabricated with 3/8″ lexan polycarbonate and supported on a mobile assembly that is positioned directly in front of the patient after configuring the patient on the harness and stool. Angle iron is placed on the sides of the beam spoiler away from the beam to provide additional rigidity when the blocks are added. Again, detailed drawings are available from the authors upon request.

The cerrobend partial transmission blocks are affixed to a separate ¼″ lexan tray. The blocking tray is supported on a tray slot placed on each side of the bam spoiler. The thickness of the transmission blocks is calculated utilizing attenuation properties measured previously. The block thickness also varies with the patient separation and the desired transmitted dose, 8 or 10Gy. Typical thickness varies between 2-4cm of cerrobend and is determined using a simple spreadsheet calculation.

The positioning of the block is verified with imaging. In our case, we utilize the Kodak ACR 2000 CR system. However, a film cassette requiring chemical processing could also be used. Fig. 4 also shows a cassette holder attached to the rear of the platform. This spring-loaded cassette holder allows easy height adjustment and was obtained from a medical equipment reclamation service for less than $50. If lateral adjustment in block placement is necessary after imaging, the blocking tray can be adjusted horizontally using a top-loaded bearing system. This adjustment provides +/- 7cm adjustment. Refer to the appendix for details. Two worm screws are added to the sides of the block assembly and vertical adjustment is accomplished by cranking up or down along this mechanism. After an acceptable image is obtained, the block shadow is traced onto the patient's surface for subsequent fractions.

As with the opposed lateral TBI treatment, the accelerator output rate is adjusted such that the midline dose rate is less than 10cGy/minute. Entrance and exit in-vivo dosimeters are placed to verify dose uniformity. Since the hands and forearms are not placed at the patient's side, but on the cushioned arm supports, there was a concern about dose uniformity in this region. Measurements confirm uniformity within +/- 5% as the hands and forearms are closer to the beam during the anterior field treatment and further from the beam during the posterior field delivery.

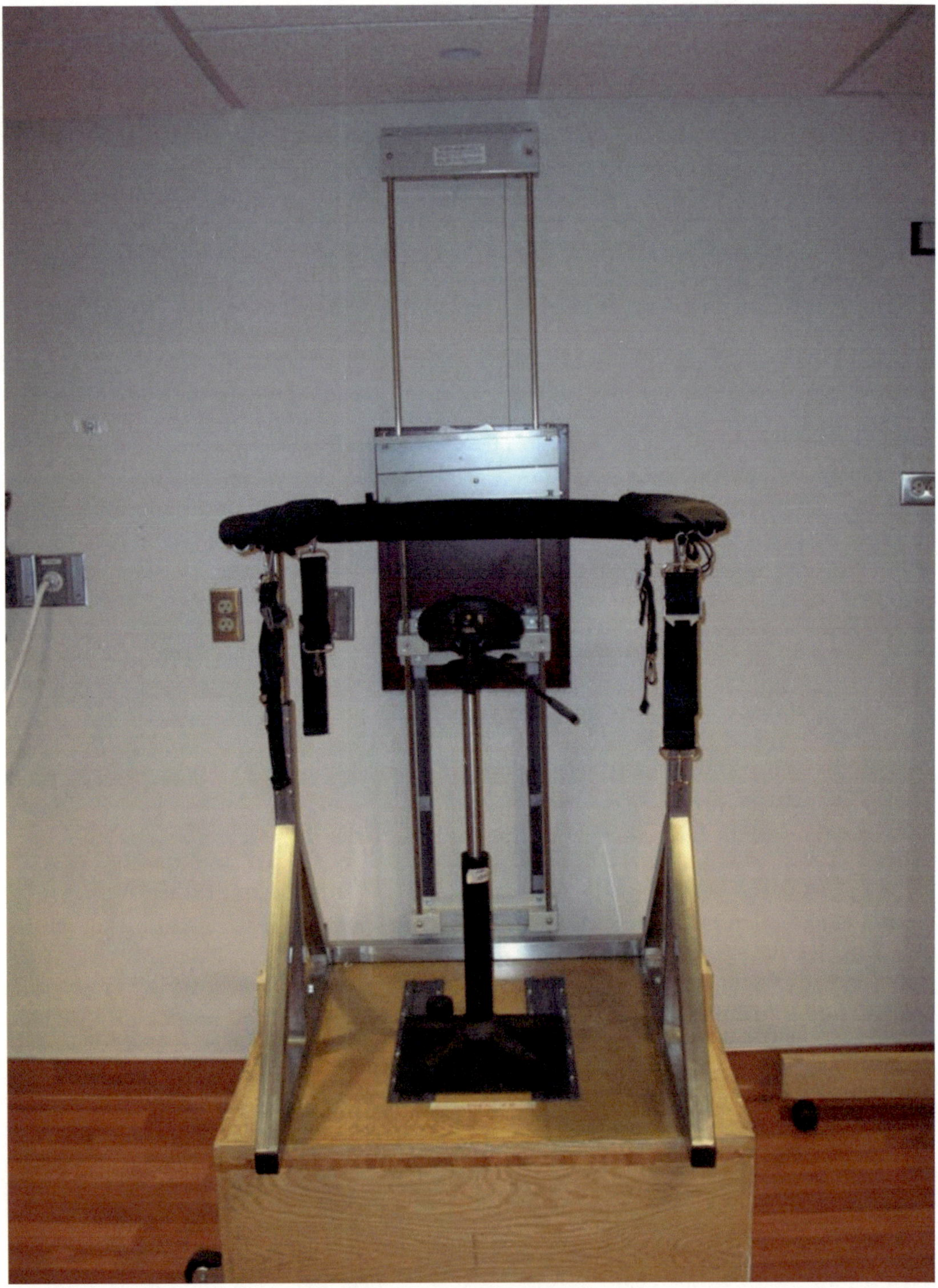

Fig. 4. Front view of TBI stand used for AP/PA fields.

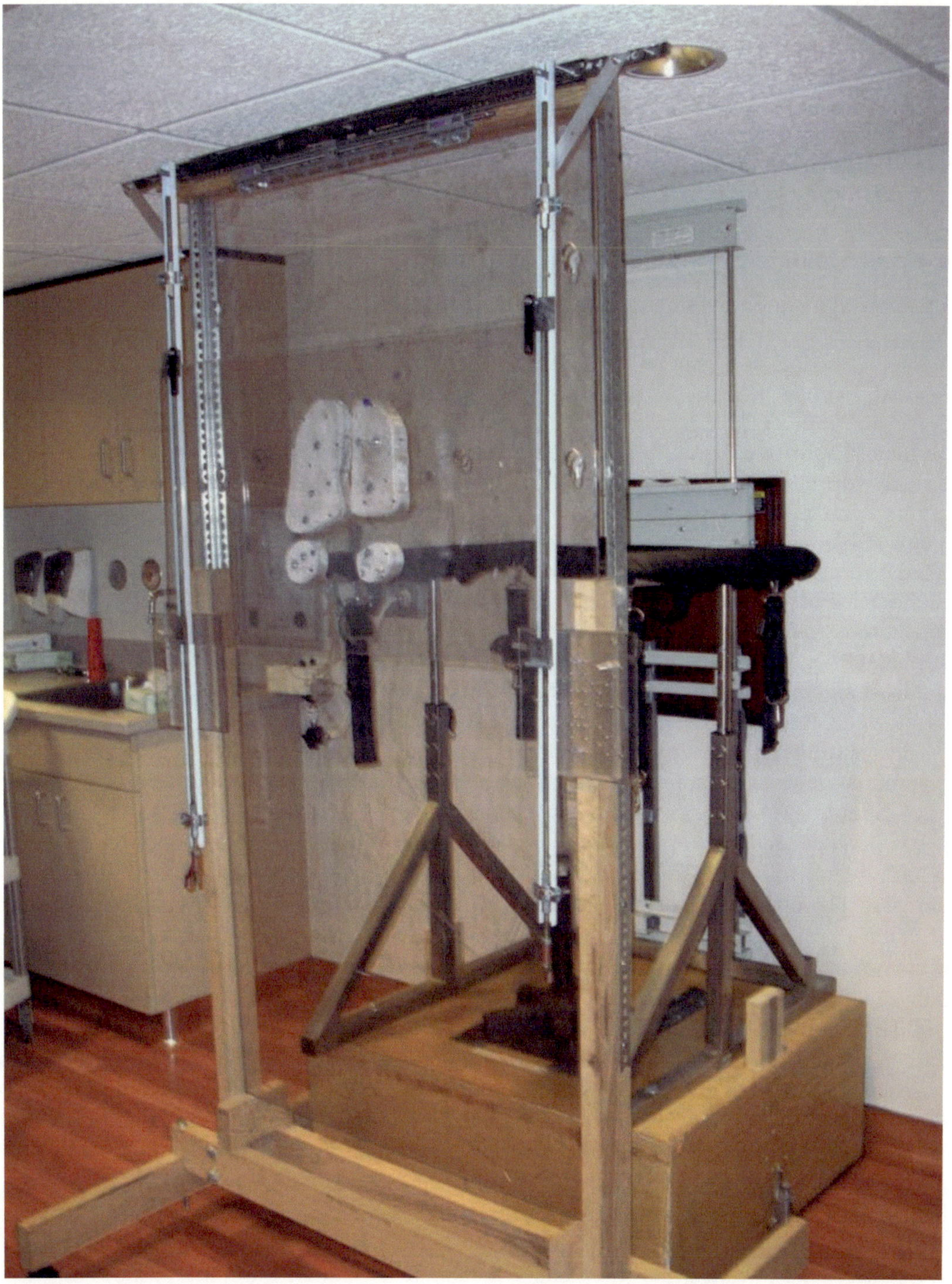

Fig. 5. Front view of mobile spoiler and blocking mechanism used in conjunction with TBI stand.

### 3.4 Combination of treatment methods

Despite efforts to provide a comfortable treatment in the TBI stand, the opposed lateral TBI table still is viewed as the most comfortable for patients and easy to set up. Patients receiving TBI that requires dose reduction to the lungs and/or liver are treated using a combination of these two techniques. All current protocols requiring dose reduction to these organs require treatments to be administered over four days or 8 fractions. We routinely treat 4 fractions with the AP/PA TBI stand technique and 4 fractions with the opposed lateral TBI table option.

## 4. Radiobiological considerations for Total Body Irradiation

The techniques and methodology described in the previous section account for the physical criteria and limitations for the TBI procedure. The actual dose prescription and dose delivery schedule also play an important role in the success of the procedure (Shank, 1999). Normal lymphocytes are among the most radiosensitive cells and become profoundly depleted with TBI (Shank, 1999). In addition to finding that TBI was more immunosuppressive than CY, Shank describes early animal studies that found the degree of immunosuppression was a function of the total radiation dose. Dividing the treatment into multiple fractions over several days required an increase in total dose to achieve consistent results. Shank states the need for an increased dose over a fractionated schedule implies repair processes occurring between fractions.

Radiobiologists categorize the repair process from fractionated radiation treatments as repair, reoxygenation, redistribution and repopulation (Evans, 2000). In the context of TBI as applied to bone marrow transplantation, Evans states repair and repopulation are probably the most significant of these processes and can be best explained with a cell survival curve as shown in Figure 6. The slope of a survival curve can describe the radiation sensitivity of a particular cell type. The slope of the curve, termed $D_o$ and the shoulder region, termed $D_q$, quantify significant parameters of a cells response to radiation. Cells from different tissues have different $D_o$'s and $D_q$'s as illustrated in Figure 6.

It has been generally accepted that a small shoulder ($D_q$) is typical of bone marrow stem cells and leukemia cells (Evans, 2002). Therefore, these cells have a limited ability to repair damage. In contrast, cells of lung tissue and intestinal epithelial cells have survival curves with must broader shoulders ($D_q$), implying a greater repair capacity. The second important repair process is repopulation. Evans defines repopulation as the proliferation of cells between dose fractions. Rapidly dividing tissues, like the intestine, can increase their normal proliferation rate after a radiation treatment. Slowly dividing tissues such as the lung and vascular tissues tend not to proliferate at a higher rate after radiation. Therefore, during a fractionated radiation therapy regimen, Evans speculates that both repair and repopulation may occur between fractions. Repair of the leukemia cells is minimal. The separation of the leukemia cell survival curve from the lung cell survival curve increases the therapeutic ratio and supports fractionation. Shank (1998) attempted to calculate the optimal TBI schedule including fraction dose, number of fractions, and total dose. In addition, Shank reviews some clinical trials with regards to percentage relapse with different TBI schedules. Shank summarizes her findings that the greatest leukemia cell kill with minimum morbidity will occur with a highly fractionated radiotherapy regimen. A total dose of 1400-1500 cGy delivered over 10-13 fractions may be optimal.

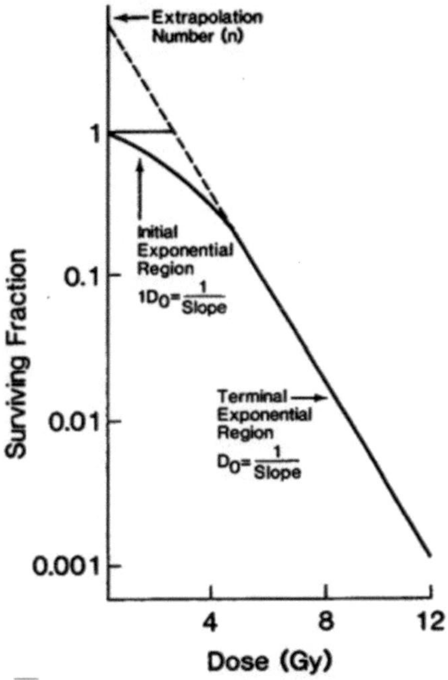


Fig. 6. A typical survival curve for mammalian cells exhibiting an initial shoulder followed by an exponential region. An initial shoulder characterizes the curve with some slope to it ($1D_o$), the exponential slope ($D_o$), n (extrapolation number) and $D_q$.

## 5. Effectiveness of TBI for various leukemias

Leukemia is a broad classification for several types of this disease. This variety of leukemias differs based on pathological examination of cell definition. Bredeson et al. (2002) provide a summary and results of clinical trials including TBI. Patients with acute myeloid leukemia (AML) have shown to be fairly responsive to stem cell transplants with TBI preparation. Results of randomized studies comparing TBI containing regimens with total chemotherapy preparatory regimens indicate a 75% actuarial survival with TBI compared to 51% without. Relapse rates are lower with the TBI regimens as well. 14% relapsed within 2 years with TBI while 34% relapsed under chemotherapy regimens.

Bredeson et al. (2002) reports acute lymphoblastic leukemia (ALL) results show significant improvement with TBI regimens. 52% disease-free survival rates are reported when TBI is utilized as compared to 37% with chemotherapy alone. The percentage relapse is nearly identical from both types of regimens. Studies of treatments for chronic myeloid leukemia patients show fairly high yet identical disease-free survival rates. Nearly 80% survival rates were reported for both protocols. Relapse rates were indistinguishably different.

## 6. Discussion and summary

Leukemia is a disease classification for an imbalance within the hemopoietic system. Acute leukemias are characterized with unregulated cell growth while chronic leukemias exhibit incomplete maturation of cells and some increase proliferation. Bone marrow or stem cell transplantation is a viable treatment option for the leukemia patient. Stem cells collected from an HLA matching donor or cells collected from the patient while in remission are provided to the leukemia recipient. The clinical desire of the transplant is repopulation and re-growth of the stem cells triggering a balanced regulated hemopoietic system.

Preparative regimens for marrow transplantation are required to rid the leukemia patient of any microscopic disease. Rigorous protocols of chemotherapy or radiation therapy combined with chemotherapy are provided prior to transplantation to reduce relapse. Radiotherapy includes fractionated treatments delivered to the total body (TBI). TBI treatments pose several concern issues in methodology and fractionation. High-energy fields with opposing beam arrangements lead to improved dose uniformity. Acrylic plates can serve as beam spoilers to increase the dose to an adequate dose for shallow depths. The lung tissue is sensitive to radiation and limits the dose delivered to the rest of the body. Accurate lung dose calculations are necessary to determine if attenuators are necessary to reduce the total lung dose. Fractionation of the TBI dose requires an increase in the total dose delivered as repair and repopulation occurs between fractions. Repair processes are minimal for the leukemia cell and therefore the therapeutic ratio is enhanced. Analysis of the disease-free survival rates and evaluation of the percentage of patients relapsing or recurring measure the effect of these preparatory regimens. TBI shows a marked improvement in both factors for AML and ALL. Studies reviewing the effects of treatments for CML show excellent results for both chemotherapy only protocols and TBI-chemotherapy combined protocols.

Over the last 35 years, TBI delivery protocols have evolved due to toxicity concerns. Radiation-induced toxicity is influenced by the dose rate and total dose. The total dose was predominantly restricted by pulmonary toxicity from interstitial pneumonitis. Single fraction TBI was replaced with fractionated and hyperfractionated techniques. Radiobiological principles of preferential normal tissue repair with fractionation forecast improved anti-leukemic effects without increasing toxicity. Dose rate was considered a strong factor in the causation of interstitial pneumonitis and most protocols restrict the delivery dose rate to less than 10 cGy/min. TBI protocols vary with the primary malignancy and complementary chemotherapy conditioning regimen. Current TBI protocols include: a single fraction of 200 Gy; two BID fractions of 2 Gy/fraction; eight BID fractions of 1.5 Gy/fraction with or without lung and liver dose reduction to 8-10 Gy; and eight BID fractions of 1.65 Gy/fraction with or without partial transmission blocking of the lung and liver.

Factors influencing large field treatment technique choice include dose homogeneity, accurate and reproducible delivery, ease of set up, treatment room limitations, and the treatment protocol used. For example, if a reduced organ dose is required with blocking, an AP/PA treatment technique is required. Different techniques have been described recently including those utilizing tomotherapy or translational couch options. Two methods of comfortable total body irradiation using conventional linear accelerators without machine modifications are presented here. A technique for lateral treatments and a process for AP/PA treatments with blocking are described. Techniques described here enhance other reported design specifications. The technique options represent an evolution in our process and should aid facilities looking to begin a TBI program or facilities desiring modifications to adjust to different treatment protocols.

Dose uniformity is the primary criterion when creating a treatment technique. The use of beam spoilers, strategically placed bolus, missing tissue compensators, and opposed fields with high energy x-rays will accomplish the uniformity goal. While dose uniformity is the major priority in developing a suitable treatment technique, patient comfort and support are equally important. Patients presenting for TBI are often weak and recovering from other chemotherapy treatments as part of the preparatory program for transplant. Two treatment options, opposed laterals and AP/PA fields and associated apparatus have been presented. The limitation of dose delivered to the lung/liver is specified in several protocols and is accomplished with partial transmission blocks placed in conjunction with AP/PA fields. Both techniques were designed to insure accurate dose delivery, comfortable patient support, and easy patient setup. Calculation spreadsheets referenced in this manuscript are available by contacting the authors.

## 7. Appendix

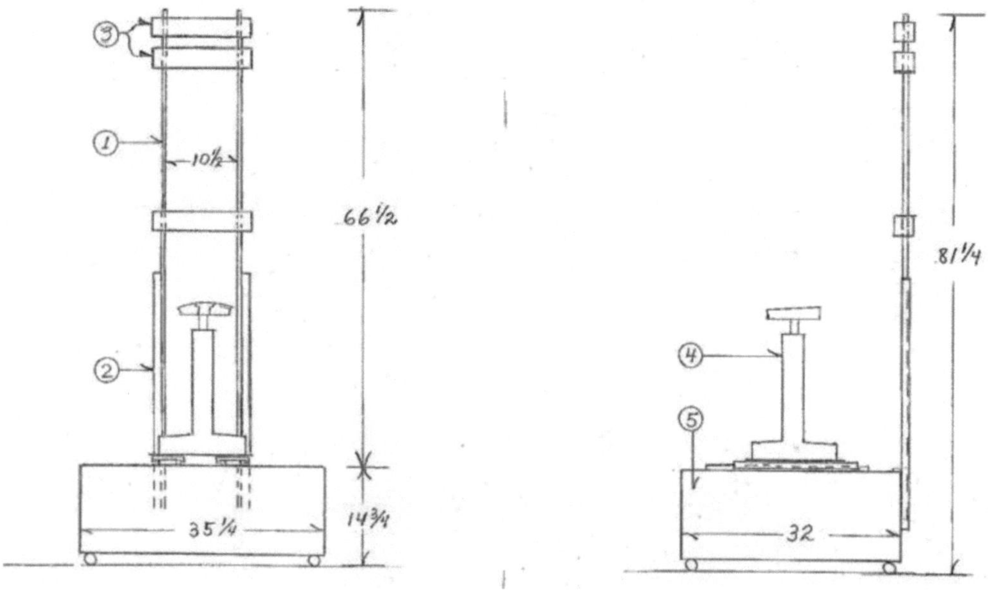


Legend: 1. 5/8" stainless steel rod, 2. Angle iron for stabilization and support, 3. Adjustable cassette holder, 4. Double track system support for bicycle seat placement, 5. Platform with ¾"plywood on oak framework

Fig. A-1 Front and side view of AP/PA stand .

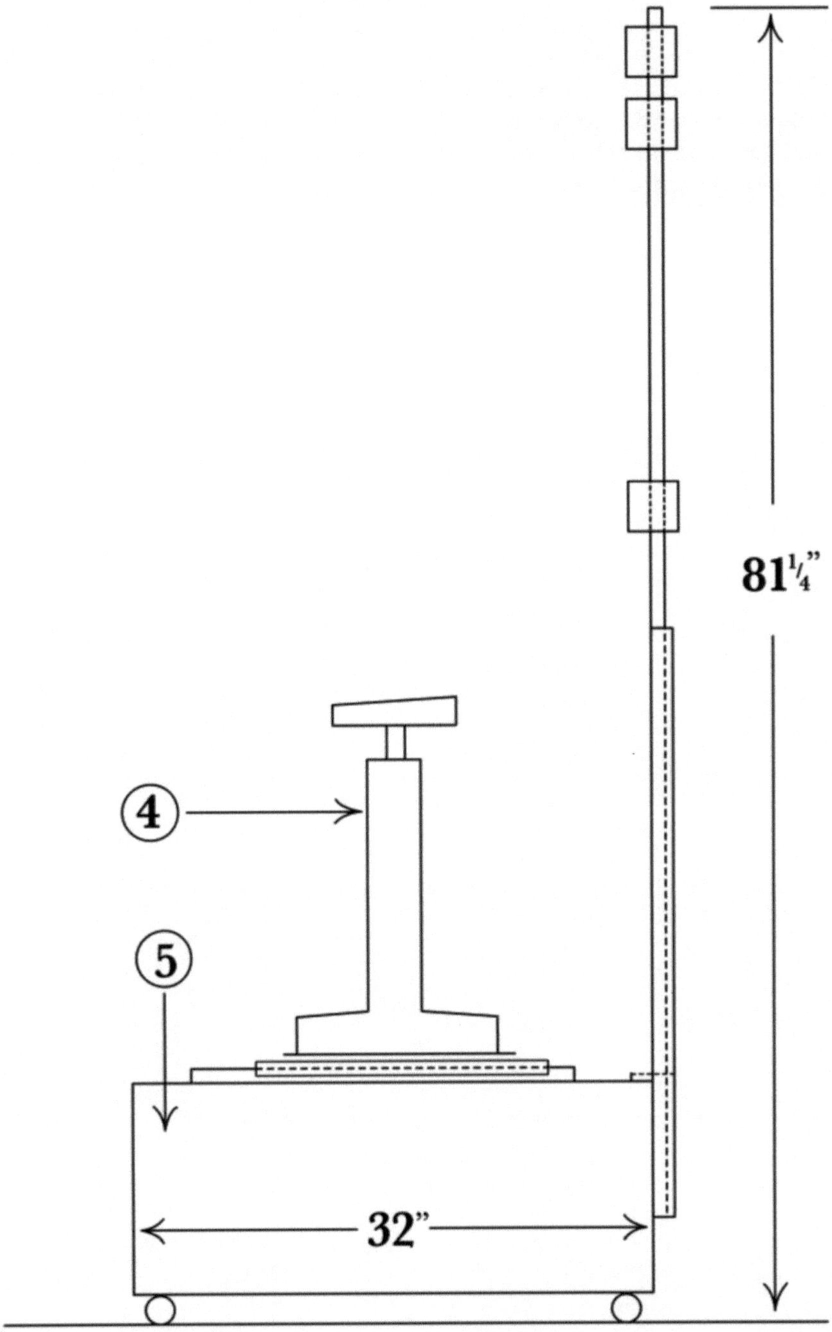


Legend: 1. 5/8" stainless steel rod, 2. Angle iron for stabilization and support, 3. Adjustable cassette holder, 4. Double track system support for bicycle seat placement, 5. Platform with ¾"plywood on oak framework

Fig. A-2 AP/PA Stand Side View

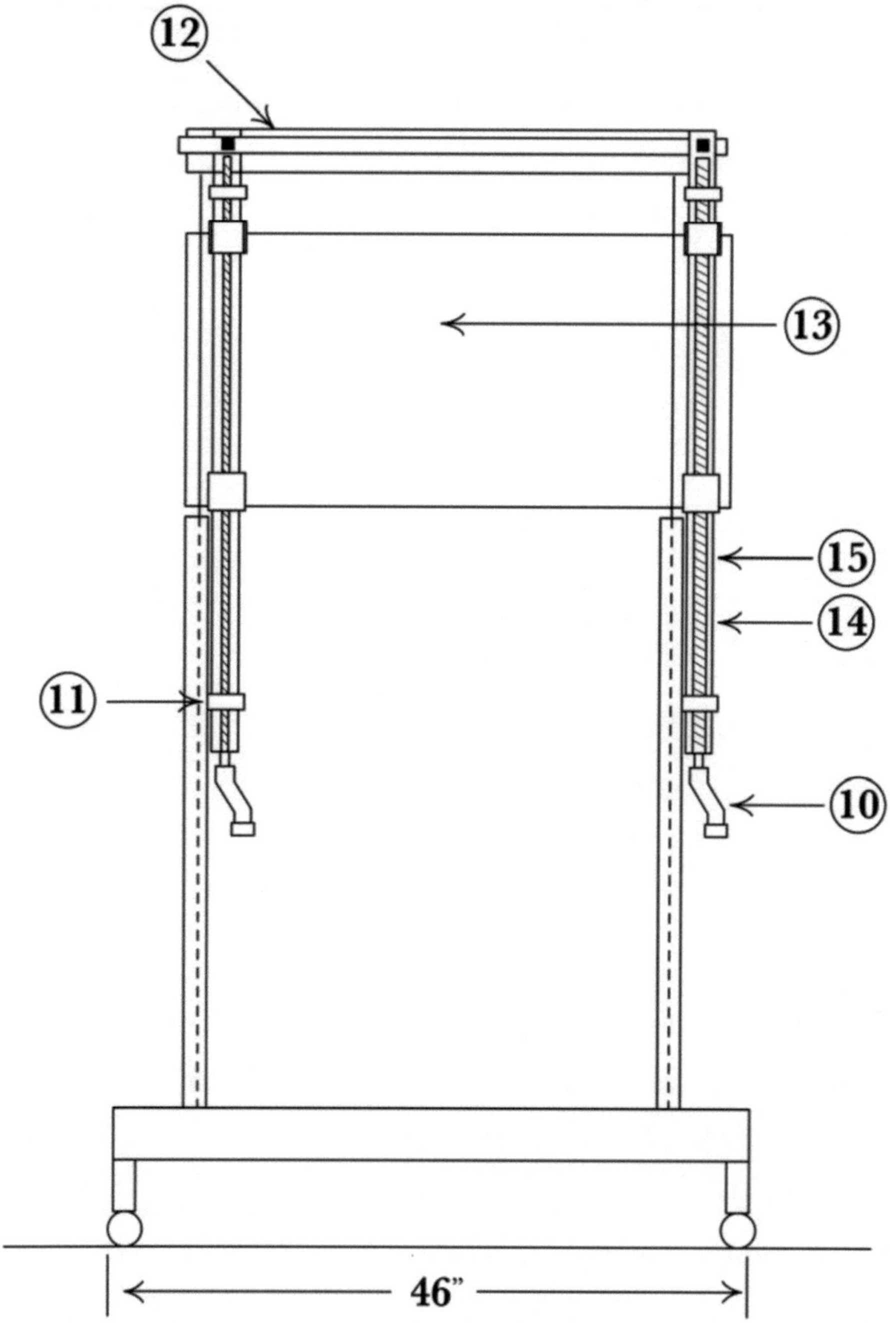


Legend: 6. 1-1/2"x3-1/2" Oak frame support, 7. Lexan beam spoiler, 8. Support for block tray with galvanized metal support, 9. Galvanized metal lock, 10. Crank, 11. Bearing location & cap (2 bearings/crank), 12. Ball bearing track for horizontal block adjustment, 13. ¼" block tray, 14. 7/16" thread rod, 15. ¼" channel for rod adjustment system

Fig. A-3 AP/PA Beam Spoiler and Blocking Support Front View

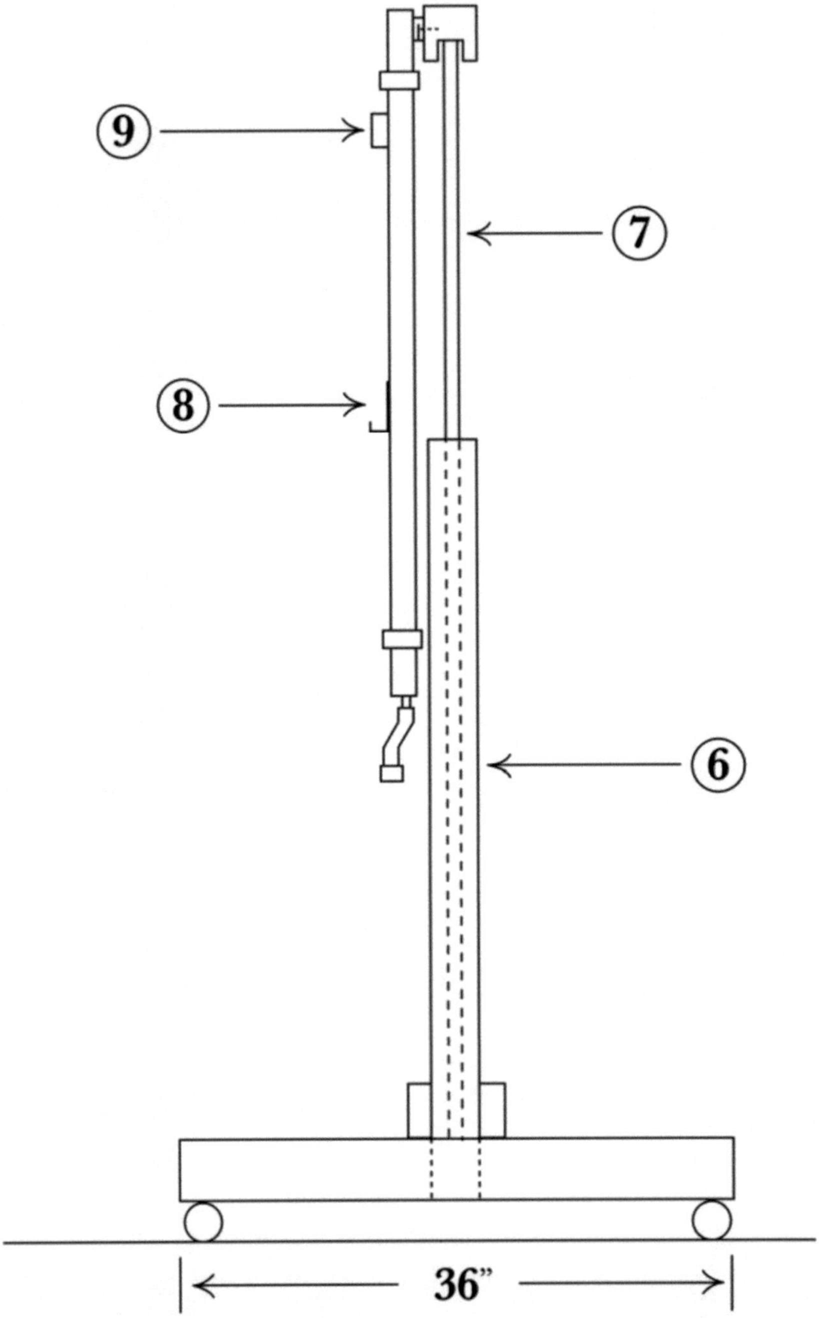


Legend: 6. 1-1/2"x3-1/2" Oak frame support, 7. Lexan beam spoiler, 8. Support for block tray with galvanized metal support, 9. Galvanized metal lock, 10. Crank, 11. Bearing location & cap (2 bearings/crank), 12. Ball bearing track for horizontal block adjustment, 13. ¼" block tray, 14. 7/16" thread rod, 15. ¼" channel for rod adjustment system

Fig. A-4 AP/PA Beam Spoiler and Blocking Support Side View

## 8. Acknowledgement

The authors express their gratitude to Craig Nicholson for his thoughtful efforts and insight in the construction of the AP/PA stand and the beam spoiler/block support system.

## 9. References

Bentel, G. (1992). *Radiation Therapy Planning* (4th ed.). New York, NY: Macmillan.

Bradley, J., Reft, C., Goldman, S., Rubin, C., Nachman, J., Larson, R., et al. (1998). High-energy total body irradiation as preparation for bone marrow transplantation in leukemia patients: treatment technique and related complications. *International Journal of Radiation Oncology, Biology and Physics, 40,* 391-396.

Bredeson, C., Perry G., Martens C., McDiarmid S., Bence-Bruckler, I. Atkins, H., et al. (2002). Outpatient total body irradiation as a component of a comprehensive outpatient transplant program. *Bone Marrow Transplantation, 29,* 667-671.

Corns, R., Evans, M., Olivares M., Syke, L., & Pogorsak, E. (2000). Designing attenuators for total body irradiation using virtual simulation. *Medical Dosimetry, 25,* 27-31.

Evans, R. (2000). Radiobiological considerations in magna-field irradiation. *International Journal of Radiation, Oncology, Biology and Physics, 43,* 1907-1911.

Galvin, J., D'Angio, G., & Walsh, G. (1999). Use of tissue compensators to improve dose uniformity for total body irradiation. *International Journal of Radiation Oncology, Biology and Physics, 42,* 767-771.

Lin, J., & Chu, T. (2001). Dose compensation of the total body irradiation therapy. *Applied Radiation Isotopes, 55,* 623-630.

Lindsley, K. & Deeg, H.J. (1998). Total body irradiation for marrow or stem-cell transplantation. *Cancer Investigation, 16,* 424-425.

Serota, F., Burkey, E., August, C., & D'Angio, G. (1998). Total body irradiation as preparation for bone marrow transplantation in treatment of acute leukemia and aplastic anemia. *International Journal of Radiation Oncology, Biology and Physics, 12,* 1941-1949.

Shank, B. (1999). Techniques of magna-field irradiation. *International Journal of Radiation Oncology, Biology and Physics, 42,* 1925-1931.

Shank, B. (1998). Total body irradiation for marrow or stem-cell transplantation. *Cancer Investigation, 16,* 397-404.

Scheinberg, D., Maslak, P., & Weiss, M. (2001). Acute leukemias. In V.T. DeVita & S. Hellman & S. Rosenberg (Eds.), *Cancer-Principles and Practice of Oncology,* (6th ed.), (pp. 2404-2432). Philadelphia, PA: J.B. Lippincott.

Urbano-Ispizua, A., Schmitz, N., de Witte, T., Frassoni, F., Rosti, G., Schrezenmeier, H., et al. (2002). Allogenic and autologous transplantation for hematologic diseases, solid tumors, and immune disorders: definitions and current practice. *Bone Marrow Transplantation, 29,* 639-646.

Van Dyk, J. (2000). Magna-field irradiation: physical considerations. *International Journal of Radiation Oncology, Biology and Physics, 43*, 1913-1918.

# 25

# Radio-Photoluminescence Glass Dosimeter (RPLGD)

David Y.C. Huang[1] and Shih-Ming Hsu[2]
[1]*Memorial Sloan-Kettering Cancer Center*
[2]*China Medical University*
[1]*USA*
[2]*Taiwan (ROC)*

## 1. Introduction

Radiation is a type of the energy transport. It produces ionization, scintillation, and luminescence when radiation interacts with matter. By detecting these phenomena from the response of the dosimeter after exposure, one can acquire an understanding on the types and the intensity of the radiation.

Solid state dosimeters can be divided into two categories, active dosimeters and passive dosimeters. When radiation interacts with medium inside the dosimeter, the active dosimeter transfers radiation intensity into the pulse of electric signals. Based on those signals, users can determine the types and the intensity of the radiation. As for passive dosimeters, radiation interaction is detected through certain physical processes after radiation interacts with medium in the dosimeter. From the physical processes, users can also determine the types and the intensity of the radiation. Active dosimeters are used for dose measurements in areas with unknown radiation level to gather the radiation information immediately. Therefore, the proper radiation protection actions can be initialized. The common active dosimeters in the market are gas-filled counters, scintillation counters, and semi-conductor detectors…etc. On the other hands, passive dosimeters are often used as periodic radiation monitor for people work in the radiation environment to monitor the cumulated dose and the types of radiation. They can be used as personal dose measurement, long-term environmental radiation dose monitor…etc. The film badge, Thermoluminescence Dosimeter (TLD), Optically Stimulated Luminescence Dosimeter (OSLD), and Radio-photoluminescence Glass Dosimeter (RPLGD) are commonly used passive dosimeters. In clinics, many different kinds of dosimeters are applied in the procedures to verify dose delivery accuracy, to obtain dose to critical areas or organs, and to verify machine output for QA purposes.

For TLD, OSLD, and RPLGD, when radiation interacts with the medium in the dosimeters, part of the absorbed energy are first stored in a metastable energy state of the medium. Then some of this energy can be recovered later as visible light after proper physical process, such as heating.

## 2. Radio-Photoluminescence Glass Dosimeter (RPLGD)

OSLD is made of the same luminescent material as one used in TLD. The only differences are different excitation source and different readout technique used. However, RPLGD uses glass compound as the luminescent material and applies different excitation method along with different readout technique. In 1949, Wely, Schulman, Ginther, and Evans manufactured the first RPLGD system (Yokota). Schulman applied this system in radiation dose measurement in 1951 (Yasuda, Troncalli). The luminescent material used by Schulman was a compound glass of 25% of $KPO_3$, 25% of Ba $(PO_3)_2$ and 50% of Al $(PO_3)_2$, with proper amount of $AgPO_3$ to form silver activated phosphate glass. It is very difficult to measure dose under 1 mGy with Schulman's RPLGD system, because it has a high pre-dose (residual dose). Pre-dose is the phosphorescence light emitted from RPLGD without any irradiation and excitation process. It is the minimum radiation can be measured with RPLGD. Besides, because of the pre-mature luminescence measurement technique and the poor quality of excitation source for color centers, the measurement accuracy with Schulman's RPLGD is very poor. Therefore, RPLGD is not a popular dosimeter in day to day applications in those days.

However, there are many researchers continue to devote in the developments of RPLGD and its readout system; including people at Asahi Techno Glass Corporation (ATGC) in Japan, at Toshiba Corporation in Japan, and at Karlsruhe Nuclear Research Center (KNRC) in Germany. The developments of new generation RPLGD and readout system were completed in 1990 (Piesch). Table 1 shows the types and compositions of the glass luminescent material developed by ATGC and Toshiba. The excitation source was changed from ultra-violet into pulse ultraviolet laser. The improvements in the glass material and in readout system make the RPLGD capable for lower dose (10 μGy) measurement with excellent accuracy (A. T. G., Corporation Chiyoda Technol).

TLD is still the major dosimeter used for personal dose monitor and for dose verification in diagnostic radiology and in radiotherapy in nowadays. The major problem with TLD is its non-repeatable readout for the measurements. Based on the preliminary report by Hsu et al on the study of the characteristics of RPLGD in radiation measurement, it proves that the radiation detection characteristics of RPLGD are superior to that of TLD (Hsu). Therefore, in the near future, RPGLD will become one of the important dosimeters for dose measurement and radiation detection in the field.

The work on the radiation measurement with self-manufactured RPLGD by Schulman in 1951 opened the history of RPLGD applications in dose measurement (Yasuda, Troncalli). After exposed to radiation, stable color centers are formed in the glass and more color centers are formed with increasing radiation intensity. After irradiated by ultraviolet light, color centers are excited and emit 600 nm to 700 nm visible orange light (Burgkhardt). It is called radio-photoluminescence phenomenon. The amount of orange light emitted from RPLGD is linearly proportional to the radiation received; therefore, it is suitable for long term personal dose monitor or environmental radiation monitor. RPLGD is used in Japan for over 80% of radiation workers as an external dosimeter (Corporation Chiyoda Technol).

## 3. Principle of RPLGD and its readout methods

The basic principle of RPLGD is that the color centers are formed when the luminescent material inside the glass compound exposed to radiation and fluorescence are emitted from the color centers after irradiated with ultra-violet light. The excited electrons generated from the color centers return to the original color centers after emitting the fluorescence. This process is called radio-photoluminescence phenomena. Because the electrons in the color centers return to the electron traps after emitting the fluorescence, it can be re-readout for a single irradiation.

| glass series | composition ratios (mol%) | | | | | | | |
|---|---|---|---|---|---|---|---|---|
| | Li | Na | P | O | Al | Ag | Mg | Ba |
| FD-1 | 3.7 | - | 33.4 | 53.7 | 4.6 | 3.7 | - | 0.9 |
| FD-3 | 3.6 | - | 34.5 | 53.5 | 5.1 | 3.3 | - | - |
| FD-4 | 3.5 | - | 34.0 | 52.7 | 5.0 | 4.8 | - | - |
| FD-5 | - | 9.0 | 33.1 | 51.3 | 6.1 | 0.5 | - | - |
| FD-6 | - | 6.6 | 33.2 | 51.4 | 5.5 | 1.4 | 1.9 | - |
| FD-7 | - | 11.0 | 31.5 | 51.2 | 6.1 | 0.2 | - | - |

Table 1. The types and compositions of silver activated phosphate glass

Figure 1 shows the old RPLGD readout technique (Piesch). The pre-dose $M_0$ ($M_0$ ($t_0$) = $I_2$ x $\Delta t$) was obtained with photomultiplier tube (PMT) first. After RPLGD irradiated by the radiation, the total light intensity is $M_1$ ($M_1$ = $I_1$ x $\Delta t$). The "actual" light intensity from the irradiation, M, is $M_1$ - $M_0$ = ($I_1$ x $\Delta t$) – ($I_2$ x $\Delta t$). The radiation dose can then be estimated from M. The traditional way to calculate the light intensity is to subtract the pre-dose reading ($M_0$) from the total reading (M). With the traditional readout technique, if the glass surface is covered with dust or other material the pre-dose reading ($M_0$) and the total dose reading (M) are both affected and results in a large error for dose estimation. Therefore the old RPLGD readout technique will not measure the dose accurately.

In 1990, a new RPLGD readout system was developed by the cooperation of ATGC (Japan) and KNRC (Germany). The major modification in this new system is to use pulse ultra-violet laser as excitation source, instead of ultra-violet light. The intensity, the excitation time and position of the pulse ultra-violet laser can be accurately controlled. Traditionally, it takes seconds for the unit to count the excitation time; however, it has changed to micro second (μs) for the new system. The readout time is decreased rapidly with the new system. Furthermore, with a collimated laser beam, the laser can be delivered to the exact position in the glass. The radiation energy can also be estimated accurately with the energy compensator filter.

With the pulse ultra-violet laser excitation system, decay curve of fluorescence can be divided into three portions according to the fluorescence decay time of RPLGD. They are (1) pre-dose or the light signal emitted from the impurity covering the glass surface, (2) the light signal from color centers formed by radiation, and (3) the light signal emitted from pre-dose after long time decay.

Any signal detected within the fluorescence decay time between 0 to 1 μs, the readout system mark it as the light signal from pre-dose or from the impurity on the glass surface.

The readout system takes light signal emitted in the fluorescence decay time between 1 to 40 μs as the signal from radiation exposure. For light signal emitted in the fluorescence decay time up to 1 ms, the readout system takes it as the signal produced by pre-dose with long decay time characteristics. The characteristics of the fluorescence decay curve are illustrated in figure 2.

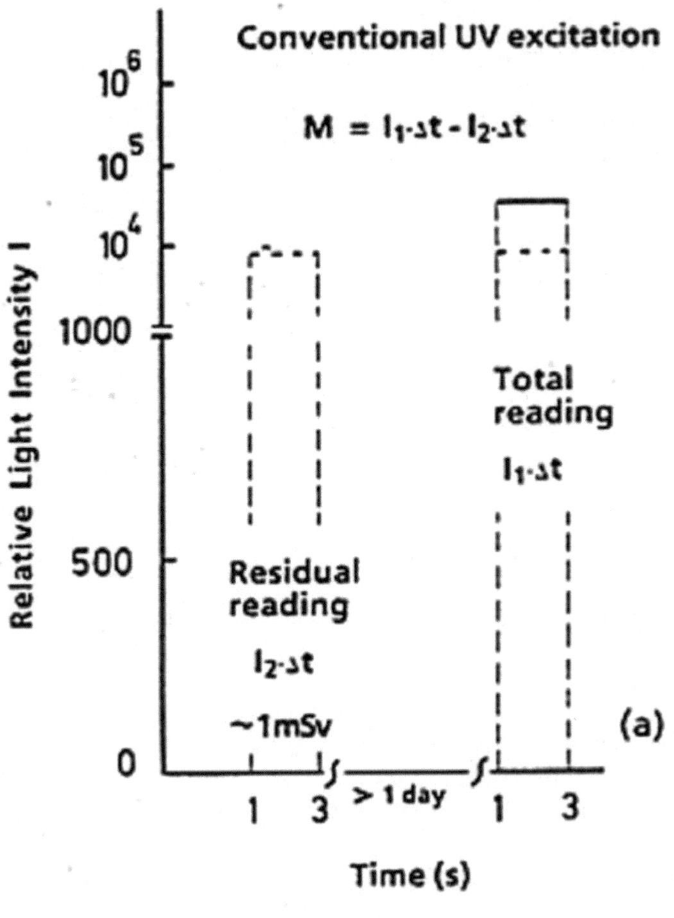


Fig. 1. Old readout technique for RPLGD (Piesch)

In figure 3, the area of $F_1$ is the integral of fluorescence decay curve between $t_1$ (1 μs) and $t_2$ (40 μs) and it is the luminescence signal produced by radiation. However, there are pre-dose signals included in the lower half part of $F_1$, therefore, one should subtract this portion from $F_1$ to obtain the "actual" luminescence signal emitted by exposure. The way to subtract the pre-dose signal is to find $F_2$ from the longer fluorescence decay curve of pre- dose. The area of $F_2$ is the integral between $t_3$ and $t_4$ where time between $t_3$ and $t_4$ and $t_1$ and $t_2$ is the same, 39 μs. From the proportional relationship of trapezium area, it shows the area of pre-dose in $F_1$ is $F_2$ x $f_{ps}$ ($f_{ps}$ is the conversion factor for trapezium area). Therefore, the actual luminescence signal from the color centers is $F_1$ - $F_2$ x $f_{ps}$. The exposure received by RPLGD can be obtained from the luminescence signal emitted.

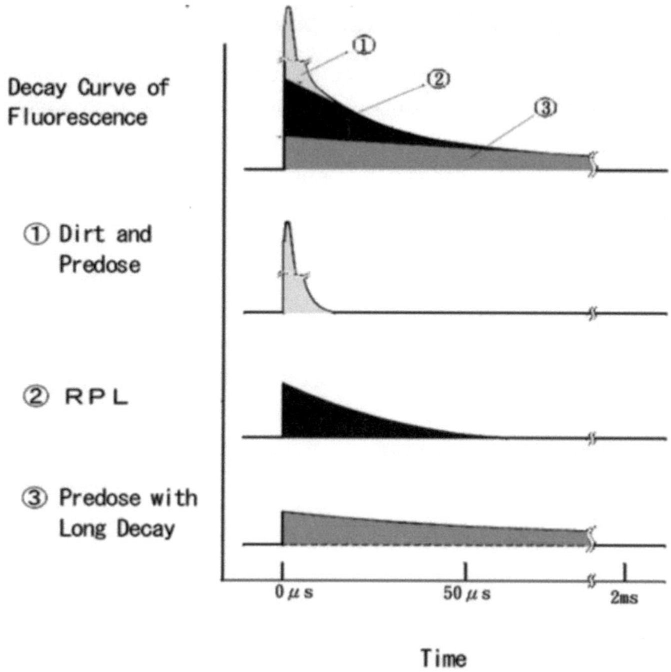


Fig. 2. The luminescence decay curve of RPLGD (A. T. G.)

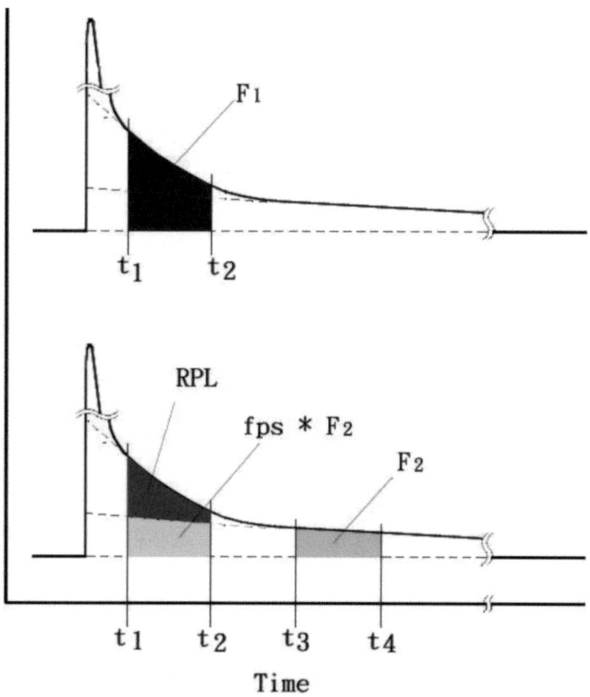


Fig. 3. The readout technique with pulse ultra-violet laser (A. T. G.).

## 4. Chemical characteristics of the silver ions

The color centers were structured at the silver activated phosphate glass. The numbers of ionic silver relate to energy levels in color centers and the numbers of electron trap(s). The numbers of electron trap(s) increase with increasing numbers of ionic silvers. However, excessive numbers of ionic silver decrease the penetration efficiency of the pulse ultra-violet laser and increases energy dependence. Therefore, a proper ratio of ionic silver is required for the best luminescence and excitation efficiency (Yokota).

At present, the most common type of glass in RPLGD for radiation dose measurement is FD-7. The $AgPO_4$ in silver activated phosphate glass of FD-7 can be viewed as $Ag^+$ and $PO_4^-$. When the tetrahedron of $PO_4^-$ is exposed to the radiation, it loses one electron and forms a "positron hole". The electron released from the $PO_4^-$ will combine with $Ag^+$ to form an $Ag^0$. Similarly, $hPO_4$ ("hole" formed after $PO_4^-$ loses one electron) will combine with $Ag^+$, and then gains a "positron hole" to become an $Ag^{2+}$. Both $Ag^0$ and $Ag^{2+}$ can form color centers as shown in Figure 4.

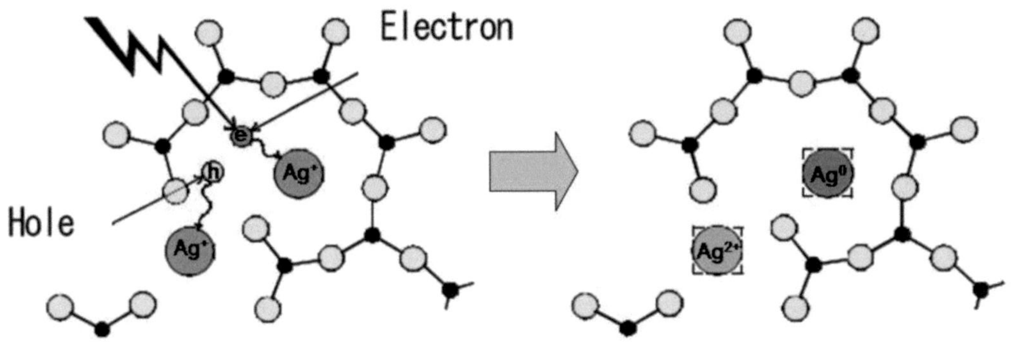


$$Ag^+ + e^- \longrightarrow Ag^o \text{ (electron trap)}$$
$$Ag^+ + hPO_4 \longrightarrow PO_4 + Ag^{2+} \text{ (hole trap)}$$

Fig. 4. The color centers formation mechanism of FD-7 (A. T. G.)

After exposure, the $Ag^+$ at valence band of silver activated phosphate glass combines with electron released from both $PO_4^-$ and $hPO_4$ (formed by $PO_4^-$) to become color centers ($Ag^0$ and $Ag^{2+}$). When these color centers excited by 337.1 nm pulse ultra-violet laser, the electrons in $Ag^0$ and $Ag^{2+}$ excited to higher energy levels and emit 600 – 700 nm visible orange light, then return to the original color centers. Energy gained by electrons from the pulse ultra-violet laser is not high enough to let electron escape from color centers. Therefore these electrons will not return to the valence band of the glass material directly. For electrons to gain enough energy to return to the valence band, we need to anneal RPLGD at 400°C for one hour. The color centers won't disappear after readout; hence, RPLGD can be read repeatedly. Figure 5 shows the energy levels of RPLGD.

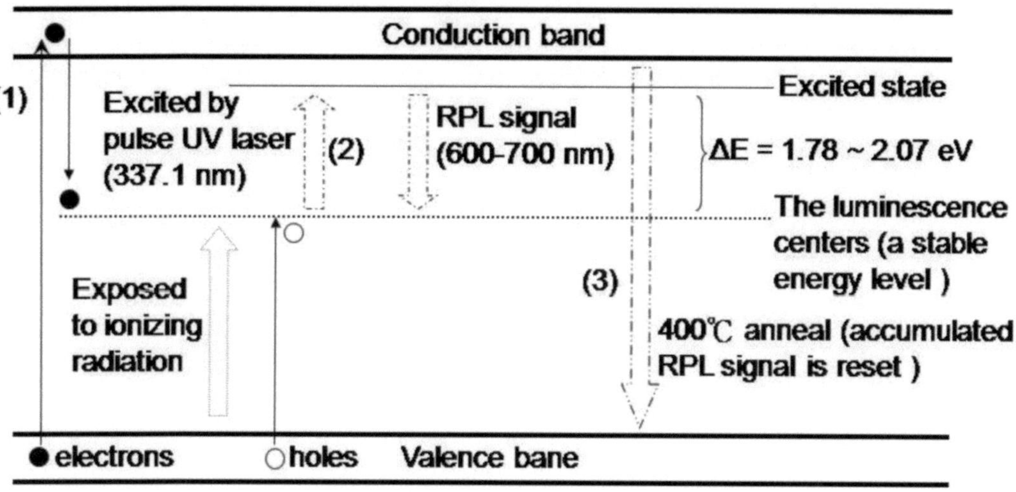


Fig. 5. The energy levels of RPLGD. (1) After RPLGD being exposed, $Ag^+$ at the valence band combines with electron released from $PO_4^-$ and $hPO_4$ formed by $PO_4^-$ to become a color center. (2) After electron at color center excited by 337.1 nm pulse ultra-violet laser, it will be excited and emits 600 – 700 nm visible orange light, then return to the original color centers (3)After annealing at 400ºC for one hour, the electron at color centers returns to the valence band of luminescence material (Hsu).

## 5. The radio-photoluminescence model

The luminescence materials used in either TLD or OSLD have an ordered crystal structure with lattice defects. From the glow curve, which is generated after annealing, one has the information on the electron distribution functions at different energy trap(s). The luminescence models for TLD and OSLD are developed based on this information. However, RPLGD is a mixture of inorganic amorphous solid and does not have lattice structure and lattice luminescence centers. Therefore we cannot get the information on electron trip(s) distribution function to establish the luminescence model for RPLGD. We can only establish the radio-photoluminescence model based on the energy of the excitation source and the energy of the released visible light.

After excited with 337.1 nm pulse ultra-violet laser, RPLGD emits 600 – 700 nm visible lights. From the emitted lights we know the energy gap between the excited energy levels which electrons jump to and the energy levels at color centers is between 1.78 and 2.07 eV. Becker assumed there are many continuous energy levels at the color centers of the RPLGD (Becker), as shown in Figure 6. It shows the electrons in the valence band are excited to the conduction band after irradiation. When electrons return to the valence band, portions of electrons are captured by the electron trap(s) located at P shell and Q shell, and then form color centers. After excitation, the electrons in color centers jump to higher energy level, emit fluoresce, then return to the original color centers. RPLGD is manufactured via the process of melting various compounds under high temperature, different from the manufacture process of TLD or OSLD which is via process of long-crystal formation. Hence, the color centers of PRLGD are not built at the lattice. There are no formal reports on the luminescence model for RPLGD. We believe that the color centers of RPLGD may be structured among the orbital electrons in the compound. The various continuous energy levels are formed with different bonding structures among elements. Those energy levels can store free electron energy which is produced by the excitation process. Therefore, its excitation energy gap has a continuous value (from 1.78 to 2.07 eV) which releases 600 nm – 700 nm visible lights.

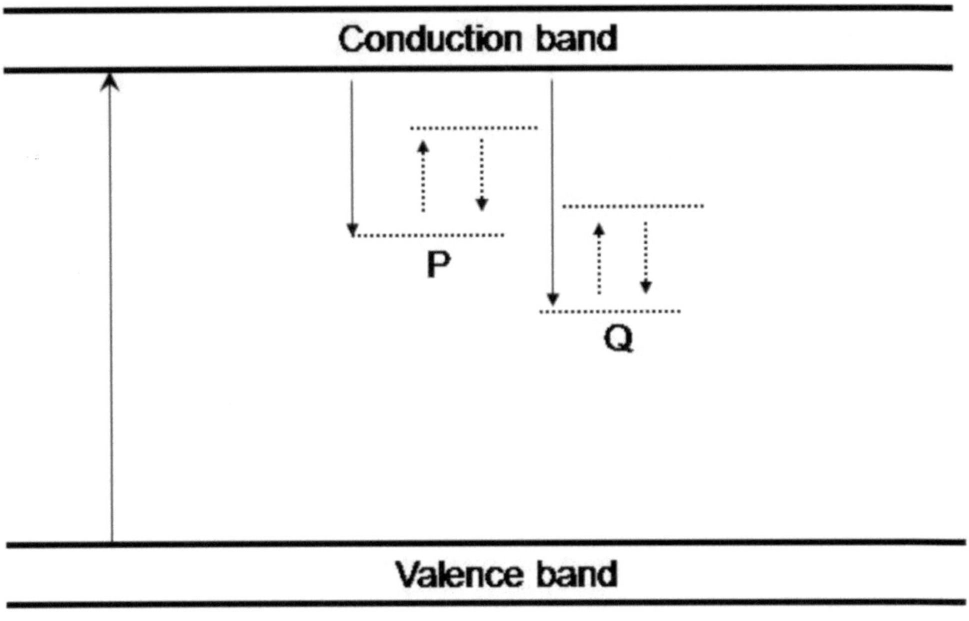


Fig. 6. There are many continuous energy levels in RPLGD color centers.

## 6. Physical characteristics of radio-photoluminescence glass dosimeter

The pulse ultra-violet laser excitation system improves the readout accuracy of RPLGD and also shortens the readout time. The improvement in the luminescent material lowers the detectable dose limit. These improvements make the applications of RPLGD in radiation measurements growing rapidly. There are three major types of RPLGD in the market; the SC-1 for environmental radiation dose monitor; the GD-450 for personal external radiation dose monitor; and the Dose Ace for research purposes. All those three types use FD-7 glass, manufactured by Asahi, Japan, as shown in Figure 7.

The SC-1 is a plate-type RPLGD with outside capsule volume of 30 x 40 x 9 $mm^3$.The dimension of FD-7 glass inside the capsule is 16 x 16 x 1.5 $mm^3$. There are two layers of tin filters, one on the top and another at the bottom, over of the capsule with a dimension of 0.75 mm and 3 mm respectively. These tin filters are used as energy compensator to estimate the radiation energy and to lower the energy dependence effect. The FD-7 in GD-450 has a dimension of 33 x 7 x 1 $mm^3$. There are five different types with different thickness of filters in the capsule of GD-450; namely, 0.2 mm acrylic plate; 0.5 mm acrylic plate; 0.7 mm aluminum filter; 0.2 mm copper filter; and 1.2 mm tin filter. The functions of these filters in

GD-450 are the same as that of SC-1; to estimate radiation energy and to lower the energy dependence effect. The GD-450 dosimeters are the major personal dosimeters used in Japan.

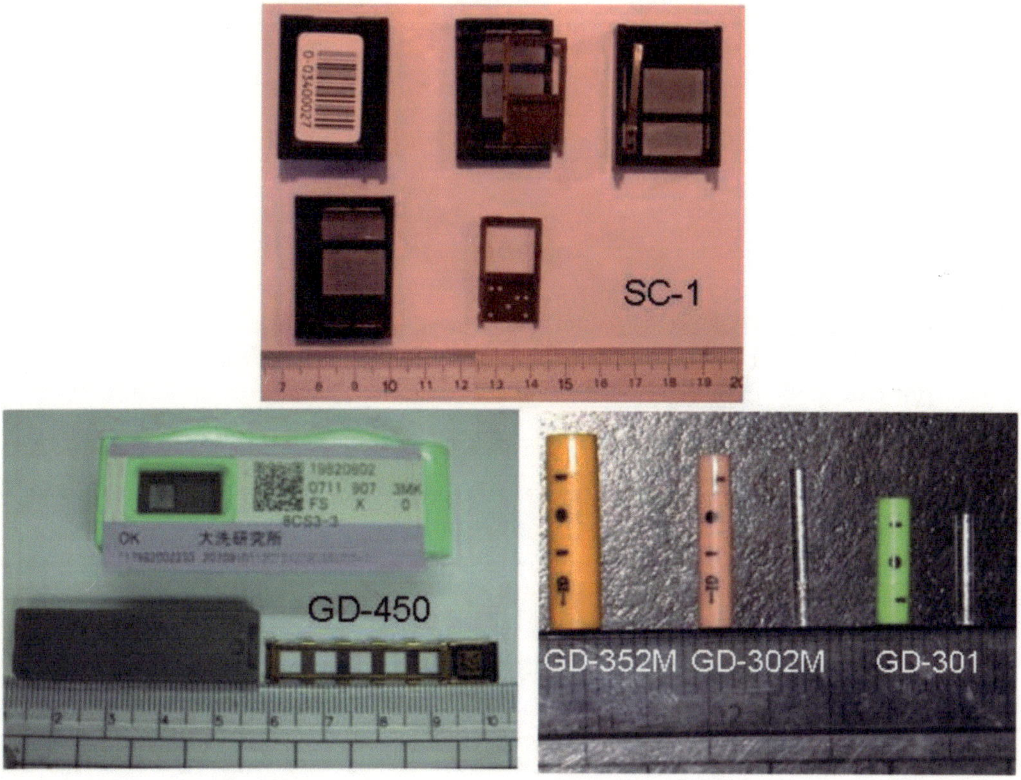


Fig. 7. Three types of RPLGD; above: SC-1 system for environmental radiation monitor; below left: GD-450 system for personal dose monitor; and below right: small volume Dose Ace system for research

The Dose Ace type RPLGD is mainly for research purposes. It is a cylindrical shape with three different models; GD-302M, GD-352M, and GD-301. The GD-302M and GD-352M have a length of 12 mm and a diameter of 1.5 mm, while GD-301 has a length of 8.5 mm and a diameter of 1.5 mm. GD-301 and GD-302M, without filters in capsule, are used to measure the dose of high energy photons as in radiotherapy. However, there is a Tin filter in the capsule for GD-352M to lower the energy dependence effect. The GD-352M can be used for measuring the dose from low energy photons as in diagnostic radiology. In the process of dose readout, based on the dose values, the dose ranges are divided into two categories, low dose range (10 μGy - 10 Gy) and high dose range (1 Gy - 500 Gy).The readout system can automatically distinguish the dose range according to different readout magazine used by the users. On the top of that, there are different readout areas in RPLGD for different dose ranges too. The readout area for high dose range is located at between 0.4 mm and 1 mm, a total length of 6 mm and a total volume of 0.47 $mm^3$, from the non-series end in the readout area (as shown in Figure 8); while the low dose range is located from 1 mm to 6 mm with a volume of 0.47 $mm^3$. The high dose readout area can be used for the measurement of dose with high gradient too. The Table 2 shows the characteristics of various RPLGDs.

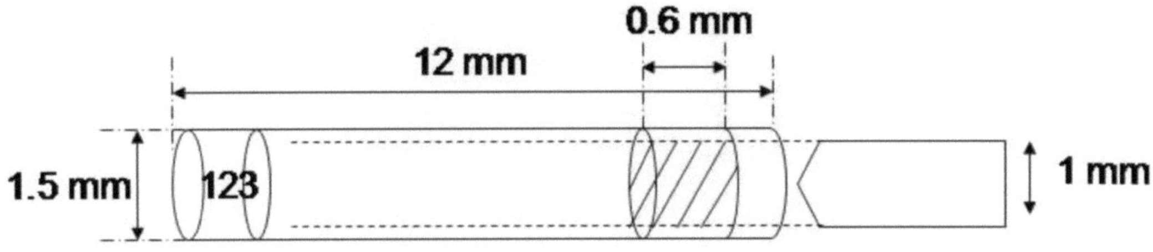


Fig. 8. The high dose readout area for GD-320M; the series end is located on the left side, the readout area is located at 0.4 mm to 1.0 mm from the non-series end, the diameter of incident pulse ultra-violet laser is 1 mm (Hsu).

| Type | SC-1 | GD-450 | Dose Ace |
|---|---|---|---|
| Effective atomic number | 12.04 | 12.04 | 12.04 |
| The dose linearity range | 10 μGy - 10 Gy | 10 μGy - 10 Gy | 10 μGy - 10 Gy<br>1 Gy - 500 Gy |
| Energy dependency (20 keV / $^{137}Cs$) | 1.2 (with energy compensator filter) | 1.2 (with energy compensator filter) | 3.4 (w/o energy compensator filter) 0.8 (with energy compensator filter) |
| Fading effect | < 5 % / yr | < 5 % / yr | < 5 % / yr |
| Repeatable readout | yes | yes | yes |
| Angular dependency | ± 8%<br>(0 ~ 80 degree) | ± 3%<br>(0 ~ 80 degree) | 0<br>(0 ~ 80 degree) |

Table 2. The characteristics of RPLGD

In Figure 9, it shows the readout reproducibility for GD-352M and TLD-100H respectively with a C.V. (coefficient of variation) of 0.46 - 3.11 for GD-325M and C.V. of 0.71 - 3.87 for TLD-100H. The figure shows that the C.V. is smaller for RPLGD as compared to that of TLD because of different manufacture methods. Each RPLGD is made after glass material melted at high temperature and results in a smaller variation among each RPLGD. On the other hand, the TLD is made with growing crystal, therefore the variation is greater.

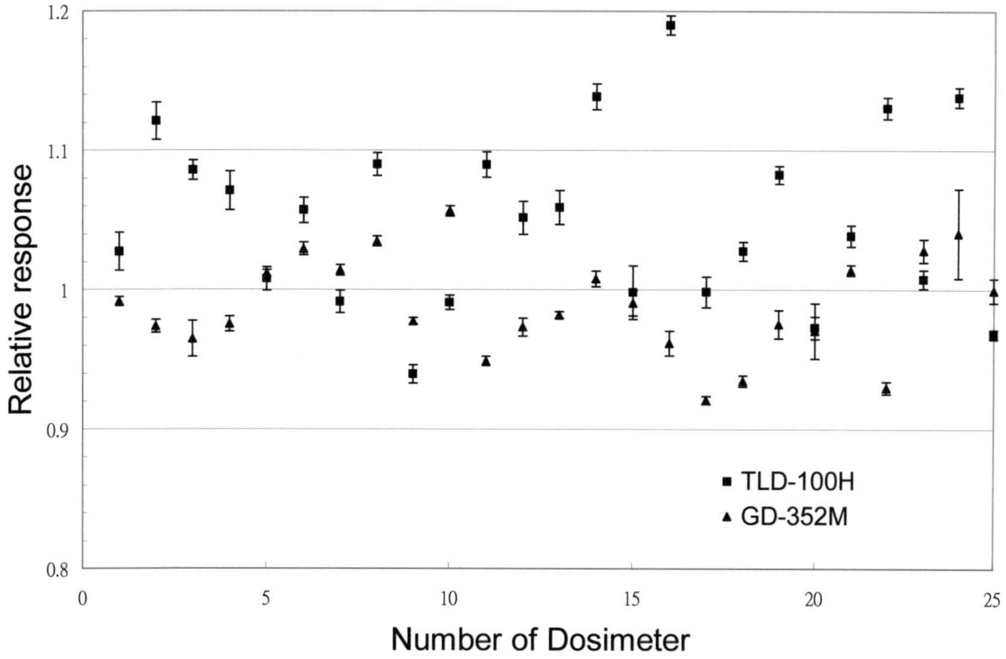


Fig. 9. The readout reproducibility of GD-352M and TLD-100H

Figure 10 shows the dose linearity for GD-352M and TLD-100H respectively in a range of 0.105 mGy and 50.4 mGy. The measured dose points are at 0.105 mGy, 0.168 mGy, 0.672 mGy, 1.05 mGy, 2.1 mGy, 6.3 mGy, 25.2 mGy, and 50.4 mGy with five RPLGDs for each measured point. The correlation coefficient is close to unity for both GD-325M and TLD-100H. It shows that the dose irradiated is proportional to the dose estimated from readout.

Figure 11 shows the energy dependence for GD-302M, GD-352M, and TLD0-100H respectively. The values shown in figure 11 are normalized to the readout from Cs-137 irradiation. When un-filtered GD-302M irradiated with low energy photons, the interactions between photons and RPLGD are increased because of the photoelectric effect. Therefore the luminescence signal is increased too. For filtered GD-352M, the Tin filter can stop the low energy photons; hence, the energy dependence effect is less.

Table 3 shows the characteristics comparisons of different passive dosimeters. It demonstrates that the physical characteristics of OSLD are better than that of TLD. And the physical characteristics of RPLGD are better than that of OSLD because of different readout system and different luminescence material. Therefore, RPLGD could become one of the important dose measurement tools in the future.

| | TLD | OSLD | RPLGD |
|---|---|---|---|
| Principe of measurement | luminescence signal | optically stimulated luminescence signal | radiophotoluminescence signal |
| Luminescence material | crystal | crystal | glass |
| Excitation source | heat | visible light | ultra-violet laser |
| Sensitivity | material-dependent | material-dependent | good |
| Repeatable readout | no | yes, but intensity reduced | yes, with the same intensity |
| Range of measurement | material-dependent (10μGy - 10 Gy) | material-dependent (10μGy - 10 Gy) | 10μGy - 10 Gy<br>1 Gy - 500 Gy |
| Geometrical shape | chip and powder | powder | various shapes |
| Fading effect | material-dependent (5 - 20 % / quarter) | material-dependent (0 - 10 %/year) | less than 5%/year |
| Energy dependence | material-dependent | material-dependent | ± 20% (having energy compensation filter) |
| Capability to distinguish the types of radiation | yes | yes | yes |
| Re-useable | yes | no | yes |

Table 3. The characteristics comparisons of TLD, OSLD, and RPLGD

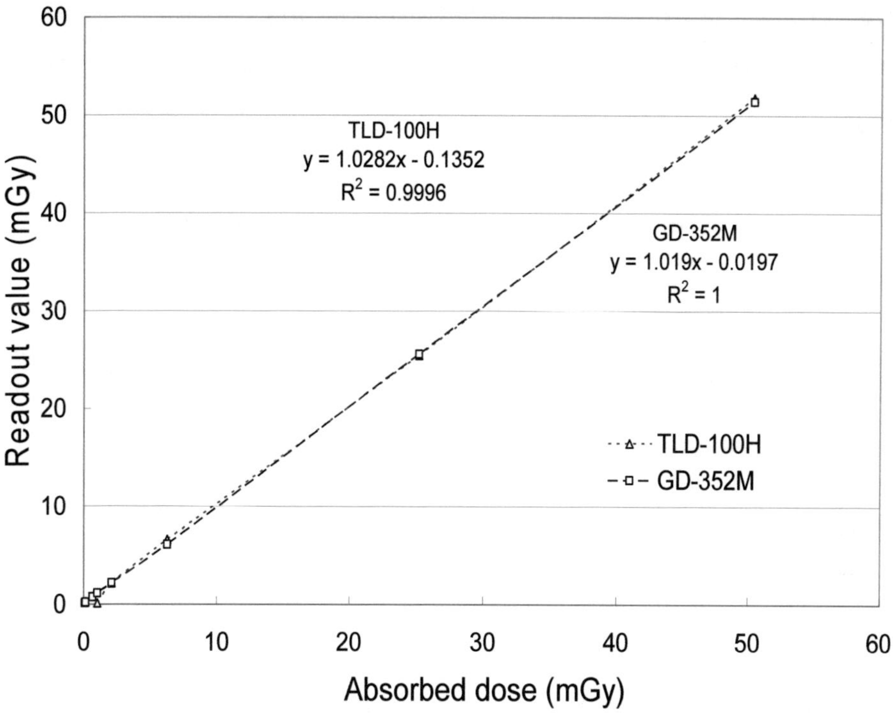


Fig. 10. The dose linearity curves for GD-352M and TLD-100H, both C.V.s are less than 3.

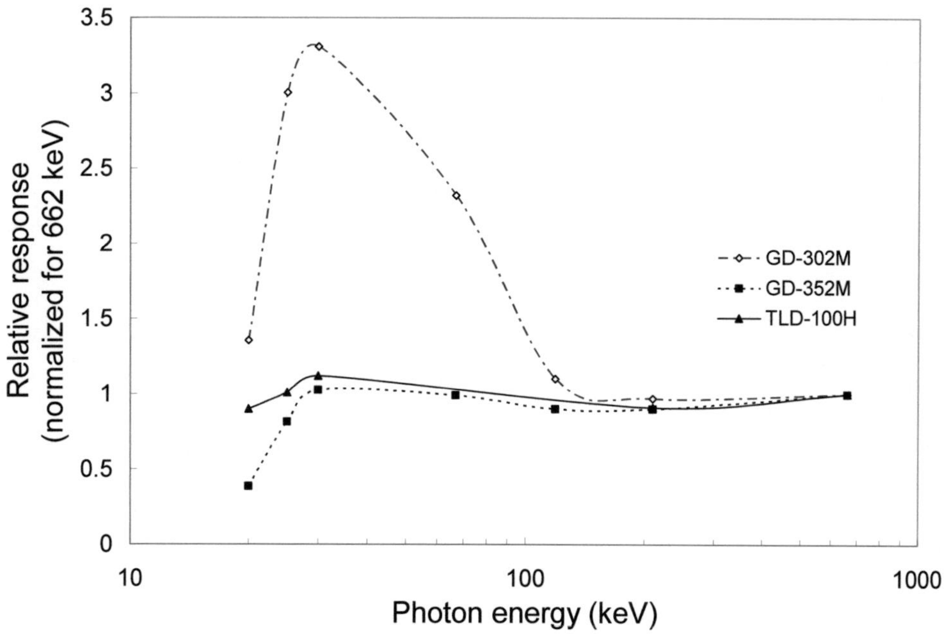


Fig. 11. The energy dependence curves for GD-302M, GD-352M, and TLD-100H

## 7. Characteristics of RPLGD for clinical applications

The clinical applications of RPLGD characteristics are summarized in the followings:

1. Repeatable readout

The luminescence signal does not disappear after readout; therefore, repeated readout for a single exposure is possible for RPLGD.

2. Small difference in individual sensitivity

The readout variation between different PRLGDs with the same exposure is small. RPLGD is manufactured with melted glass; therefore, its individual sensitivity is small as compared to that of either TLD or OSLD.

3. No correction factor needed

The luminescence single can be converted to the exposure dose directly without the need of correction factors. The exposure dose can be determined with the help of readout from reference PRLGD built-in to the readout system.

4. Small energy dependence

The energy dependence existed in FD-7 glass, if there is no energy compensator filter with it. However, energy dependence can be reduced with energy compensator filter.

5. Small fading effect

The stability of color centers in RPLGD is high. Hence the effects of environment conditions such as humidity and temperature have very little impact to color centers, hence low fading effects for RPLGD.

6. Better reproducibility

By using pulse ultra-violet laser as excited source, the accuracy of repeated readout can be maintained. Therefore, RPLGD has a very good reproducibility.

7. Wide measurable dose range

The dose linearity range for RPLGD is 0 - 500 Gy. This range covers the dose range used in the medical field. RPLGD can therefore be applied for dose verification in radiotherapy as well as in diagnostic radiology. RPLGD is also desirable for high dose gradient area, such as IMRT (Intensity Modulated Radiotherapy) procedures or HDR (High Dose Rate Remote Afterloader) procedures because of its small effective readout area.

8. Feasibility of personal dose monitor tools

The characteristics, physical and chemical, of RPLGD are equal to or better than that of TLD and OSLD because of its luminescence material and readout technique. Hence, RPLGD can be used as dose monitor for radiation field worker.

## 8. Applications of RPLGD

Araki applied the RPLGD system in Stereotactic Radiosurgery (SRS) procedure for dose measurements, including Gamma Knife, Cyberknife etc (Araki, Arakia). The results of output factors are comparable with the results from Hi-p Si Stereotactic field detector and Mote Carlo calculation. It shows RPLGD can be used for small field radiation measurements effectively. Nose designed a tube to hold RPLGDs for dose measurements for head and neck patients to verify the delivery dose against the calculated dose from treatment planning system (Nose). Although the maximum dose variation can be as high as 15%; however, those differences are mostly from the positioning errors. Based on the RPLGD physical characteristics study, the error from the RPLGD system stability is less than 3% (out of 15%). Yasuda and Iyogi applied RPLGD in space and environment radiation monitor (Yasuda, Iyogi). Hsu et al. also applied RPLGD in prostate HDR (High Dose Rate Remote Afterloader) procedure to study the dose distributions (Hsu). Many institutes in US and Europe devote into the developments and the researches in the new luminescence material and readout techniques for RPLGD (Yasuda, Araki, Arakia, Nose, Iyogi, Norimichi ,Hsu).

With its small volume, RPLGD can be used in in-vivo dose measurements; e.g. dose evaluation in animal irradiation study. RPLGD can also be placed in the anthropomorphic phantom to evaluate dose received during the clinical procedures for diagnostic radiology and radiotherapy. With its characteristics of repeatable readout and small effective readout area, RPLGD can also be used in brachytherapy procedures to evaluate the dose delivery accuracy for each procedure as well as for entire course. On the top of that, with the help of dedicated tube to hold RPLGD, one can apply RPLGD in the area of adjacent critical organs to monitor the organ dose to avoid the dose exceeding the tolerance during the radiotherapy procedure. It can improve the patient life quality after radiotherapy.

## 9. References

[1] Yokota R., Nakajima S., Improved fluoro-glass dosimeter as personnel monitoring dosimeter and micro-dosimeter. Health phys.11, 241; 1965.

[2] Yasuda H., and Ishidoya, T., Time resolved photoluminescence from a phosphate glass (GD-300) irradiated with heavy ions and gamma rays. Health Phys. 84, 373；2003.

[3] Yasuda H., and Fujitaka K., Efficiency of a radio-photoluminescence glass dosemeter for low-earth-orbit space radiation. Radiat Prot Dosimetry. 100, 545；2002.

[4] Troncalli A. J., and Chapman J., TLD linearity vs. beam energy and modality. Med Dosim. 27, 295；2002.

[5] Piesch E., Burgkhardt B., Vilgis M., Photoluminescence dosimetry: progress and present state of art. Radiat Prot Dosimetry. 33, 215; 1990.

[6] Corporation, A. T. G., RPL glass dosimeter / Small element system Dose Ace；2000.

[7] Corporation Chiyoda Technol, Personal monitoring system by glass badge；2003.

[8] Hsu S.M., Yeh S.H., Lin M.S. and Chen W.L., Comparison on Characteristics of Radio-photoluminescent Glass Dosimeters and Thermoluminescent Dosimeters. Radiat. Prot. Dosim. 119, 327；2006.

[9] Burgkhardt B., Festag J. G., Piesh E., and Ugi S., New aspects of environmental monitoring using flat phosphate glass and thermoluminescence dosimeters. Radiat Prot Dosimetry. 66, 187；1996.

[10] Yokota R., Muto Y., Silver-activated phosphate dosimeter glasses with low energy dependence and higher sensitivity. Health phys. 20, 662: 1971.

[11] Becker K., High r-dose response of recent silver-activated phosphate glasses. Health phys. 11, 523: 1964.

[12] Araki F., T. Ikegami, Measurements of Gamma-Knife helmet output factors using a radio-photoluminescent glass rod dosimeter and a diode detector. Med Phys. 30, 1976; 2003.

[13] Arakia F., Moribe N., Dosimetric properties of radio-photoluminescent glass rod detector in high-energy photon beams from a linear accelerator and cyber-knife. Med Phys. 31, 1980; 2004.

[14] Nose T., Koizumi M., Yoshida K., Nishiyama K., Sasaki J., Ohnishi T., Peiffert D., In vivo dosimetry of high-dose-rate brachytherapy: study on 61 head-and-neck cancer patients using radio-photoluminescence glass dosimeter. Int J Radiat Oncol Biol Phys. 61, 945: 2005.

[15] Iyogi T., Ueda S., Environmental gamma-ray dose rate in Aomori Prefecture, Japan. Health Phys. 82, 521; 2002.

[16] Hsu S.M., Yeh C.Y., Yeh T.C., Hong J.H., Tipton Annie Y.H., Chen W.L., Sun S.S., D.Y.C. Huang, Clinical application of radio-photoluminescent glass dosimeter on dose verification for prostate HDR procedure. Med. Phys. 35, 5558: 2008.

[17] Norimichi Juto. The large scale personal monitoring service using the latest personal monitor glass badge. Paper of proceedings of AOCRP-1-Korea, 2003.